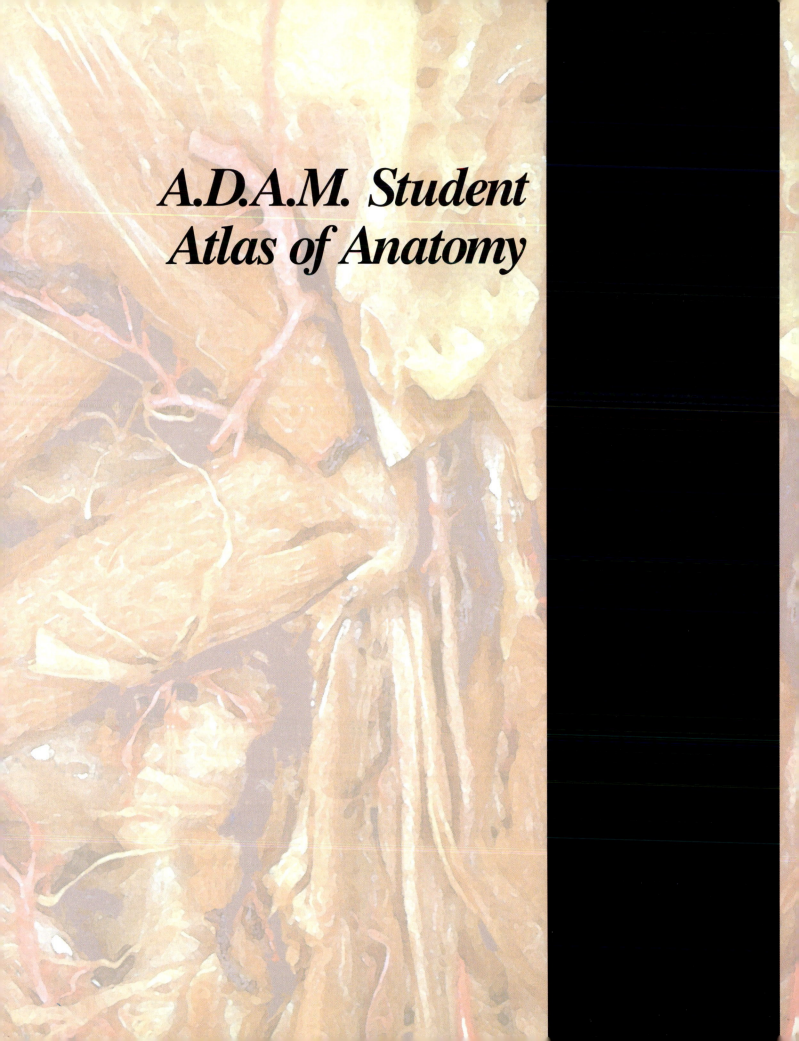

A.D.A.M. Student
Atlas of Anatomy

A.D.A.M. Student
Atlas of Anatomy

Todd R. Olson, Ph.D.
Associate Professor
Department of Anatomy & Structural Biology
Albert Einstein College of Medicine
Bronx, New York

Illustrative Art
A.D.A.M.® Software, Inc.
Atlanta, Georgia

Cadaver Photographs
The Bassett Collection
Stanford University
School of Medicine
Stanford, California

with the assistance of
Wojciech Pawlina, M.D.
Assistant Professor
Department of
Anatomy & Cell Biology
University of Florida
College of Medicine
Gainesville, Florida

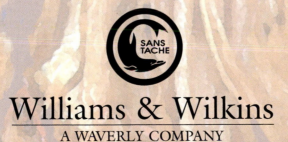

Williams & Wilkins
A WAVERLY COMPANY

BALTIMORE • PHILADELPHIA • LONDON • PARIS • BANGKOK
BUENOS AIRES • HONG KONG • MUNICH • SYDNEY • TOKYO • WROCLAW

Editor: Timothy S. Satterfield
Managing Editor: Crystal Taylor
Production Manager: Paula Huber
Project Editor: Janet M. Krejci
Illustration Planners: Mario Fernández, Wayne Hubbel, Raymond Lowman, Donna Smith
Typesetter: The Image Foundry, Ltd., Baltimore, MD
Printer: Metropole Litho, Montreal, Canada

351 West Camden Street
Baltimore, Maryland 21201-2436 USA

Rose Tree Corporate Center
1400 North Providence Road
Building II, Suite 5025
Media, Pennsylvania 19063-2043 USA

Printed in Canada

Library of Congress Cataloging-in-Publication Data

Olson, Todd R.
    A.D.A.M. student atlas of anatomy with the assistance of Wojciech Pawlina; illustrative art by
A.D.A.M. Software, Inc.; cadaver photographs from the Bassett collection.
      p.   cm.
    Includes index.
    ISBN 0-683-00042-X
    1. Human anatomy—Atlases. I. Pawlina, Wojciech. II. Title. III. Title: Student atlas of anatomy.
    [DNLM: 1. Anatomy—atlases. QS 17 052a 1996]
QM25.047 1996
611'.0022'2—dc20
DNLM/DLC
for Library of Congress   95-11593
                                                 CIP

To purchase additional copies of this book, call our customer service department at (800) 638-0672 or fax orders to (800) 447-8438. For other book services, including chapter reprints and large quantity sales, ask for the Special Sales department.

Canadian customers should call (800) 268-4178, or fax (905) 470-6780. For all other calls originating outside the United States, please call (410) 528-4223 or fax us at (410) 528-8550.

Visit Williams & Wilkins on the Internet http://www.wwilkins.com or contact our customer service department at custserv@wwilkins.com. Williams & Wilkins customer service representatives are available from 8:30am to 6:00pm, EST, Monday through Friday, for either telephone or Internet access.

96 97 98 99 00
1 2 3 4 5 6 7 8 9 10

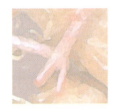

Dedication

To my family, especially my parents and my wife, Sarah, for the support and encouragement that have constantly been a part of their love; to my friends for the many pleasures and insights that I have experienced in our camaraderie; and to my teachers, colleagues, and students for having made education an exciting and rewarding lifelong endeavor.

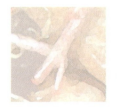

Foreword

During the course of my training in medical illustration, I relied heavily upon the most important tool a student can have in the study of gross anatomy: the anatomy atlas. The extent of my atlas collection reflected this importance; no one atlas provided the ultimate reference, so I felt I had to have them all. However, my extensive collection could not provide an adequate picture of the three-dimensional relationships within the body. In particular, superficial-to-deep relationships were a struggle to comprehend within the two-dimensional world of an anatomy atlas. Although I could discover the three-dimensional anatomical relationships in the dissection lab, standing over a cadaver all day was not a viable option. So, like most students, I relied upon the atlas as my primary tool for learning and turned to dissection for reinforcement and the three-dimensional visualization I ultimately required. The gap between the representations of the atlas and the reality of the human body eventually led me to envision and help create a computerized, multimedia version of a dissectable human body: *A.D.A.M.,* or *Animated Dissection of Anatomy for Medicine.* The first version of *A.D.A.M.* has now evolved into a family of related products: the *A.D.A.M. Scholar Series.*

In developing that first *A.D.A.M.* product, my team of medical illustrators and anatomists assembled the most comprehensive set of medical images ever created. Presenting these images through a computer allowed a user to peel away each structure of the anatomy, one layer at a time, from the skin to the bones, and from four views. This major achievement overcame many of the limitations of the anatomy atlas, allowing students to navigate through a virtual body to any depth they chose.

At about the same time A.D.A.M. Software completed the first *A.D.A.M.* product, I met Dr. Todd Olson. From the first time he saw *A.D.A.M.*, Todd appreciated its value to anatomy education. He quickly became an advocate for the product and began to experiment with ways he could use it in his courses at Albert Einstein College of Medicine. Todd recognized early on, however, that widespread student access to the rich image database would be limited by the slow pace of computerization in medical education. In response to this recognition, A.D.A.M. Software began discussions with Williams & Wilkins about the creation of a printed student atlas modeled on the strategy of the multimedia *A.D.A.M.* product: to give students the ability to explore superficial-to-deep relationships while maintaining a clear sense of orientation within the body. Further discussions led to the idea to include cadaver photographs from the world-renowned collection of David L. Bassett, M.D. As the manuscript evolved, I sensed a product with a real competitive advantage over other atlases. Some provided good illustrations but no photos; others had photos but few illustrations. I remembered my days in gross anatomy flipping from one type of atlas to the other. This product would have it all!

Todd's clear vision of what he wanted to achieve as a teacher of anatomy and the passion, talent, and commitment of A.D.A.M. medical illustrators Eric Grafman and Ed Stewart resulted in a work which, in my opinion, is one of the most impressive anatomy atlases on the market today. This atlas embodies many of the same qualities that have made the electronic *A.D.A.M.* products so valuable. From page to page, the images are arranged to give the viewer a sense of moving ever deeper into the body. Within many illustrations, a technique called "ghosting" reveals the anatomic relationships between semitransparent superficial structures and underlying structures. Additionally, *A.D.A.M. Student Atlas of Anatomy* allows side-by-side comparison of the A.D.A.M. images and the Bassett cadaver photographs. The resulting work represents a milestone in the presentation of anatomic information.

I like to think that this atlas represents human accomplishment at its best. The talent, dedication, and professionalism of those who created it can be seen on every page. It is my hope that as *A.D.A.M. Student Atlas of Anatomy* helps students more fully visualize the complexity of the human body, it can also contribute to a better understanding of ourselves as human beings, enabling us to open doors to a better educated and healthier society.

Gregory M. Swayne
President
A.D.A.M. Software, Inc.

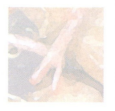

Preface

Our knowledge of human gross anatomy has changed relatively little in the past 100 years; however, the time devoted to the study of anatomy by medical students has decreased greatly. Gross anatomy was the principal course taught in the first year of medical school for the first half of this century. Today, the spectacular development of bioscience technology has resulted in first-year medical students devoting two to three times as much study to cellular, subcellular, molecular, and biochemical processes than to gross anatomy.

Anatomists have successfully responded to this new curricular challenge in two ways. Most significantly, the amount of information covered in our courses has been distilled to those aspects of anatomy that are clinically relevant and, therefore, of greatest potential value to a student's future medical practice. Second, anatomic details pertinent to specialty study are now taught in postgraduate programs and are not part of the anatomic essentials taught during the basic medical education.

Although a new generation of introductory textbooks has been written that reduce gross anatomy to essential concepts and present it within a practical, clinical context, for some time I have thought it remarkable that no one had attempted to incorporate these new perspectives into an anatomy atlas for beginning students. Then, in the winter of 1994, at the request of Williams & Wilkins, I prepared a proposal for just such a new human anatomy atlas using the electronic images in the A.D.A.M. database and the exquisite collection of dissection photographs in Dr. David Bassett's *Stereoscopic Atlas of Human Anatomy,* which is housed in the Division of Human Anatomy at Stanford University School of Medicine.

A.D.A.M. Student Atlas of Anatomy is foremost a visual guide and interactive learning resource to be used in conjunction with a clinical anatomy textbook. In the structure and content of the atlas, I have emphasized those structures that are fundamental to the clinical education of every medical student. It has not been my intention to create a comprehensive atlas nor an atlas to accompany laboratory dissection. I have included more images of fewer structures; particularly, more images of those parts of the body that present the beginning student with the greatest difficulty to comprehend and appreciate three-dimensionally. It is important that those who use this atlas understand both its distinctive emphasis and limited scope, and appreciate the necessity of a more comprehensive atlas as their knowledge of human anatomy matures.

Nowhere in *A.D.A.M. Student Atlas of Anatomy* is the emphasis on essential and difficult material more evident than in Chapter 4, which covers the pelvic contents and perineum. These topics are treated in a substantially expanded format than is normally found in traditional atlases for two reasons. First, the major clerkship of obstetrics and gynecology, and to a lesser extent the field of urology, dictate the necessity of knowing the basic anatomy of the pelvis and perineum. Second, experience indicates that this region is possibly the most difficult for first-time students to understand. The pelvis and perineum present unique problems of spatial and surface relationships, compounded by the fact that dissection of the pelvis only partially reveals its contents in situ and is difficult and time-consuming, even for an experienced prosector working on an ideal specimen.

It is ultimately the objective in teaching patient-oriented anatomy to provide the student with an understanding of the composite anatomy of all or selected regions of the body; however, experience has convinced me that many students find it easier initially to have information organized by systems. The extensive systemic sections in *A.D.A.M. Student Atlas of Anatomy* should not only make it more useful for first-year medical students, but also make it a valuable resource for allied health students who learn anatomy systemically but have never had a regional atlas that emphasized this approach. I have included lengthy systemic sections at the beginning of the chapters on the trunk (Chapter 1), pelvis and perineum (Chapter 4), limbs (Chapters 5 and 6), and head and neck (Chapter 7). Systemic descriptions were not included in the chapters on the thoracic and abdominal contents (Chapters 2 and 3) because the systemic anatomy of the body walls of these regions is covered extensively in Chapter 1 and because the distribution and pattern of deeper neurovascular structures can be clearly appreciated in the sequence of dissection images in each of these two chapters.

In organizing the atlas, I have arranged cadaveric photographs to provide beginning students with an overview of some of the more important dissections that are seen in the laboratory. In most cases, photographs are numerically labeled to facilitate their use in practical examination review. Their placement adjacent to corresponding A.D.A.M. images, which serve as the keys to the numbered structures in the photographs, offers the student a detailed artistic image (instead of a highly simplified schematic drawing) that enhances what is most important in the view. In addition, the student needs to apply anatomic knowledge in the identification of the numerically labeled structures.

The student who is using *A.D.A.M. Student Atlas of Anatomy* to the fullest advantage must identify anatomic landmarks, find these landmarks on a second figure (the key image), and then identify the structure by locating it relative to the landmarks. This is precisely the observation and orientation process that anatomists are trying to teach in the laboratory.

An appreciation of both cross-sectional and radiographic anatomy is important in many areas of basic clinical work. However, given the circumscribed scope of this atlas, it was impossible to incorporate more than a limited number of cross-sectional and radiographic images into each chapter. Those that are included either best display the distribution of a prominent structure (e.g., the peritoneum) or provide another means of visualizing the relationships within a region.

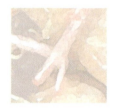

Acknowledgments

A.D.A.M. Student Atlas of Anatomy is the result of a major collective effort, and I extend my appreciation to all of the individuals who contributed to this project, in particular, Paula Huber and Tim Satterfield of Williams & Wilkins, Gregory Swayne of A.D.A.M. Software, Dr. Robert Chase of Stanford University School of Medicine, and Dr. Arthur F. Dalley II of Creighton University School of Medicine.

Dr. Wojciech Pawlina, of University of Florida College of Medicine, worked tirelessly on this project from almost its inception, and his critical advice contributed significantly to the quality of this book and, indeed, made its completion possible.

I acknowledge the talent, dedication, and professionalism of all those at A.D.A.M. Software who are responsible for the artwork in this atlas and in the original *A.D.A.M. Comprehensive*. Their efforts and commitment are clearly visible on every page of this book. I thank Ed Stewart, Eric Grafman, Lynda Leigh Levy, Lelayne Weiss, Virginia Sue Mabry, Dee Mustafa-Bowne, Bill Blakesley, Barry Golivesky, Cordero Jenkins, Cindy Quamme, Suzanne Swayne, Audra Brand, Stephanie Calabrese, Ron Collins, Mary Beth Clough, Dan Johnson, Kyle McNeir, Meredith Nienkamp, Lisa Quattrini, and Laura Petrides. In addition, I would like to extend my appreciation to Tim Brammer and Roger Jackson for their technical assistance and support.

The following individuals at Williams & Wilkins brought their expertise, enthusiasm, and commitment to quality to this project: Crystal Taylor, Mary Finch, Anne Stewart Seitz, and Janet Krejci.

I wish to thank Dottie Mims of the Image Foundry, Ltd.

My gratitude is extended to Dr. Keith Moore for use of tables from his book *Clinically Oriented Anatomy*, Third Edition, published in 1992 by Williams & Wilkins. I am grateful to Dr. Lothar Wicke for use of several radiographic images from his *Atlas of Radiographic Anatomy*, Fifth Edition, published in 1994 by Lea & Febiger.

Gregory Smith of St. Mary's College of California, Dr. Sharon Sawitzke, and Dr. Burton Dornfest provided invaluable insight and suggestions while reviewing the atlas during its production. The input of Dr. Thomas Gest into an earlier version of the project was also very helpful. Dr. Olga Malakhova of University of Florida College of Medicine deserves a special acknowledgment for the help and consultation she provided Dr. Pawlina to further his labors on the *Atlas*.

Many individuals contributed to my education as an anatomist and, thus, to this endeavor, and I extend my sincere appreciation and indebtedness to Dr. Ralph Ger, Dr. Peter Satir, Dr. Ilya Glezer, Dr. Herbert Srebnik, Professor Michael Day, and my dear friend the late Dr. Warren Kinzey.

Colleagues in the American Association of Clinical Anatomists are too numerous to name here, although I wish to acknowledge them as well as my fellow course directors here in New York: Drs. Ernest April, N. Barry Berg, Bruce Bogart, Ray Dannenhoffer, Daria Dykyj, Fakhry Girgis, Mahmood Khan, Jeffrey Laitman, Martin Levine, Leon Martino, Anthony Mercurio, Nikos Solounias, and Eugene Wenk, for the conversations that we have had about the teaching of clinical anatomy and its role in medical education.

Although all of my former and current anatomy students have contributed to my experience and insights that I developed into the concept and organization of this book, six students at Albert Einstein College of Medicine deserve recognition for their work on and support of this project: Debbie Chirnomas, Benjamin Cilento, Sharon Goldstein, Soleyman Rokhsar, Kimberly Valenti, and Christine Yuen.

Finally, I would like to thank the many students in Albert Einstein College of Medicine's Class of 1999 for their helpful comments on many of the chapters in this book.

A.D.A.M. Student Atlas of Anatomy Team

Anatomic Illustration

Eric D. Grafman, *Project Director and Medical Illustrator*

Ed M. Stewart, *Production Manager and Medical Illustrator*

Lynda Leigh Levy, *Medical Illustrator*

Lelayne Weiss, *Illustrator*

Virginia Sue Mabry, *Illustrator*

Dee Mustafa-Bowne, *Illustrator*

Photo Retouch

Bill Blakesley, *Medical Illustrator*

Barry Golivesky, *Graphic Designer*

Cordero D. Jenkins, *Illustrator*

Cindy Quamme, *Graphic Designer*

Post Production

Suzanne Swayne

Lelayne Weiss

Audra Brand

Product Manager

Stephanie Calabrese

A.D.A.M. Software Comprehensive Team

Gregory M. Swayne, *Executive Producer and Medical Illustrator*

Ron Collins, *Project Director and Medical Illustrator*

Mary Beth Clough, *Medical Illustrator*

Dan Johnson, *Medical Illustrator*

Kyle McNeir, *Medical Illustrator*

Meredith Nienkamp, *Medical Illustrator*

Lisa Quattrini, *Medical Illustrator*

Lelayne Weiss, *Illustrator*

Virginia Sue Mabry, *Illustrator*

Dee Mustafa-Bowne, *Illustrator*

Cindy Quamme, *Graphic Designer*

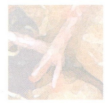

Contents

Credits

Many of the tables and all of the radiographs appearing in this atlas are used with permission from the following:

Moore, KL, Clinically Oriented Anatomy, 3rd ed. Baltimore: Williams & Wilkins, 1992.
Tables 1.1, 1.2, 1.3, 1.4, 4.1, 4.2, 5.1, 5.2, 5.3, 5.6, 6.1, 6.2, 6.3, 6.4, 6.5, 6.6, 7.1, 7.2, 7.3, 7.4, 7.5, 7.6, 7.7, 7.8, 7.9, 8.1, and 8.2.

Wicke L, Röntgen-Anatomie Normalbefund, 4th German ed. München-Wein-Baltimore: Urban & Schwarzenberg, 1992.
Radiographs in Plates 2.20, 2.36, 3.12, 3.22, 3.26, 3.28, 3.36, 5.42, 5.52, 5.58, 6.36, 6.46, 6.62, 7.1, 7.6, and 7.8.

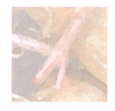

User's Guide

A.D.A.M. Student Atlas of Anatomy was designed to be an interactive pictorial guide for the beginning student to master both basic human anatomic methodology and terminology as well as the three-dimensional relationships of the body's constituent parts. The next few pages explain how to use the illustrations and special features of the atlas to their fullest advantage.

Three-Dimensional Anatomy

Among the problems faced by the beginning anatomy student, none is more universally perplexing than acquiring an appreciation of the three-dimensional relationships within the human body. Recent anatomy books have addressed this problem largely through the inclusion of cross sections and computed tomographic (CT) and magnetic resonance imaging (MRI) scans. Typically, anatomy atlases and textbooks illustrate a region from only one of the four traditional vertical perspectives (i.e., anterior, posterior, medial, lateral), and students are left to extrapolate the anatomy of the third dimension from a two-dimensional picture.

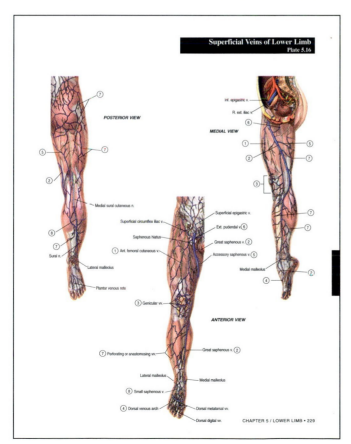

One of the most effective ways to overcome this problem is to illustrate the region in question from an orientation that is at right angles to the original perspective. Using the distinctive ability of *A.D.A.M.* illustrations to view the body from any one of the four vertical perspectives, included are at least two, sometimes more, orientations in many of the plates. For example, the medial, anterior, and posterior views of the leg in Plate 5.16 make visualizing the location, distribution, and relationships of the superficial veins, especially the clinically important saphenous vein, and cutaneous nerves of the lower limb much easier. The extensive use of these multiple views is one of the most striking and valuable characteristics of *A.D.A.M. Student Atlas of Anatomy.*

Labels and Key and Test Images

The two figures here from Plate 1.48 demonstrate the **three ways that structures are labeled in the atlas** and the rationale for the labeling.

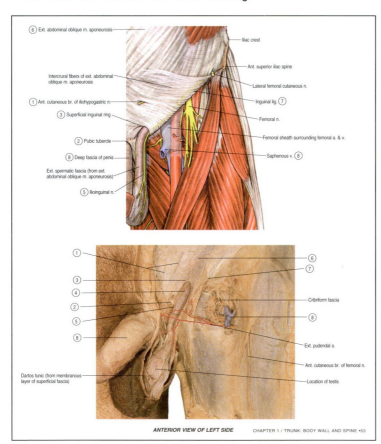

First, the ***iliac crest*** in the *top* figure and the ***cribriform fascia*** in the *lower* are **identified simply by** name because both of these structures are not present in both figures.

Second, the ***superficial inguinal ring*** and ***deep fascia of penis*** are identified by name in the *top* figure and are associated with a *circled number.* The presence of **circled numbers next to structure names** indicates that the figure is a **key image.** A key image should be used in identifying structures **labeled only by a circled number on a test image,** which is the third type of labeling used in the atlas.

Third, a **test image** is typically located on the plate to the *right* of a key image; however, sometimes a test image is placed on the *same* plate as a key image, as occurs in Plate 1.48, the example used here.

Circled numbers are placed randomly on test images to emphasize the importance of associating structural landmarks on corresponding key images and test images. The correlation of a particular number with a particular structure is valid only within a plate or within adjacent plates. For example, the ***ilioinguinal n.*** is labeled (13) in the key image on Plate 1.48, but it is labeled (4) on Plate 1.50. The only exception to this pattern is the series of plates on the perineum (Plates 4.39–4.50) where a number is consistently assigned to a structure throughout the series.

Anatomical Nomenclature

The anglicized and classical terminology used in *A.D.A.M. Student Atlas of Anatomy* follows the sixth edition of *Nomina Anatomica.* In some cases, the use of brackets [ ] and parentheses ( ) has formal meaning in the internationally recognized code of anatomical nomenclature.

> **Brackets** signify:
> 1.   An officially recognized alternative name or synonym.
>   Fibularis [Peroneus] longus m.
>   L. vagus n. [CN X], where CN refers to a cranial nerve
>   L. gastro-omental [gastroepiploic] v.
> 2.   An equivalent anatomical name.
>   Subcostal n. [T12], where T12 = 12th thoracic spinal n.
>   C1 [Atlas]

> **Parentheses** identify:
> 1.   An official name of inconsistent structures.
>   (Accessory parotid gland)
>   (Frontal suture)
>
> 2.   Eponyms and alternative names that are not officially recognized as appropriate in contemporary usage.
>   L. colic (splenic) flexure
>   Costoaxillary (ext. mammary) v.
>   Hepatopancreatic ampulla (of Vater)
>
> 3.   Additional components of a name that are usually omitted but have been added for clarification or that are supplemental to the name.
>   Greater tuberosity (of humerus)
>   Acromion (process of scapula)
>   Posterior basal bronchopulmonary segment (S10)

4. Motor and sensory segmental and spinal nerve levels of a peripheral nerve.
   Femoral n. (L2–L4)
   Lat. femoral cutaneous n. (L2, L3)
   Middle cluneal nn. (dorsal rami of S1–S3)

   Two adjacent spinal nn., are separated by a comma; however, when more than two spinal nn. are involved, only the cranial and caudal-most are listed, separated by a dash.

5. Conditions specific or unique to the image or dissection.
   L. rectus abdominis m. (reflected medially)
   R. primary bronchus (pulled to L.)

6. In some names, long dashes replace or are used in conjunction with parentheses.
   Biceps femoris m.—long head tendon
   Vestibular bulb of vagina—corpus spongiosum
   Superficial perineal fascia—membranous layer (Colles')
   Urinary bladder—empty

Abbreviations

The following abbreviations are used in this atlas. **Bold** entries are abbreviated everywhere they appear, other entries are sometimes abbreviated in order to save space.

&	**= and**	inf.	= inferior	nn.	= nerves
a.	**= artery**	int.	= internal	pt.	= part
aa.	**= arteries**	**L.**	**= Left**	port.	= portion
ant.	= anterior	lat.	= lateral	post.	= posterior
asc.	= ascending	**lig.**	**= ligament**	proc.	= process
br.	**= branch**	**ligg.**	**= ligaments**	**R.**	**= Right**
brr.	**= branches**	**m.**	**= muscle**	sup.	= superior
comm.	**= communicating**	**mm.**	**= muscles**	trib.	= tributary
desc.	= descending	med.	= medial	**v.**	**= vein**
ext.	= external	**n.**	**= nerve**	**vv.**	**= veins**

Another system of abbreviation is used when labels for segmental structures (i.e., vertebrae, spinal or intercostal nerves, ribs) are superimposed on or immediately adjacent to the structure. Thus, **C6** on or next to a vertebra identifies the sixth cervical vertebra; the "C" distinguishes the vertebral type and the number its segmental location. Abbreviations used this way are:

   C = Cervical
   Cc = Coccygeal
   L = Lumbar
   R = Rib
   S = Sacral
   T = Thoracic

Trunk:
Body Wall and Spine

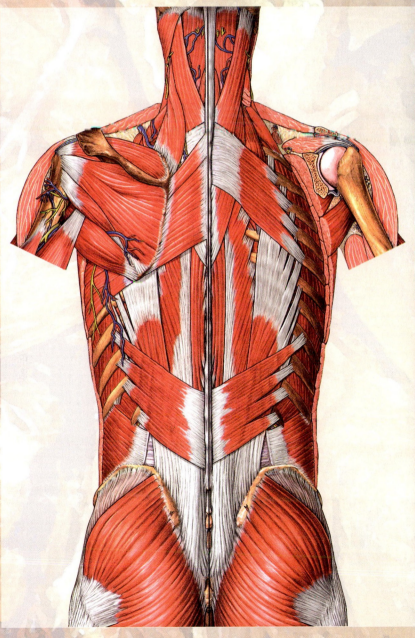

Chapter **1**

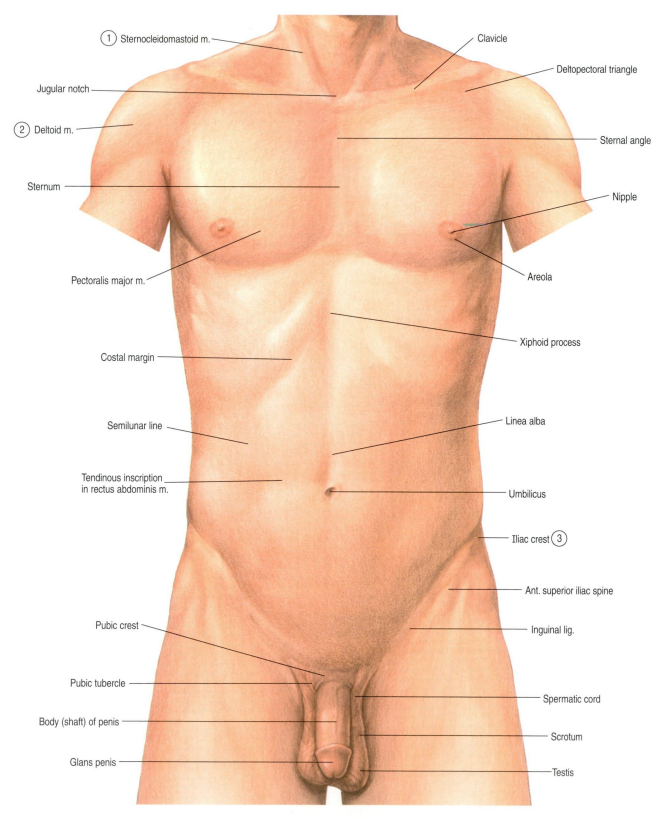

1 Sternocleidomastoid m.

Clavicle

Jugular notch

Deltopectoral triangle

2 Deltoid m.

Sternal angle

Sternum

Nipple

Pectoralis major m.

Areola

Xiphoid process

Costal margin

Semilunar line

Linea alba

Tendinous inscription in rectus abdominis m.

Umbilicus

Iliac crest 3

Ant. superior iliac spine

Pubic crest

Inguinal lig.

Pubic tubercle

Spermatic cord

Body (shaft) of penis

Scrotum

Glans penis

Testis

ANTERIOR VIEW

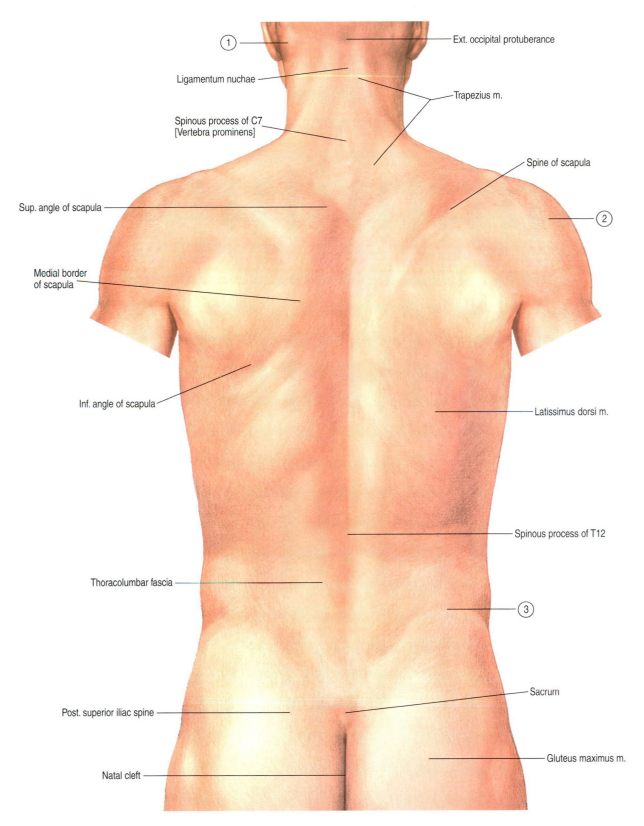

① Ext. occipital protuberance

Ligamentum nuchae

Trapezius m.

Spinous process of C7
[Vertebra prominens]

Spine of scapula

Sup. angle of scapula

②

Medial border
of scapula

Inf. angle of scapula

Latissimus dorsi m.

Spinous process of T12

Thoracolumbar fascia

③

Sacrum

Post. superior iliac spine

Gluteus maximus m.

Natal cleft

POSTERIOR VIEW

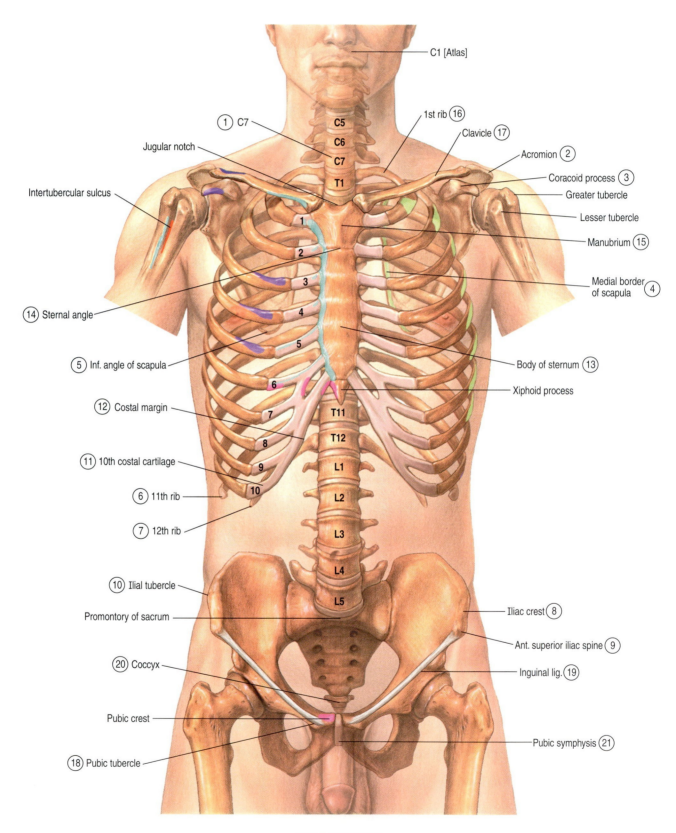

C1 [Atlas]

① C7

C5
C6
C7
T1

Jugular notch

1st rib ⑯

Clavicle ⑰

Acromion ②

Coracoid process ③

Greater tubercle

Intertubercular sulcus

Lesser tubercle

1

2

Manubrium ⑮

3

Medial border
of scapula ④

⑭ Sternal angle

4

5

Body of sternum ⑬

⑤ Inf. angle of scapula

6

Xiphoid process

⑫ Costal margin

7

T11

8

T12

⑪ 10th costal cartilage

9

L1

⑥ 11th rib

10

L2

⑦ 12th rib

L3

L4

⑩ Ilial tubercle

L5

Iliac crest ⑧

Promontory of sacrum

Ant. superior iliac spine ⑨

⑳ Coccyx

Inguinal lig. ⑲

Pubic crest

Pubic symphysis ㉑

⑱ Pubic tubercle

ANTERIOR VIEW

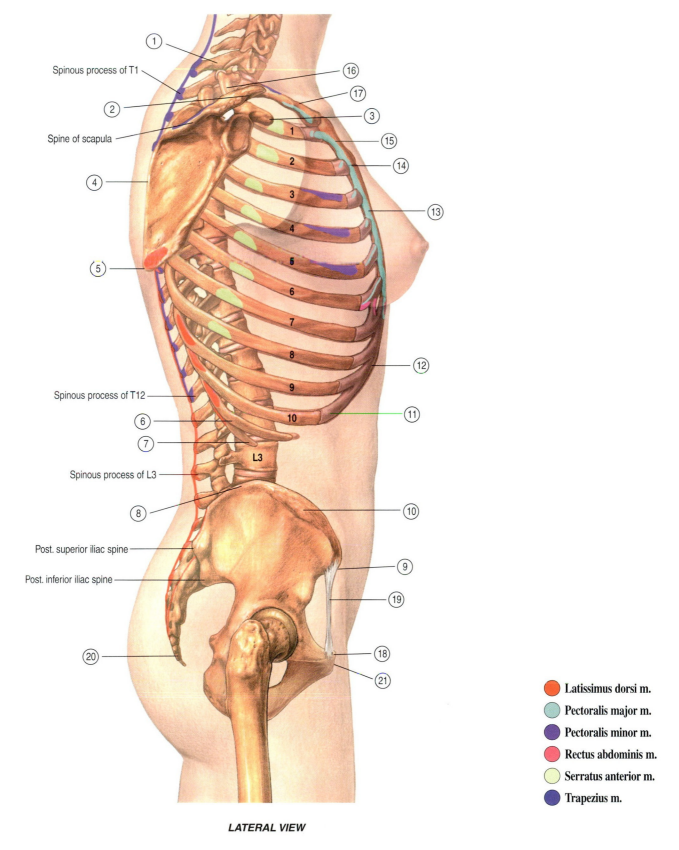

Spinous process of T1

Spine of scapula

Spinous process of T12

Spinous process of L3

Post. superior iliac spine

Post. inferior iliac spine

LATERAL VIEW

🔴 Latissimus dorsi m.
🟢 Pectoralis major m.
🟣 Pectoralis minor m.
🩷 Rectus abdominis m.
🟡 Serratus anterior m.
🔵 Trapezius m.

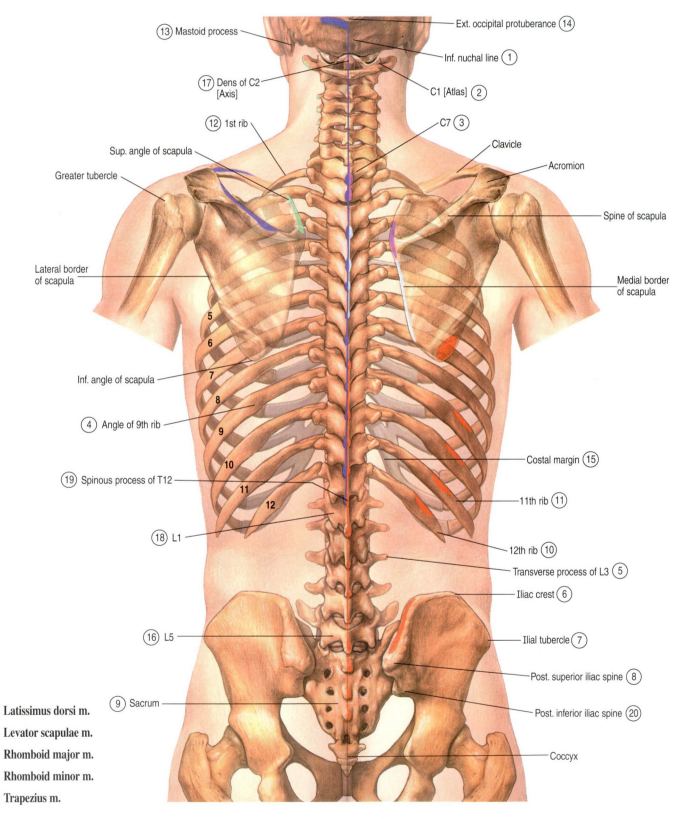

⑬ Mastoid process

Ext. occipital protuberance ⑭

Inf. nuchal line ①

⑰ Dens of C2 [Axis]

C1 [Atlas] ②

⑫ 1st rib

C7 ③

Sup. angle of scapula

Clavicle

Greater tubercle

Acromion

Spine of scapula

Lateral border of scapula

Medial border of scapula

5

6

Inf. angle of scapula

7

8

④ Angle of 9th rib

9

10

Costal margin ⑮

⑲ Spinous process of T12

11

12

11th rib ⑪

⑱ L1

12th rib ⑩

Transverse process of L3 ⑤

Iliac crest ⑥

⑯ L5

Ilial tubercle ⑦

Post. superior iliac spine ⑧

⑨ Sacrum

Post. inferior iliac spine ⑳

Coccyx

🔴 **Latissimus dorsi m.**

🟢 **Levator scapulae m.**

🟣 **Rhomboid major m.**

🔵 **Rhomboid minor m.**

🟪 **Trapezius m.**

POSTERIOR VIEW

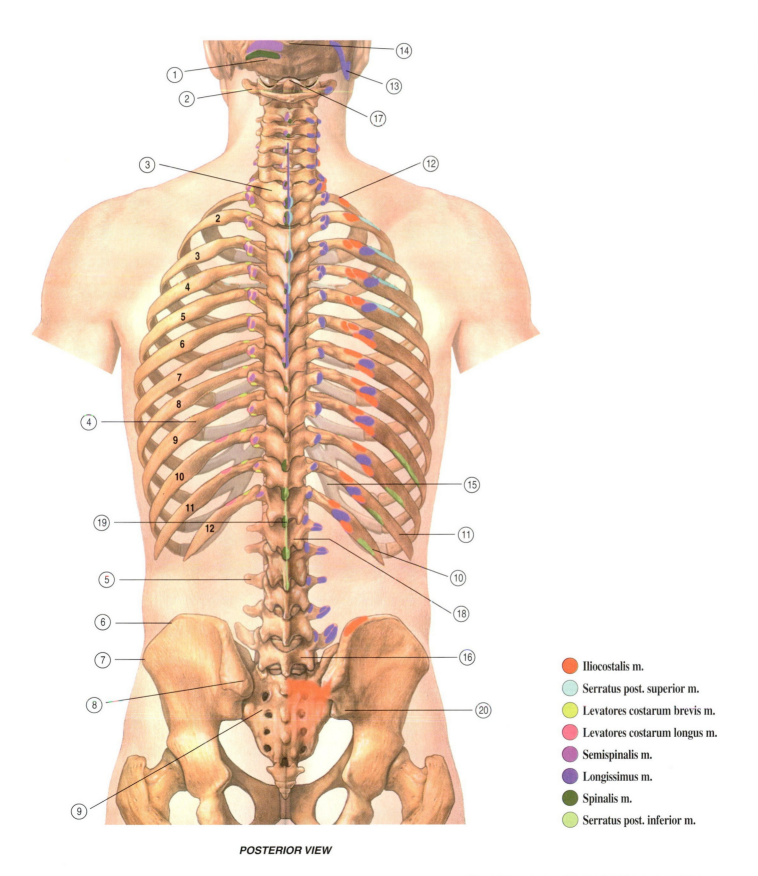

POSTERIOR VIEW

- 🔴 Iliocostalis m.
- 🔵 Serratus post. superior m.
- 🟡 Levatores costarum brevis m.
- 🩷 Levatores costarum longus m.
- 🟣 Semispinalis m.
- 🟪 Longissimus m.
- 🟢 Spinalis m.
- 🟩 Serratus post. inferior m.

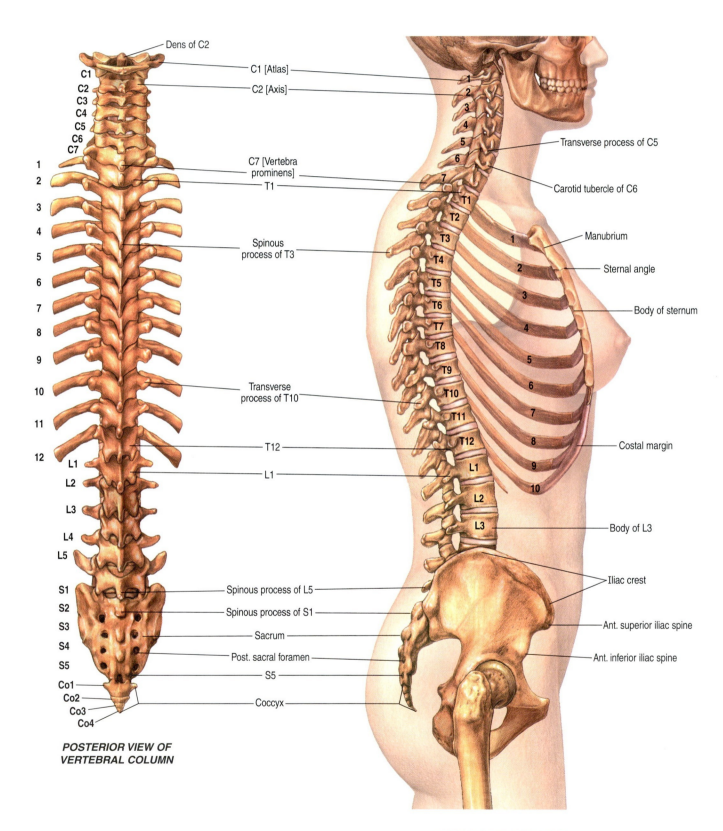

POSTERIOR VIEW OF VERTEBRAL COLUMN

LATERAL VIEW OF RIGHT HALF OF SKELETON

Dens of C2

C1 [Atlas]

C2 [Axis]

C7 [Vertebra prominens]

T1

Spinous process of T3

Transverse process of T10

T12

L1

Spinous process of L5

Spinous process of S1

Sacrum

Post. sacral foramen

S5

Coccyx

Transverse process of C5

Carotid tubercle of C6

Manubrium

Sternal angle

Body of sternum

Costal margin

Body of L3

Iliac crest

Ant. superior iliac spine

Ant. inferior iliac spine

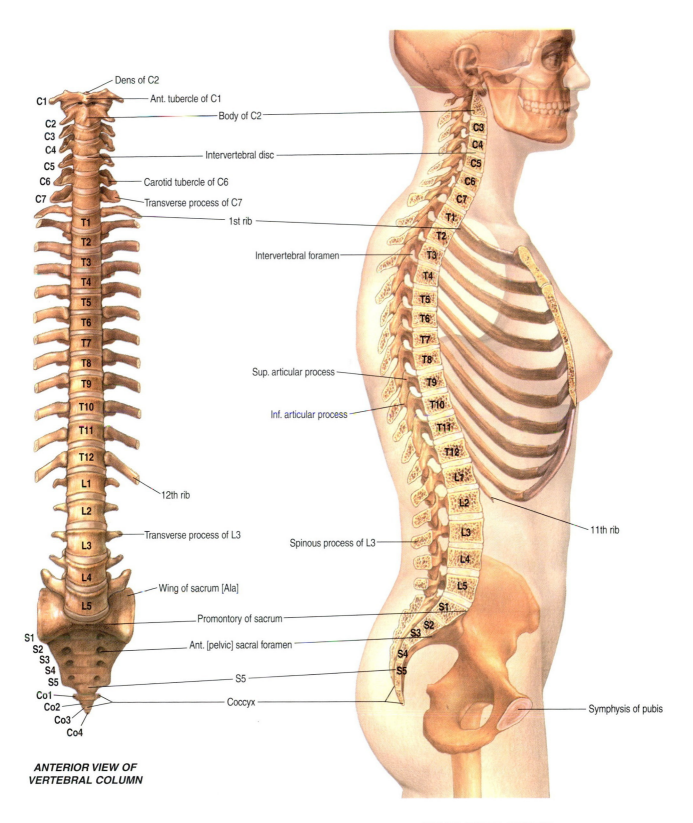

Dens of C2
Ant. tubercle of C1
Body of C2
Intervertebral disc
Carotid tubercle of C6
Transverse process of C7
1st rib

C1
C2
C3
C4
C5
C6
C7
T1
T2
T3
T4
T5
T6
T7
T8
T9
T10
T11
T12
L1
L2
L3
L4
L5
S1
S2
S3
S4
S5
Co1
Co2
Co3
Co4

12th rib

Transverse process of L3

Wing of sacrum [Ala]

Promontory of sacrum

Ant. [pelvic] sacral foramen

S5

Coccyx

**ANTERIOR VIEW OF
VERTEBRAL COLUMN**

Intervertebral foramen

Sup. articular process

Inf. articular process

Spinous process of L3

C3
C4
C5
C6
C7
T1
T2
T3
T4
T5
T6
T7
T8
T9
T10
T11
T12
L1
L2
L3
L4
L5
S1
S2
S3
S4
S5

11th rib

Symphysis of pubis

**RIGHT LATERAL VIEW OF
MEDIAN SECTIONED SKELETON**

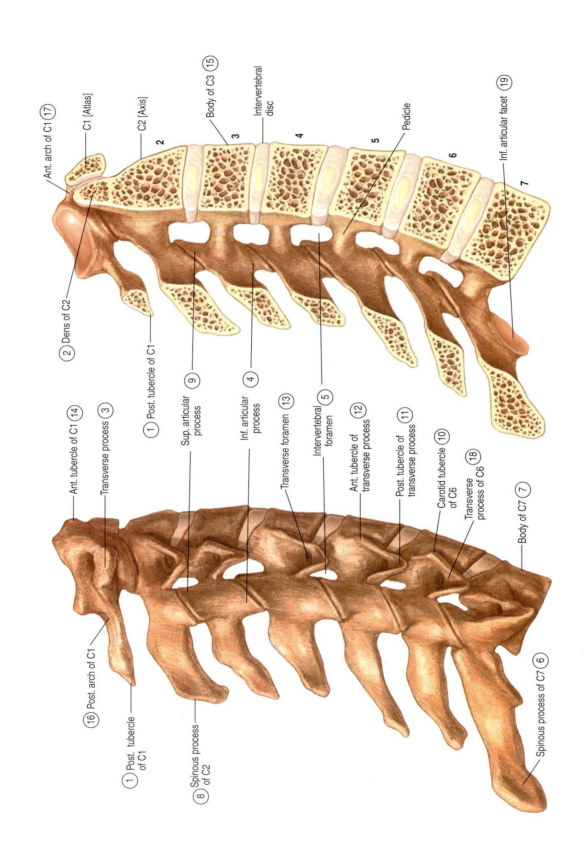

Ant. arch of C1 ⑰

C1 [Atlas]

C2 [Axis]

Body of C3 ⑮

Intervertebral disc

Pedicle

Inf. articular facet ⑲

② Dens of C2

① Post. tubercle of C1

Ant. tubercle of C1 ⑭

Transverse process ③

① Post. tubercle of C1

⑯ Post. arch of C1

① Post. tubercle of C1

⑧ Spinous process of C2

Sup. articular process ⑨

Inf. articular process ④

Transverse foramen ⑬

Intervertebral foramen ⑤

Ant. tubercle of transverse process ⑫

Post. tubercle of transverse process ⑪

Carotid tubercle of C6 ⑩

Transverse process of C6 ⑱

Body of C7 ⑦

Spinous process of C7 ⑥

MEDIAN SECTION OF CERVICAL VERTEBRAE

LATERAL VIEW OF CERVICAL VERTEBRAE

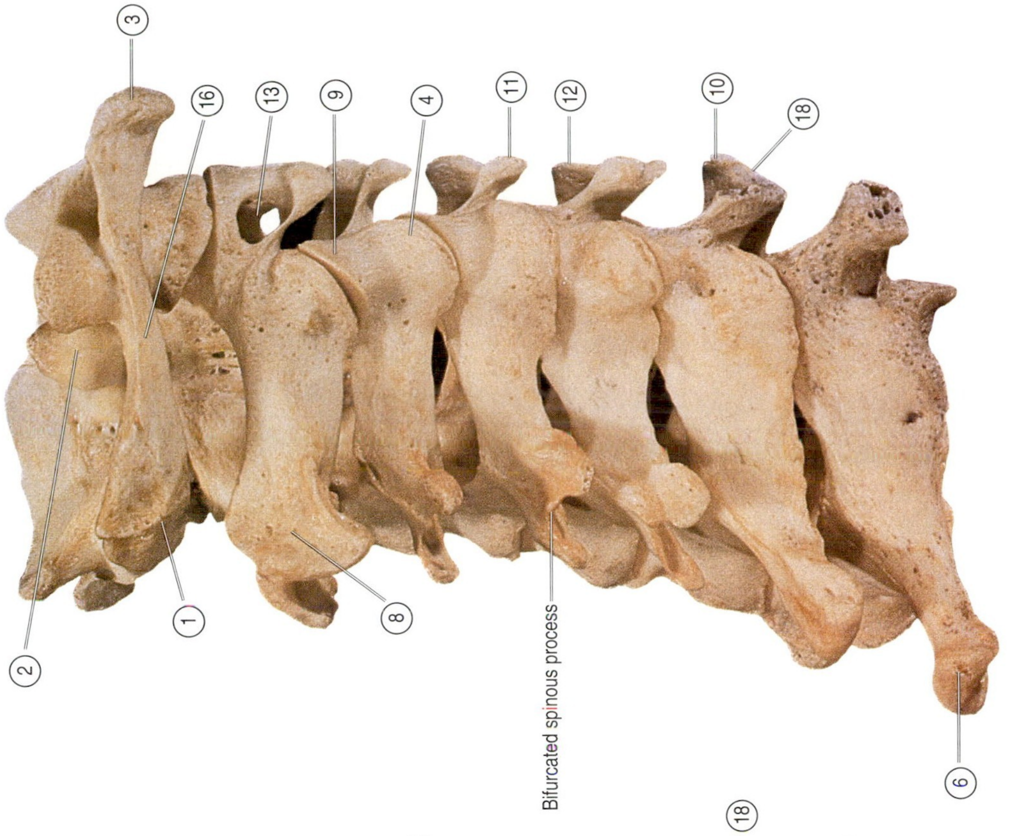
3
16
13
9
4
11
12
10
18
2
1
8
Bifurcated spinous process
6

POSTEROLATERAL VIEW OF CERVICAL VERTEBRAE

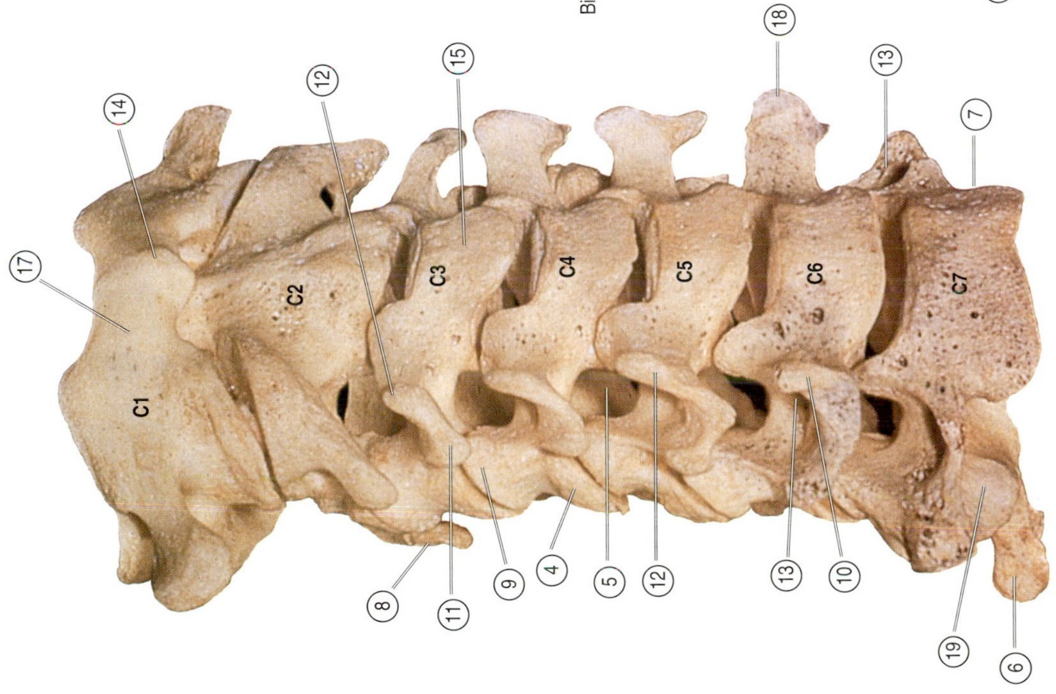
17
14
12
15
18
13
7
C1
C2
C3
C4
C5
C6
C7
8
11
9
4
5
12
13
10
19
6

ANTEROLATERAL VIEW OF CERVICAL VERTEBRAE

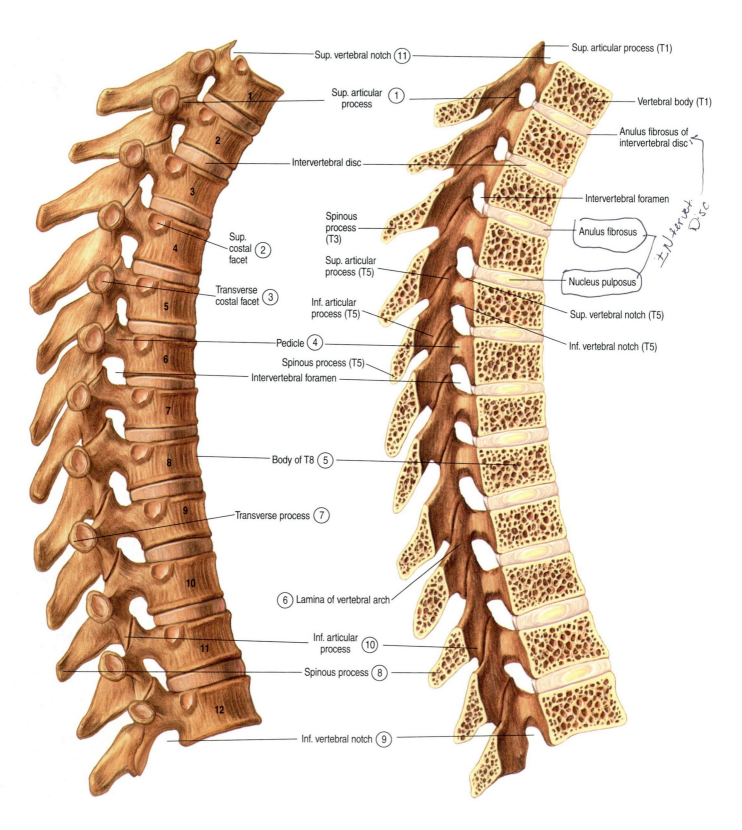

Sup. vertebral notch ⑪

Sup. articular process ①

Intervertebral disc

Sup. costal facet ②

Transverse costal facet ③

Pedicle ④

Spinous process (T5)

Intervertebral foramen

Body of T8 ⑤

Transverse process ⑦

⑥ Lamina of vertebral arch

Inf. articular process ⑩

Spinous process ⑧

Inf. vertebral notch ⑨

Sup. articular process (T1)

Vertebral body (T1)

Anulus fibrosus of intervertebral disc

Intervertebral foramen

Anulus fibrosus

Nucleus pulposus

Sup. vertebral notch (T5)

Inf. vertebral notch (T5)

Spinous process (T3)

Sup. articular process (T5)

Inf. articular process (T5)

Intervet. Disc

**LATERAL VIEW OF
THORACIC VERTEBRAE**

**MIDSAGITTAL SECTION OF
THORACIC VERTEBRAE**

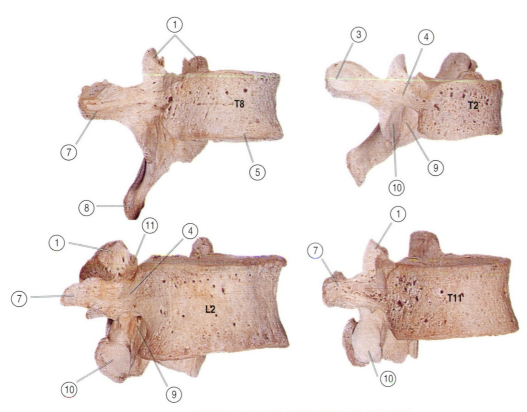

ANTEROLATERAL VIEW OF T8, T2, L2 & T11

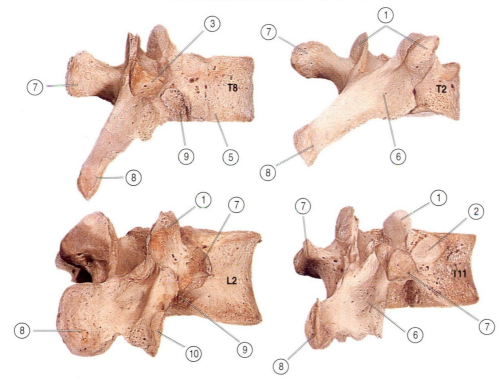

POSTEROLATERAL VIEW OF T8, T2, L2 & T11

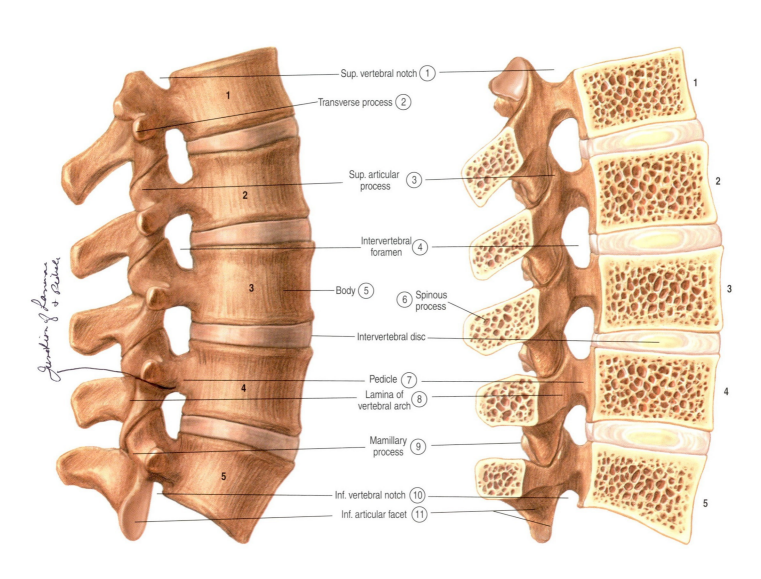

Sup. vertebral notch (1)

Transverse process (2)

Sup. articular process (3)

Intervertebral foramen (4)

Body (5)

(6) Spinous process

Intervertebral disc

Pedicle (7)

Lamina of vertebral arch (8)

Mamillary process (9)

Inf. vertebral notch (10)

Inf. articular facet (11)

Junction of lamina & pedicle

**LATERAL VIEW OF
LUMBAR VERTEBRAE**

**MEDIAN SECTION
OF LUMBAR VERTEBRAE**

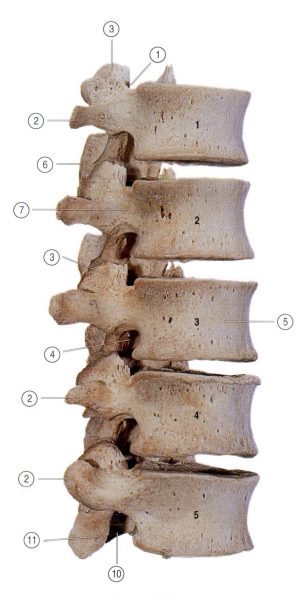

ANTEROLATERAL VIEW
OF LUMBAR VERTEBRAE

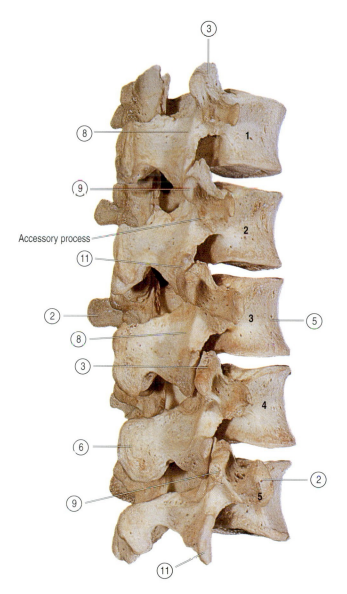

Accessory process

POSTEROLATERAL VIEW
OF LUMBAR VERTEBRAE

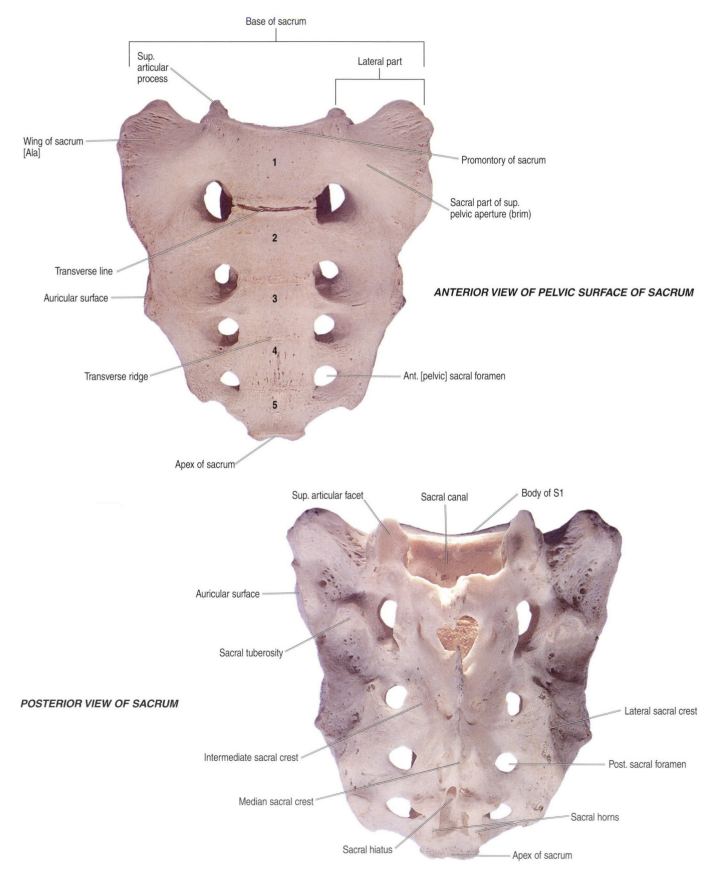

Base of sacrum

Sup. articular process

Lateral part

Wing of sacrum [Ala]

Promontory of sacrum

Sacral part of sup. pelvic aperture (brim)

1

2

Transverse line

3

Auricular surface

4

Transverse ridge

Ant. [pelvic] sacral foramen

5

ANTERIOR VIEW OF PELVIC SURFACE OF SACRUM

Apex of sacrum

Sup. articular facet

Sacral canal

Body of S1

Auricular surface

Sacral tuberosity

POSTERIOR VIEW OF SACRUM

Lateral sacral crest

Post. sacral foramen

Intermediate sacral crest

Median sacral crest

Sacral horns

Sacral hiatus

Apex of sacrum

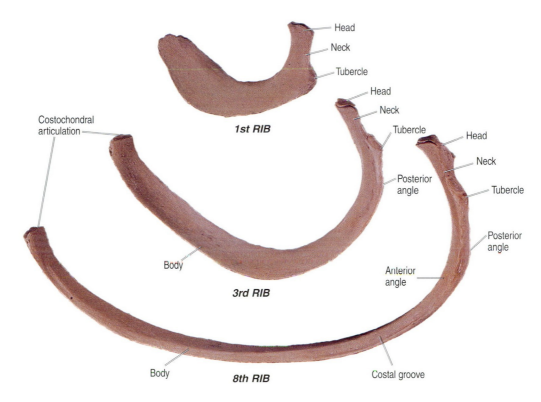

Head

Neck

Tubercle

Head

Neck

Costochondral
articulation

Tubercle

Head

Neck

Posterior
angle

Tubercle

1st RIB

Posterior
angle

Body

Anterior
angle

3rd RIB

Body

Costal groove

8th RIB

INFERIOR VIEW OF RIBS 1, 3 & 8 (RIGHT SIDE)

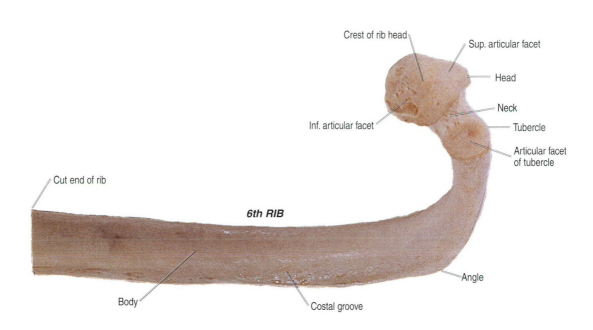

Crest of rib head

Sup. articular facet

Head

Neck

Inf. articular facet

Tubercle

Articular facet
of tubercle

Cut end of rib

6th RIB

Angle

Body

Costal groove

MEDIAL VIEW OF PROXIMAL END OF RIGHT 6TH RIB

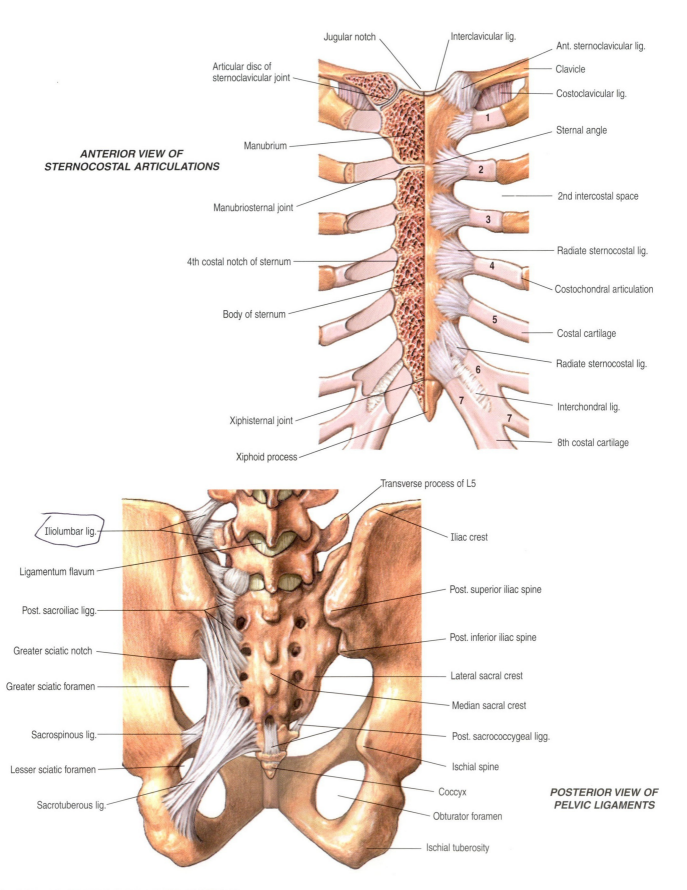

Jugular notch

Interclavicular lig.

Ant. sternoclavicular lig.

Articular disc of sternoclavicular joint

Clavicle

Costoclavicular lig.

1

Sternal angle

ANTERIOR VIEW OF STERNOCOSTAL ARTICULATIONS

Manubrium

2

2nd intercostal space

Manubriosternal joint

3

4th costal notch of sternum

Radiate sternocostal lig.

4

Costochondral articulation

Body of sternum

5

Costal cartilage

Radiate sternocostal lig.

6

Xiphisternal joint

7

7

Interchondral lig.

Xiphoid process

8th costal cartilage

Transverse process of L5

Iliolumbar lig.

Iliac crest

Ligamentum flavum

Post. superior iliac spine

Post. sacroiliac ligg.

Post. inferior iliac spine

Greater sciatic notch

Lateral sacral crest

Greater sciatic foramen

Median sacral crest

Sacrospinous lig.

Post. sacrococcygeal ligg.

Lesser sciatic foramen

Ischial spine

Sacrotuberous lig.

Coccyx

Obturator foramen

POSTERIOR VIEW OF PELVIC LIGAMENTS

Ischial tuberosity

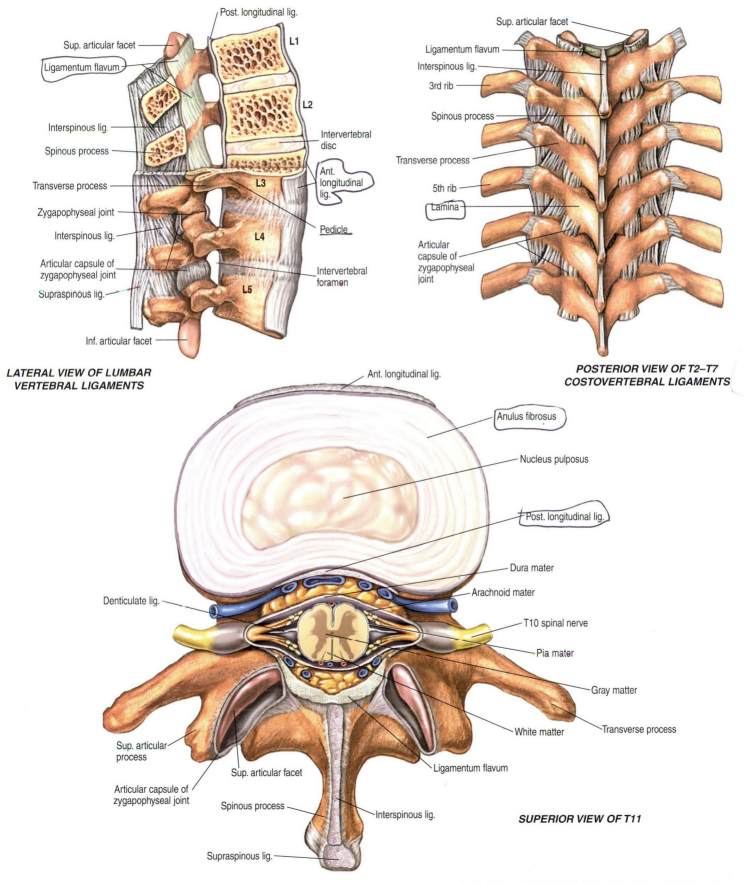

LATERAL VIEW OF LUMBAR VERTEBRAL LIGAMENTS

Sup. articular facet
Ligamentum flavum
Interspinous lig.
Spinous process
Transverse process
Zygapophyseal joint
Interspinous lig.
Articular capsule of zygapophyseal joint
Supraspinous lig.
Inf. articular facet

Post. longitudinal lig.
L1
L2
Intervertebral disc
Ant. longitudinal lig.
L3
Pedicle
L4
Intervertebral foramen
L5

POSTERIOR VIEW OF T2–T7 COSTOVERTEBRAL LIGAMENTS

Sup. articular facet
Ligamentum flavum
Interspinous lig.
3rd rib
Spinous process
Transverse process
5th rib
Lamina
Articular capsule of zygapophyseal joint

SUPERIOR VIEW OF T11

Ant. longitudinal lig.
Anulus fibrosus
Nucleus pulposus
Post. longitudinal lig.
Dura mater
Denticulate lig.
Arachnoid mater
T10 spinal nerve
Pia mater
Gray matter
White matter
Transverse process
Ligamentum flavum
Sup. articular process
Sup. articular facet
Articular capsule of zygapophyseal joint
Spinous process
Interspinous lig.
Supraspinous lig.

Muscle	Superior or Medial Attachment	Inferior or Lateral Attachment	Innervation	Action(s)
External intercostal	Inf. border of rib that bounds intercostal space cranially	Sup. border of rib bounding intercostal space caudally, muscular from costal tubercle to end of rib with membranous connection to sternum	1st to 11th intercostal nn. & subcostal n.	Elevate ribs in inspiration
Internal intercostal		Sup. border of rib bounding intercostal space caudally, muscular from angle to sternum		
Innermost intercostal		Separated from int. intercostal mm. only by neurovascular bundle		
Subcostal	Inf. border lateral to angle of rib that bounds intercostal space cranially	Int. surface near angle of rib that bounds intercostal space caudally, best developed between ribs 6 & 12, may cross 2 intercostal spaces		Depress ribs in expiration
Transversus thoracis	Int. surface of body & xiphoid of sternum	Inf. border of 2nd to 6th costal cartilages	1st to 11th intercostal nn.	Depress costal cartilages in expiration
Levatores costarum L. c. brevis m. L. c. longus m.	Transverse processes of C7 to T11	Between tubercle & angle on ext. surface of rib caudal to vertebral attachment	Dorsal primary rami of C8 & T1 to T11 spinal nn.	Elevate ribs in inspiration; laterally flex spine
Serratus posterior superior	Inf. part of ligamentum nuchae & spinous process from C7 to T2/T3	Sup. border of 2nd to 5th ribs just lateral to angles	2nd to 5th intercostal nn.	Elevate ribs in inspiration
Serratus posterior inferior	Spinous processes & thoracolumbar fascia from T11/T12 to L3	Inf. border of 9th/10th to 12th ribs just lateral to angles	9th to 11th intercostal nn. & subcostal n.	Depress ribs in expiration

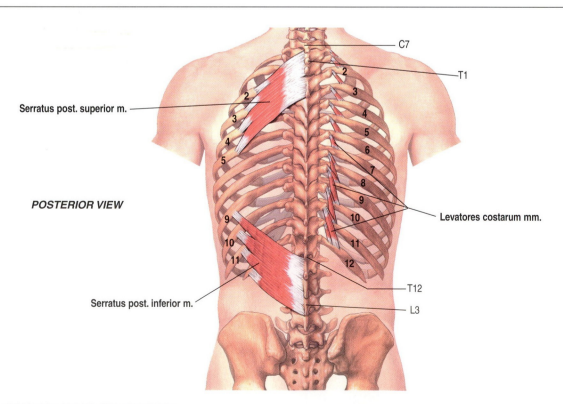

POSTERIOR VIEW

Serratus post. superior m.

Serratus post. inferior m.

Levatores costarum mm.

C7

T1

T12

L3

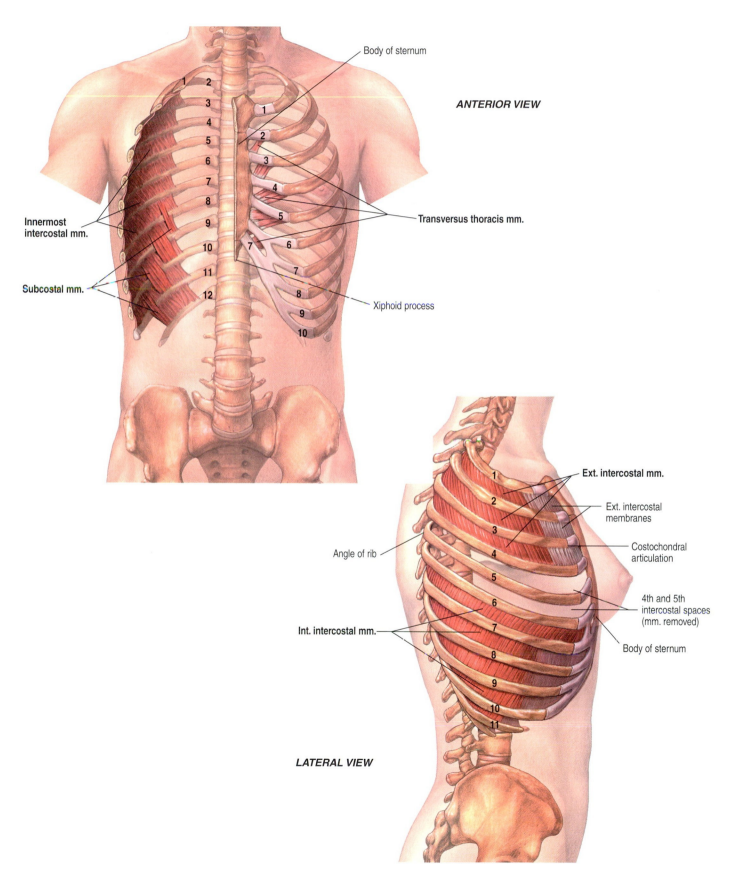

Body of sternum

ANTERIOR VIEW

1 2
3
4
5
6
7
8
9
10
11
12

1
2
3
4
5
6
7
8
9
10

Innermost intercostal mm.

Transversus thoracis mm.

Subcostal mm.

Xiphoid process

Ext. intercostal mm.

Ext. intercostal membranes

Costochondral articulation

4th and 5th intercostal spaces (mm. removed)

Body of sternum

Angle of rib

Int. intercostal mm.

LATERAL VIEW

1
2
3
4
5
6
7
8
9
10
11

Muscles—Abdominal Wall
Table 1.2

Muscle	Lateral or Superior Attachment	Medial or Inferior Attachment	Innervation	Action(s)
External oblique	Ext. surfaces of 5th to 12th ribs	Linea alba, pubic tubercle & ant. half of iliac crest	Inf. six thoracic nn. & subcostal n.	Compress & support abdominal viscera; flex & rotate trunk
Internal oblique	Thoracolumbar fascia, ant. two-thirds of iliac crest & lateral half of inguinal lig.	Inf. borders of 10th to 12th ribs, linea alba & pubis via the conjoint tendon	Ventral rami of inf. six thoracic & first lumbar nn.	
Transversus abdominis	Int. surfaces of 7th to 12th costal cartilages, thoracolumbar fascia, iliac crest & lateral third of inguinal lig.	Linea alba with aponeurosis of int. oblique, pubic crest & pecten pubis via conjoint tendon		Compress & support abdominal viscera
Rectus abdominis	Xiphoid process & 5th to 7th costal cartilages	Pubic symphysis & pubic crest	Ventral rami of inf. six thoracic nn.	Flex trunk & compress abdominal viscera
Quadratus lumborum	Medial half of inf. border of 12th rib & tips of lumbar transverse processes	Iliolumbar lig. & int. lip of iliac crest	Ventral rami of T12 & L1 to L4	Extend & laterally fixes the vertebral column; flex 12th rib during inspiration
Cremaster	Inf. edge of int. abdominal oblique, inguinal lig., pubic tubercle & pubic crest	Invest spermatic cord and testis	Genital br. of genitofemoral n. (L1 & L2)	Retract testis

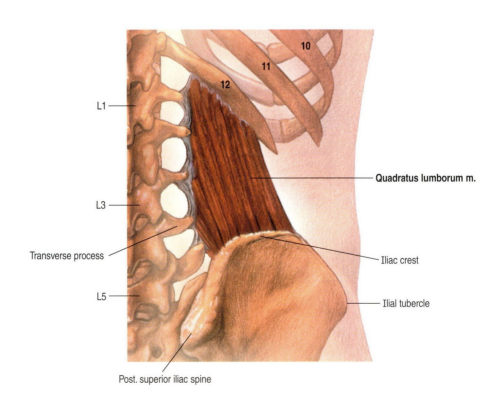

POSTERIOR VIEW

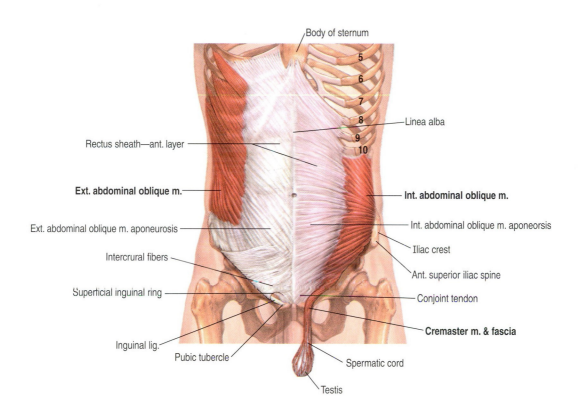

Body of sternum

5
6
7
8
9
10

Linea alba

Rectus sheath—ant. layer

Ext. abdominal oblique m.

Int. abdominal oblique m.

Ext. abdominal oblique m. aponeurosis

Int. abdominal oblique m. aponeorsis

Iliac crest

Intercrural fibers

Ant. superior iliac spine

Superficial inguinal ring

Conjoint tendon

Cremaster m. & fascia

Inguinal lig.

Pubic tubercle

Spermatic cord

Testis

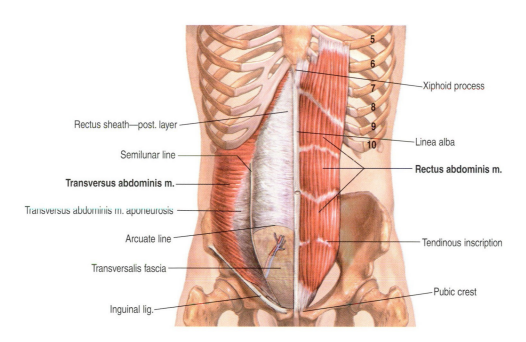

Rectus sheath—post. layer

5
6
7
8
9
10

Xiphoid process

Semilunar line

Linea alba

Transversus abdominis m.

Rectus abdominis m.

Transversus abdominis m. aponeurosis

Arcuate line

Transversalis fascia

Tendinous inscription

Inguinal lig.

Pubic crest

ANTERIOR VIEWS

Intrinsic Muscles of the Back
Table 1.3

Intrinsic Muscles of the Back[a]

Muscle	Inferior or Medial Attachment	Superior or Lateral Attachment	Innervation	Action(s)
SUPERFICIAL—SPINOTRANSVERSE GROUP				
Splenius capitis	Inf. half of ligamentum nuchae, spinous processes of C7 to T3/T4	Mastoid process, lateral third of the sup. nuchal line	Dorsal primary rami of middle cervical spinal nn.	Unilaterally, rotate & laterally flex neck to same side; bilaterally, extend the neck & head
Splenius cervicis	Spinous processes of T3/T4 to T6	Post. tubercles of transverse processes of C1 to C3	Dorsal primary rami of lower cervical spinal nn.	
INTERMEDIATE LAYER—ERECTOR SPINAE GROUP				
Iliocostalis m. *I. cervicis* *I. thoracis* *I. lumborum*	Sacrum, medial part of iliac crest, 12th to 3rd ribs	Angles of all ribs, transverse processes of C7 to C4		
Longissimus m. *L. capitis* *L. cervicis* *L. thoracis*	Sacrum, transverse processes of all vertebrae from L5 to C7, transverse & articular processes of C6 to C4	Transverse processes of all vertebrae from T12 to C2; angles of all ribs, mastoid process	Dorsal primary rami of all cervical, thoracic & lumbar spinal nn.	Unilaterally, flex vertebral column to same side; bilaterally, extend vertebral column; important in maintaining erect posture while standing or walking
Spinalis m. *S. capitis* *S. cervicis* *S. thoracis*	Spinous processes of L2/L3 to T11, ligamentum nuchae & spinous processes of T2 to C7, transverse processes of C7/C6 to C2, articular processes of C6 to C4	Spinous processes from T9/T8 to C7/C6, spinous processes of C3/C4 & C2, occipital bone between sup. & inf. nuchal lines with semispinalis m.		
DEEP LAYER—TRANSVERSOSPINAL GROUP				
Semispinalis m. *S. capitis* *S. cervicis* *S. thoracis*	Transverse processes of all vertebrae from T10 to C3, articular processes of C6 to C4	Spinous processes from T4 to C2, occipital bone between sup. & inf. nuchal lines; usually includes spinalis capitis m.	Dorsal primary rami of T6 to T1, all cervical spinal nn.	Unilaterally, lateral flex and/or rotate vertebral column & head to opposite side; bilaterally, extend vertebral column & head
Multifidus	All lamina from S4 to C2, transverse processes L5 to T1, articular processes C7 to C3	Spinous process of all vertebrae; spans 1 to 3 vertebrae	Dorsal primary rami of T6 to C1 spinal nn.	Unilaterally, lateral flex and/or rotate vertebral column to opposite side; bilaterally, extend or stabilize vertebral column
Rotatores	Transverse processes of all vertebrae L5 to T2	Lamina & roots of spinous process of next vertebra superiorly; best developed in thoracic region	Dorsal primary rami of L4 to T1 spinal nn.	

[a]The most superficial layer also includes the trapezius, latissimus dorsi, levator scapulae & rhomboid muscles which move the upper limb. The intermediate layer is formed by the serratus posterior muscles. The muscles of both of these layers are considered extrinsic to the back. The intrinsic muscles of the back form the deepest three back muscle layers.

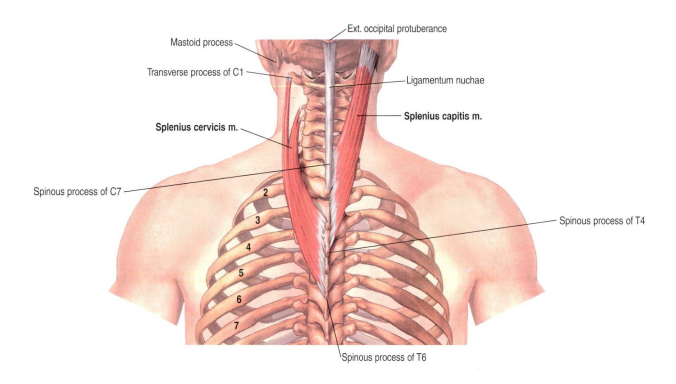

Ext. occipital protuberance

Mastoid process

Transverse process of C1

Ligamentum nuchae

Splenius capitis m.

Splenius cervicis m.

Spinous process of C7

Spinous process of T4

2

3

4

5

6

7

Spinous process of T6

POSTERIOR VIEWS

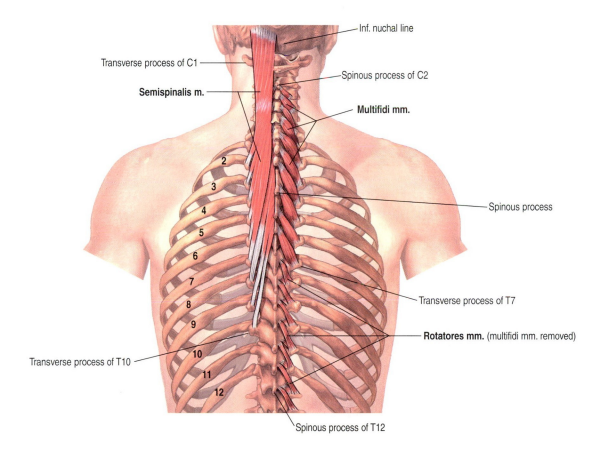

Inf. nuchal line

Transverse process of C1

Spinous process of C2

Semispinalis m.

Multifidi mm.

2

3

4

5

6

Spinous process

7

8

Transverse process of T7

9

Rotatores mm. (multifidi mm. removed)

10

Transverse process of T10

11

12

Spinous process of T12

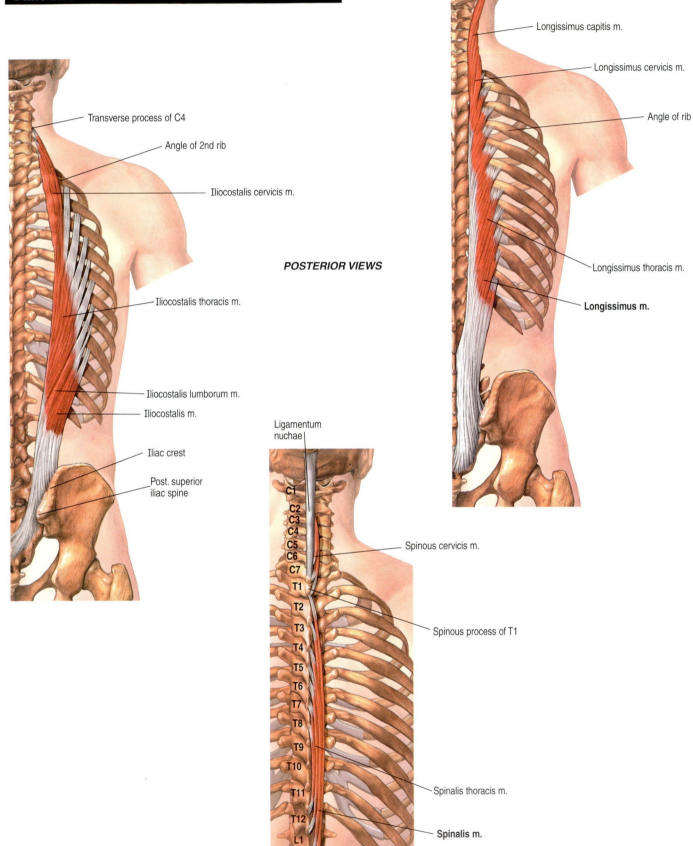

Mastoid process

Longissimus capitis m.

Longissimus cervicis m.

Angle of rib

Transverse process of C4

Angle of 2nd rib

Iliocostalis cervicis m.

POSTERIOR VIEWS

Longissimus thoracis m.

Iliocostalis thoracis m.

Longissimus m.

Iliocostalis lumborum m.

Iliocostalis m.

Iliac crest

Post. superior
iliac spine

Ligamentum
nuchae

C1
C2
C3
C4
C5
C6
C7
T1
T2
T3
T4
T5
T6
T7
T8
T9
T10
T11
T12
L1
L2

Spinous cervicis m.

Spinous process of T1

Spinalis thoracis m.

Spinalis m.

Spinous process of L2

Muscle	Inferior or Medial Attachment	Superior or Lateral Attachment	Innervation	Action(s)
DEEP LAYER—SUBOCCIPITAL GROUP				
Rectus capitis posterior major	Spinous process of C2	Lateral part of inf. nuchal line	Dorsal primary ramus of C1 [suboccipital] n.	Unilaterally, rotate head to same side; bilaterally, extend head at atlanto-occipital joint
Rectus capitis posterior minor	Post. tubercle of C1	Medial part of inf. nuchal line		
Obliquus capitis superior	Transverse process of C1	Sup. to inf. nuchal line		Unilaterally, rotate C1 & head to same side around odontoid process; bilaterally, extend head at atlanto-axial joint
Obliquus capitis inferior	Spinous process of C2	Transverse process of C1		

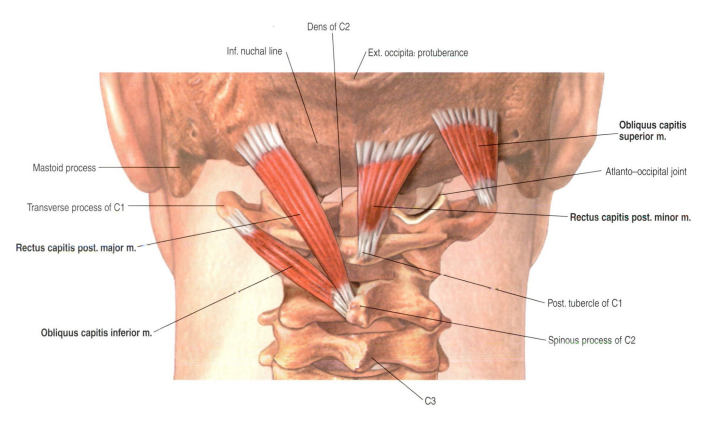

POSTERIOR VIEW

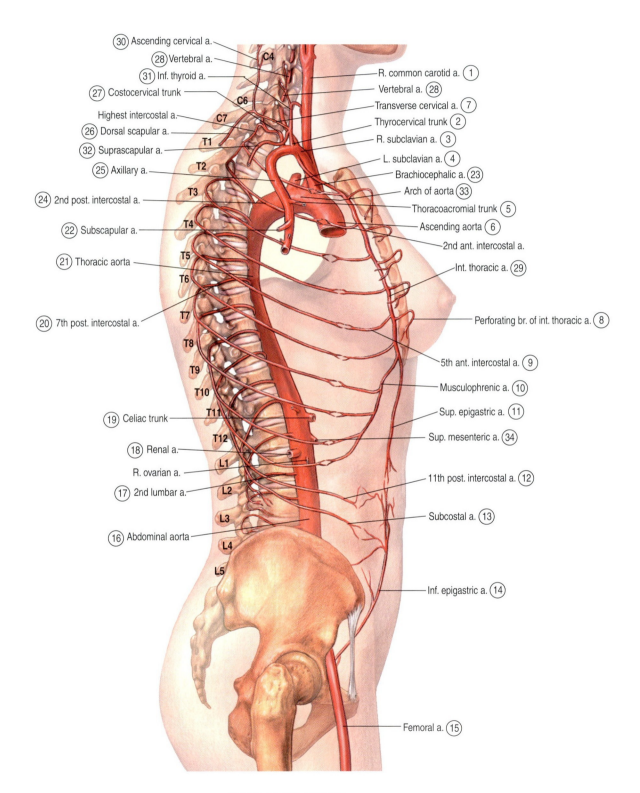

- (30) Ascending cervical a.
- (28) Vertebral a.
- (31) Inf. thyroid a.
- (27) Costocervical trunk
- Highest intercostal a.
- (26) Dorsal scapular a.
- (32) Suprascapular a.
- (25) Axillary a.
- (24) 2nd post. intercostal a.
- (22) Subscapular a.
- (21) Thoracic aorta
- (20) 7th post. intercostal a.
- (19) Celiac trunk
- (18) Renal a.
- R. ovarian a.
- (17) 2nd lumbar a.
- (16) Abdominal aorta

C4, C6, C7, T1, T2, T3, T4, T5, T6, T7, T8, T9, T10, T11, T12, L1, L2, L3, L4, L5

- R. common carotid a. (1)
- Vertebral a. (28)
- Transverse cervical a. (7)
- Thyrocervical trunk (2)
- R. subclavian a. (3)
- L. subclavian a. (4)
- Brachiocephalic a. (23)
- Arch of aorta (33)
- Thoracoacromial trunk (5)
- Ascending aorta (6)
- 2nd ant. intercostal a.
- Int. thoracic a. (29)
- Perforating br. of int. thoracic a. (8)
- 5th ant. intercostal a. (9)
- Musculophrenic a. (10)
- Sup. epigastric a. (11)
- Sup. mesenteric a. (34)
- 11th post. intercostal a. (12)
- Subcostal a. (13)
- Inf. epigastric a. (14)
- Femoral a. (15)

RIGHT LATERAL VIEW

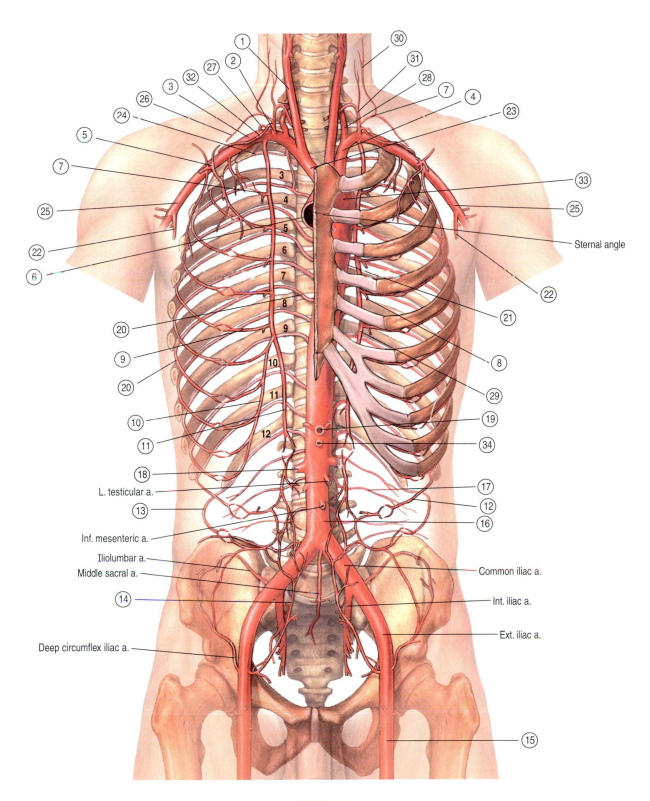

L. testicular a.

Inf. mesenteric a.

Iliolumbar a.

Middle sacral a.

Deep circumflex iliac a.

Sternal angle

Common iliac a.

Int. iliac a.

Ext. iliac a.

ANTERIOR VIEW

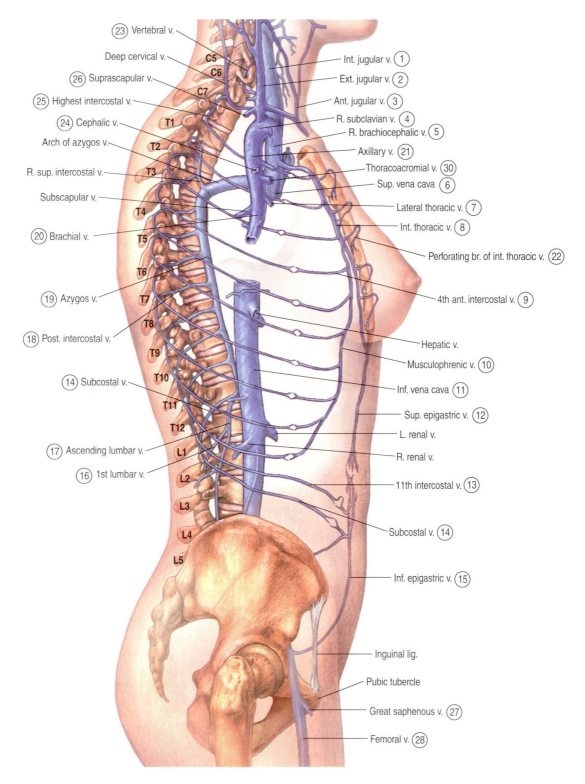

㉓ Vertebral v.

Deep cervical v.

㉖ Suprascapular v.

㉕ Highest intercostal v.

㉔ Cephalic v.

Arch of azygos v.

R. sup. intercostal v.

Subscapular v.

⑳ Brachial v.

⑲ Azygos v.

⑱ Post. intercostal v.

⑭ Subcostal v.

⑰ Ascending lumbar v.

⑯ 1st lumbar v.

Int. jugular v. ①
Ext. jugular v. ②
Ant. jugular v. ③
R. subclavian v. ④
R. brachiocephalic v. ⑤
Axillary v. ㉑
Thoracoacromial v. ㉚
Sup. vena cava ⑥
Lateral thoracic v. ⑦
Int. thoracic v. ⑧
Perforating br. of int. thoracic v. ㉒
4th ant. intercostal v. ⑨
Hepatic v.
Musculophrenic v. ⑩
Inf. vena cava ⑪
Sup. epigastric v. ⑫
L. renal v.
R. renal v.
11th intercostal v. ⑬
Subcostal v. ⑭
Inf. epigastric v. ⑮
Inguinal lig.
Pubic tubercle
Great saphenous v. ㉗
Femoral v. ㉘

C5
C6
C7
T1
T2
T3
T4
T5
T6
T7
T8
T9
T10
T11
T12
L1
L2
L3
L4
L5

RIGHT LATERAL VIEW

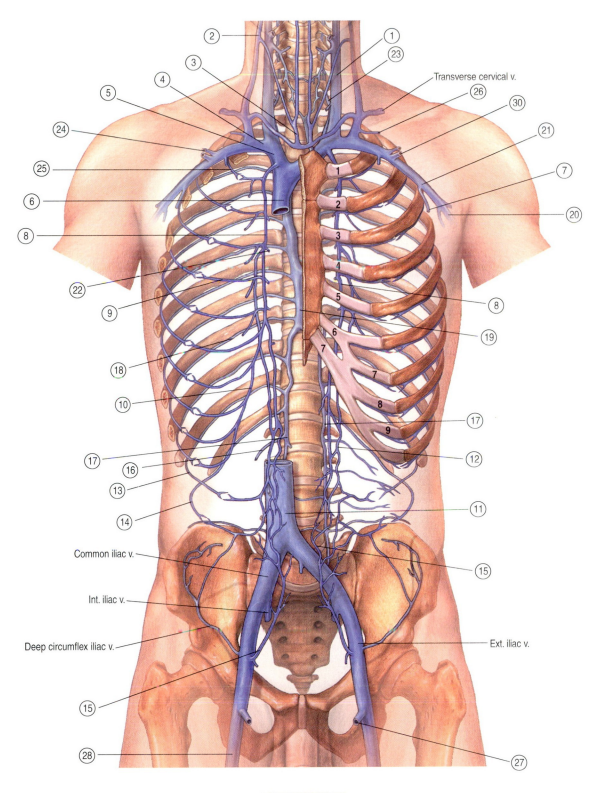

Transverse cervical v.

Common iliac v.

Int. iliac v.

Deep circumflex iliac v.

Ext. iliac v.

ANTERIOR VIEW

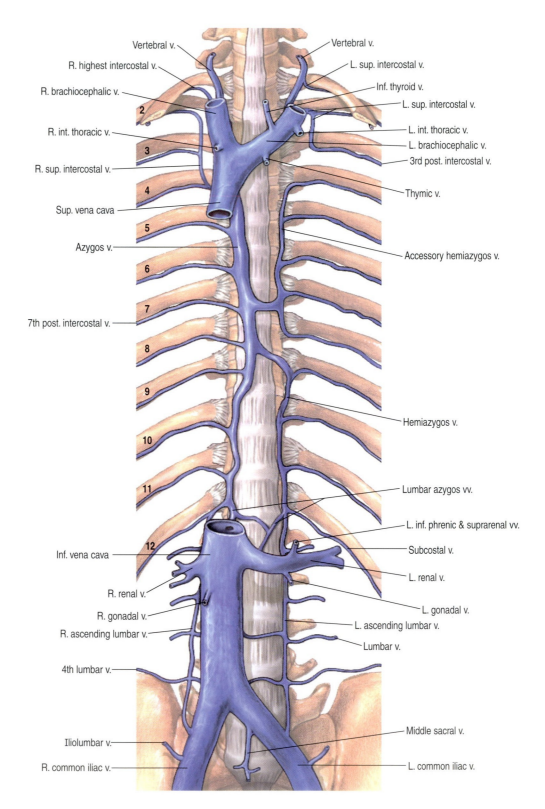

Vertebral v.
Vertebral v.
R. highest intercostal v.
L. sup. intercostal v.
R. brachiocephalic v.
Inf. thyroid v.
L. sup. intercostal v.
R. int. thoracic v.
L. int. thoracic v.
L. brachiocephalic v.
R. sup. intercostal v.
3rd post. intercostal v.
Thymic v.
Sup. vena cava
Azygos v.
Accessory hemiazygos v.
7th post. intercostal v.
Hemiazygos v.
Lumbar azygos vv.
L. inf. phrenic & suprarenal vv.
Subcostal v.
Inf. vena cava
L. renal v.
R. renal v.
R. gonadal v.
L. gonadal v.
R. ascending lumbar v.
L. ascending lumbar v.
Lumbar v.
4th lumbar v.
Middle sacral v.
Iliolumbar v.
R. common iliac v.
L. common iliac v.

ANTERIOR VIEW

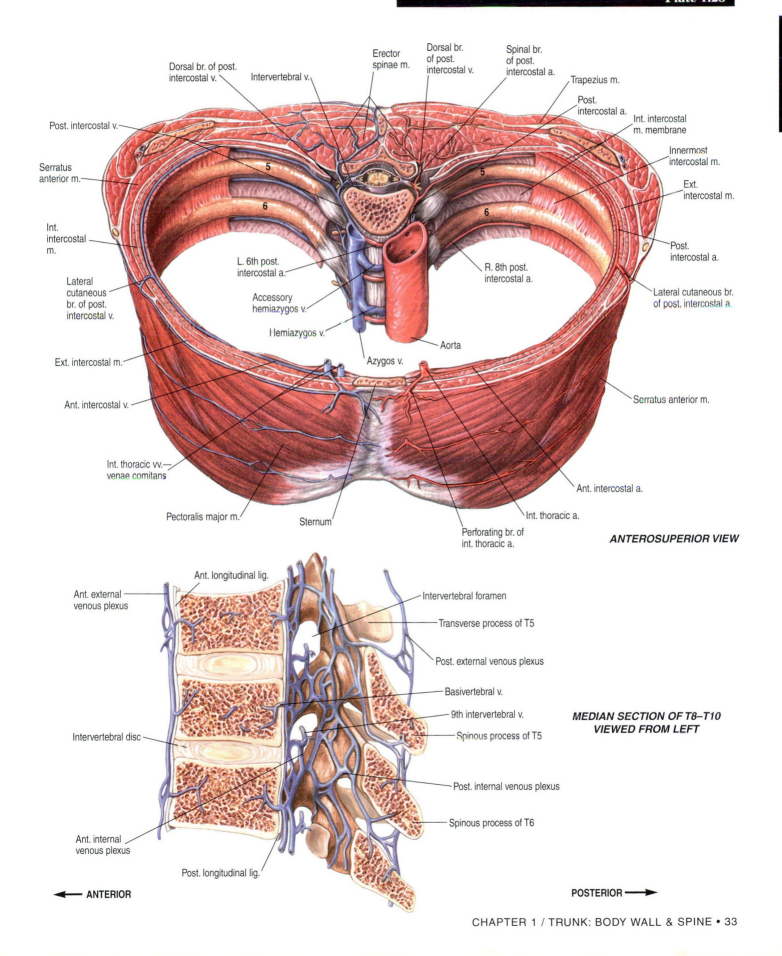

Dorsal br. of post. intercostal v.

Intervertebral v.

Erector spinae m.

Dorsal br. of post. intercostal v.

Spinal br. of post. intercostal a.

Trapezius m.

Post. intercostal a.

Int. intercostal m. membrane

Innermost intercostal m.

Ext. intercostal m.

Post. intercostal v.

Serratus anterior m.

Int. intercostal m.

Lateral cutaneous br. of post. intercostal v.

Ext. intercostal m.

Ant. intercostal v.

L. 6th post. intercostal a.

Accessory hemiazygos v.

Hemiazygos v.

Azygos v.

R. 8th post. intercostal a.

Post. intercostal a.

Lateral cutaneous br. of post. intercostal a.

Aorta

Int. thoracic vv. venae comitans

Pectoralis major m.

Sternum

Serratus anterior m.

Ant. intercostal a.

Int. thoracic a.

Perforating br. of int. thoracic a.

ANTEROSUPERIOR VIEW

Ant. longitudinal lig.

Ant. external venous plexus

Intervertebral foramen

Transverse process of T5

Post. external venous plexus

Basivertebral v.

9th intervertebral v.

Spinous process of T5

MEDIAN SECTION OF T8–T10 VIEWED FROM LEFT

Intervertebral disc

Post. internal venous plexus

Ant. internal venous plexus

Spinous process of T6

Post. longitudinal lig.

◄— **ANTERIOR**

POSTERIOR —►

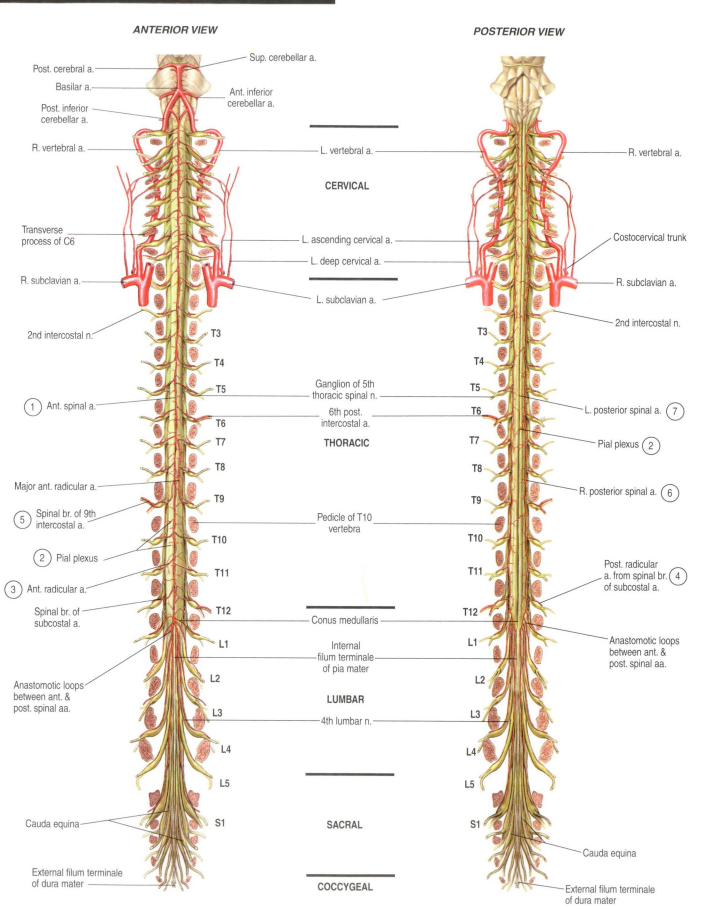

ANTERIOR VIEW

POSTERIOR VIEW

Post. cerebral a.

Sup. cerebellar a.

Basilar a.

Ant. inferior cerebellar a.

Post. inferior cerebellar a.

R. vertebral a.

L. vertebral a.

R. vertebral a.

CERVICAL

Transverse process of C6

L. ascending cervical a.

Costocervical trunk

L. deep cervical a.

R. subclavian a.

R. subclavian a.

L. subclavian a.

2nd intercostal n.

2nd intercostal n.

T3

T3

2nd intercostal n.

T4

T4

T5

Ganglion of 5th thoracic spinal n.

T5

① Ant. spinal a.

6th post. intercostal a.

T6

T6

L. posterior spinal a. ⑦

T7

THORACIC

T7

Pial plexus ②

T8

T8

Major ant. radicular a.

T9

T9

R. posterior spinal a. ⑥

⑤ Spinal br. of 9th intercostal a.

Pedicle of T10 vertebra

T10

T10

② Pial plexus

T11

T11

Post. radicular a. from spinal br. of subcostal a. ④

③ Ant. radicular a.

Spinal br. of subcostal a.

T12

T12

Conus medullaris

Anastomotic loops between ant. & post. spinal aa.

L1

L1

Anastomotic loops between ant. & post. spinal aa.

Internal filum terminale of pia mater

L2

L2

LUMBAR

L3

4th lumbar n.

L3

L4

L4

L5

L5

Cauda equina

S1

SACRAL

S1

Cauda equina

External filum terminale of dura mater

COCCYGEAL

External filum terminale of dura mater

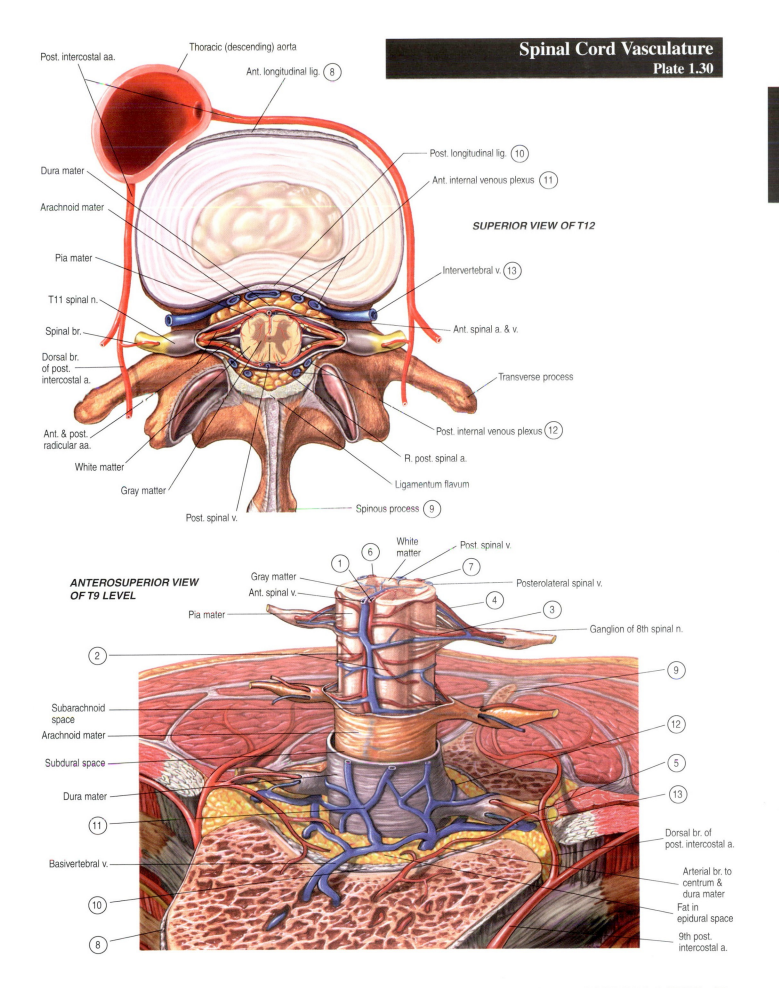

Post. intercostal aa.

Thoracic (descending) aorta

Ant. longitudinal lig. (8)

Dura mater

Arachnoid mater

Pia mater

T11 spinal n.

Spinal br.

Dorsal br.
of post.
intercostal a.

Ant. & post.
radicular aa.

White matter

Gray matter

Post. spinal v.

Post. longitudinal lig. (10)

Ant. internal venous plexus (11)

SUPERIOR VIEW OF T12

Intervertebral v. (13)

Ant. spinal a. & v.

Transverse process

Post. internal venous plexus (12)

R. post. spinal a.

Ligamentum flavum

Spinous process (9)

**ANTEROSUPERIOR VIEW
OF T9 LEVEL**

White
matter

Post. spinal v.

Gray matter

Ant. spinal v.

Pia mater

(1) (6)

(7)

(4)

(3)

Posterolateral spinal v.

Ganglion of 8th spinal n.

(2)

(9)

Subarachnoid
space

Arachnoid mater

Subdural space

Dura mater

(11)

Basivertebral v.

(10)

(8)

(12)

(5)

(13)

Dorsal br. of
post. intercostal a.

Arterial br. to
centrum &
dura mater

Fat in
epidural space

9th post.
intercostal a.

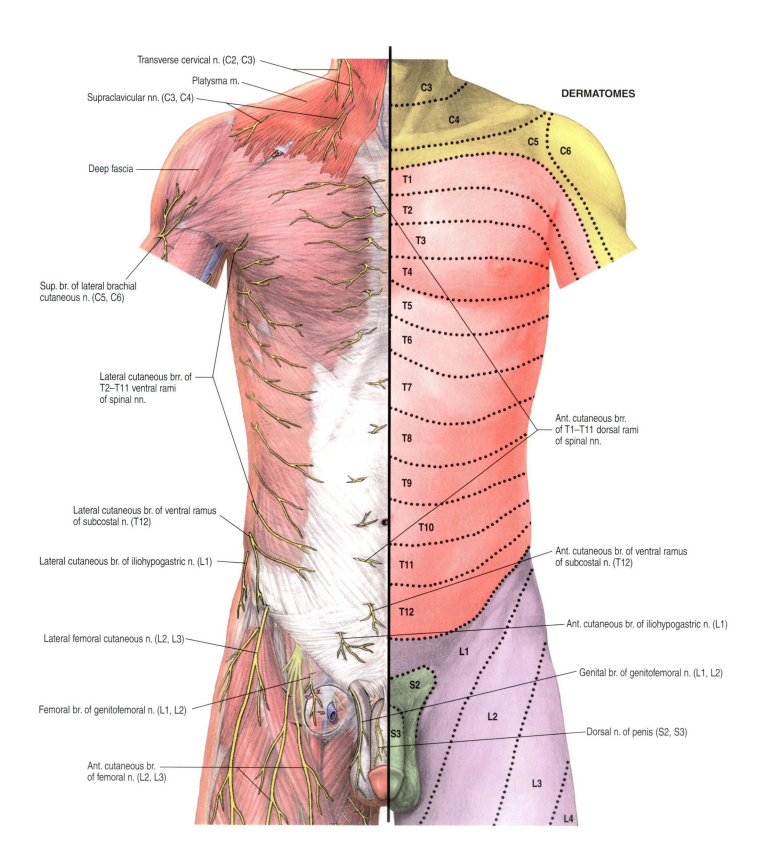

Transverse cervical n. (C2, C3)

Platysma m.

Supraclavicular nn. (C3, C4)

Deep fascia

Sup. br. of lateral brachial cutaneous n. (C5, C6)

Lateral cutaneous brr. of T2–T11 ventral rami of spinal nn.

Lateral cutaneous br. of ventral ramus of subcostal n. (T12)

Lateral cutaneous br. of iliohypogastric n. (L1)

Lateral femoral cutaneous n. (L2, L3)

Femoral br. of genitofemoral n. (L1, L2)

Ant. cutaneous br. of femoral n. (L2, L3)

DERMATOMES

C3
C4
C5
C6
T1
T2
T3
T4
T5
T6
T7
T8
T9
T10
T11
T12
L1
S2
S3
L2
L3
L4

Ant. cutaneous brr. of T1–T11 dorsal rami of spinal nn.

Ant. cutaneous br. of ventral ramus of subcostal n. (T12)

Ant. cutaneous br. of iliohypogastric n. (L1)

Genital br. of genitofemoral n. (L1, L2)

Dorsal n. of penis (S2, S3)

ANTERIOR VIEW

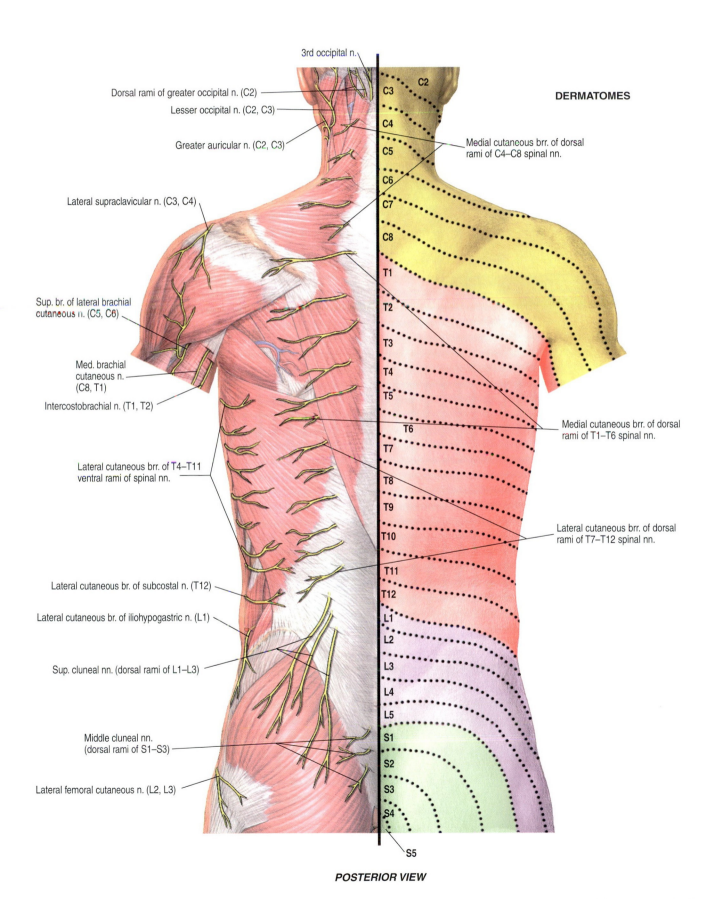

3rd occipital n.

Dorsal rami of greater occipital n. (C2)

Lesser occipital n. (C2, C3)

Greater auricular n. (C2, C3)

Lateral supraclavicular n. (C3, C4)

Sup. br. of lateral brachial cutaneous n. (C5, C6)

Med. brachial cutaneous n. (C8, T1)

Intercostobrachial n. (T1, T2)

Lateral cutaneous brr. of T4–T11 ventral rami of spinal nn.

Lateral cutaneous br. of subcostal n. (T12)

Lateral cutaneous br. of iliohypogastric n. (L1)

Sup. cluneal nn. (dorsal rami of L1–L3)

Middle cluneal nn. (dorsal rami of S1–S3)

Lateral femoral cutaneous n. (L2, L3)

DERMATOMES

Medial cutaneous brr. of dorsal rami of C4–C8 spinal nn.

Medial cutaneous brr. of dorsal rami of T1–T6 spinal nn.

Lateral cutaneous brr. of dorsal rami of T7–T12 spinal nn.

C2 C3 C4 C5 C6 C7 C8 T1 T2 T3 T4 T5 T6 T7 T8 T9 T10 T11 T12 L1 L2 L3 L4 L5 S1 S2 S3 S4 S5

POSTERIOR VIEW

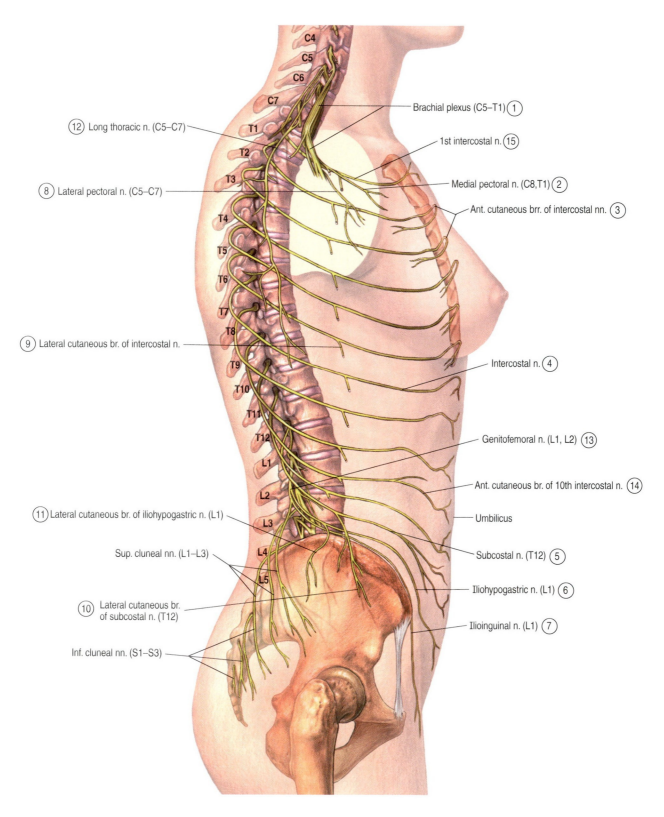

C4
C5
C6
C7
T1
T2
T3
T4
T5
T6
T7
T8
T9
T10
T11
T12
L1
L2
L3
L4
L5

⑫ Long thoracic n. (C5–C7)

⑧ Lateral pectoral n. (C5–C7)

⑨ Lateral cutaneous br. of intercostal n.

⑪ Lateral cutaneous br. of iliohypogastric n. (L1)

Sup. cluneal nn. (L1–L3)

⑩ Lateral cutaneous br. of subcostal n. (T12)

Inf. cluneal nn. (S1–S3)

Brachial plexus (C5–T1) ①

1st intercostal n. ⑮

Medial pectoral n. (C8,T1) ②

Ant. cutaneous brr. of intercostal nn. ③

Intercostal n. ④

Genitofemoral n. (L1, L2) ⑬

Ant. cutaneous br. of 10th intercostal n. ⑭

Umbilicus

Subcostal n. (T12) ⑤

Iliohypogastric n. (L1) ⑥

Ilioinguinal n. (L1) ⑦

RIGHT LATERAL VIEW

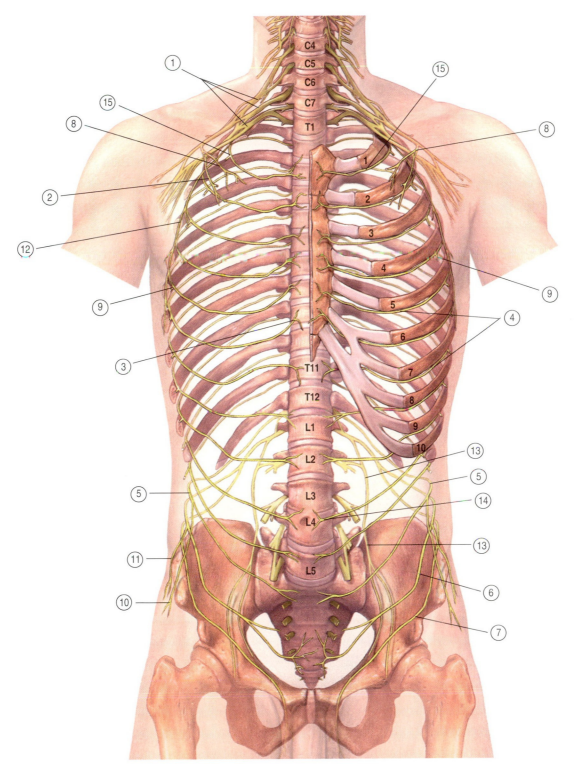

ANTERIOR VIEW

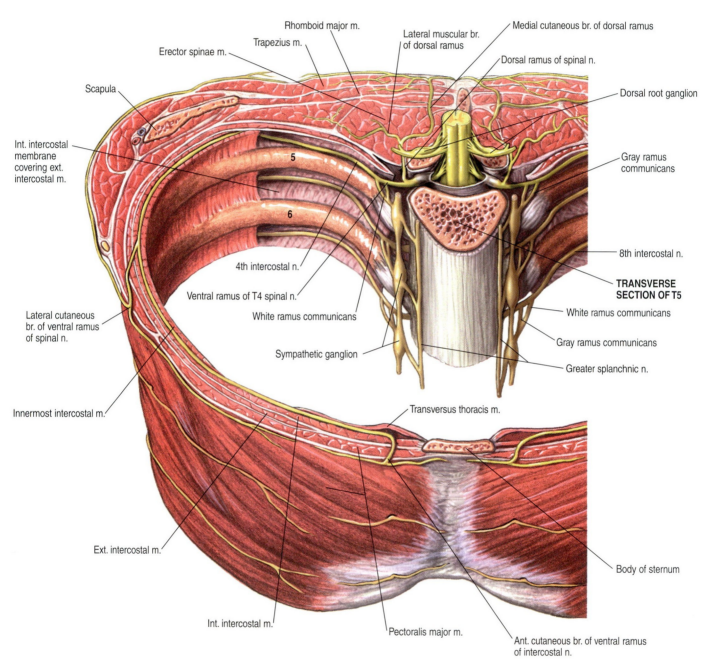

Rhomboid major m.

Lateral muscular br. of dorsal ramus

Medial cutaneous br. of dorsal ramus

Trapezius m.

Erector spinae m.

Dorsal ramus of spinal n.

Scapula

Dorsal root ganglion

Int. intercostal membrane covering ext. intercostal m.

Gray ramus communicans

5

6

4th intercostal n.

8th intercostal n.

Ventral ramus of T4 spinal n.

TRANSVERSE SECTION OF T5

White ramus communicans

White ramus communicans

Lateral cutaneous br. of ventral ramus of spinal n.

Sympathetic ganglion

Gray ramus communicans

Greater splanchnic n.

Innermost intercostal m.

Transversus thoracis m.

Ext. intercostal m.

Body of sternum

Int. intercostal m.

Pectoralis major m.

Ant. cutaneous br. of ventral ramus of intercostal n.

ANTEROSUPERIOR

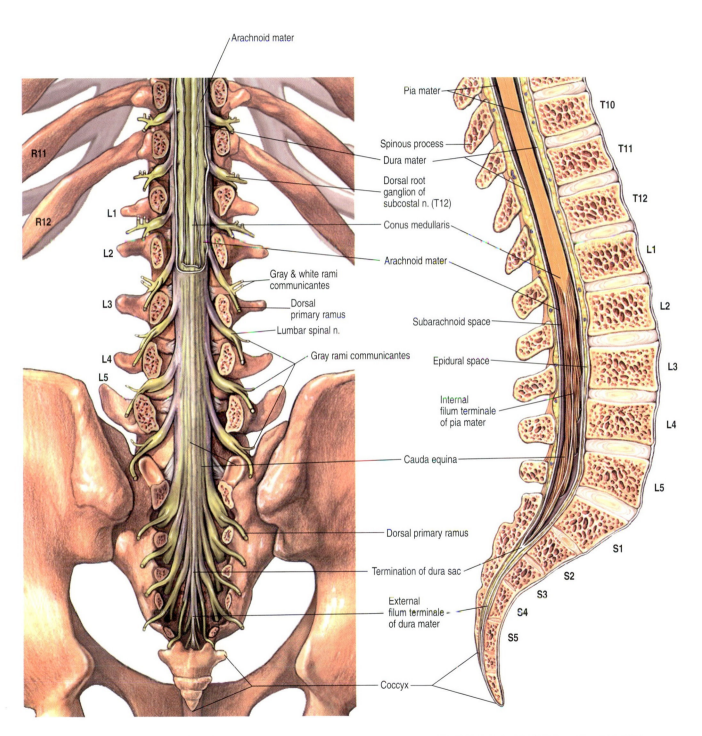

Arachnoid mater

R11

R12

L1

L2

L3

L4

L5

Gray & white rami communicantes

Dorsal primary ramus

Lumbar spinal n.

Gray rami communicantes

Pia mater

Spinous process

Dura mater

Dorsal root ganglion of subcostal n. (T12)

Conus medullaris

Arachnoid mater

Subarachnoid space

Epidural space

Internal filum terminale of pia mater

Cauda equina

Dorsal primary ramus

Termination of dura sac

External filum terminale of dura mater

Coccyx

T10

T11

T12

L1

L2

L3

L4

L5

S1

S2

S3

S4

S5

POSTERIOR VIEW

MEDIAN SECTION VIEWED FROM RIGHT

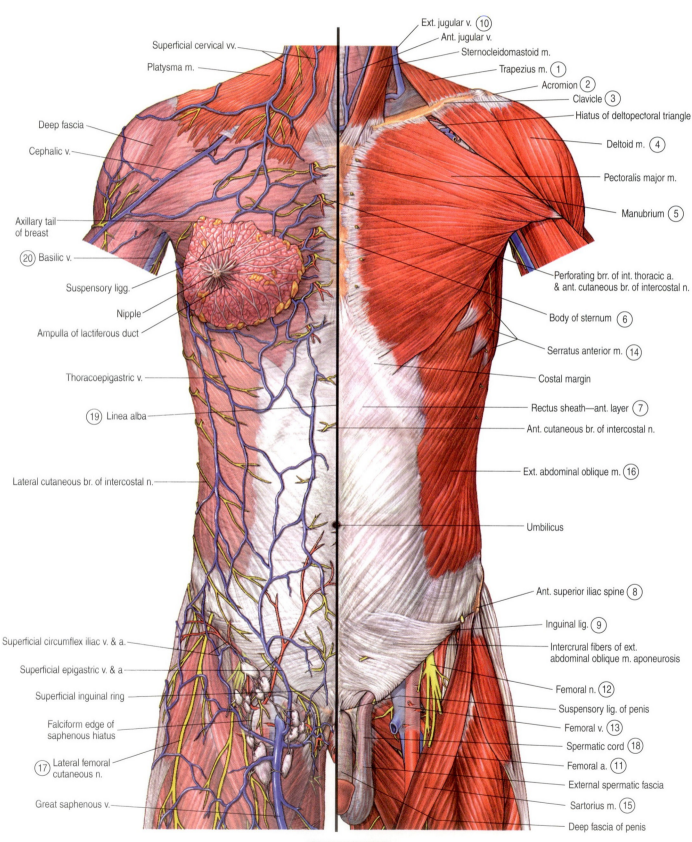

Ext. jugular v. (10)
Ant. jugular v.
Sternocleidomastoid m.
Trapezius m. (1)
Acromion (2)
Clavicle (3)
Hiatus of deltopectoral triangle
Deltoid m. (4)
Pectoralis major m.
Manubrium (5)
Perforating brr. of int. thoracic a. & ant. cutaneous br. of intercostal n.
Body of sternum (6)
Serratus anterior m. (14)
Costal margin
Rectus sheath—ant. layer (7)
Ant. cutaneous br. of intercostal n.
Ext. abdominal oblique m. (16)
Umbilicus
Ant. superior iliac spine (8)
Inguinal lig. (9)
Intercrural fibers of ext. abdominal oblique m. aponeurosis
Femoral n. (12)
Suspensory lig. of penis
Femoral v. (13)
Spermatic cord (18)
Femoral a. (11)
External spermatic fascia
Sartorius m. (15)
Deep fascia of penis

Superficial cervical vv.
Platysma m.
Deep fascia
Cephalic v.
Axillary tail of breast
(20) Basilic v.
Suspensory ligg.
Nipple
Ampulla of lactiferous duct
Thoracoepigastric v.
(19) Linea alba
Lateral cutaneous br. of intercostal n.
Superficial circumflex iliac v. & a.
Superficial epigastric v. & a
Superficial inguinal ring
Falciform edge of saphenous hiatus
(17) Lateral femoral cutaneous n.
Great saphenous v.

ANTERIOR VIEW

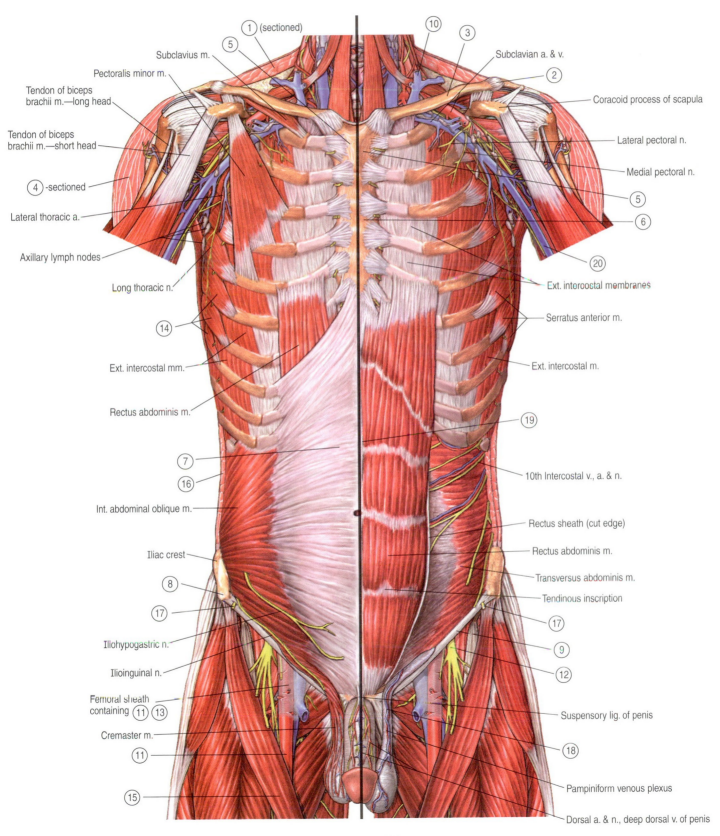

Subclavius m.

Pectoralis minor m.

Tendon of biceps
brachii m.—long head

Tendon of biceps
brachii m.—short head

④ -sectioned

Lateral thoracic a.

Axillary lymph nodes

Long thoracic n.

⑭

Ext. intercostal mm.

Rectus abdominis m.

⑦

⑯

Int. abdominal oblique m.

Iliac crest

⑧

⑰

Iliohypogastric n.

Ilioinguinal n.

Femoral sheath
containing ⑪ ⑬

Cremaster m.

⑪

⑮

① (sectioned)

⑤

⑩

③

Subclavian a. & v.

②

Coracoid process of scapula

Lateral pectoral n.

Medial pectoral n.

⑤

⑥

⑳

Ext. intercostal membranes

Serratus anterior m.

Ext. intercostal m.

⑲

10th Intercostal v., a. & n.

Rectus sheath (cut edge)

Rectus abdominis m.

Transversus abdominis m.

Tendinous inscription

⑰

⑨

⑫

Suspensory lig. of penis

⑱

Pampiniform venous plexus

Dorsal a. & n., deep dorsal v. of penis

ANTERIOR VIEW

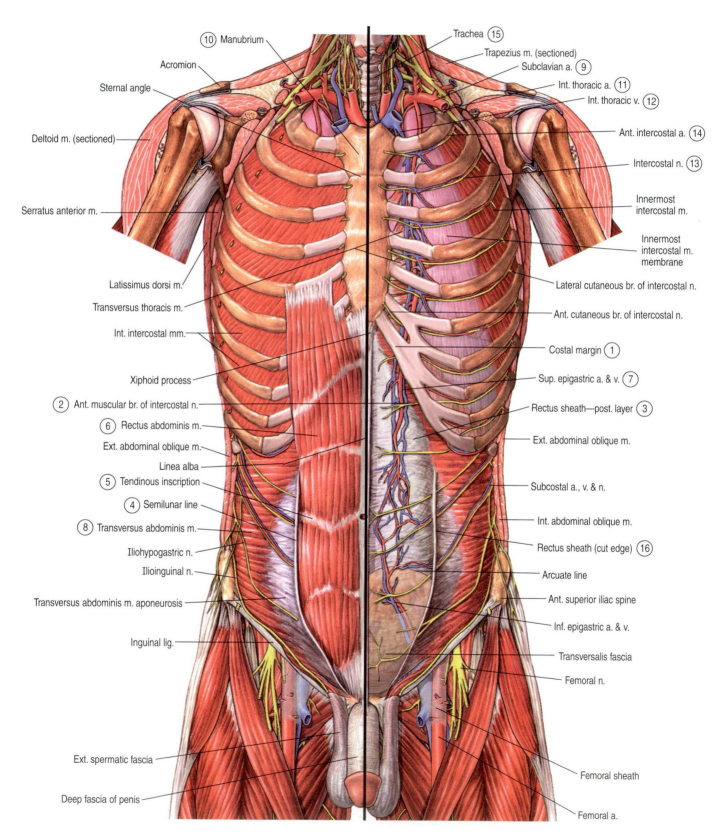

Manubrium ⑩

Acromion

Sternal angle

Deltoid m. (sectioned)

Serratus anterior m.

Latissimus dorsi m.

Transversus thoracis m.

Int. intercostal mm.

Xiphoid process

② Ant. muscular br. of intercostal n.

⑥ Rectus abdominis m.

Ext. abdominal oblique m.

Linea alba

⑤ Tendinous inscription

④ Semilunar line

⑧ Transversus abdominis m.

Iliohypogastric n.

Ilioinguinal n.

Transversus abdominis m. aponeurosis

Inguinal lig.

Ext. spermatic fascia

Deep fascia of penis

Trachea ⑮

Trapezius m. (sectioned)

Subclavian a. ⑨

Int. thoracic a. ⑪

Int. thoracic v. ⑫

Ant. intercostal a. ⑭

Intercostal n. ⑬

Innermost intercostal m.

Innermost intercostal m. membrane

Lateral cutaneous br. of intercostal n.

Ant. cutaneous br. of intercostal n.

Costal margin ①

Sup. epigastric a. & v. ⑦

Rectus sheath—post. layer ③

Ext. abdominal oblique m.

Subcostal a., v. & n.

Int. abdominal oblique m.

Rectus sheath (cut edge) ⑯

Arcuate line

Ant. superior iliac spine

Inf. epigastric a. & v.

Transversalis fascia

Femoral n.

Femoral sheath

Femoral a.

ANTERIOR VIEW

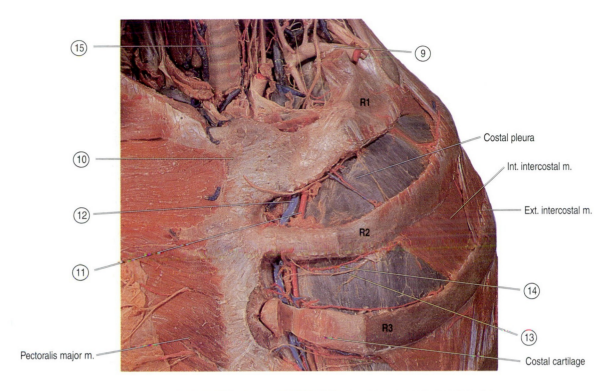

Costal pleura

Int. intercostal m.

Ext. intercostal m.

R1

R2

R3

Pectoralis major m.

Costal cartilage

ANTERIOR VIEW OF LEFT SUPERIOR PORTION OF THORACIC WALL

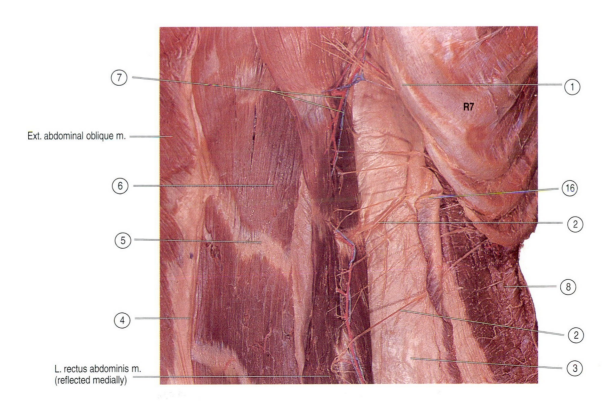

Ext. abdominal oblique m.

R7

L. rectus abdominis m.
(reflected medially)

ANTERIOR VIEW OF SUBCOSTAL PORTION OF ABDOMINAL WALL

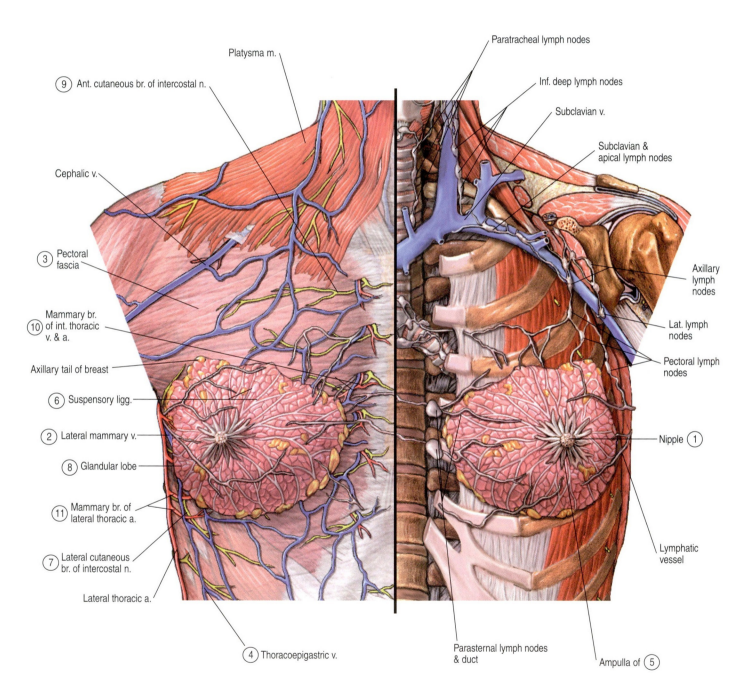

Platysma m.

⑨ Ant. cutaneous br. of intercostal n.

Cephalic v.

③ Pectoral fascia

Mammary br.
⑩ of int. thoracic v. & a.

Axillary tail of breast

⑥ Suspensory ligg.

② Lateral mammary v.

⑧ Glandular lobe

⑪ Mammary br. of lateral thoracic a.

⑦ Lateral cutaneous br. of intercostal n.

Lateral thoracic a.

④ Thoracoepigastric v.

Paratracheal lymph nodes

Inf. deep lymph nodes

Subclavian v.

Subclavian & apical lymph nodes

Axillary lymph nodes

Lat. lymph nodes

Pectoral lymph nodes

Nipple ①

Lymphatic vessel

Parasternal lymph nodes & duct

Ampulla of ⑤

ANTERIOR VIEW

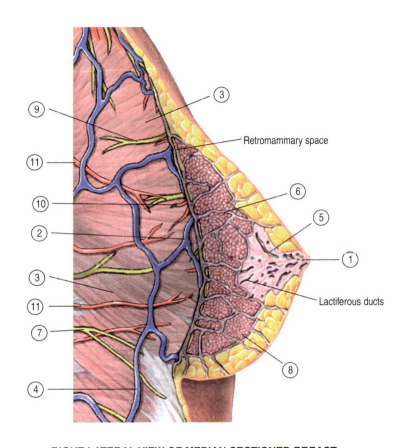

Retromammary space

Lactiferous ducts

RIGHT LATERAL VIEW OF MEDIAN SECTIONED BREAST

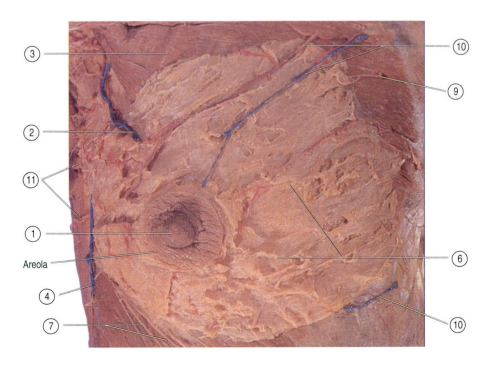

Areola

ANTERIOR VIEW OF RIGHT BREAST

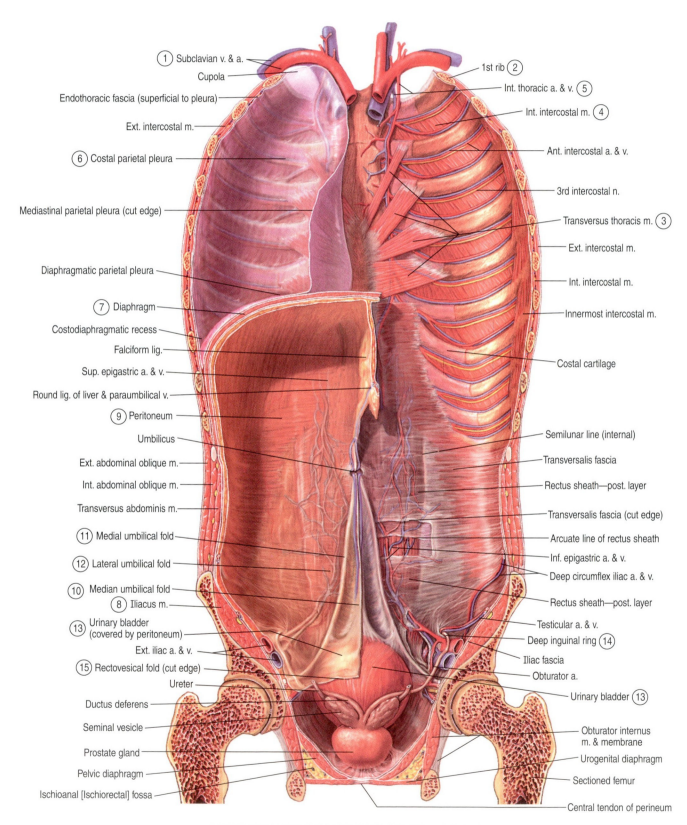

1. Subclavian v. & a.
Cupola
Endothoracic fascia (superficial to pleura)
Ext. intercostal m.
6. Costal parietal pleura
Mediastinal parietal pleura (cut edge)
Diaphragmatic parietal pleura
7. Diaphragm
Costodiaphragmatic recess
Falciform lig.
Sup. epigastric a. & v.
Round lig. of liver & paraumbilical v.
9. Peritoneum
Umbilicus
Ext. abdominal oblique m.
Int. abdominal oblique m.
Transversus abdominis m.
11. Medial umbilical fold
12. Lateral umbilical fold
10. Median umbilical fold
8. Iliacus m.
13. Urinary bladder (covered by peritoneum)
Ext. iliac a. & v.
15. Rectovesical fold (cut edge)
Ureter
Ductus deferens
Seminal vesicle
Prostate gland
Pelvic diaphragm
Ischioanal [Ischiorectal] fossa

1st rib 2.
Int. thoracic a. & v. 5.
Int. intercostal m. 4.
Ant. intercostal a. & v.
3rd intercostal n.
Transversus thoracis m. 3.
Ext. intercostal m.
Int. intercostal m.
Innermost intercostal m.
Costal cartilage
Semilunar line (internal)
Transversalis fascia
Rectus sheath—post. layer
Transversalis fascia (cut edge)
Arcuate line of rectus sheath
Inf. epigastric a. & v.
Deep circumflex iliac a. & v.
Rectus sheath—post. layer
Testicular a. & v.
Deep inguinal ring 14.
Iliac fascia
Obturator a.
Urinary bladder 13.
Obturator internus m. & membrane
Urogenital diaphragm
Sectioned femur
Central tendon of perineum

POSTERIOR (INTERNAL) VIEW OF ANTERIOR BODY WALL

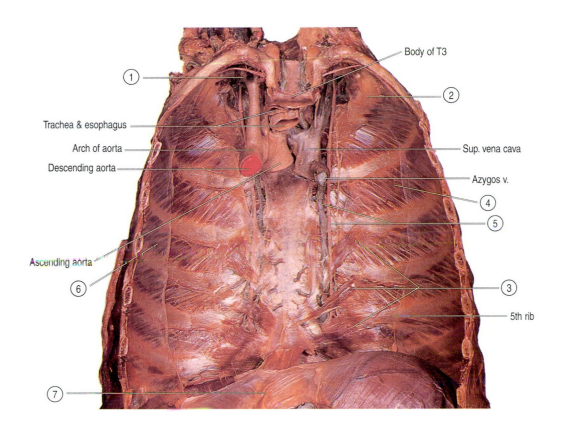

Body of T3

Trachea & esophagus

Arch of aorta

Descending aorta

Sup. vena cava

Azygos v.

Ascending aorta

5th rib

POSTERIOR (INTERNAL) VIEW OF ANTERIOR THORACIC WALL

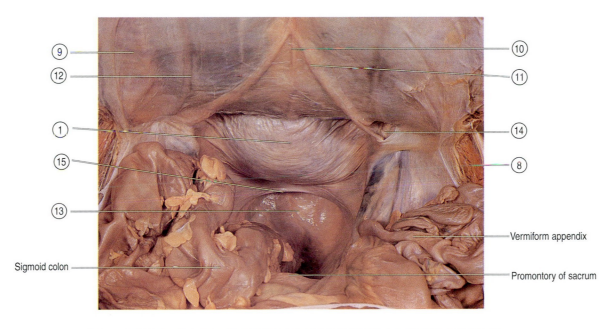

Vermiform appendix

Sigmoid colon

Promontory of sacrum

POSTEROSUPERIOR VIEW OF ANTERIOR ABDOMINAL WALL & PELVIC CONTENTS

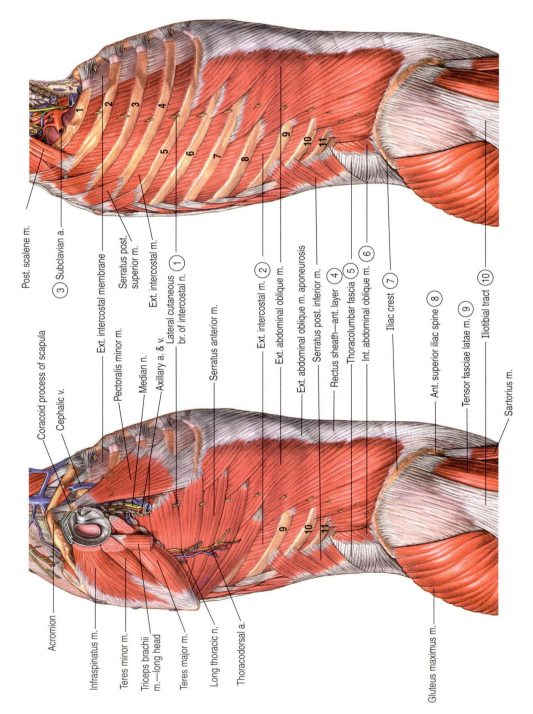

RIGHT LATERAL VIEWS

Post. scalene m.

③ Subclavian a.

Ext. intercostal membrane

Serratus post. superior m.

Ext. intercostal m.

Lateral cutaneous br. of intercostal n. ①

Serratus anterior m.

Ext. intercostal m. ②

Ext. abdominal oblique m.

Ext. abdominal oblique m. aponeurosis

Serratus post. inferior m.

Rectus sheath—ant. layer ④

Thoracolumbar fascia ⑤

Int. abdominal oblique m. ⑥

Iliac crest ⑦

Ant. superior iliac spine ⑧

Tensor fasciae latae m. ⑨

Iliotibial tract ⑩

Sartorius m.

Coracoid process of scapula

Cephalic v.

Pectoralis minor m.

Median n.

Axillary a. & v.

Acromion

Infraspinatus m.

Teres minor m.

Triceps brachii m.—long head

Teres major m.

Long thoracic n.

Thoracodorsal a.

Gluteus maximus m.

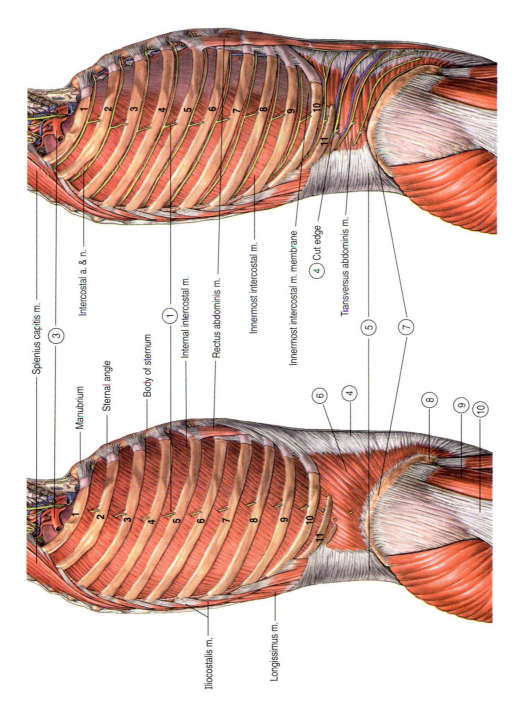

Splenius capitis m.

Intercostal a. & n.

Manubrium

Sternal angle

Body of sternum

Internal intercostal m.

Rectus abdominis m.

Innermost intercostal m.

Innermost intercostal m. membrane

Cut edge

Transversus abdominis m.

Iliocostalis m.

Longissimus m.

RIGHT LATERAL VIEWS

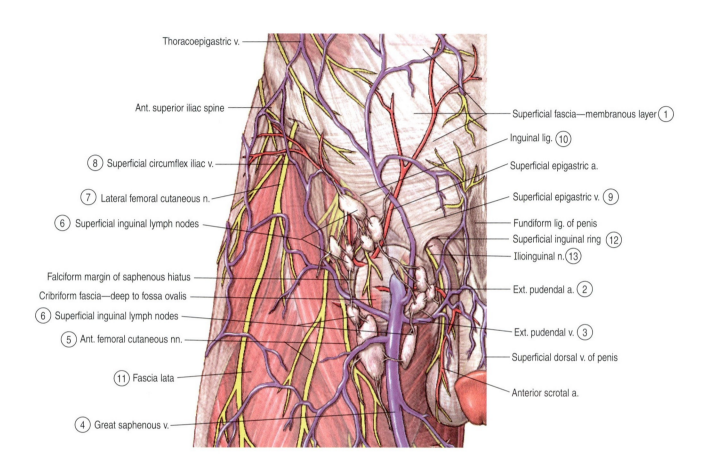

Thoracoepigastric v.

Ant. superior iliac spine

⑧ Superficial circumflex iliac v.

⑦ Lateral femoral cutaneous n.

⑥ Superficial inguinal lymph nodes

Falciform margin of saphenous hiatus

Cribriform fascia—deep to fossa ovalis

⑥ Superficial inguinal lymph nodes

⑤ Ant. femoral cutaneous nn.

⑪ Fascia lata

④ Great saphenous v.

Superficial fascia—membranous layer ①

Inguinal lig. ⑩

Superficial epigastric a.

Superficial epigastric v. ⑨

Fundiform lig. of penis

Superficial inguinal ring ⑫

Ilioinguinal n. ⑬

Ext. pudendal a. ②

Ext. pudendal v. ③

Superficial dorsal v. of penis

Anterior scrotal a.

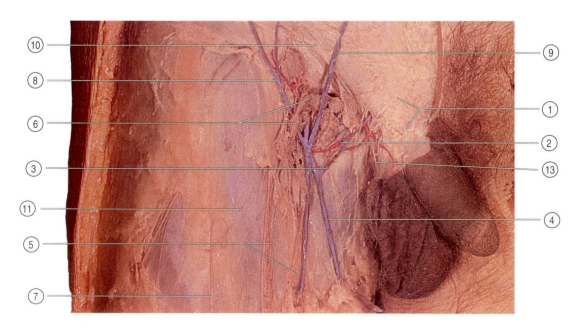

ANTERIOR VIEWS OF RIGHT SIDE

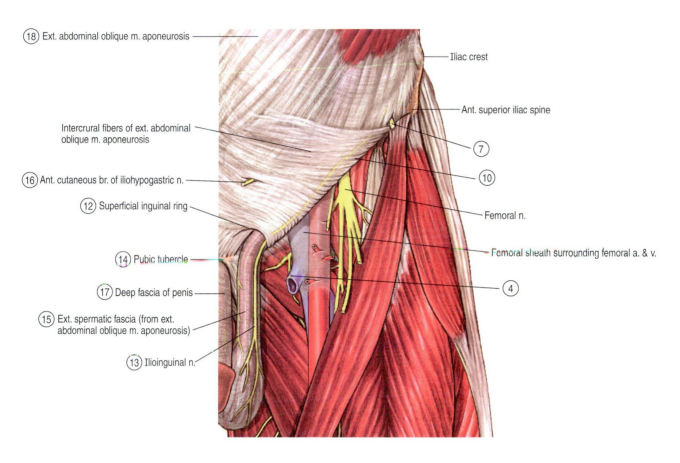

(18) Ext. abdominal oblique m. aponeurosis

Iliac crest

Intercrural fibers of ext. abdominal oblique m. aponeurosis

Ant. superior iliac spine

(7)

(10)

(16) Ant. cutaneous br. of iliohypogastric n.

(12) Superficial inguinal ring

Femoral n.

(14) Pubic tubercle

Femoral sheath surrounding femoral a. & v.

(17) Deep fascia of penis

(4)

(15) Ext. spermatic fascia (from ext. abdominal oblique m. aponeurosis)

(13) Ilioinguinal n.

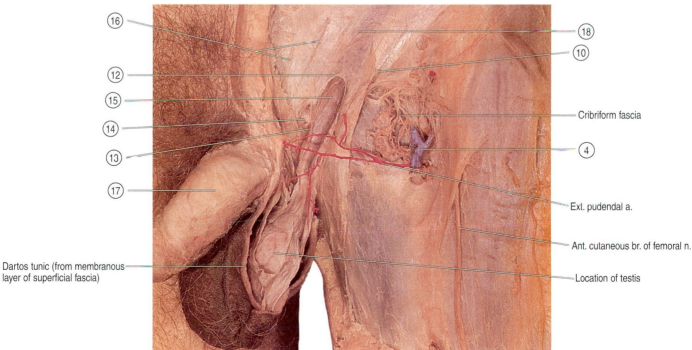

(16)

(18)

(10)

(12)

(15)

Cribriform fascia

(14)

(4)

(13)

(17)

Ext. pudendal a.

Ant. cutaneous br. of femoral n.

Dartos tunic (from membranous layer of superficial fascia)

Location of testis

ANTERIOR VIEWS OF LEFT SIDE

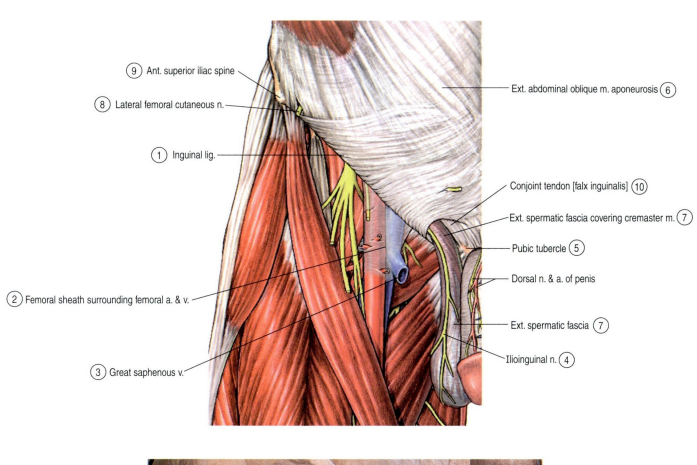

⑨ Ant. superior iliac spine

⑧ Lateral femoral cutaneous n.

① Inguinal lig.

② Femoral sheath surrounding femoral a. & v.

③ Great saphenous v.

Ext. abdominal oblique m. aponeurosis ⑥

Conjoint tendon [falx inguinalis] ⑩

Ext. spermatic fascia covering cremaster m. ⑦

Pubic tubercle ⑤

Dorsal n. & a. of penis

Ext. spermatic fascia ⑦

Ilioinguinal n. ④

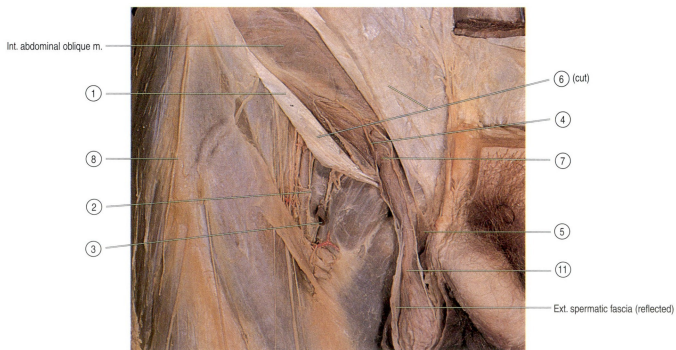

Int. abdominal oblique m.

①
⑧
②
③

⑥ (cut)

④

⑦

⑤

⑪

Ext. spermatic fascia (reflected)

ANTERIOR VIEWS OF RIGHT SIDE

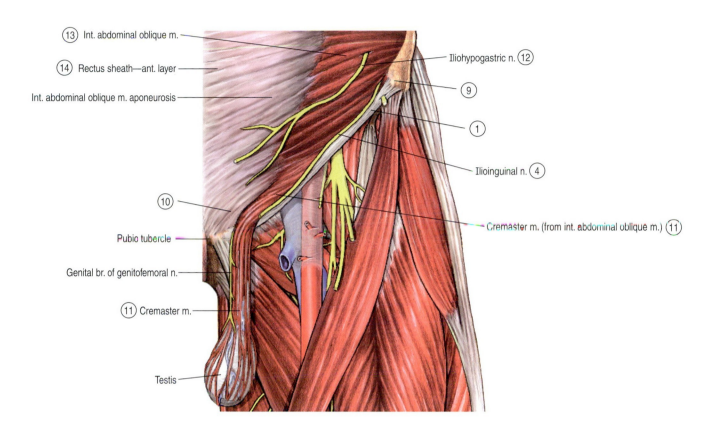

(13) Int. abdominal oblique m.

(14) Rectus sheath—ant. layer

Int. abdominal oblique m. aponeurosis

(10)

Pubic tubercle

Genital br. of genitofemoral n.

(11) Cremaster m.

Testis

Iliohypogastric n. (12)

(9)

(1)

Ilioinguinal n. (4)

Cremaster m. (from int. abdominal oblique m.) (11)

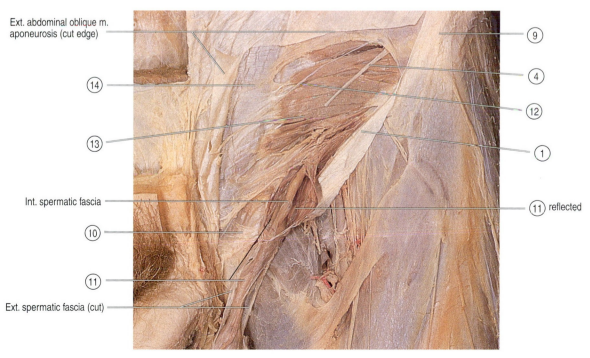

Ext. abdominal oblique m.
aponeurosis (cut edge)

(14)

(13)

Int. spermatic fascia

(10)

(11)

Ext. spermatic fascia (cut)

(9)

(4)

(12)

(1)

(11) reflected

ANTERIOR VIEWS OF LEFT SIDE

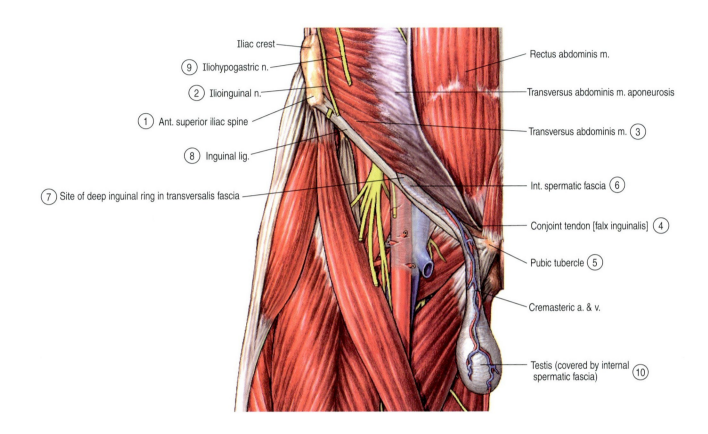

Iliac crest

⑨ Iliohypogastric n.

② Ilioinguinal n.

① Ant. superior iliac spine

⑧ Inguinal lig.

⑦ Site of deep inguinal ring in transversalis fascia

Rectus abdominis m.

Transversus abdominis m. aponeurosis

Transversus abdominis m. ③

Int. spermatic fascia ⑥

Conjoint tendon [falx inguinalis] ④

Pubic tubercle ⑤

Cremasteric a. & v.

Testis (covered by internal spermatic fascia) ⑩

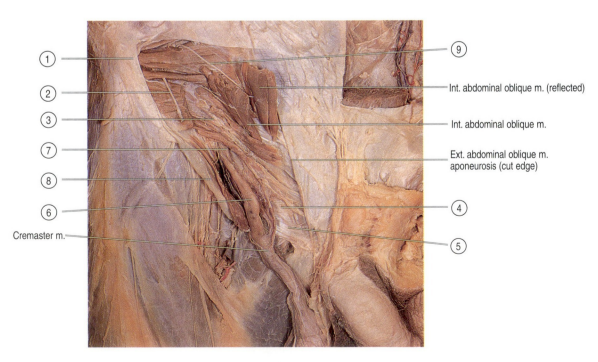

① ② ③ ⑦ ⑧ ⑥

Cremaster m.

⑨ Int. abdominal oblique m. (reflected)

Int. abdominal oblique m.

Ext. abdominal oblique m. aponeurosis (cut edge)

④ ⑤

ANTERIOR VIEWS

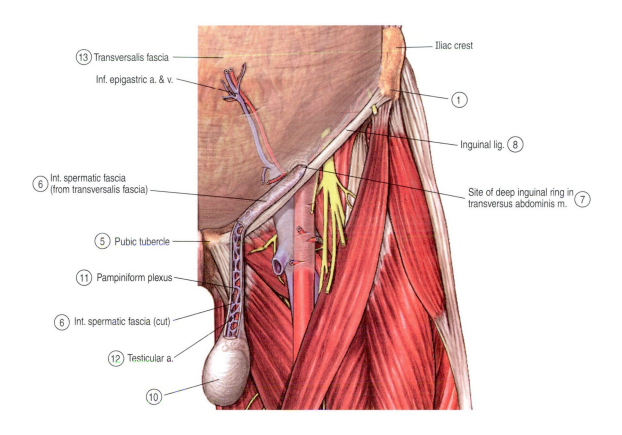

13 Transversalis fascia

Inf. epigastric a. & v.

Iliac crest

1

Inguinal lig. 8

6 Int. spermatic fascia
(from transversalis fascia)

Site of deep inguinal ring in
transversus abdominis m. 7

5 Pubic tubercle

11 Pampiniform plexus

6 Int. spermatic fascia (cut)

12 Testicular a.

10

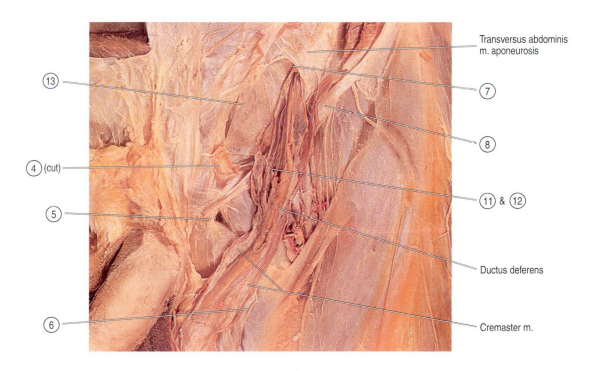

Transversus abdominis
m. aponeurosis

13

7

8

4 (cut)

11 & 12

5

Ductus deferens

6

Cremaster m.

ANTERIOR VIEWS

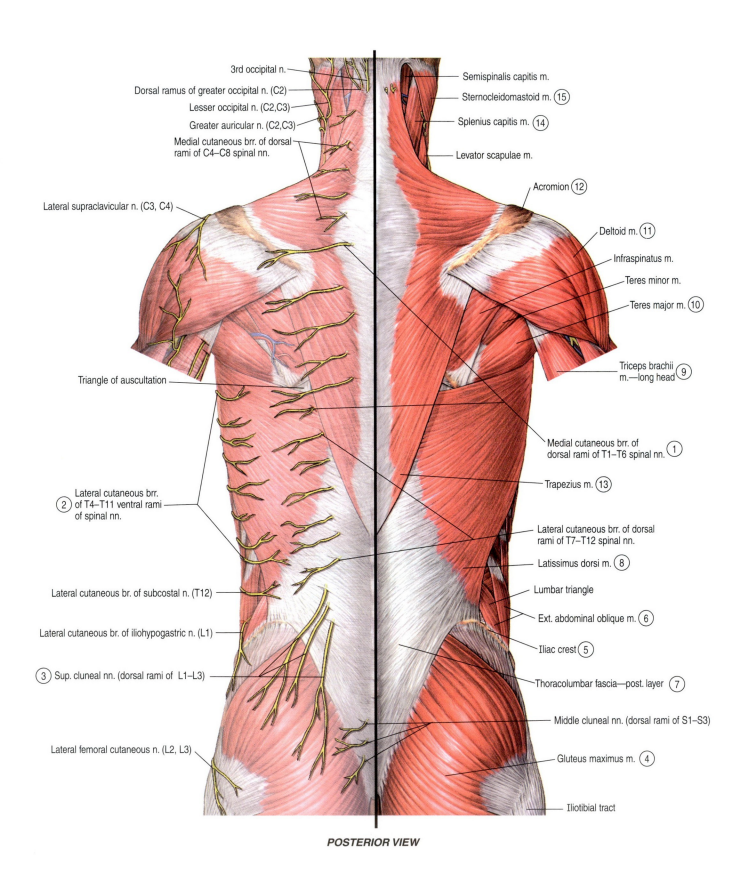

3rd occipital n.

Dorsal ramus of greater occipital n. (C2)

Lesser occipital n. (C2,C3)

Greater auricular n. (C2,C3)

Medial cutaneous brr. of dorsal rami of C4–C8 spinal nn.

Lateral supraclavicular n. (C3, C4)

Triangle of auscultation

Lateral cutaneous brr. of T4–T11 ventral rami of spinal nn. ②

Lateral cutaneous br. of subcostal n. (T12)

Lateral cutaneous br. of iliohypogastric n. (L1)

③ Sup. cluneal nn. (dorsal rami of L1–L3)

Lateral femoral cutaneous n. (L2, L3)

Semispinalis capitis m.

Sternocleidomastoid m. ⑮

Splenius capitis m. ⑭

Levator scapulae m.

Acromion ⑫

Deltoid m. ⑪

Infraspinatus m.

Teres minor m.

Teres major m. ⑩

Triceps brachii m.—long head ⑨

Medial cutaneous brr. of dorsal rami of T1–T6 spinal nn. ①

Trapezius m. ⑬

Lateral cutaneous brr. of dorsal rami of T7–T12 spinal nn.

Latissimus dorsi m. ⑧

Lumbar triangle

Ext. abdominal oblique m. ⑥

Iliac crest ⑤

Thoracolumbar fascia—post. layer ⑦

Middle cluneal nn. (dorsal rami of S1–S3)

Gluteus maximus m. ④

Iliotibial tract

POSTERIOR VIEW

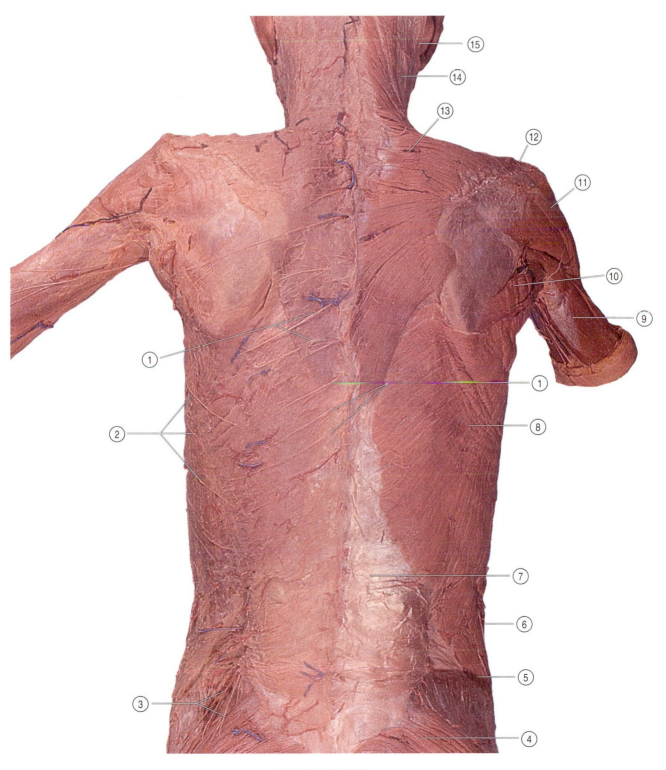

POSTERIOR VIEW

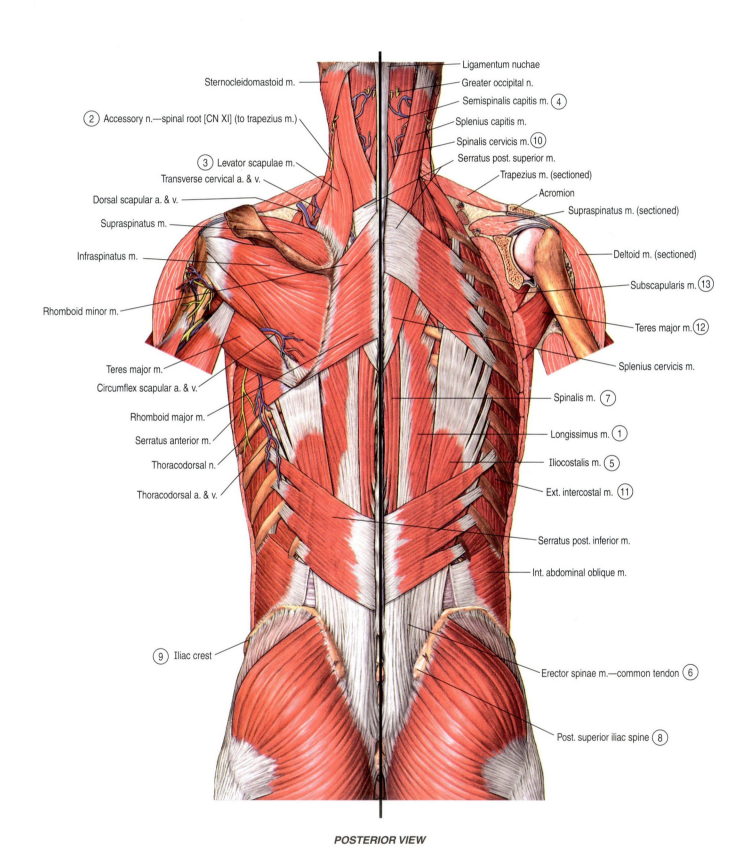

Sternocleidomastoid m.

(2) Accessory n.—spinal root [CN XI] (to trapezius m.)

(3) Levator scapulae m.

Transverse cervical a. & v.

Dorsal scapular a. & v.

Supraspinatus m.

Infraspinatus m.

Rhomboid minor m.

Teres major m.

Circumflex scapular a. & v.

Rhomboid major m.

Serratus anterior m.

Thoracodorsal n.

Thoracodorsal a. & v.

(9) Iliac crest

Ligamentum nuchae

Greater occipital n.

Semispinalis capitis m. (4)

Splenius capitis m.

Spinalis cervicis m. (10)

Serratus post. superior m.

Trapezius m. (sectioned)

Acromion

Supraspinatus m. (sectioned)

Deltoid m. (sectioned)

Subscapularis m. (13)

Teres major m. (12)

Splenius cervicis m.

Spinalis m. (7)

Longissimus m. (1)

Iliocostalis m. (5)

Ext. intercostal m. (11)

Serratus post. inferior m.

Int. abdominal oblique m.

Erector spinae m.—common tendon (6)

Post. superior iliac spine (8)

POSTERIOR VIEW

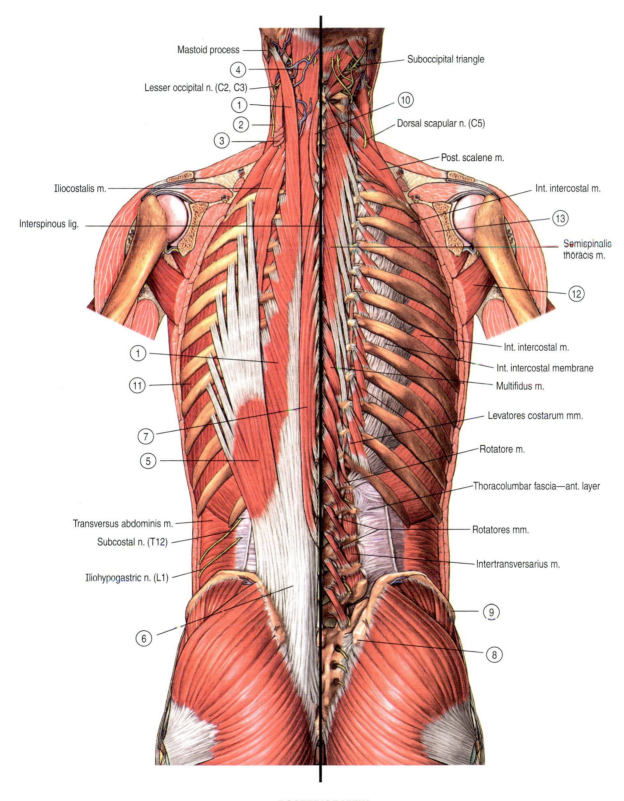

Mastoid process

④

Lesser occipital n. (C2, C3)

①

②

③

Iliocostalis m.

Interspinous lig.

①

⑪

⑦

⑤

Transversus abdominis m.

Subcostal n. (T12)

Iliohypogastric n. (L1)

⑥

Suboccipital triangle

⑩

Dorsal scapular n. (C5)

Post. scalene m.

Int. intercostal m.

⑬

Semispinalis thoracis m.

⑫

Int. intercostal m.

Int. intercostal membrane

Multifidus m.

Levatores costarum mm.

Rotatore m.

Thoracolumbar fascia—ant. layer

Rotatores mm.

Intertransversarius m.

⑨

⑧

POSTERIOR VIEW

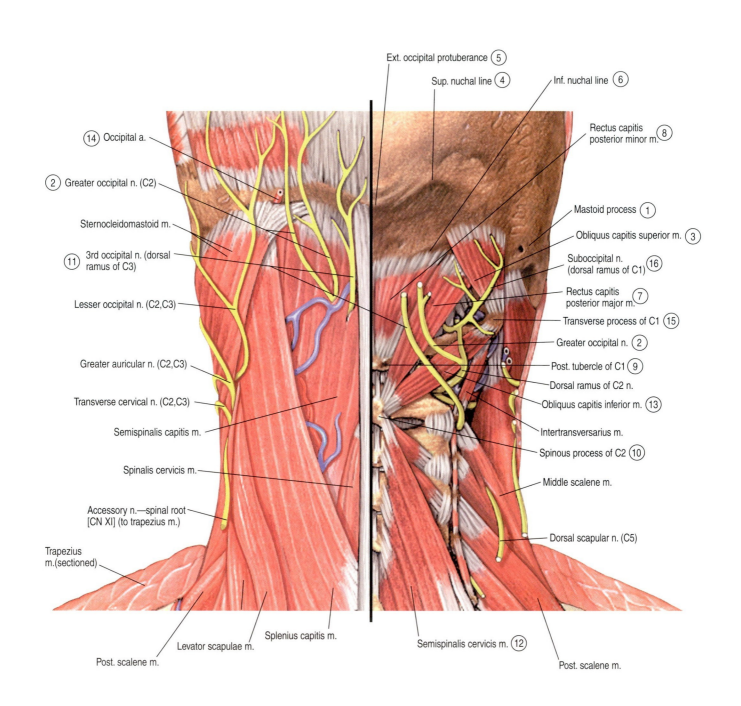

Ext. occipital protuberance ⑤

Sup. nuchal line ④

Inf. nuchal line ⑥

⑭ Occipital a.

② Greater occipital n. (C2)

Sternocleidomastoid m.

⑪ 3rd occipital n. (dorsal ramus of C3)

Lesser occipital n. (C2,C3)

Greater auricular n. (C2,C3)

Transverse cervical n. (C2,C3)

Semispinalis capitis m.

Spinalis cervicis m.

Accessory n.—spinal root [CN XI] (to trapezius m.)

Trapezius m.(sectioned)

Post. scalene m.

Levator scapulae m.

Splenius capitis m.

Rectus capitis posterior minor m. ⑧

Mastoid process ①

Obliquus capitis superior m. ③

Suboccipital n. (dorsal ramus of C1) ⑯

Rectus capitis posterior major m. ⑦

Transverse process of C1 ⑮

Greater occipital n. ②

Post. tubercle of C1 ⑨

Dorsal ramus of C2 n.

Obliquus capitis inferior m. ⑬

Intertransversarius m.

Spinous process of C2 ⑩

Middle scalene m.

Dorsal scapular n. (C5)

Semispinalis cervicis m. ⑫

Post. scalene m.

POSTERIOR VIEW

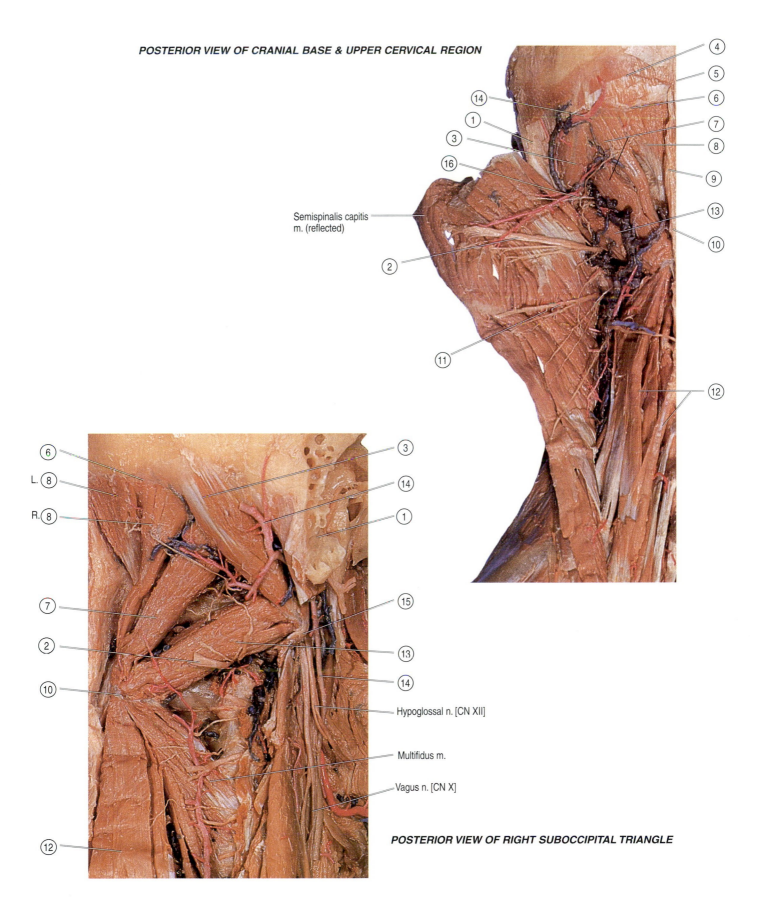

POSTERIOR VIEW OF CRANIAL BASE & UPPER CERVICAL REGION

Semispinalis capitis m. (reflected)

L.

R.

Hypoglossal n. [CN XII]

Multifidus m.

Vagus n. [CN X]

POSTERIOR VIEW OF RIGHT SUBOCCIPITAL TRIANGLE

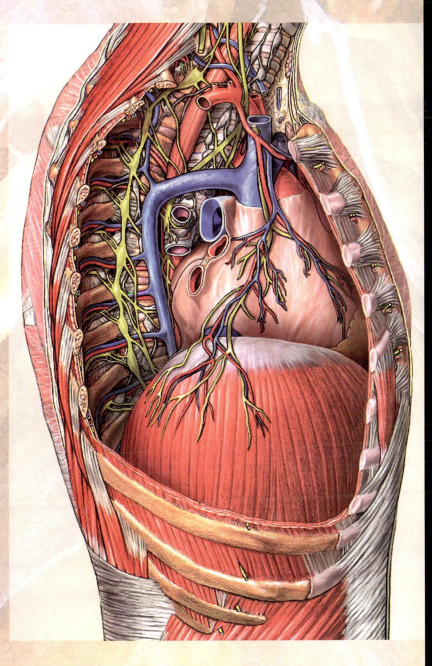

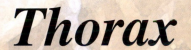

Thorax

Chapter 2

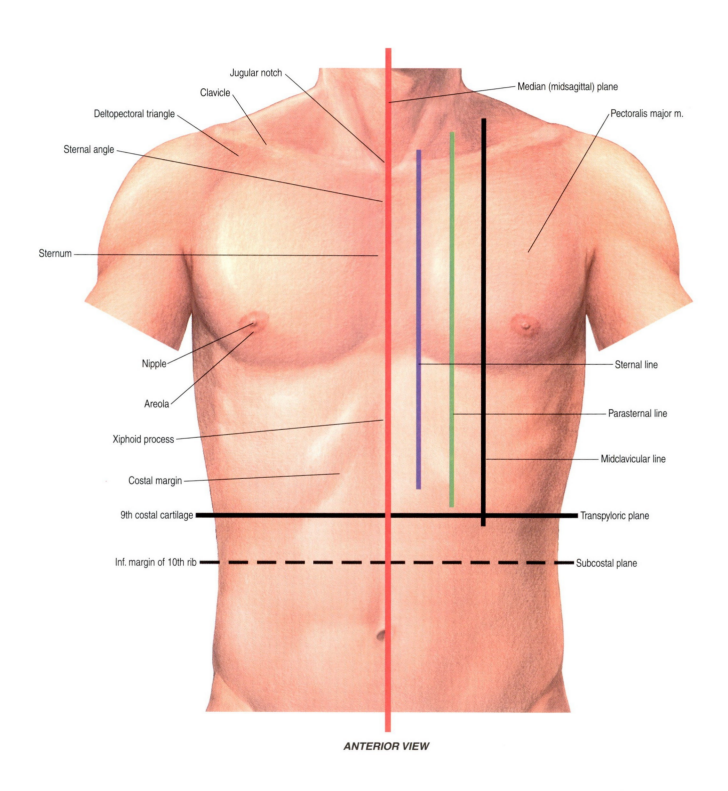

Jugular notch

Clavicle

Deltopectoral triangle

Sternal angle

Sternum

Nipple

Areola

Xiphoid process

Costal margin

9th costal cartilage

Inf. margin of 10th rib

Median (midsagittal) plane

Pectoralis major m.

Sternal line

Parasternal line

Midclavicular line

Transpyloric plane

Subcostal plane

ANTERIOR VIEW

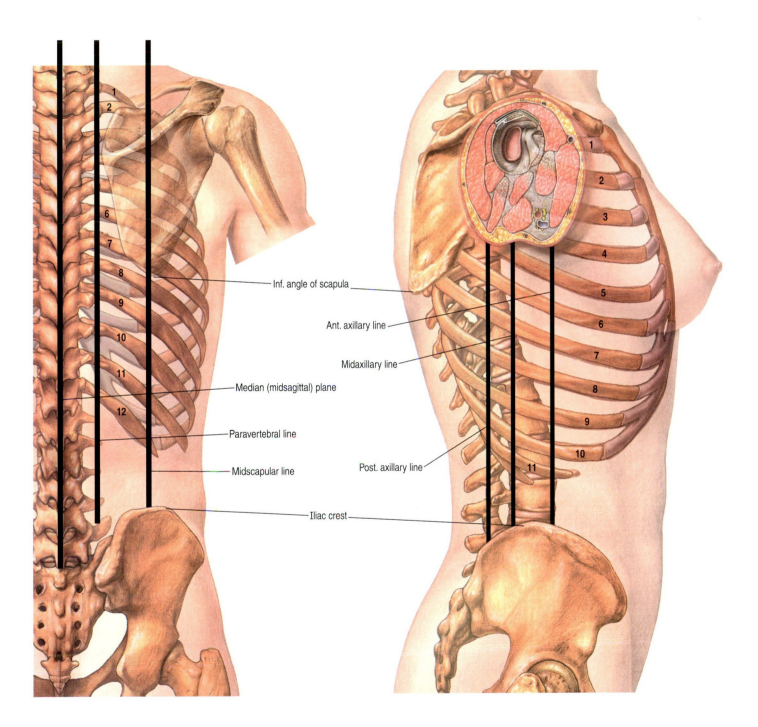

1
2

6
7
8
9
10
11
12

Inf. angle of scapula

Ant. axillary line

Midaxillary line

Median (midsagittal) plane

Paravertebral line

Post. axillary line

Midscapular line

Iliac crest

1
2
3
4
5
6
7
8
9
10
11

POSTERIOR VIEW

RIGHT LATERAL VIEW

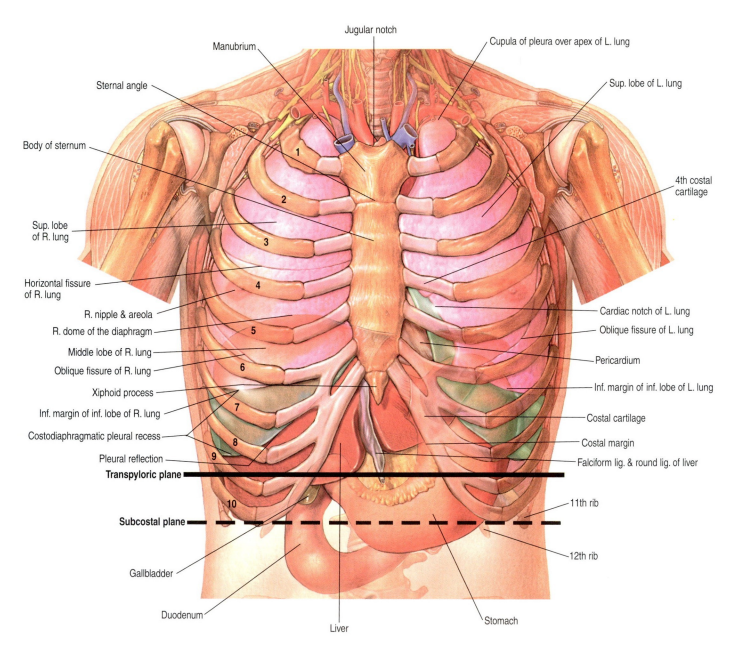

Jugular notch

Manubrium

Sternal angle

Cupula of pleura over apex of L. lung

Sup. lobe of L. lung

Body of sternum

4th costal cartilage

Sup. lobe of R. lung

Horizontal fissure of R. lung

R. nipple & areola

Cardiac notch of L. lung

R. dome of the diaphragm

Oblique fissure of L. lung

Middle lobe of R. lung

Pericardium

Oblique fissure of R. lung

Xiphoid process

Inf. margin of inf. lobe of L. lung

Inf. margin of inf. lobe of R. lung

Costal cartilage

Costodiaphragmatic pleural recess

Costal margin

Pleural reflection

Falciform lig. & round lig. of liver

Transpyloric plane

Subcostal plane

11th rib

12th rib

Gallbladder

Duodenum

Liver

Stomach

ANTERIOR VIEW

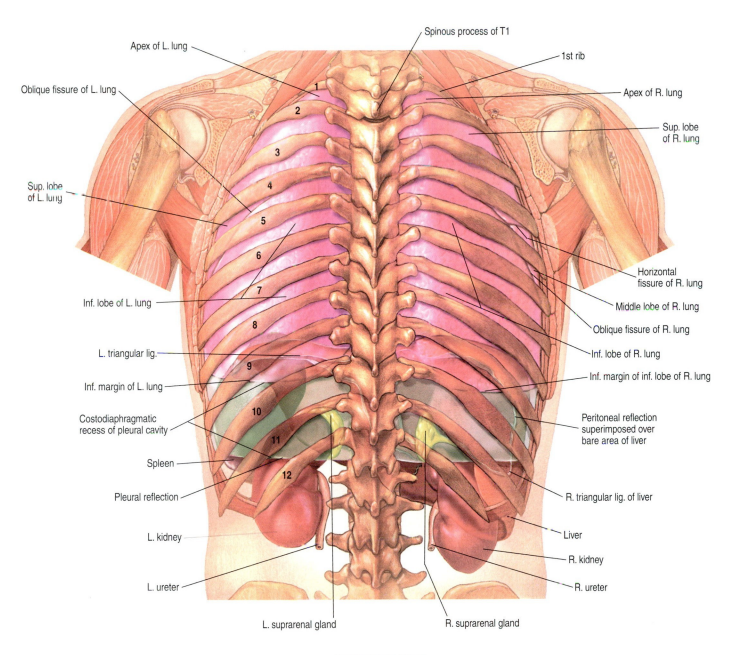

Spinous process of T1

Apex of L. lung

1st rib

Oblique fissure of L. lung

Apex of R. lung

Sup. lobe
of R. lung

Sup. lobe
of L. lung

Horizontal
fissure of R. lung

Inf. lobe of L. lung

Middle lobe of R. lung

Oblique fissure of R. lung

L. triangular lig.

Inf. lobe of R. lung

Inf. margin of L. lung

Inf. margin of inf. lobe of R. lung

Costodiaphragmatic
recess of pleural cavity

Peritoneal reflection
superimposed over
bare area of liver

Spleen

R. triangular lig. of liver

Pleural reflection

L. kidney

Liver

R. kidney

L. ureter

R. ureter

L. suprarenal gland

R. suprarenal gland

POSTERIOR VIEW

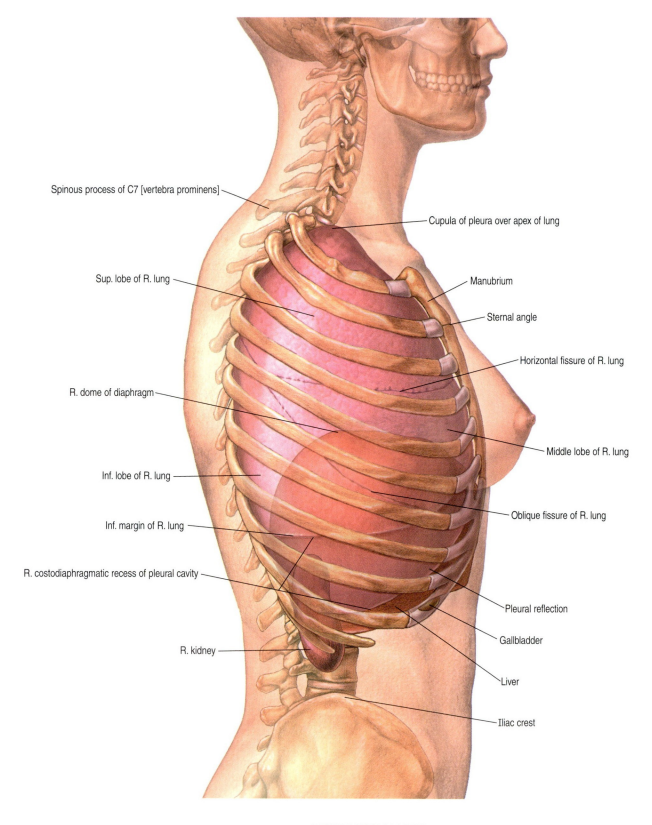

Spinous process of C7 [vertebra prominens]

Cupula of pleura over apex of lung

Sup. lobe of R. lung

Manubrium

Sternal angle

Horizontal fissure of R. lung

R. dome of diaphragm

Middle lobe of R. lung

Inf. lobe of R. lung

Oblique fissure of R. lung

Inf. margin of R. lung

R. costodiaphragmatic recess of pleural cavity

Pleural reflection

Gallbladder

R. kidney

Liver

Iliac crest

RIGHT LATERAL VIEW

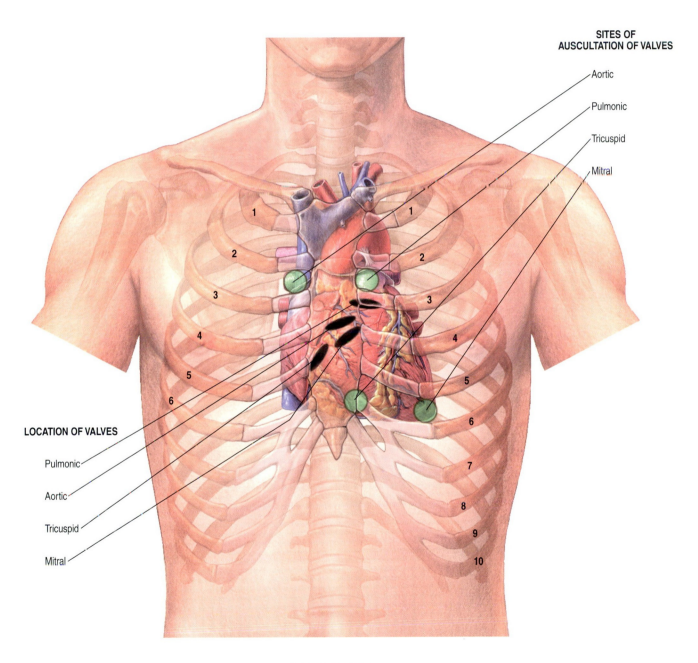

SITES OF
AUSCULTATION OF VALVES

Aortic

Pulmonic

Tricuspid

Mitral

LOCATION OF VALVES

Pulmonic

Aortic

Tricuspid

Mitral

ANTERIOR VIEW

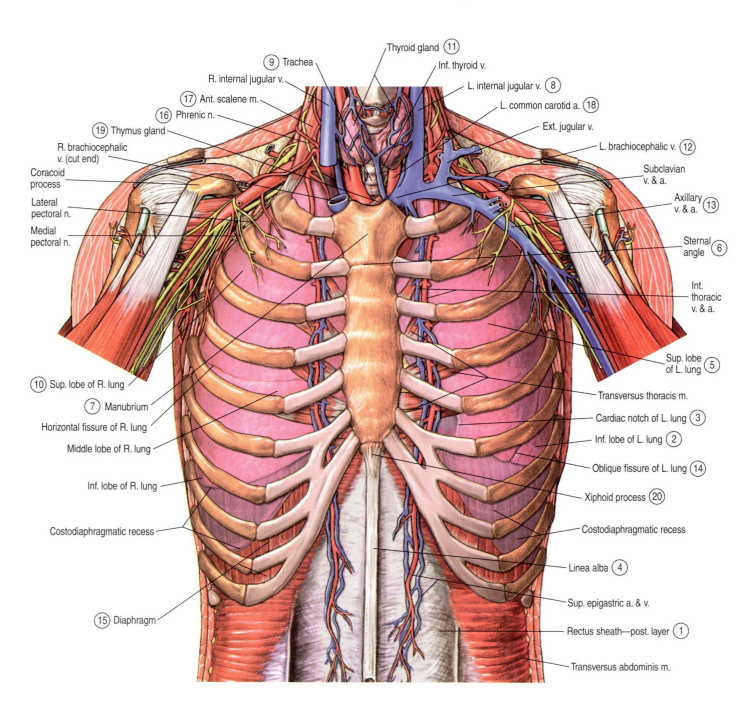

Thyroid gland (11)

(9) Trachea

Inf. thyroid v.

R. internal jugular v.

L. internal jugular v. (8)

(17) Ant. scalene m.

L. common carotid a. (18)

(16) Phrenic n.

Ext. jugular v.

(19) Thymus gland

L. brachiocephalic v. (12)

R. brachiocephalic v. (cut end)

Subclavian v. & a.

Coracoid process

Axillary v. & a. (13)

Lateral pectoral n.

Sternal angle (6)

Medial pectoral n.

Int. thoracic v. & a.

Sup. lobe of L. lung (5)

(10) Sup. lobe of R. lung

Transversus thoracis m.

(7) Manubrium

Cardiac notch of L. lung (3)

Horizontal fissure of R. lung

Inf. lobe of L. lung (2)

Middle lobe of R. lung

Oblique fissure of L. lung (14)

Inf. lobe of R. lung

Xiphoid process (20)

Costodiaphragmatic recess

Costodiaphragmatic recess

Linea alba (4)

Sup. epigastric a. & v.

(15) Diaphragm

Rectus sheath—post. layer (1)

Transversus abdominis m.

ANTERIOR VIEW

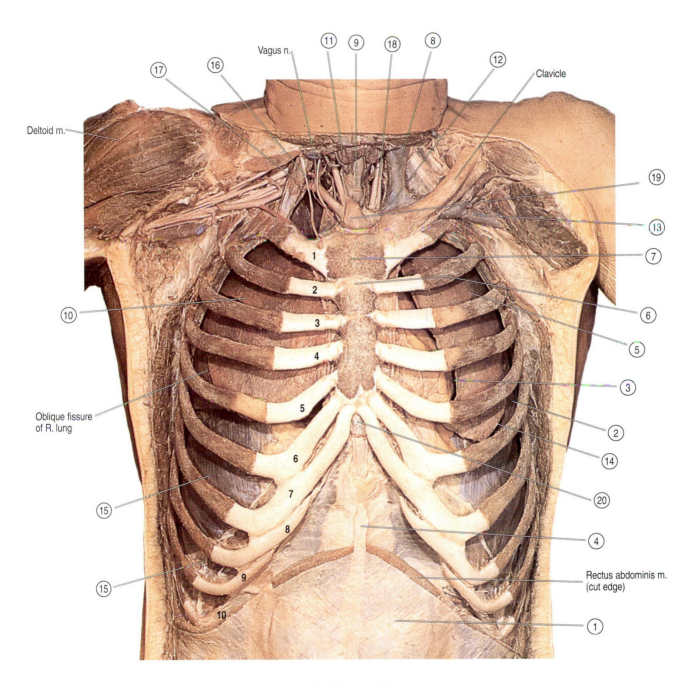

Vagus n.

Clavicle

Deltoid m.

Oblique fissure
of R. lung

Rectus abdominis m.
(cut edge)

ANTERIOR VIEW

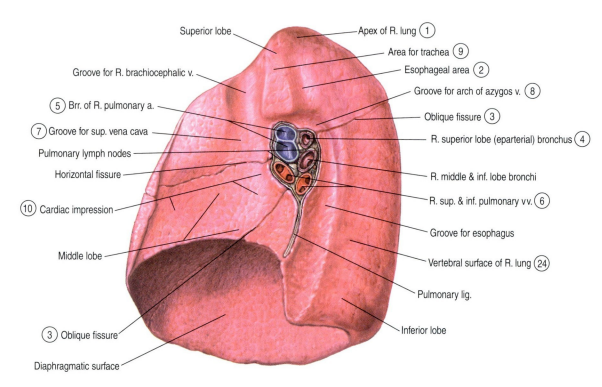

Superior lobe

Groove for R. brachiocephalic v.

⑤ Brr. of R. pulmonary a.

⑦ Groove for sup. vena cava

Pulmonary lymph nodes

Horizontal fissure

⑩ Cardiac impression

Middle lobe

③ Oblique fissure

Diaphragmatic surface

Apex of R. lung ①

Area for trachea ⑨

Esophageal area ②

Groove for arch of azygos v. ⑧

Oblique fissure ③

R. superior lobe (eparterial) bronchus ④

R. middle & inf. lobe bronchi

R. sup. & inf. pulmonary v v. ⑥

Groove for esophagus

Vertebral surface of R. lung ㉔

Pulmonary lig.

Inferior lobe

MEDIAL VIEW OF RIGHT LUNG

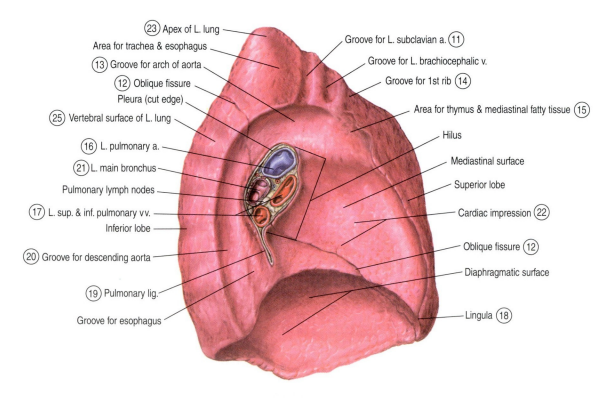

㉓ Apex of L. lung

Area for trachea & esophagus

⑬ Groove for arch of aorta

⑫ Oblique fissure

Pleura (cut edge)

㉕ Vertebral surface of L. lung

⑯ L. pulmonary a.

㉑ L. main bronchus

Pulmonary lymph nodes

⑰ L. sup. & inf. pulmonary v v.

Inferior lobe

⑳ Groove for descending aorta

⑲ Pulmonary lig.

Groove for esophagus

Groove for L. subclavian a. ⑪

Groove for L. brachiocephalic v.

Groove for 1st rib ⑭

Area for thymus & mediastinal fatty tissue ⑮

Hilus

Mediastinal surface

Superior lobe

Cardiac impression ㉒

Oblique fissure ⑫

Diaphragmatic surface

Lingula ⑱

MEDIAL VIEW OF LEFT LUNG

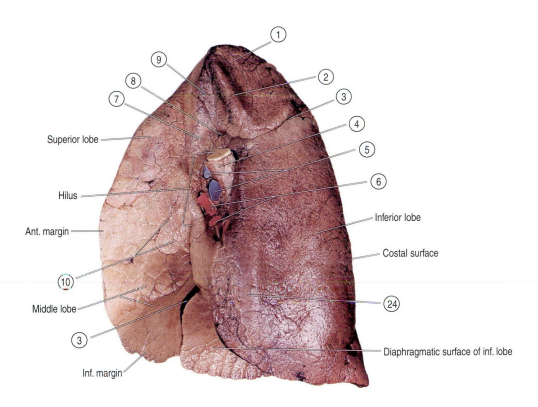

Superior lobe

Hilus

Ant. margin

Middle lobe

Inf. margin

Inferior lobe

Costal surface

Diaphragmatic surface of inf. lobe

POSTEROMEDIAL VIEW OF RIGHT LUNG

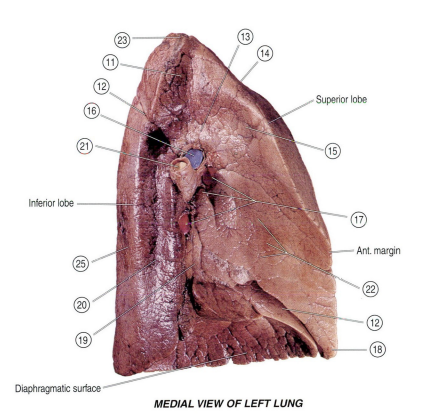

Superior lobe

Inferior lobe

Ant. margin

Diaphragmatic surface

MEDIAL VIEW OF LEFT LUNG

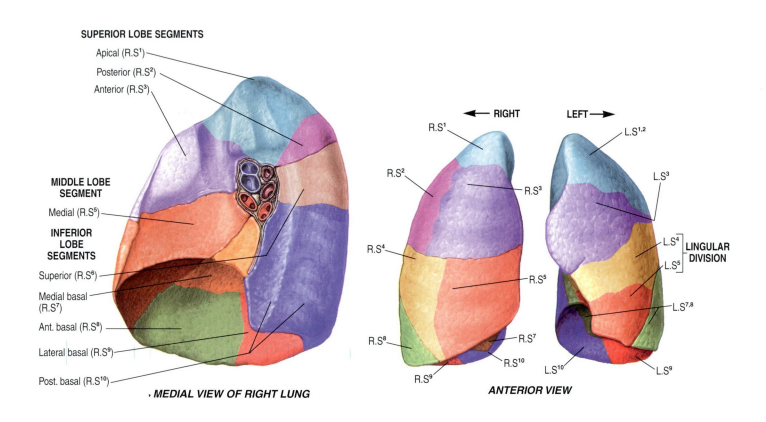

SUPERIOR LOBE SEGMENTS

Apical (R.S¹)

Posterior (R.S²)

Anterior (R.S³)

MIDDLE LOBE SEGMENT

Medial (R.S⁵)

INFERIOR LOBE SEGMENTS

Superior (R.S⁶)

Medial basal (R.S⁷)

Ant. basal (R.S⁸)

Lateral basal (R.S⁹)

Post. basal (R.S¹⁰)

MEDIAL VIEW OF RIGHT LUNG

← RIGHT   LEFT →

R.S¹

R.S²

R.S³

R.S⁴

R.S⁵

R.S⁸

R.S⁷

R.S⁹

R.S¹⁰

L.S¹,²

L.S³

L.S⁴   **LINGULAR DIVISION**

L.S⁵

L.S⁷,⁸

L.S¹⁰

L.S⁹

ANTERIOR VIEW

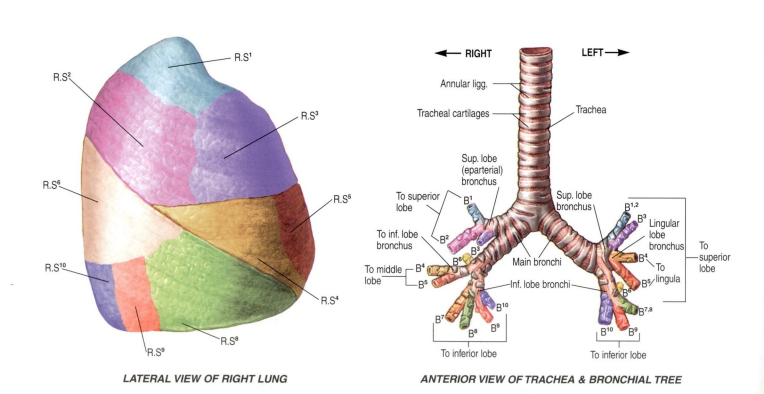

R.S¹

R.S²

R.S³

R.S⁶

R.S⁵

R.S⁴

R.S¹⁰

R.S⁸

R.S⁹

LATERAL VIEW OF RIGHT LUNG

← RIGHT   LEFT →

Annular ligg.

Tracheal cartilages

Trachea

Sup. lobe (eparterial) bronchus

Sup. lobe bronchus

To superior lobe

B¹

B¹,²

B³

Lingular lobe bronchus

B²

B³

B⁴

To lingula

To inf. lobe bronchus

B⁴

B⁶

Main bronchi

To middle lobe

B⁵

Inf. lobe bronchi

B⁵

To superior lobe

B⁶

B⁷

B¹⁰

B⁷,⁸

B⁸   B⁹

B¹⁰   B⁹

To inferior lobe

To inferior lobe

ANTERIOR VIEW OF TRACHEA & BRONCHIAL TREE

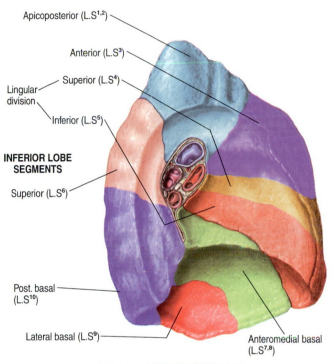

SUPERIOR LOBE SEGMENTS

Apicoposterior (L.S^{1,2})

Anterior (L.S^3)

Superior (L.S^4)

Lingular division

Inferior (L.S^5)

INFERIOR LOBE SEGMENTS

Superior (L.S^6)

Post. basal (L.S^{10})

Lateral basal (L.S^9)

Anteromedial basal (L.S^{7,8})

MEDIAL VIEW OF LEFT LUNG

← **LEFT**   **RIGHT** →

L.S^{1,2}

L.S^3

L.S^4

L.S^6

L.S^9

L.S^{10}

R.S^1

R.S^2

R.S^3

R.S^6

R.S^4

R.S^9

R.S^{10}

POSTERIOR VIEW

L.S^{1,2}

L.S^3

L.S^6

L.S^4

L.S^5

L.S^{10}

L.S^{7,8}

L.S^9

LATERAL VIEW OF LEFT LUNG

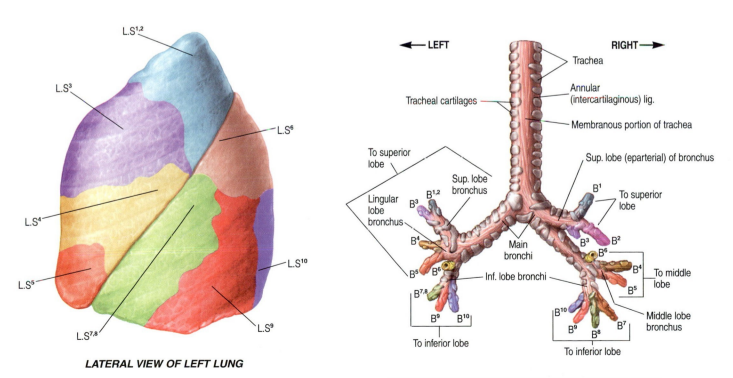

← **LEFT**   **RIGHT** →

Trachea

Annular (intercartilaginous) lig.

Tracheal cartilages

Membranous portion of trachea

To superior lobe

Sup. lobe bronchus

Sup. lobe (eparterial) of bronchus

Lingular lobe bronchus

Main bronchi

Inf. lobe bronchi

To superior lobe

To middle lobe

Middle lobe bronchus

To inferior lobe

To inferior lobe

B^{1,2} B^3 B^4 B^5 B^6 B^{7,8} B^9 B^{10}

B^1 B^2 B^3 B^4 B^5 B^6 B^7 B^8 B^9 B^{10}

POSTERIOR VIEW OF TRACHEA & BRONCHIAL TREE

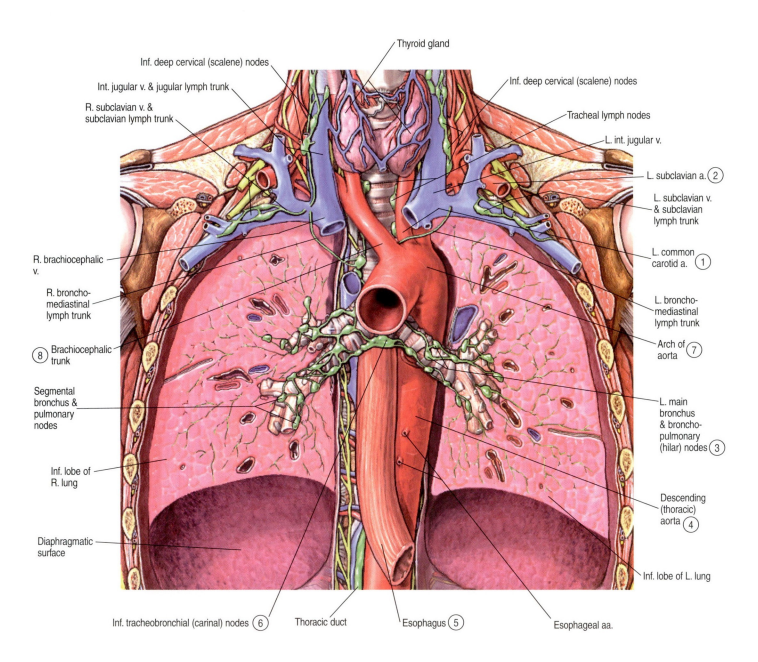

Thyroid gland

Inf. deep cervical (scalene) nodes

Int. jugular v. & jugular lymph trunk

R. subclavian v. & subclavian lymph trunk

Inf. deep cervical (scalene) nodes

Tracheal lymph nodes

L. int. jugular v.

L. subclavian a. ②

L. subclavian v. & subclavian lymph trunk

L. common carotid a. ①

R. brachiocephalic v.

R. broncho-mediastinal lymph trunk

L. broncho-mediastinal lymph trunk

Arch of aorta ⑦

⑧ Brachiocephalic trunk

Segmental bronchus & pulmonary nodes

L. main bronchus & broncho-pulmonary (hilar) nodes ③

Inf. lobe of R. lung

Descending (thoracic) aorta ④

Diaphragmatic surface

Inf. lobe of L. lung

Inf. tracheobronchial (carinal) nodes ⑥

Thoracic duct

Esophagus ⑤

Esophageal aa.

ANTERIOR VIEW WITH CORONALLY SECTIONED LUNGS

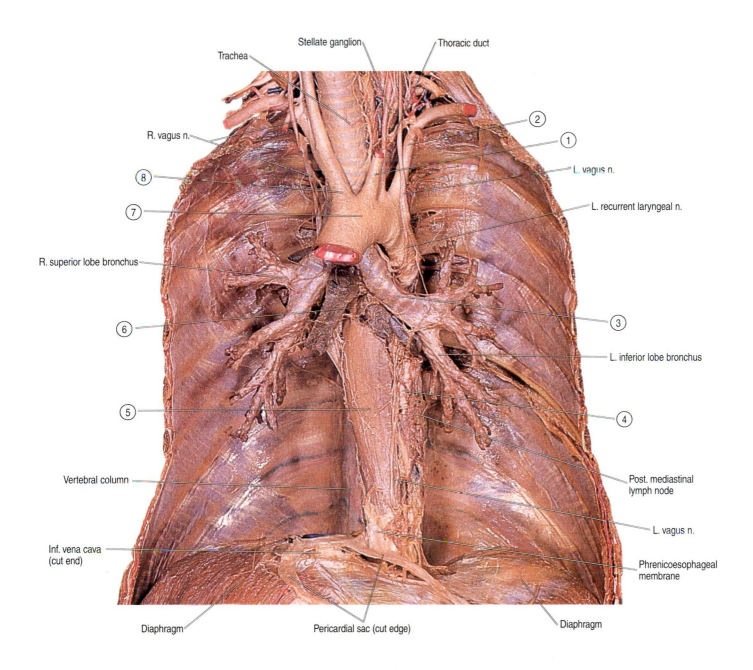

Stellate ganglion

Thoracic duct

Trachea

R. vagus n.

2

1

L. vagus n.

8

L. recurrent laryngeal n.

7

R. superior lobe bronchus

3

6

L. inferior lobe bronchus

5

4

Vertebral column

Post. mediastinal
lymph node

Inf. vena cava
(cut end)

L. vagus n.

Phrenicoesophageal
membrane

Diaphragm

Pericardial sac (cut edge)

Diaphragm

ANTERIOR VIEW

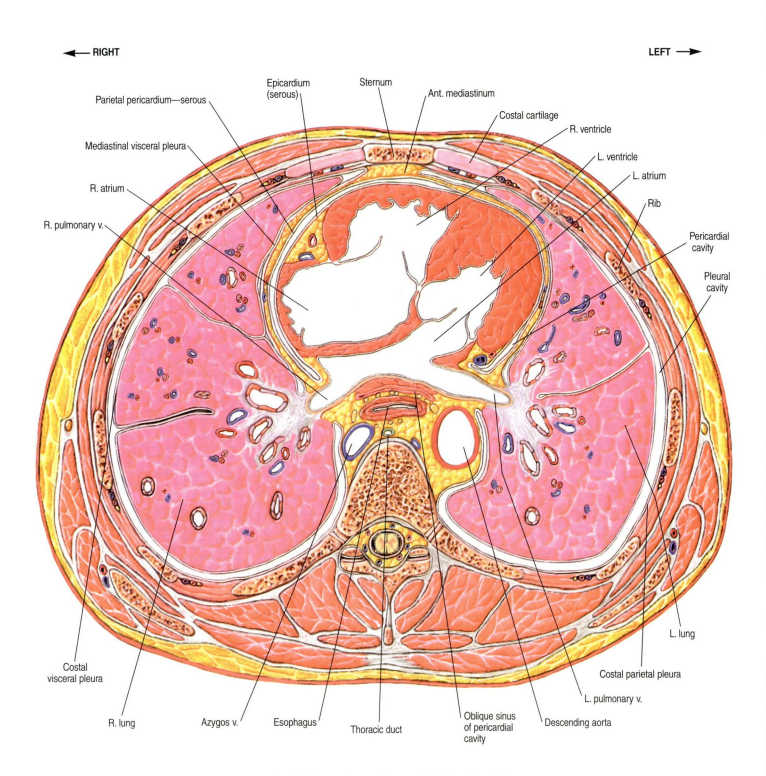

RIGHT ←   LEFT →

Epicardium (serous)

Sternum

Ant. mediastinum

Parietal pericardium—serous

Costal cartilage

R. ventricle

Mediastinal visceral pleura

L. ventricle

R. atrium

L. atrium

Rib

R. pulmonary v.

Pericardial cavity

Pleural cavity

Costal visceral pleura

R. lung

Azygos v.

Esophagus

Thoracic duct

Oblique sinus of pericardial cavity

Descending aorta

L. pulmonary v.

Costal parietal pleura

L. lung

TRANSVERSE SECTION AT T8—INFERIOR VIEW

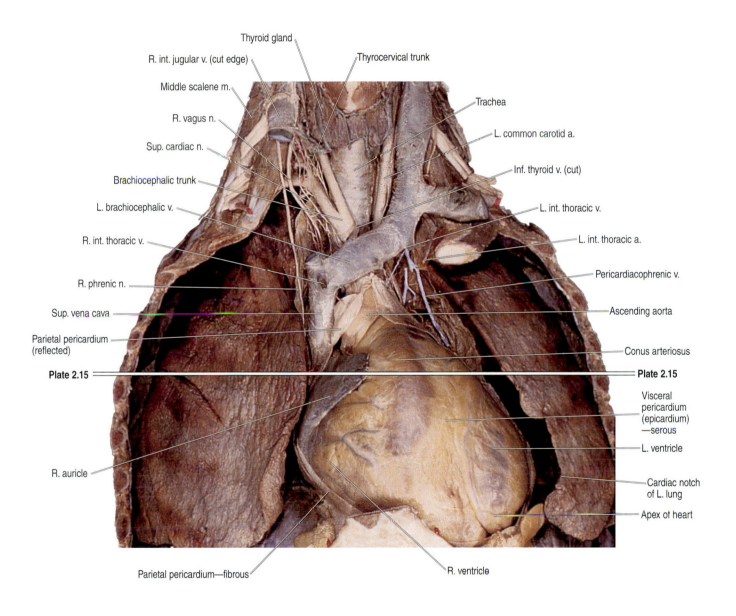

Thyroid gland

R. int. jugular v. (cut edge)

Thyrocervical trunk

Middle scalene m.

Trachea

R. vagus n.

L. common carotid a.

Sup. cardiac n.

Inf. thyroid v. (cut)

Brachiocephalic trunk

L. brachiocephalic v.

L. int. thoracic v.

R. int. thoracic v.

L. int. thoracic a.

R. phrenic n.

Pericardiacophrenic v.

Sup. vena cava

Ascending aorta

Parietal pericardium (reflected)

Conus arteriosus

Plate 2.15

Plate 2.15

Visceral pericardium (epicardium) —serous

L. ventricle

R. auricle

Cardiac notch of L. lung

Apex of heart

Parietal pericardium—fibrous

R. ventricle

ANTERIOR VIEW

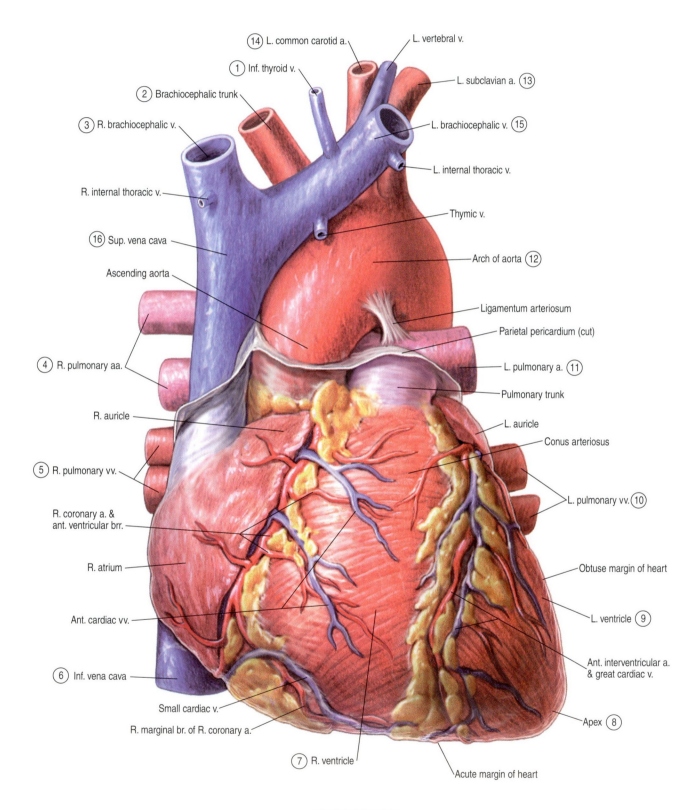

14 L. common carotid a.

L. vertebral v.

1 Inf. thyroid v.

2 Brachiocephalic trunk

L. subclavian a. 13

3 R. brachiocephalic v.

L. brachiocephalic v. 15

R. internal thoracic v.

L. internal thoracic v.

Thymic v.

16 Sup. vena cava

Ascending aorta

Arch of aorta 12

Ligamentum arteriosum

Parietal pericardium (cut)

4 R. pulmonary aa.

L. pulmonary a. 11

Pulmonary trunk

R. auricle

L. auricle

Conus arteriosus

5 R. pulmonary vv.

L. pulmonary vv. 10

R. coronary a. &
ant. ventricular brr.

R. atrium

Obtuse margin of heart

Ant. cardiac vv.

L. ventricle 9

6 Inf. vena cava

Ant. interventricular a.
& great cardiac v.

Small cardiac v.

Apex 8

R. marginal br. of R. coronary a.

7 R. ventricle

Acute margin of heart

ANTERIOR VIEW

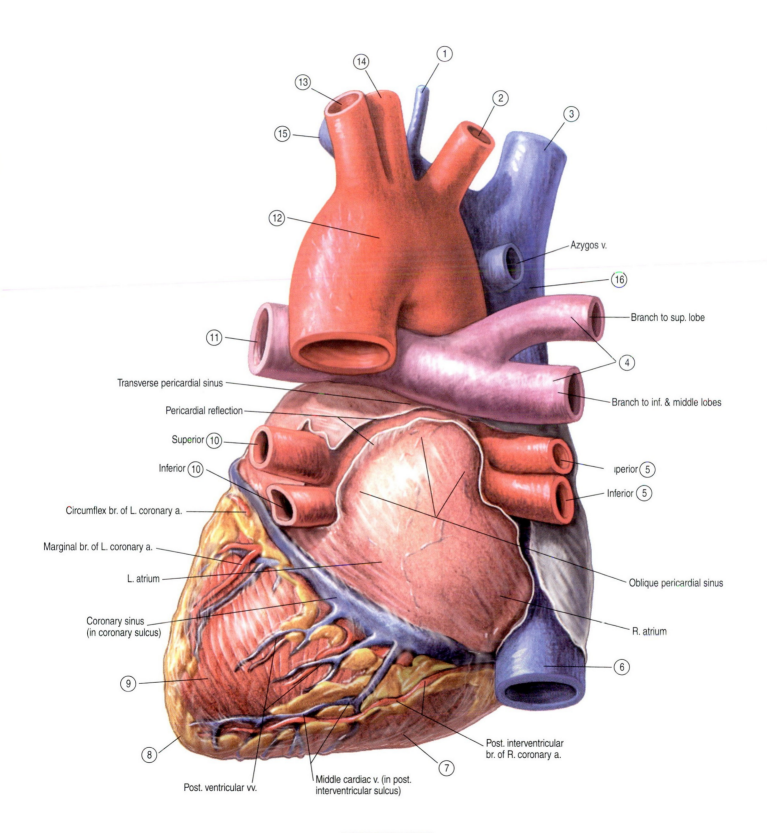

Azygos v.

Branch to sup. lobe

Branch to inf. & middle lobes

Transverse pericardial sinus

Pericardial reflection

Superior ⑩

Inferior ⑩

Circumflex br. of L. coronary a.

Marginal br. of L. coronary a.

L. atrium

Coronary sinus
(in coronary sulcus)

ıperior ⑤

Inferior ⑤

Oblique pericardial sinus

R. atrium

⑥

Post. interventricular
br. of R. coronary a.

Post. ventricular vv.

Middle cardiac v. (in post.
interventricular sulcus)

POSTERIOR VIEW

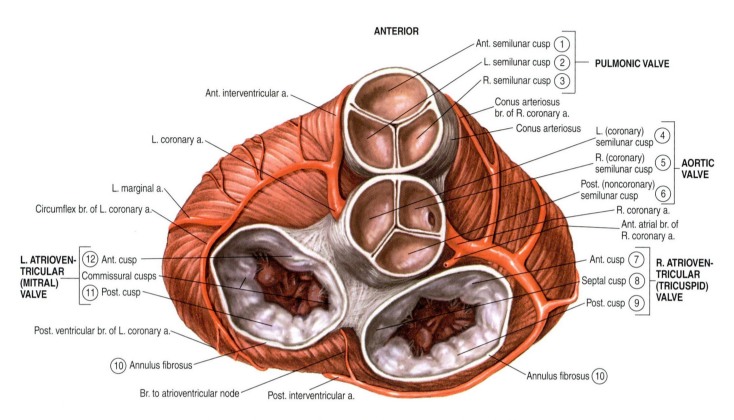

ANTERIOR

Ant. interventricular a.

Ant. semilunar cusp ①
L. semilunar cusp ② — **PULMONIC VALVE**
R. semilunar cusp ③

Conus arteriosus
br. of R. coronary a.

Conus arteriosus

L. coronary a.

L. (coronary) ④
semilunar cusp
R. (coronary) ⑤ **AORTIC
semilunar cusp   VALVE**
Post. (noncoronary) ⑥
semilunar cusp

L. marginal a.

Circumflex br. of L. coronary a.

R. coronary a.

Ant. atrial br. of
R. coronary a.

**L. ATRIOVEN-
TRICULAR
(MITRAL)
VALVE**

⑫ Ant. cusp
Commissural cusps
⑪ Post. cusp

Ant. cusp ⑦ **R. ATRIOVEN-
Septal cusp ⑧ TRICULAR
(TRICUSPID)
Post. cusp ⑨ VALVE**

Post. ventricular br. of L. coronary a.

Annulus fibrosus ⑩

⑩ Annulus fibrosus

Br. to atrioventricular node

Post. interventricular a.

HEART IN DIASTOLE VIEWED FROM BASE WITH ATRIA REMOVED

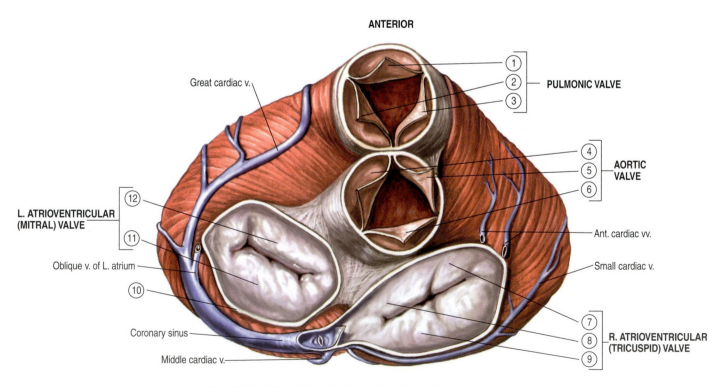

ANTERIOR

Great cardiac v.

①
② **PULMONIC VALVE**
③

④
⑤ **AORTIC
⑥ VALVE**

**L. ATRIOVENTRICULAR
(MITRAL) VALVE**

⑫

⑪

Ant. cardiac vv.

Oblique v. of L. atrium

Small cardiac v.

⑩

⑦
⑧ **R. ATRIOVENTRICULAR
(TRICUSPID) VALVE**
⑨

Coronary sinus

Middle cardiac v.

HEART IN SYSTOLE VIEWED FROM BASE WITH ATRIA REMOVED

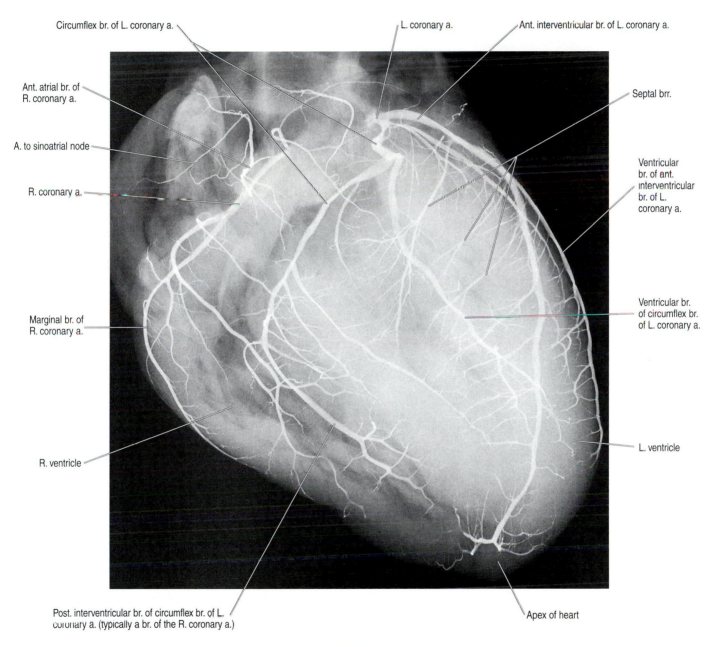

Circumflex br. of L. coronary a.

L. coronary a.

Ant. interventricular br. of L. coronary a.

Ant. atrial br. of
R. coronary a.

Septal brr.

A. to sinoatrial node

R. coronary a.

Ventricular
br. of ant.
interventricular
br. of L.
coronary a.

Marginal br. of
R. coronary a.

Ventricular br.
of circumflex br.
of L. coronary a.

L. ventricle

R. ventricle

Post. interventricular br. of circumflex br. of L.
coronary a. (typically a br. of the R. coronary a.)

Apex of heart

ANTEROPOSTERIOR VIEW

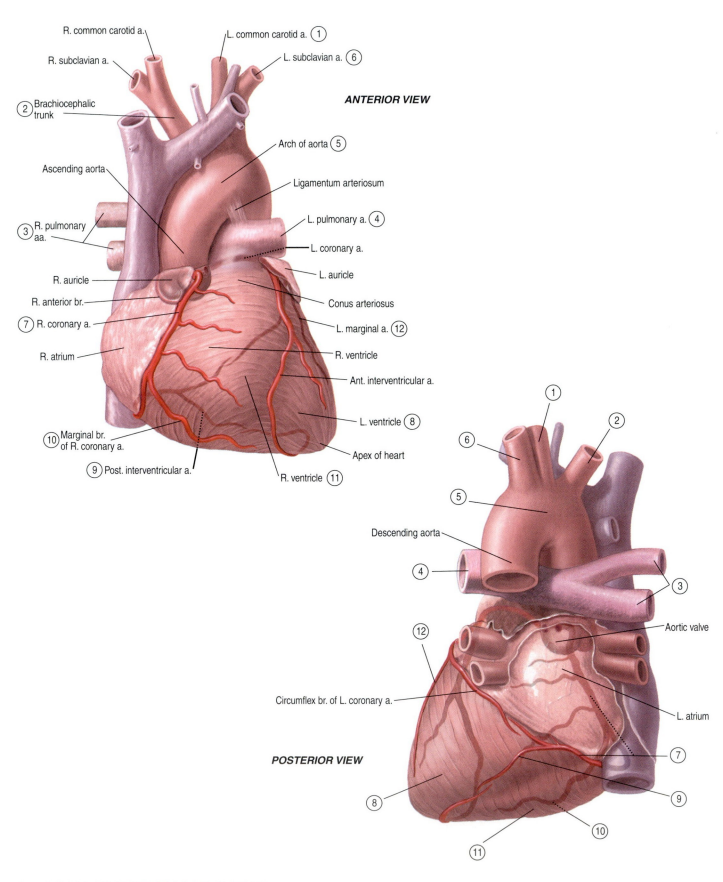

R. common carotid a. L. common carotid a. ①

R. subclavian a. L. subclavian a. ⑥

② Brachiocephalic trunk

ANTERIOR VIEW

Arch of aorta ⑤

Ascending aorta Ligamentum arteriosum

③ R. pulmonary aa. L. pulmonary a. ④

L. coronary a.

R. auricle L. auricle

R. anterior br. Conus arteriosus

⑦ R. coronary a. L. marginal a. ⑫

R. atrium R. ventricle

Ant. interventricular a.

L. ventricle ⑧

⑩ Marginal br. of R. coronary a. Apex of heart

⑨ Post. interventricular a. R. ventricle ⑪

Descending aorta

Aortic valve

⑫

Circumflex br. of L. coronary a. L. atrium

⑦

POSTERIOR VIEW ⑨

⑧ ⑩

⑪

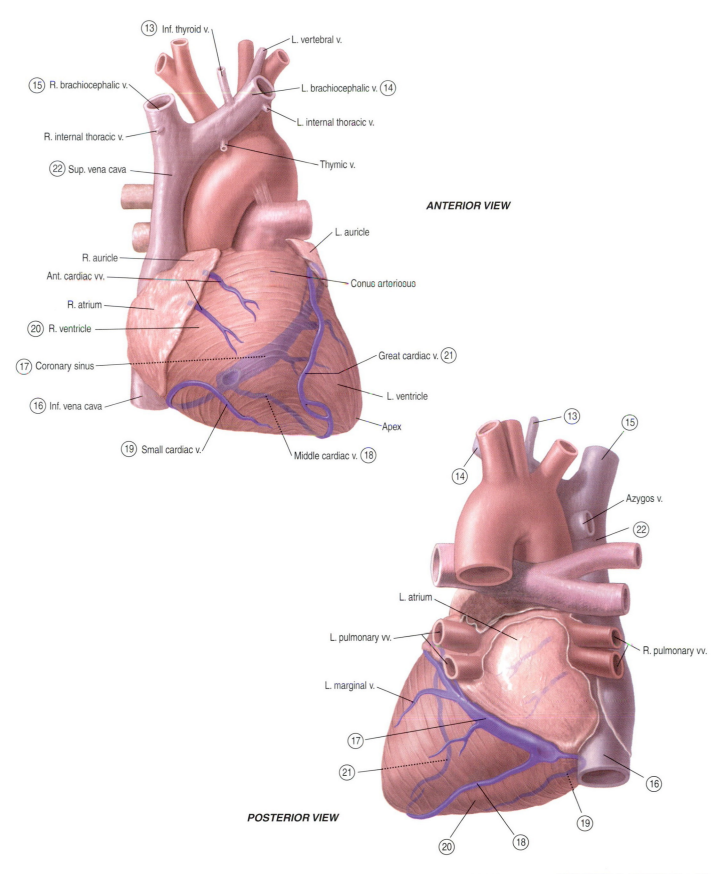

13 Inf. thyroid v.
L. vertebral v.
15 R. brachiocephalic v.
L. brachiocephalic v. 14
L. internal thoracic v.
R. internal thoracic v.
Thymic v.
22 Sup. vena cava

ANTERIOR VIEW

L. auricle
R. auricle
Ant. cardiac vv.
Conus arteriosus
R. atrium
20 R. ventricle
17 Coronary sinus
Great cardiac v. 21
L. ventricle
16 Inf. vena cava
Apex
19 Small cardiac v.
Middle cardiac v. 18

13
15
14
Azygos v.
22
L. atrium
L. pulmonary vv.
R. pulmonary vv.
L. marginal v.
17
21
16
19
20
18

POSTERIOR VIEW

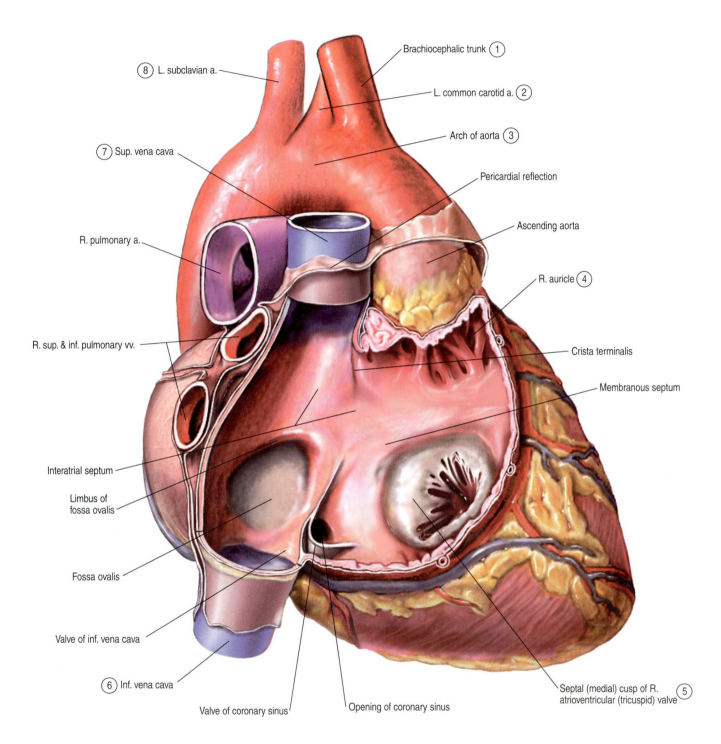

⑧ L. subclavian a.

Brachiocephalic trunk ①

L. common carotid a. ②

Arch of aorta ③

Pericardial reflection

⑦ Sup. vena cava

Ascending aorta

R. pulmonary a.

R. auricle ④

Crista terminalis

R. sup. & inf. pulmonary vv.

Membranous septum

Interatrial septum

Limbus of
fossa ovalis

Fossa ovalis

Valve of inf. vena cava

⑥ Inf. vena cava

Valve of coronary sinus

Opening of coronary sinus

Septal (medial) cusp of R.
atrioventricular (tricuspid) valve ⑤

LATERAL VIEW OF OPENED RIGHT ATRIUM

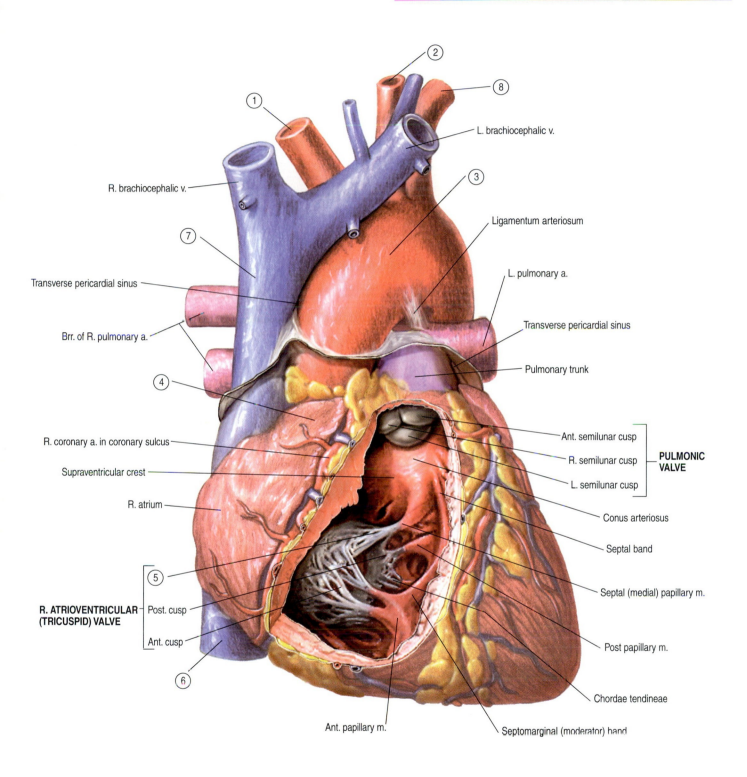

R. brachiocephalic v.

L. brachiocephalic v.

Ligamentum arteriosum

L. pulmonary a.

Transverse pericardial sinus

Transverse pericardial sinus

Brr. of R. pulmonary a.

Pulmonary trunk

R. coronary a. in coronary sulcus

Ant. semilunar cusp

R. semilunar cusp

PULMONIC VALVE

Supraventricular crest

L. semilunar cusp

R. atrium

Conus arteriosus

Septal band

Septal (medial) papillary m.

R. ATRIOVENTRICULAR (TRICUSPID) VALVE

Post. cusp

Ant. cusp

Post papillary m.

Chordae tendineae

Ant. papillary m.

Septomarginal (moderator) band

ANTERIOR VIEW OF OPENED RIGHT VENTRICLE

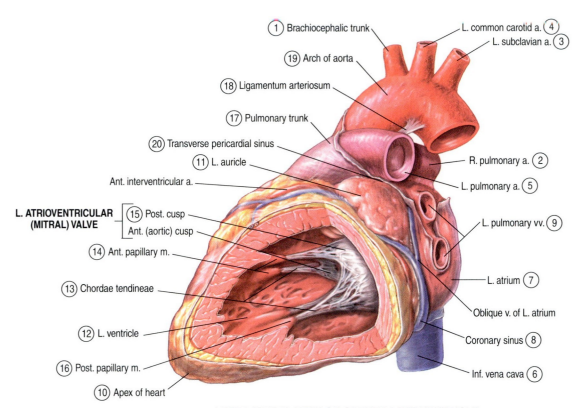

① Brachiocephalic trunk
L. common carotid a. ④
L. subclavian a. ③
⑲ Arch of aorta
⑱ Ligamentum arteriosum
⑰ Pulmonary trunk
⑳ Transverse pericardial sinus
⑪ L. auricle
Ant. interventricular a.
R. pulmonary a. ②
L. pulmonary a. ⑤

L. ATRIOVENTRICULAR (MITRAL) VALVE { ⑮ Post. cusp
Ant. (aortic) cusp

⑭ Ant. papillary m.
L. pulmonary vv. ⑨
⑬ Chordae tendineae
L. atrium ⑦
Oblique v. of L. atrium
⑫ L. ventricle
Coronary sinus ⑧
⑯ Post. papillary m.
Inf. vena cava ⑥
⑩ Apex of heart

LEFT LATERAL VIEW OF OPENED LEFT VENTRICLE

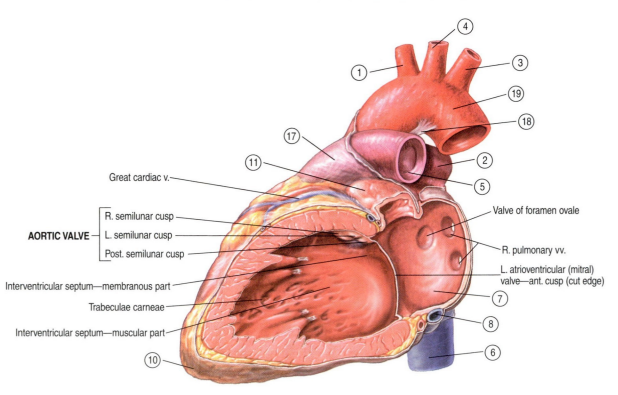

④
③
⑲
⑱
⑰
①
⑪
②
⑤
Great cardiac v.
Valve of foramen ovale

AORTIC VALVE { R. semilunar cusp
L. semilunar cusp
Post. semilunar cusp

R. pulmonary vv.
L. atrioventricular (mitral) valve—ant. cusp (cut edge)
Interventricular septum—membranous part
⑦
Trabeculae carneae
⑧
Interventricular septum—muscular part
⑥
⑩

LEFT LATERAL VIEW OF LEFT VENTRICLE & ATRIUM WITH MITRAL VALVE REMOVED

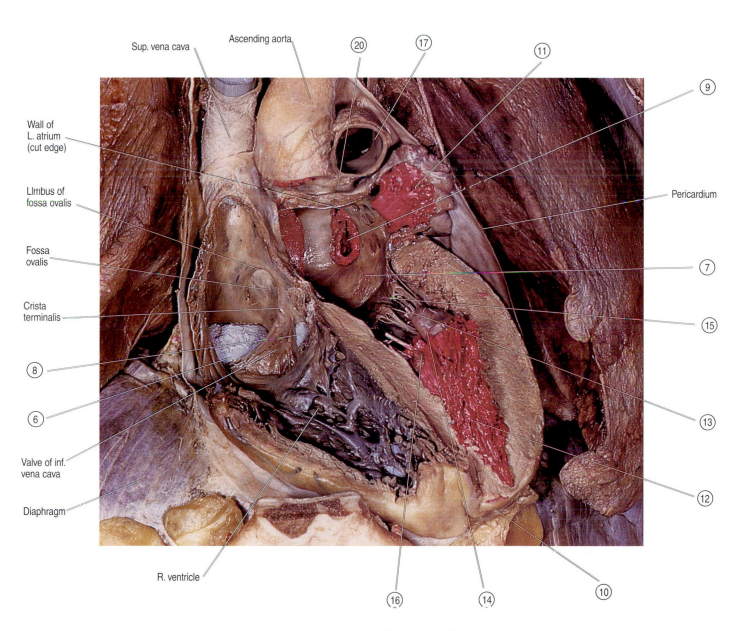

Sup. vena cava

Ascending aorta

20

17

11

9

Wall of
L. atrium
(cut edge)

Pericardium

Limbus of
fossa ovalis

Fossa
ovalis

7

Crista
terminalis

15

8

6

13

Valve of inf.
vena cava

12

Diaphragm

R. ventricle

16

14

10

INTERIOR OF ANTERIOR VIEW OF HEART

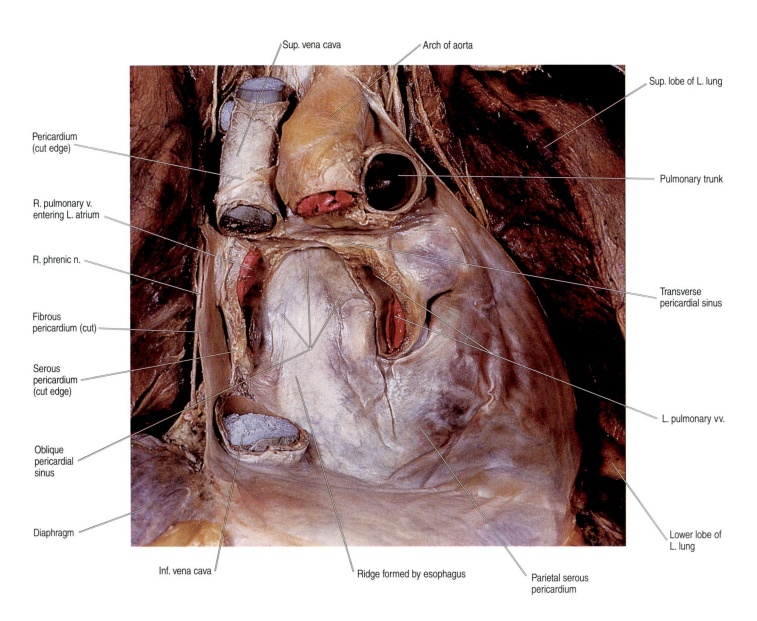

Sup. vena cava

Arch of aorta

Sup. lobe of L. lung

Pericardium (cut edge)

Pulmonary trunk

R. pulmonary v. entering L. atrium

R. phrenic n.

Transverse pericardial sinus

Fibrous pericardium (cut)

Serous pericardium (cut edge)

L. pulmonary vv.

Oblique pericardial sinus

Diaphragm

Lower lobe of L. lung

Inf. vena cava

Ridge formed by esophagus

Parietal serous pericardium

ANTERIOR VIEW OF PERICARDIAL CAVITY WITH HEART REMOVED

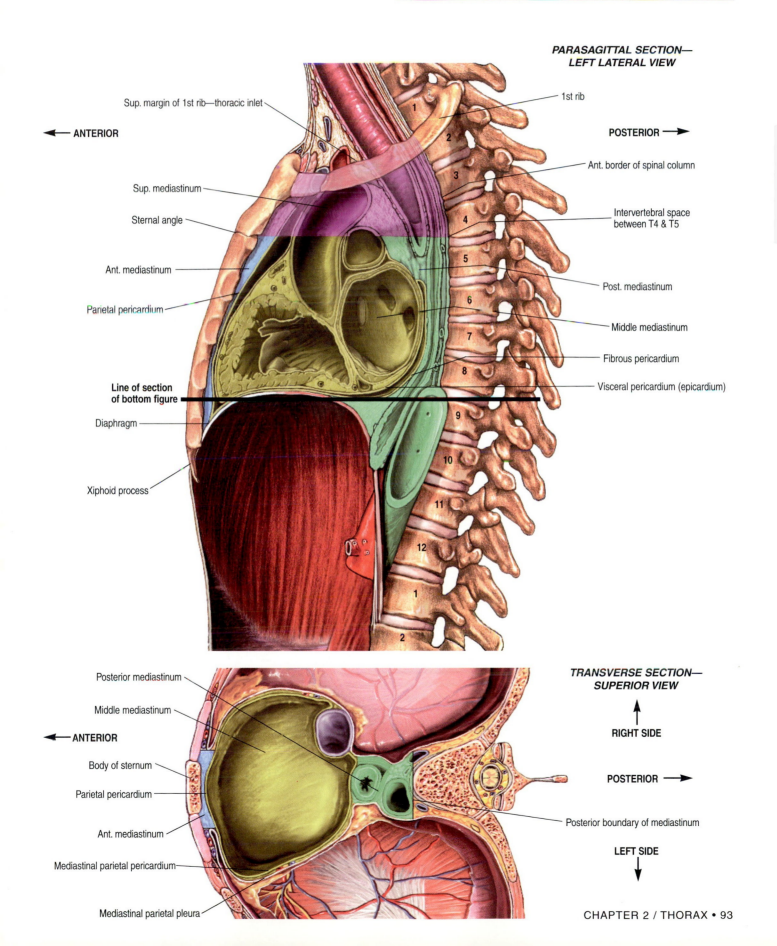

PARASAGITTAL SECTION—
LEFT LATERAL VIEW

Sup. margin of 1st rib—thoracic inlet

1st rib

◄ ANTERIOR

POSTERIOR ►

Sup. mediastinum

Ant. border of spinal column

Sternal angle

Intervertebral space between T4 & T5

Ant. mediastinum

Post. mediastinum

Parietal pericardium

Middle mediastinum

Fibrous pericardium

Visceral pericardium (epicardium)

Line of section of bottom figure

Diaphragm

Xiphoid process

TRANSVERSE SECTION—
SUPERIOR VIEW

Posterior mediastinum

Middle mediastinum

RIGHT SIDE

◄ ANTERIOR

Body of sternum

POSTERIOR ►

Parietal pericardium

Ant. mediastinum

Posterior boundary of mediastinum

Mediastinal parietal pericardium

LEFT SIDE

Mediastinal parietal pleura

CHAPTER 2 / THORAX • 93

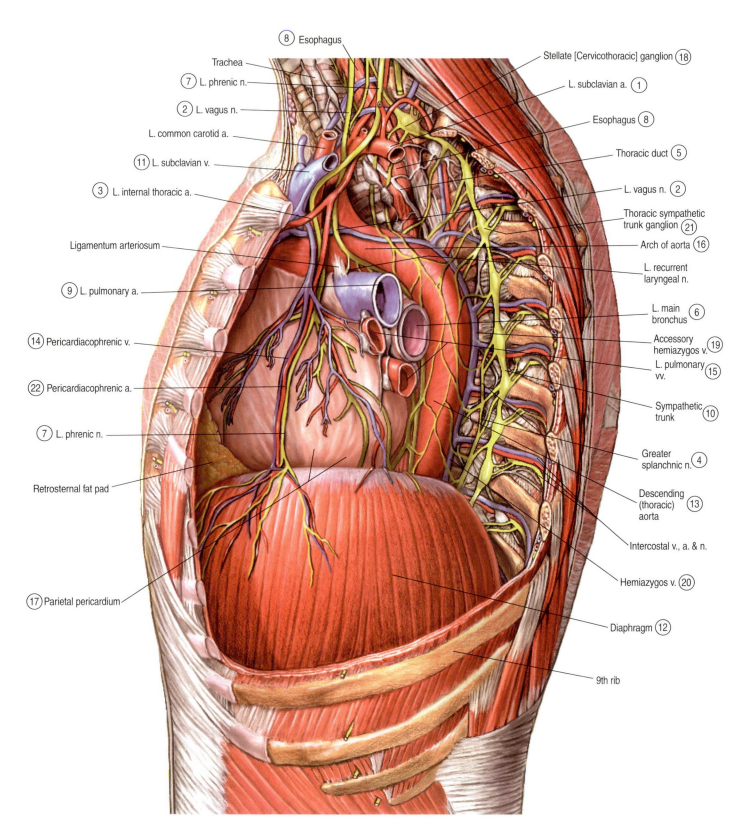

(8) Esophagus

Trachea

(7) L. phrenic n.

(2) L. vagus n.

L. common carotid a.

(11) L. subclavian v.

(3) L. internal thoracic a.

Ligamentum arteriosum

(9) L. pulmonary a.

(14) Pericardiacophrenic v.

(22) Pericardiacophrenic a.

(7) L. phrenic n.

Retrosternal fat pad

(17) Parietal pericardium

Stellate [Cervicothoracic] ganglion (18)

L. subclavian a. (1)

Esophagus (8)

Thoracic duct (5)

L. vagus n. (2)

Thoracic sympathetic trunk ganglion (21)

Arch of aorta (16)

L. recurrent laryngeal n.

L. main bronchus (6)

Accessory hemiazygos v. (19)

L. pulmonary vv. (15)

Sympathetic trunk (10)

Greater splanchnic n. (4)

Descending (thoracic) aorta (13)

Intercostal v., a. & n.

Hemiazygos v. (20)

Diaphragm (12)

9th rib

LEFT LATERAL VIEW OF MEDIASTINUM

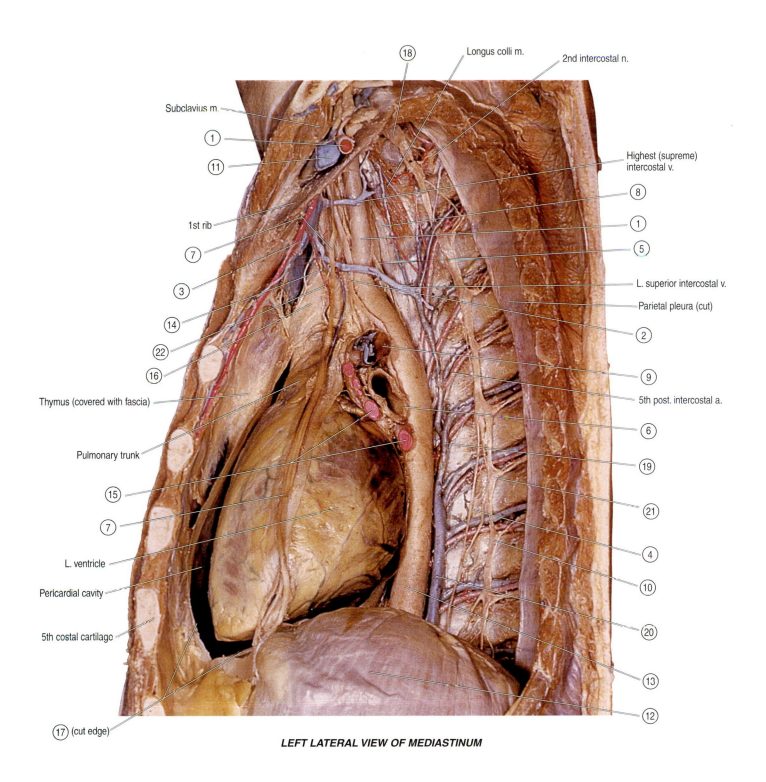

Subclavius m.

Longus colli m.

2nd intercostal n.

Highest (supreme) intercostal v.

1st rib

L. superior intercostal v.

Parietal pleura (cut)

Thymus (covered with fascia)

5th post. intercostal a.

Pulmonary trunk

L. ventricle

Pericardial cavity

5th costal cartilago

(17) (cut edge)

LEFT LATERAL VIEW OF MEDIASTINUM

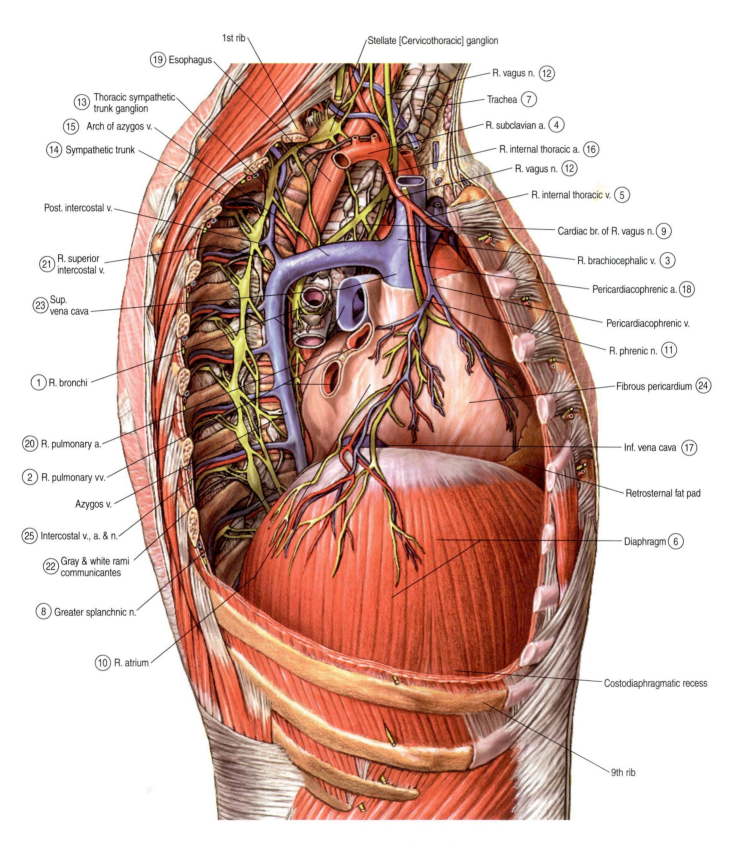

1st rib

Stellate [Cervicothoracic] ganglion

(19) Esophagus

(13) Thoracic sympathetic trunk ganglion

(15) Arch of azygos v.

(14) Sympathetic trunk

Post. intercostal v.

(21) R. superior intercostal v.

(23) Sup. vena cava

(1) R. bronchi

(20) R. pulmonary a.

(2) R. pulmonary vv.

Azygos v.

(25) Intercostal v., a. & n.

(22) Gray & white rami communicantes

(8) Greater splanchnic n.

(10) R. atrium

R. vagus n. (12)

Trachea (7)

R. subclavian a. (4)

R. internal thoracic a. (16)

R. vagus n. (12)

R. internal thoracic v. (5)

Cardiac br. of R. vagus n. (9)

R. brachiocephalic v. (3)

Pericardiacophrenic a. (18)

Pericardiacophrenic v.

R. phrenic n. (11)

Fibrous pericardium (24)

Inf. vena cava (17)

Retrosternal fat pad

Diaphragm (6)

Costodiaphragmatic recess

9th rib

RIGHT LATERAL VIEW OF MEDIASTINUM

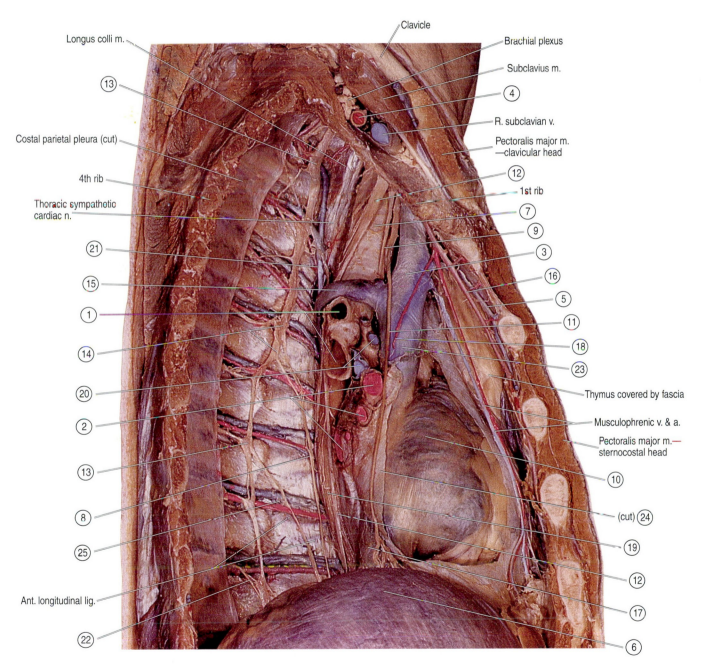

Longus colli m.

Clavicle

Brachial plexus

Subclavius m.

(13)

(4)

R. subclavian v.

Costal parietal pleura (cut)

Pectoralis major m. —clavicular head

4th rib

(12)

1st rib

Thoracic sympathetic cardiac n.

(7)

(9)

(21)

(3)

(15)

(16)

(1)

(5)

(14)

(11)

(20)

(18)

(2)

(23)

Thymus covered by fascia

(13)

Musculophrenic v. & a.

(8)

Pectoralis major m.— sternocostal head

(25)

(10)

Ant. longitudinal lig.

(cut) (24)

(22)

(19)

(12)

(17)

(6)

RIGHT LATERAL VIEW OF MEDIASTINUM

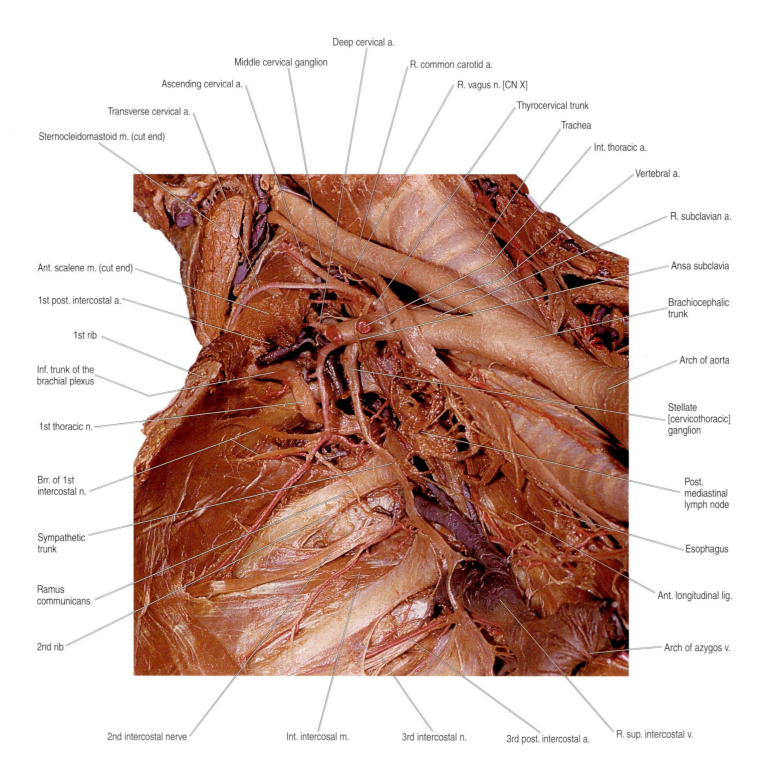

Deep cervical a.

Middle cervical ganglion

R. common carotid a.

Ascending cervical a.

R. vagus n. [CN X]

Transverse cervical a.

Thyrocervical trunk

Trachea

Sternocleidomastoid m. (cut end)

Int. thoracic a.

Vertebral a.

R. subclavian a.

Ant. scalene m. (cut end)

Ansa subclavia

1st post. intercostal a.

Brachiocephalic trunk

1st rib

Inf. trunk of the brachial plexus

Arch of aorta

1st thoracic n.

Stellate [cervicothoracic] ganglion

Brr. of 1st intercostal n.

Post. mediastinal lymph node

Sympathetic trunk

Esophagus

Ramus communicans

Ant. longitudinal lig.

2nd rib

Arch of azygos v.

2nd intercostal nerve   Int. intercosal m.   3rd intercostal n.   3rd post. intercostal a.   R. sup. intercostal v.

RIGHT ANTEROLATERAL INFERIOR OBLIQUE VIEW

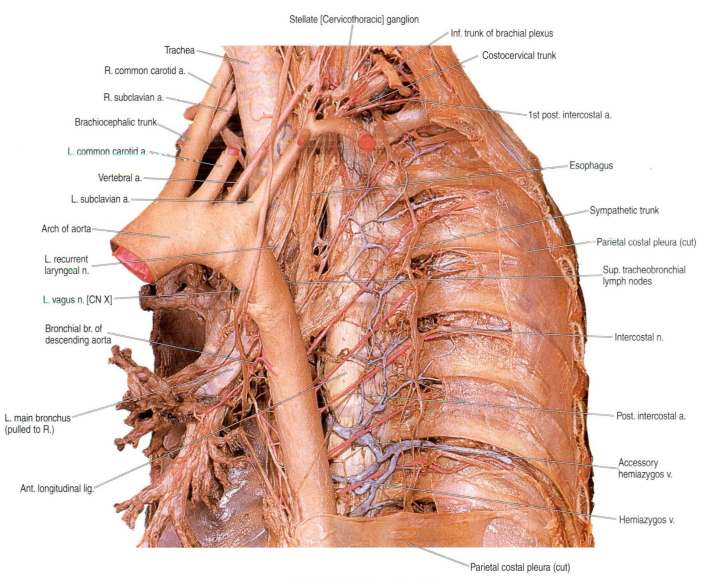

Stellate [Cervicothoracic] ganglion

Inf. trunk of brachial plexus

Costocervical trunk

Trachea

R. common carotid a.

R. subclavian a.

Brachiocephalic trunk

L. common carotid a.

1st post. intercostal a.

Vertebral a.

Esophagus

L. subclavian a.

Sympathetic trunk

Arch of aorta

Parietal costal pleura (cut)

L. recurrent laryngeal n.

Sup. tracheobronchial lymph nodes

L. vagus n. [CN X]

Bronchial br. of descending aorta

Intercostal n.

L. main bronchus (pulled to R.)

Post. intercostal a.

Accessory hemiazygos v.

Ant. longitudinal lig.

Hemiazygos v.

Parietal costal pleura (cut)

LEFT ANTEROLATERAL VIEW

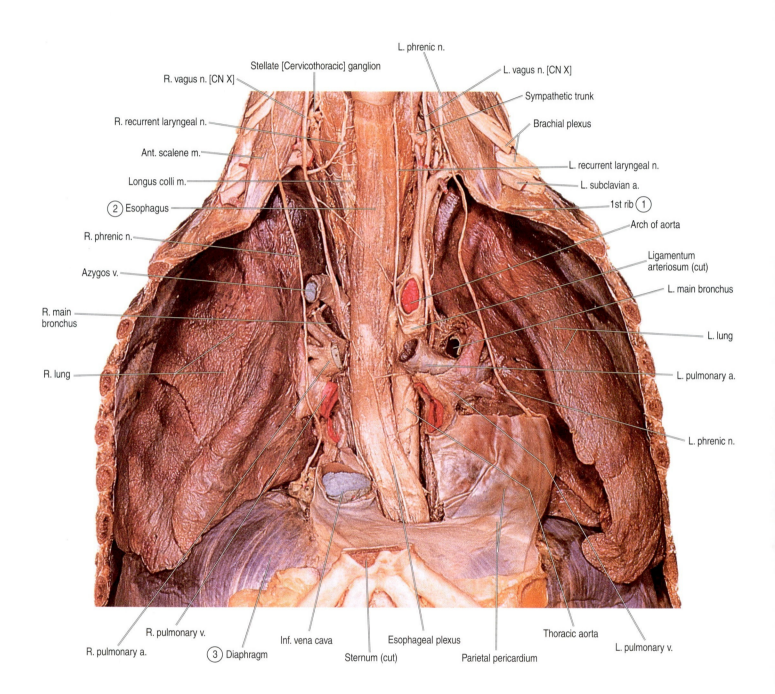

L. phrenic n.

Stellate [Cervicothoracic] ganglion

R. vagus n. [CN X]

L. vagus n. [CN X]

Sympathetic trunk

R. recurrent laryngeal n.

Brachial plexus

Ant. scalene m.

L. recurrent laryngeal n.

Longus colli m.

L. subclavian a.

② Esophagus

1st rib ①

R. phrenic n.

Arch of aorta

Azygos v.

Ligamentum arteriosum (cut)

R. main bronchus

L. main bronchus

R. lung

L. lung

L. pulmonary a.

L. phrenic n.

R. pulmonary v.

Inf. vena cava

Esophageal plexus

Thoracic aorta

R. pulmonary a.

③ Diaphragm

Sternum (cut)

Parietal pericardium

L. pulmonary v.

ANTERIOR VIEW OF POSTERIOR MEDIASTINAL STRUCTURES

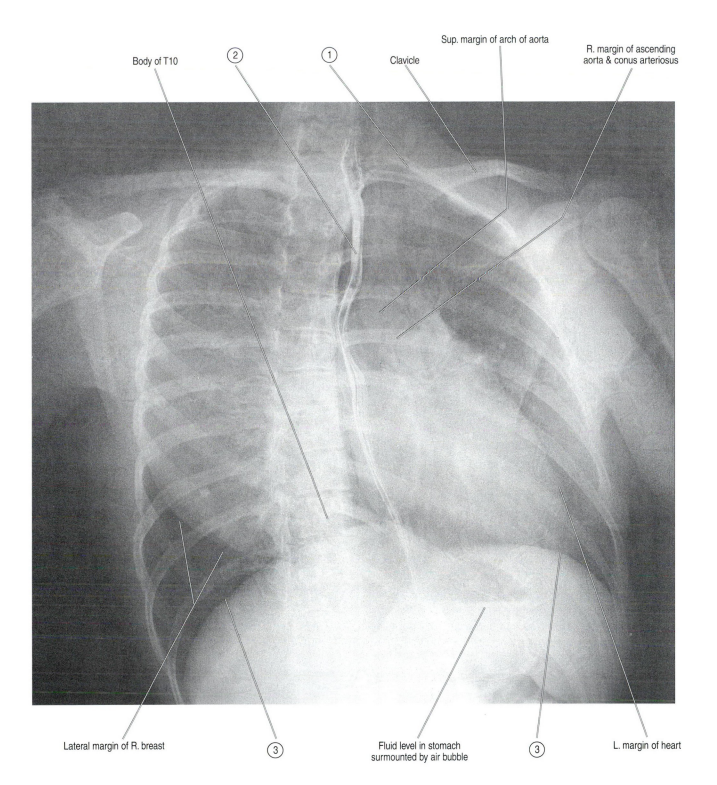

Body of T10

②

①

Clavicle

Sup. margin of arch of aorta

R. margin of ascending aorta & conus arteriosus

Lateral margin of R. breast

③

Fluid level in stomach surmounted by air bubble

③

L. margin of heart

RIGHT ANTERIOR OBLIQUE VIEW OF ESOPHAGUS

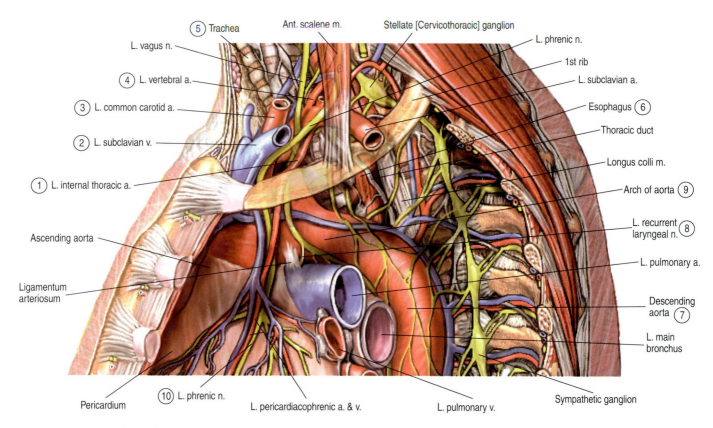

Trachea (5)

Ant. scalene m.

Stellate [Cervicothoracic] ganglion

L. phrenic n.

1st rib

L. subclavian a.

Esophagus (6)

Thoracic duct

Longus colli m.

Arch of aorta (9)

L. recurrent laryngeal n. (8)

L. pulmonary a.

Descending aorta (7)

L. main bronchus

L. vagus n.

L. vertebral a. (4)

L. common carotid a. (3)

L. subclavian v. (2)

L. internal thoracic a. (1)

Ascending aorta

Ligamentum arteriosum

Pericardium

L. phrenic n. (10)

L. pericardiacophrenic a. & v.

L. pulmonary v.

Sympathetic ganglion

LEFT LATERAL VIEW OF MEDIASTINUM

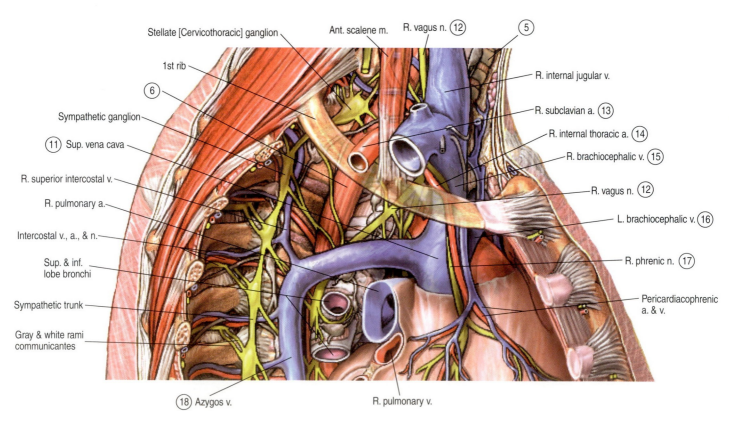

Stellate [Cervicothoracic] ganglion

Ant. scalene m.

R. vagus n. (12)

(5)

1st rib

6

Sympathetic ganglion

Sup. vena cava (11)

R. superior intercostal v.

R. pulmonary a.

Intercostal v., a., & n.

Sup. & inf. lobe bronchi

Sympathetic trunk

Gray & white rami communicantes

R. internal jugular v.

R. subclavian a. (13)

R. internal thoracic a. (14)

R. brachiocephalic v. (15)

R. vagus n. (12)

L. brachiocephalic v. (16)

R. phrenic n. (17)

Pericardiacophrenic a. & v.

Azygos v. (18)

R. pulmonary v.

RIGHT LATERAL VIEW OF MEDIASTINUM

ANTERIOR

◄— RIGHT SIDE

LEFT SIDE —►

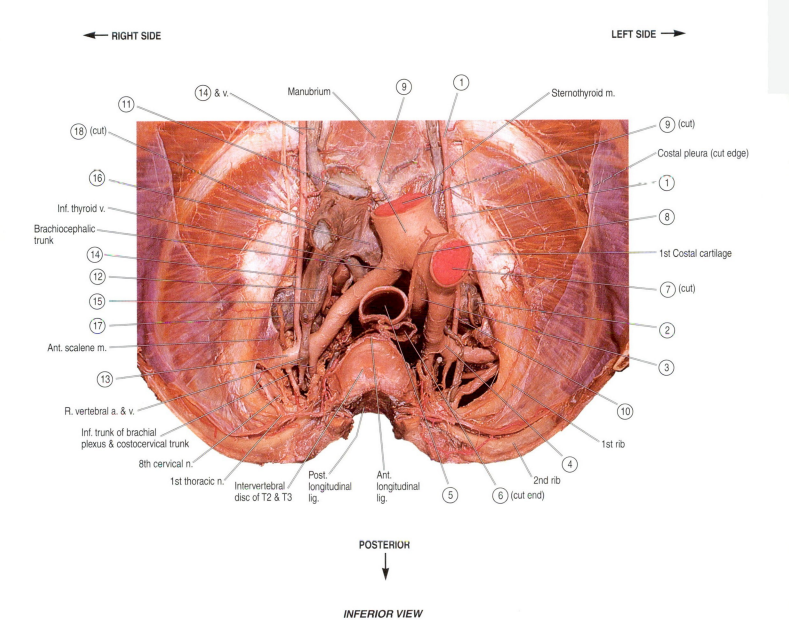

(14) & v.   Manubrium   (9)   (1)   Sternothyroid m.

(11)

(18) (cut)   (9) (cut)

(16)   Costal pleura (cut edge)

(1)

Inf. thyroid v.   (8)

Brachiocephalic
trunk   1st Costal cartilage

(14)   (7) (cut)

(12)

(15)   (2)

(17)   (3)

Ant. scalene m.

(13)   (10)

R. vertebral a. & v.   1st rib

Inf. trunk of brachial
plexus & costocervical trunk   (4)

8th cervical n.   2nd rib

1st thoracic n.   Intervertebral   Post.   Ant.   (5)   (6) (cut end)
disc of T2 & T3   longitudinal   longitudinal
lig.   lig.

POSTERIOR

INFERIOR VIEW

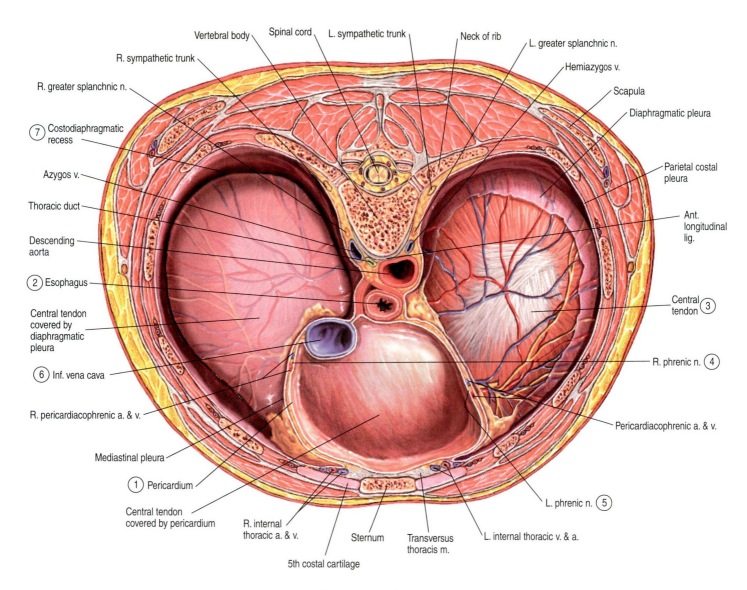

Vertebral body
Spinal cord
L. sympathetic trunk
Neck of rib
L. greater splanchnic n.
R. sympathetic trunk
Hemiazygos v.
R. greater splanchnic n.
Scapula
⑦ Costodiaphragmatic recess
Diaphragmatic pleura
Azygos v.
Parietal costal pleura
Thoracic duct
Descending aorta
Ant. longitudinal lig.
② Esophagus
Central tendon covered by diaphragmatic pleura
Central tendon ③
⑥ Inf. vena cava
R. phrenic n. ④
R. pericardiacophrenic a. & v.
Pericardiacophrenic a. & v.
Mediastinal pleura
① Pericardium
L. phrenic n. ⑤
Central tendon covered by pericardium
R. internal thoracic a. & v.
Sternum
Transversus thoracis m.
L. internal thoracic v. & a.
5th costal cartilage

SUPERIOR SURFACE

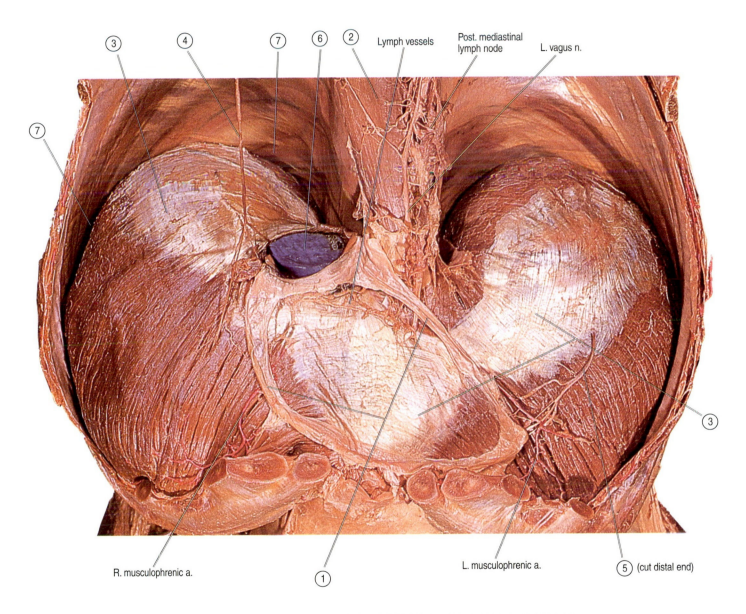

③ ④ ⑦ ⑥ ② Lymph vessels   Post. mediastinal lymph node   L. vagus n.

⑦

③

⑥

③

R. musculophrenic a.   ① L. musculophrenic a.   ⑤ (cut distal end)

ANTERIOR SUPERIOR OBLIQUE VIEW OF SUPERIOR SURFACE OF DIAPHRAGM

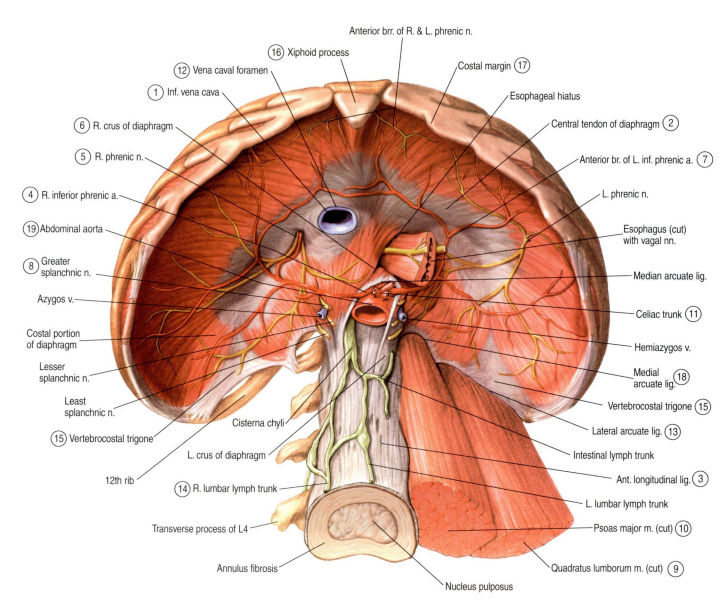

Anterior brr. of R. & L. phrenic n.

(16) Xiphoid process

(12) Vena caval foramen

Costal margin (17)

(1) Inf. vena cava

Esophageal hiatus

(6) R. crus of diaphragm

Central tendon of diaphragm (2)

(5) R. phrenic n.

Anterior br. of L. inf. phrenic a. (7)

(4) R. inferior phrenic a.

L. phrenic n.

(19) Abdominal aorta

Esophagus (cut) with vagal nn.

(8) Greater splanchnic n.

Median arcuate lig.

Azygos v.

Celiac trunk (11)

Costal portion of diaphragm

Hemiazygos v.

Lesser splanchnic n.

Medial arcuate lig. (18)

Least splanchnic n.

Vertebrocostal trigone (15)

(15) Vertebrocostal trigone

Lateral arcuate lig. (13)

12th rib

Intestinal lymph trunk

Cisterna chyli

Ant. longitudinal lig. (3)

(14) R. lumbar lymph trunk

L. crus of diaphragm

L. lumbar lymph trunk

Transverse process of L4

Psoas major m. (cut) (10)

Annulus fibrosis

Quadratus lumborum m. (cut) (9)

Nucleus pulposus

INFERIOR VIEW

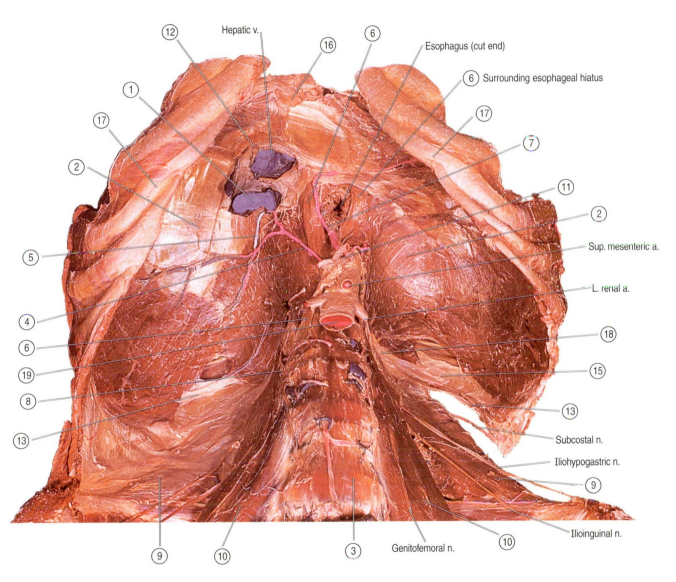

Hepatic v.

Esophagus (cut end)

Surrounding esophageal hiatus

Sup. mesenteric a.

L. renal a.

Subcostal n.

Iliohypogastric n.

Ilioinguinal n.

Genitofemoral n.

INFERIOR VIEW

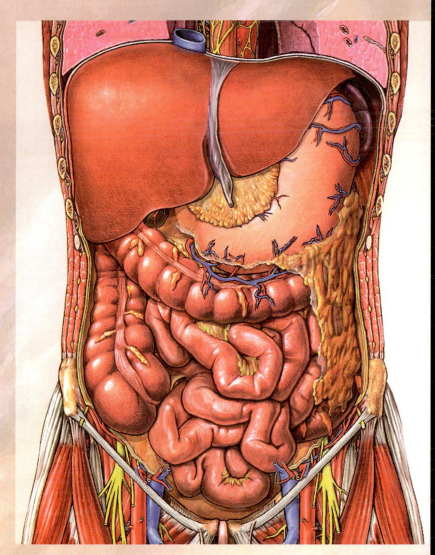

Abdomen

Chapter 3

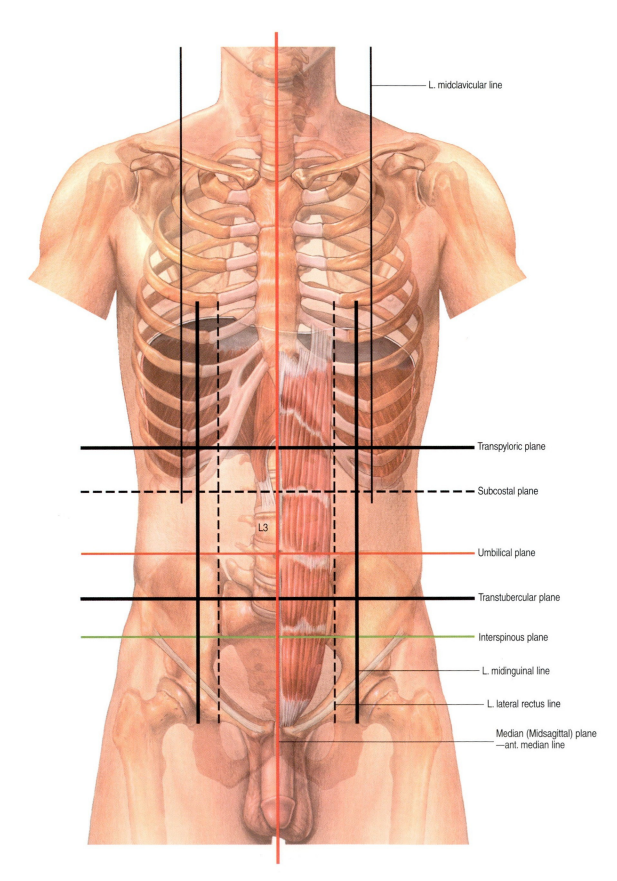

L. midclavicular line

Transpyloric plane

Subcostal plane

L3

Umbilical plane

Transtubercular plane

Interspinous plane

L. midinguinal line

L. lateral rectus line

Median (Midsagittal) plane
—ant. median line

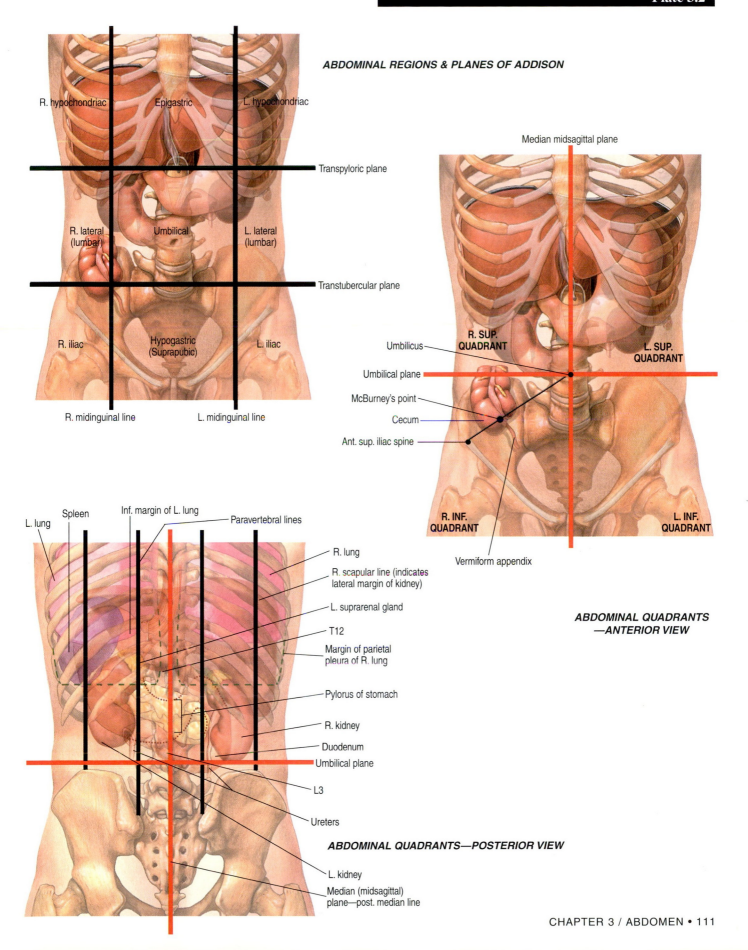

ABDOMINAL REGIONS & PLANES OF ADDISON

R. hypochondriac — Epigastric — L. hypochondriac

Transpyloric plane

R. lateral (lumbar) — Umbilical — L. lateral (lumbar)

Transtubercular plane

R. iliac — Hypogastric (Suprapubic) — L. iliac

R. midinguinal line — L. midinguinal line

Median midsagittal plane

Umbilicus

Umbilical plane

McBurney's point

Cecum

Ant. sup. iliac spine

R. SUP. QUADRANT — L. SUP. QUADRANT

R. INF. QUADRANT — L. INF. QUADRANT

Vermiform appendix

ABDOMINAL QUADRANTS —ANTERIOR VIEW

L. lung — Spleen — Inf. margin of L. lung — Paravertebral lines

R. lung

R. scapular line (indicates lateral margin of kidney)

L. suprarenal gland

T12

Margin of parietal pleura of R. lung

Pylorus of stomach

R. kidney

Duodenum

Umbilical plane

L3

Ureters

ABDOMINAL QUADRANTS—POSTERIOR VIEW

L. kidney

Median (midsagittal) plane—post. median line

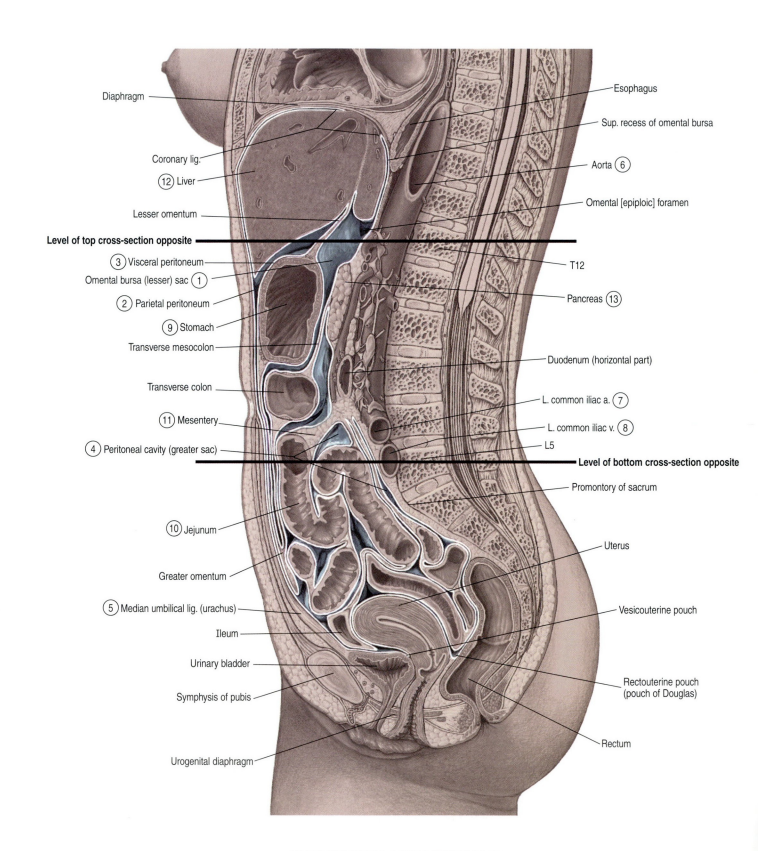

Diaphragm

Coronary lig.

(12) Liver

Lesser omentum

Level of top cross-section opposite

(3) Visceral peritoneum

Omental bursa (lesser) sac (1)

(2) Parietal peritoneum

(9) Stomach

Transverse mesocolon

Transverse colon

(11) Mesentery

(4) Peritoneal cavity (greater sac)

(10) Jejunum

Greater omentum

(5) Median umbilical lig. (urachus)

Ileum

Urinary bladder

Symphysis of pubis

Urogenital diaphragm

Esophagus

Sup. recess of omental bursa

Aorta (6)

Omental [epiploic] foramen

T12

Pancreas (13)

Duodenum (horizontal part)

L. common iliac a. (7)

L. common iliac v. (8)

L5

Level of bottom cross-section opposite

Promontory of sacrum

Uterus

Vesicouterine pouch

Rectouterine pouch
(pouch of Douglas)

Rectum

MEDIAN SECTION—LEFT LATERAL VIEW

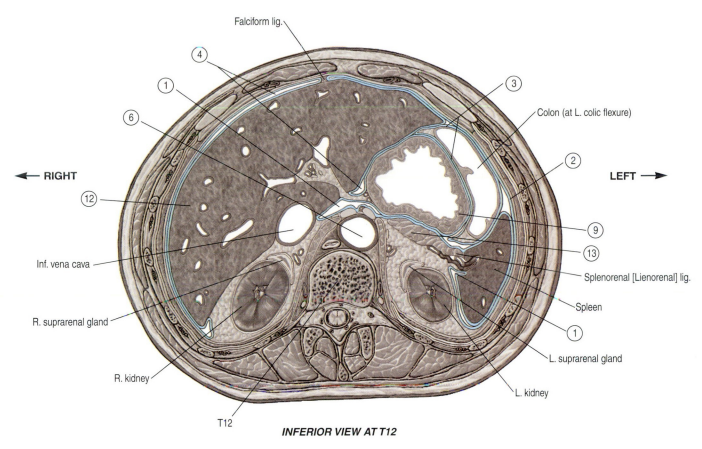

Falciform lig.

Colon (at L. colic flexure)

◄— RIGHT

LEFT —►

Inf. vena cava

Splenorenal [Lienorenal] lig.

Spleen

R. suprarenal gland

L. suprarenal gland

R. kidney

L. kidney

T12

INFERIOR VIEW AT T12

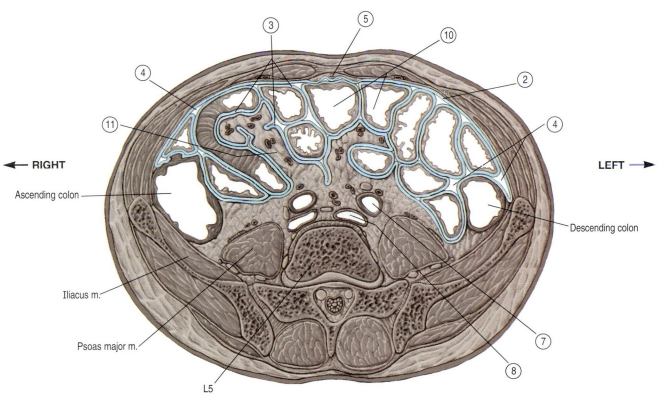

◄— RIGHT

LEFT —►

Ascending colon

Descending colon

Iliacus m.

Psoas major m.

L5

INFERIOR VIEW AT L5

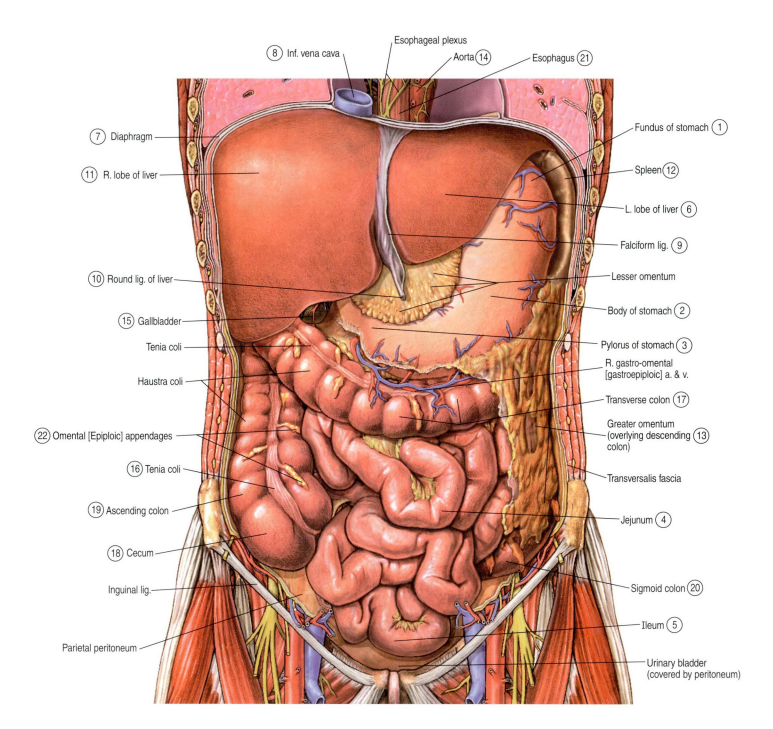

(8) Inf. vena cava — Esophageal plexus — Aorta (14) — Esophagus (21)

(7) Diaphragm

(11) R. lobe of liver

(10) Round lig. of liver

(15) Gallbladder

Tenia coli

Haustra coli

(22) Omental [Epiploic] appendages

(16) Tenia coli

(19) Ascending colon

(18) Cecum

Inguinal lig.

Parietal peritoneum

Fundus of stomach (1)

Spleen (12)

L. lobe of liver (6)

Falciform lig. (9)

Lesser omentum

Body of stomach (2)

Pylorus of stomach (3)

R. gastro-omental [gastroepiploic] a. & v.

Transverse colon (17)

Greater omentum (overlying descending (13) colon)

Transversalis fascia

Jejunum (4)

Sigmoid colon (20)

Ileum (5)

Urinary bladder (covered by peritoneum)

ANTERIOR VIEW

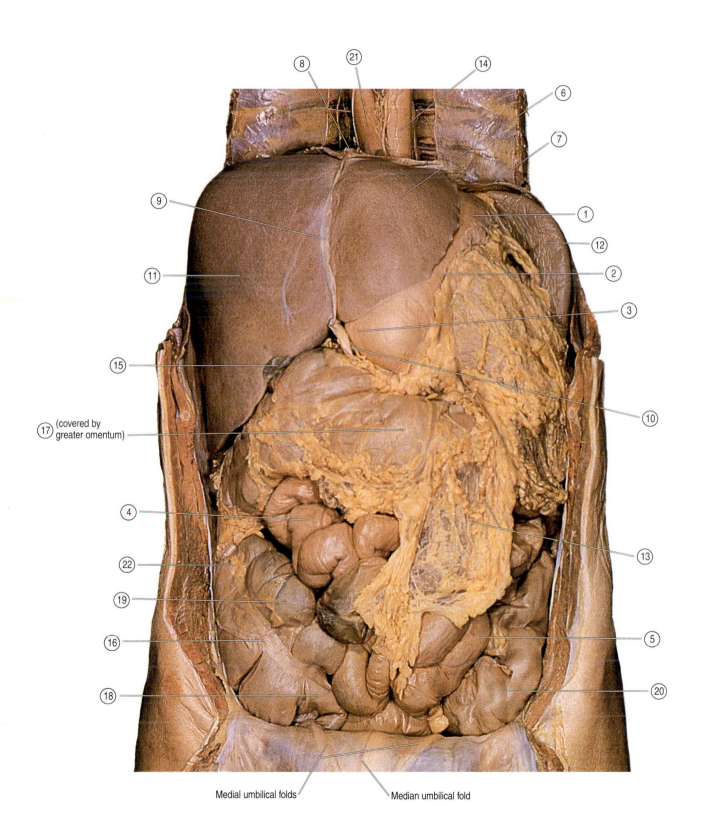

9

8   21   14

6

7

1

12

2

3

11

15

10

17 (covered by
    greater omentum)

4

22

19

16   5

18   20

13

Medial umbilical folds   Median umbilical fold

ANTERIOR VIEW

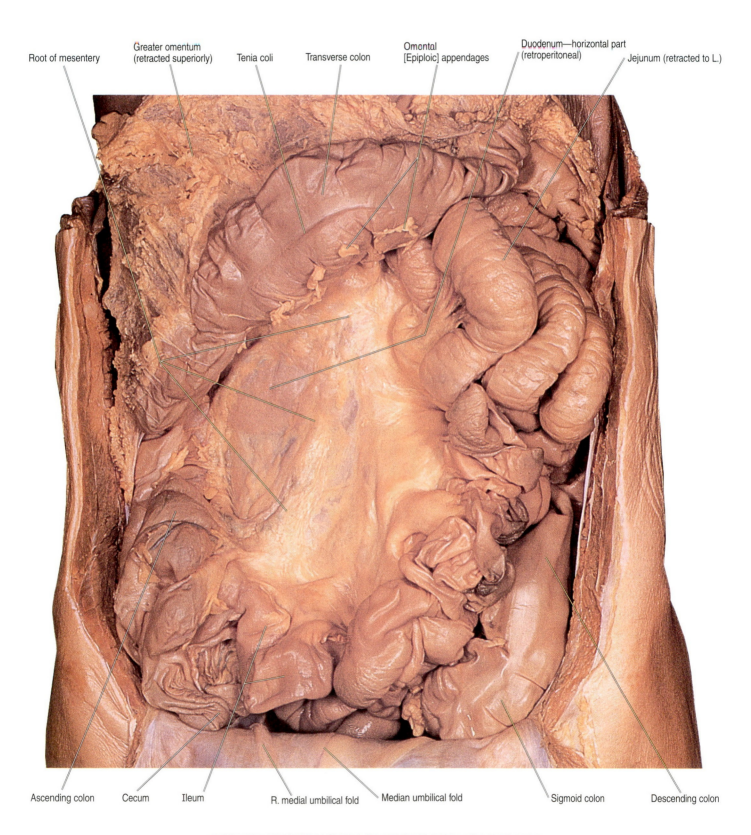

Root of mesentery

Greater omentum (retracted superiorly)

Tenia coli

Transverse colon

Omental [Epiploic] appendages

Duodenum—horizontal part (retroperitoneal)

Jejunum (retracted to L.)

Ascending colon

Cecum

Ileum

R. medial umbilical fold

Median umbilical fold

Sigmoid colon

Descending colon

ANTERIOR VIEW WITH SMALL INTESTINES RETRACTED TO LEFT

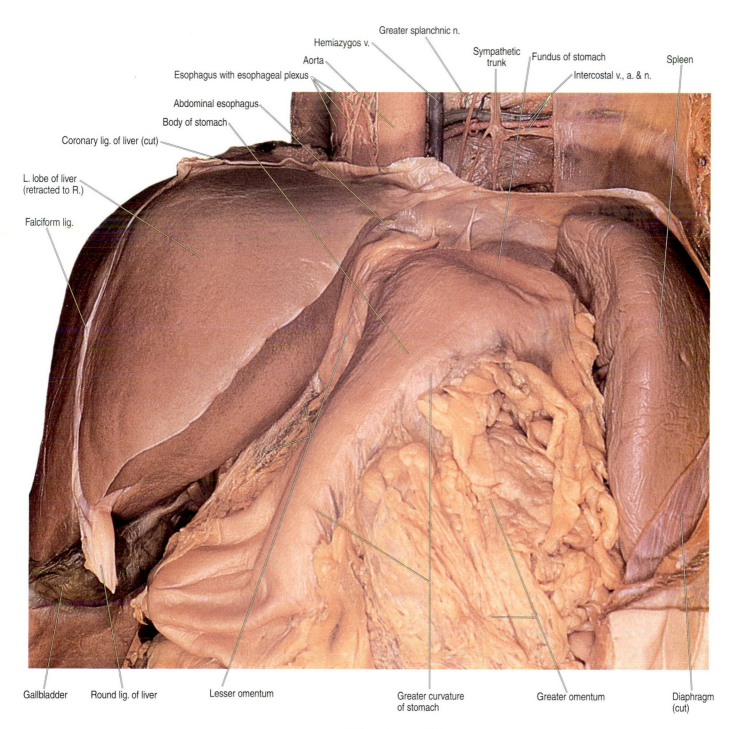

Greater splanchnic n.

Hemiazygos v.

Aorta

Sympathetic trunk

Fundus of stomach

Spleen

Esophagus with esophageal plexus

Intercostal v., a. & n.

Abdominal esophagus

Body of stomach

Coronary lig. of liver (cut)

L. lobe of liver (retracted to R.)

Falciform lig.

Gallbladder

Round lig. of liver

Lesser omentum

Greater curvature of stomach

Greater omentum

Diaphragm (cut)

LEFT ANTEROLATERAL VIEW

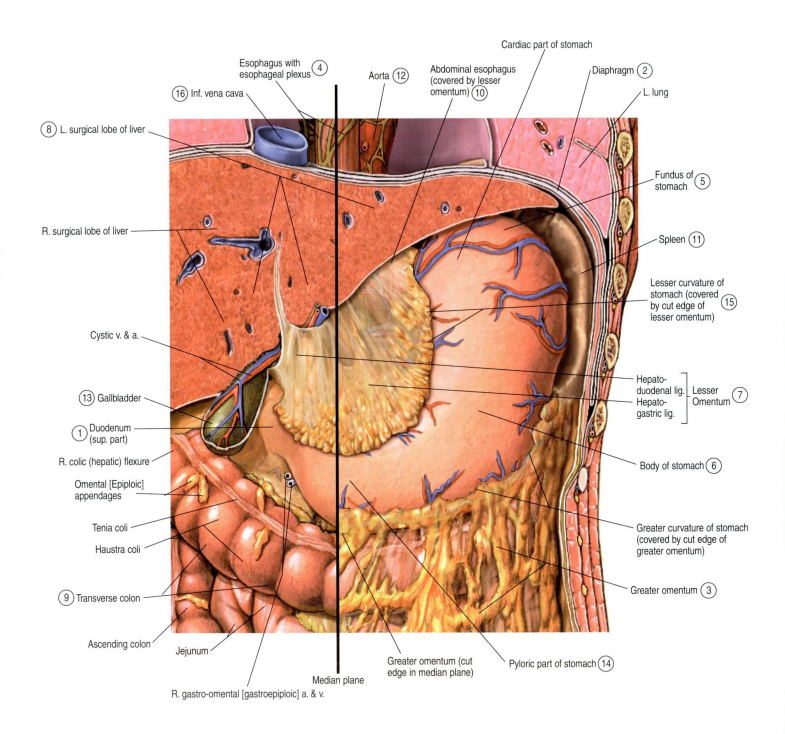

Esophagus with esophageal plexus ④

⑯ Inf. vena cava

Aorta ⑫

Cardiac part of stomach

Abdominal esophagus (covered by lesser omentum) ⑩

Diaphragm ②

L. lung

⑧ L. surgical lobe of liver

Fundus of stomach ⑤

R. surgical lobe of liver

Spleen ⑪

Lesser curvature of stomach (covered by cut edge of lesser omentum) ⑮

Cystic v. & a.

Hepato-duodenal lig.
Hepato-gastric lig.

Lesser Omentum ⑦

⑬ Gallbladder

① Duodenum (sup. part)

Body of stomach ⑥

R. colic (hepatic) flexure

Omental [Epiploic] appendages

Tenia coli

Greater curvature of stomach (covered by cut edge of greater omentum)

Haustra coli

Greater omentum ③

⑨ Transverse colon

Ascending colon

Jejunum

Median plane

Greater omentum (cut edge in median plane)

Pyloric part of stomach ⑭

R. gastro-omental [gastroepiploic] a. & v.

ANTERIOR VIEW

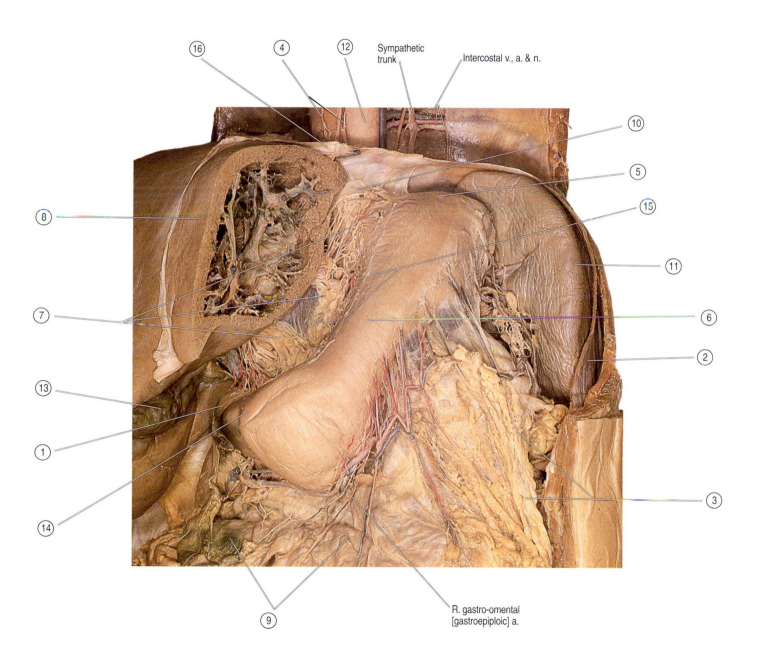

16 4 12 Sympathetic trunk Intercostal v., a. & n.

10

5

8

15

7

11

6

2

13

1

3

14

9

R. gastro-omental [gastroepiploic] a.

LEFT ANTEROLATERAL VIEW—LATERAL SEGMENT OF L. LOBE OF LIVER PARTIALLY REMOVED

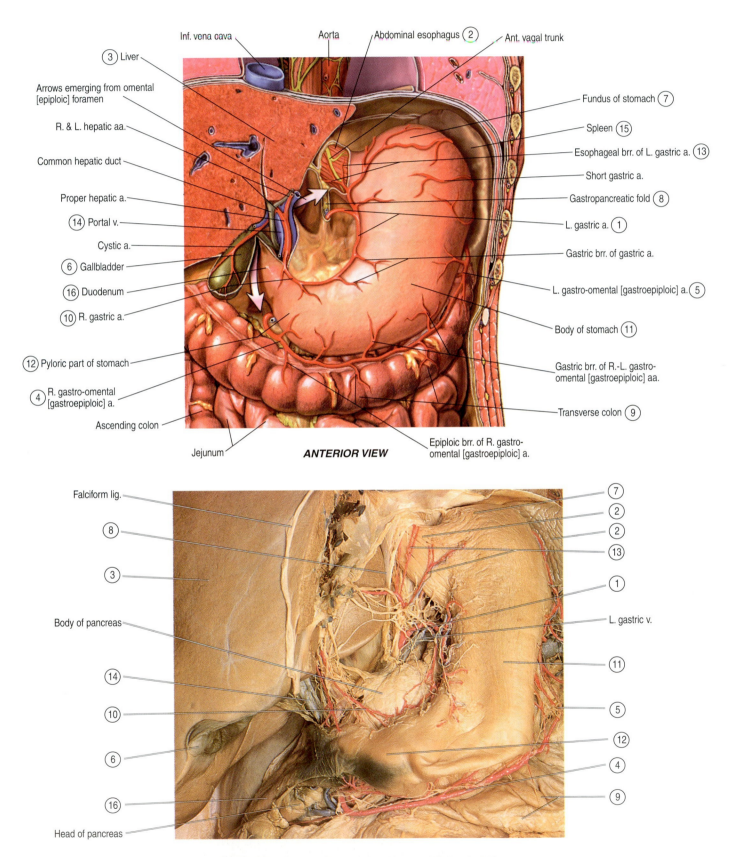

Inf. vena cava
Aorta
Abdominal esophagus ②
Ant. vagal trunk

③ Liver

Arrows emerging from omental [epiploic] foramen

R. & L. hepatic aa.

Common hepatic duct

Proper hepatic a.

⑭ Portal v.

Cystic a.

⑥ Gallbladder

⑯ Duodenum

⑩ R. gastric a.

⑫ Pyloric part of stomach

④ R. gastro-omental [gastroepiploic] a.

Ascending colon

Jejunum

ANTERIOR VIEW

Fundus of stomach ⑦

Spleen ⑮

Esophageal brr. of L. gastric a. ⑬

Short gastric a.

Gastropancreatic fold ⑧

L. gastric a. ①

Gastric brr. of gastric a.

L. gastro-omental [gastroepiploic] a. ⑤

Body of stomach ⑪

Gastric brr. of R.-L. gastro-omental [gastroepiploic] aa.

Transverse colon ⑨

Epiploic brr. of R. gastro-omental [gastroepiploic] a.

Falciform lig.

⑧

③

Body of pancreas

⑭

⑩

⑥

⑯

Head of pancreas

⑦
②
②
⑬

①

L. gastric v.

⑪

⑤

⑫

④

⑨

ANTERIOR VIEW—LIVER LEFT OF FALCIFORM LIG. REMOVED

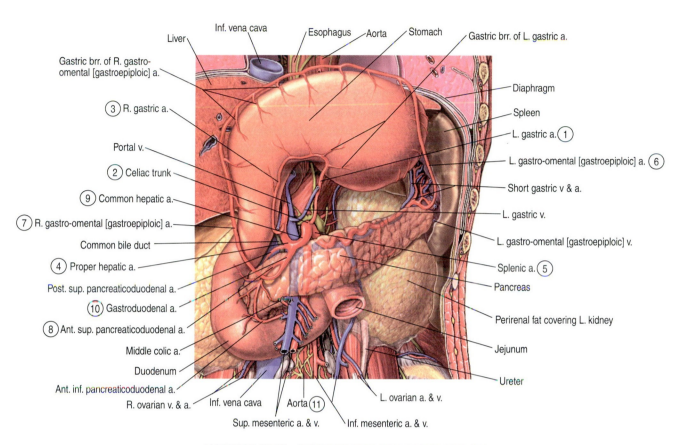

Inf. vena cava — Esophagus — Aorta — Stomach — Gastric brr. of L. gastric a.

Liver

Gastric brr. of R. gastro-omental [gastroepiploic] a.

(3) R. gastric a.

Portal v.

(2) Celiac trunk

(9) Common hepatic a.

(7) R. gastro-omental [gastroepiploic] a.

Common bile duct

(4) Proper hepatic a.

Post. sup. pancreaticoduodenal a.

(10) Gastroduodenal a.

(8) Ant. sup. pancreaticoduodenal a.

Middle colic a.

Duodenum

Ant. inf. pancreaticoduodenal a.

R. ovarian v. & a. — Inf. vena cava — Aorta (11) — L. ovarian a. & v.

Sup. mesenteric a. & v. — Inf. mesenteric a. & v.

Diaphragm

Spleen

L. gastric a. (1)

L. gastro-omental [gastroepiploic] a. (6)

Short gastric v & a.

L. gastric v.

L. gastro-omental [gastroepiploic] v.

Splenic a. (5)

Pancreas

Perirenal fat covering L. kidney

Jejunum

Ureter

ANTERIOR VIEW—STOMACH REFLECTED SUPERIORLY AND POSTERIOR PARIETAL PERITONEUM REMOVED

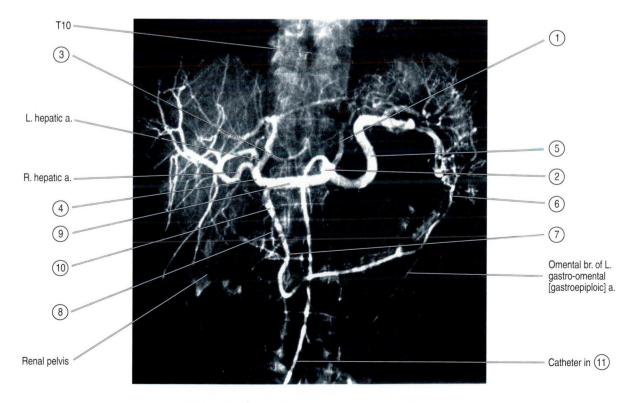

T10

(3)

L. hepatic a.

R. hepatic a.

(4)

(9)

(10)

(8)

Renal pelvis

(1)

(5)

(2)

(6)

(7)

Omental br. of L. gastro-omental [gastroepiploic] a.

Catheter in (11)

ARTERIOGRAPH OF CELIAC TRUNK & BRANCHES

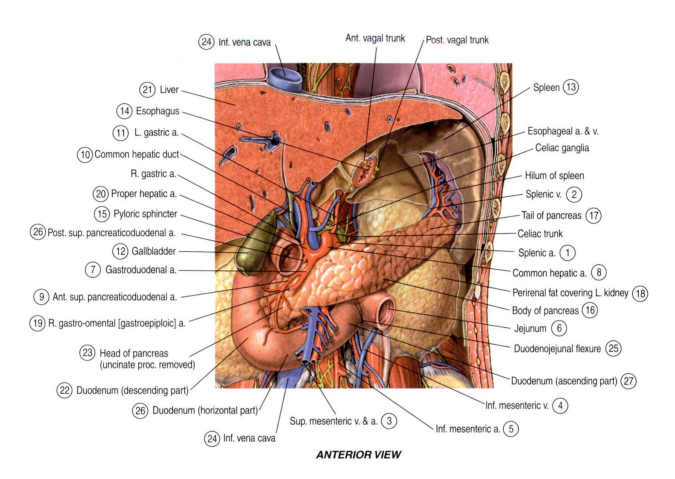

24 Inf. vena cava · Ant. vagal trunk · Post. vagal trunk

21 Liver

14 Esophagus

11 L. gastric a.

10 Common hepatic duct

R. gastric a.

20 Proper hepatic a.

15 Pyloric sphincter

26 Post. sup. pancreaticoduodenal a.

12 Gallbladder

7 Gastroduodenal a.

9 Ant. sup. pancreaticoduodenal a.

19 R. gastro-omental [gastroepiploic] a.

23 Head of pancreas (uncinate proc. removed)

22 Duodenum (descending part)

26 Duodenum (horizontal part)

Sup. mesenteric v. & a. 3

24 Inf. vena cava

Spleen 13

Esophageal a. & v.

Celiac ganglia

Hilum of spleen

Splenic v. 2

Tail of pancreas 17

Celiac trunk

Splenic a. 1

Common hepatic a. 8

Perirenal fat covering L. kidney 18

Body of pancreas 16

Jejunum 6

Duodenojejunal flexure 25

Duodenum (ascending part) 27

Inf. mesenteric v. 4

Inf. mesenteric a. 5

ANTERIOR VIEW

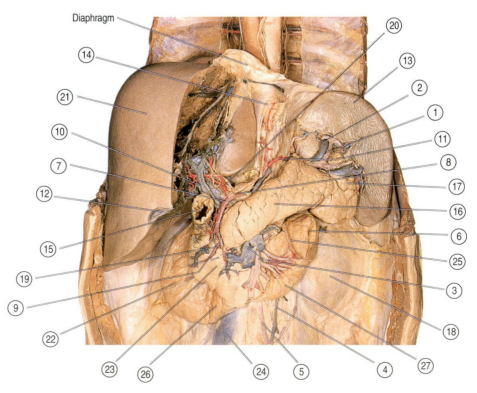

Diaphragm

14

21

10

7

12

15

19

9

22

23   26   24   5   4   27

20

13

2

1

11

8

17

16

6

25

3

18

ANTERIOR VIEW

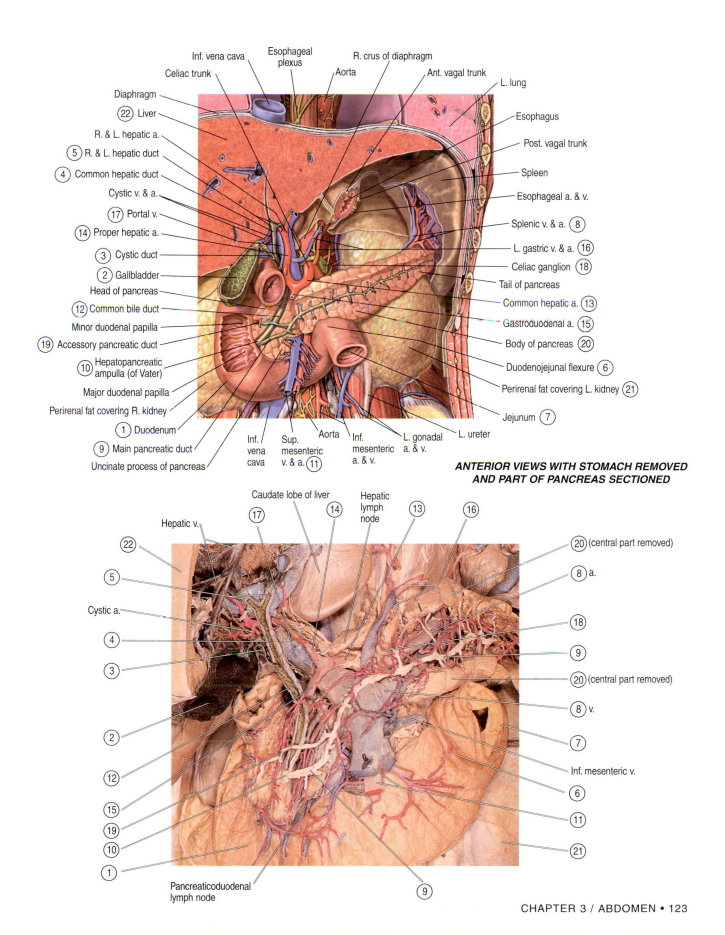

Inf. vena cava

Esophageal plexus

R. crus of diaphragm

Aorta

Ant. vagal trunk

L. lung

Celiac trunk

Diaphragm

22 Liver

5 R. & L. hepatic a.

5 R. & L. hepatic duct

4 Common hepatic duct

Cystic v. & a.

17 Portal v.

14 Proper hepatic a.

3 Cystic duct

2 Gallbladder

Head of pancreas

12 Common bile duct

Minor duodenal papilla

19 Accessory pancreatic duct

10 Hepatopancreatic ampulla (of Vater)

Major duodenal papilla

Perirenal fat covering R. kidney

1 Duodenum

9 Main pancreatic duct

Uncinate process of pancreas

Esophagus

Post. vagal trunk

Spleen

Esophageal a. & v.

Splenic v. & a. 8

L. gastric v. & a. 16

Celiac ganglion 18

Tail of pancreas

Common hepatic a. 13

Gastroduodenal a. 15

Body of pancreas 20

Duodenojejunal flexure 6

Perirenal fat covering L. kidney 21

Jejunum 7

Inf. / vena cava

Sup. mesenteric v. & a. 11

Aorta

Inf. mesenteric a. & v.

L. gonadal a. & v.

L. ureter

ANTERIOR VIEWS WITH STOMACH REMOVED AND PART OF PANCREAS SECTIONED

Caudate lobe of liver

Hepatic v.

17

14

Hepatic lymph node

13

16

22

5

Cystic a.

4

3

2

12

15

19

10

1

Pancreaticoduodenal lymph node

9

20 (central part removed)

8 a.

18

9

20 (central part removed)

8 v.

7

Inf. mesenteric v.

6

11

21

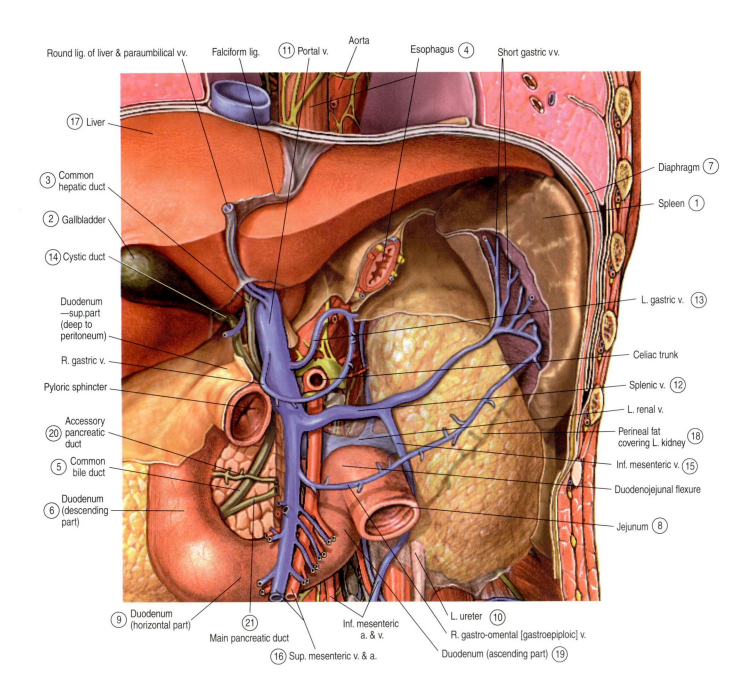

Round lig. of liver & paraumbilical vv.
Falciform lig.
(11) Portal v.
Aorta
Esophagus (4)
Short gastric vv.

(17) Liver

(3) Common hepatic duct

(2) Gallbladder

(14) Cystic duct

Duodenum —sup.part (deep to peritoneum)

R. gastric v.

Pyloric sphincter

(20) Accessory pancreatic duct

(5) Common bile duct

(6) Duodenum (descending part)

Diaphragm (7)

Spleen (1)

L. gastric v. (13)

Celiac trunk

Splenic v. (12)

L. renal v.

Perineal fat covering L. kidney (18)

Inf. mesenteric v. (15)

Duodenojejunal flexure

Jejunum (8)

(9) Duodenum (horizontal part)

(21) Main pancreatic duct

Inf. mesenteric a. & v.

L. ureter (10)

R. gastro-omental [gastroepiploic] v.

(16) Sup. mesenteric v. & a.

Duodenum (ascending part) (19)

ANTERIOR VIEW WITH STOMACH REMOVED

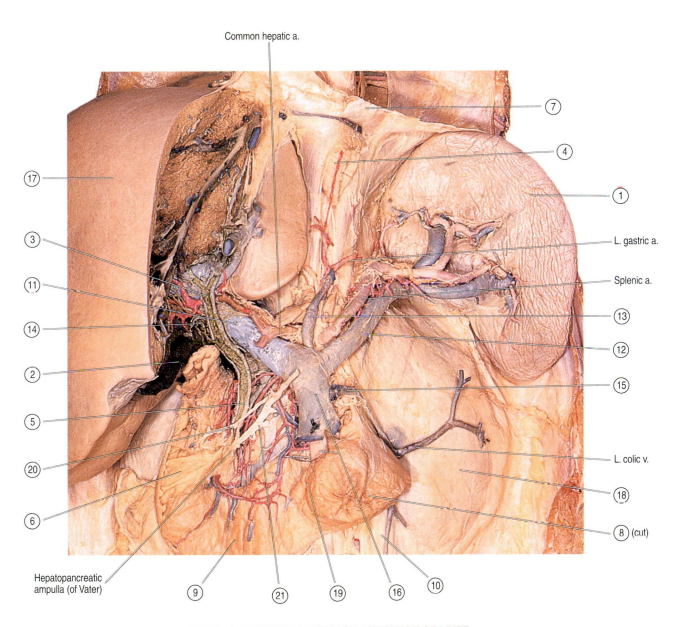

Common hepatic a.

L. gastric a.

Splenic a.

L. colic v.

Hepatopancreatic
ampulla (of Vater)

(7)
(4)
(1)
(13)
(12)
(15)
(18)
(8) (cut)

(17)
(3)
(11)
(14)
(2)
(5)
(20)
(6)

(9)
(21)
(19)
(16)
(10)

**ANTERIOR VIEW WITH STOMACH, LEFT HALF OF LIVER,
AND PANCREAS REMOVED**

Liver
Plate 3.17

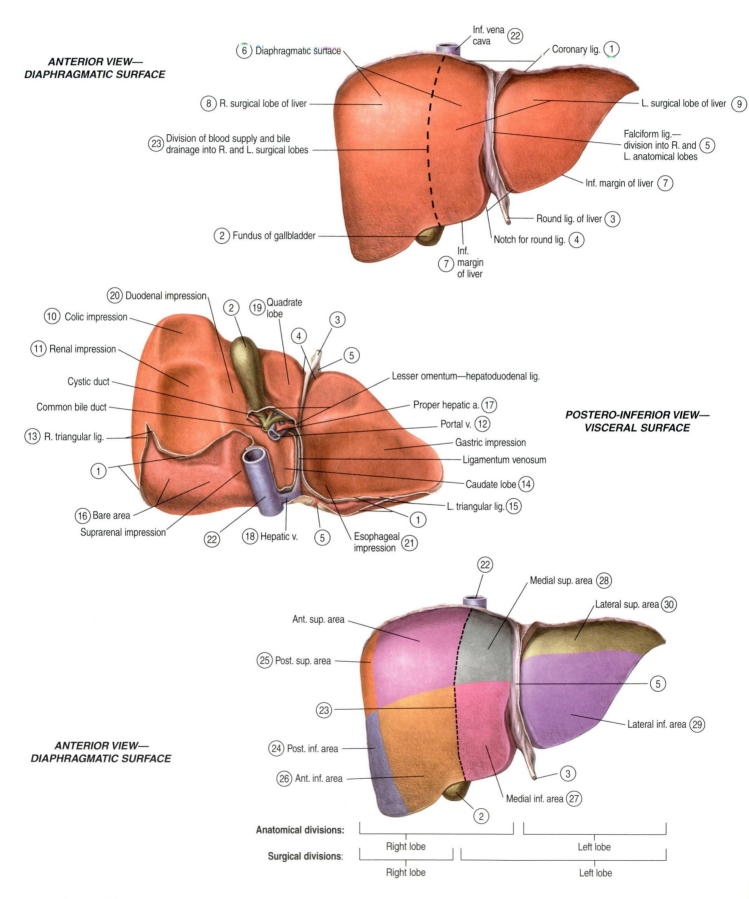

**ANTERIOR VIEW—
DIAPHRAGMATIC SURFACE**

(6) Diaphragmatic surface

Inf. vena cava (22)

Coronary lig. (1)

(8) R. surgical lobe of liver

L. surgical lobe of liver (9)

(23) Division of blood supply and bile drainage into R. and L. surgical lobes

Falciform lig.— division into R. and L. anatomical lobes (5)

Inf. margin of liver (7)

Round lig. of liver (3)

(2) Fundus of gallbladder

Notch for round lig. (4)

Inf. margin of liver (7)

(20) Duodenal impression

(10) Colic impression

(2)

(19) Quadrate lobe

(3)

(11) Renal impression

(4)

(5)

Cystic duct

Lesser omentum—hepatoduodenal lig.

Common bile duct

Proper hepatic a. (17)

Portal v. (12)

(13) R. triangular lig.

Gastric impression

(1)

Ligamentum venosum

Caudate lobe (14)

L. triangular lig. (15)

(16) Bare area

(1)

Suprarenal impression

(22)

(18) Hepatic v.

(5)

Esophageal impression (21)

**POSTERO-INFERIOR VIEW—
VISCERAL SURFACE**

(22)

Medial sup. area (28)

Ant. sup. area

Lateral sup. area (30)

(25) Post. sup. area

(5)

(23)

Lateral inf. area (29)

**ANTERIOR VIEW—
DIAPHRAGMATIC SURFACE**

(24) Post. inf. area

(26) Ant. inf. area

(3)

Medial inf. area (27)

(2)

Anatomical divisions:

Right lobe | Left lobe

Surgical divisions:

Right lobe | Left lobe

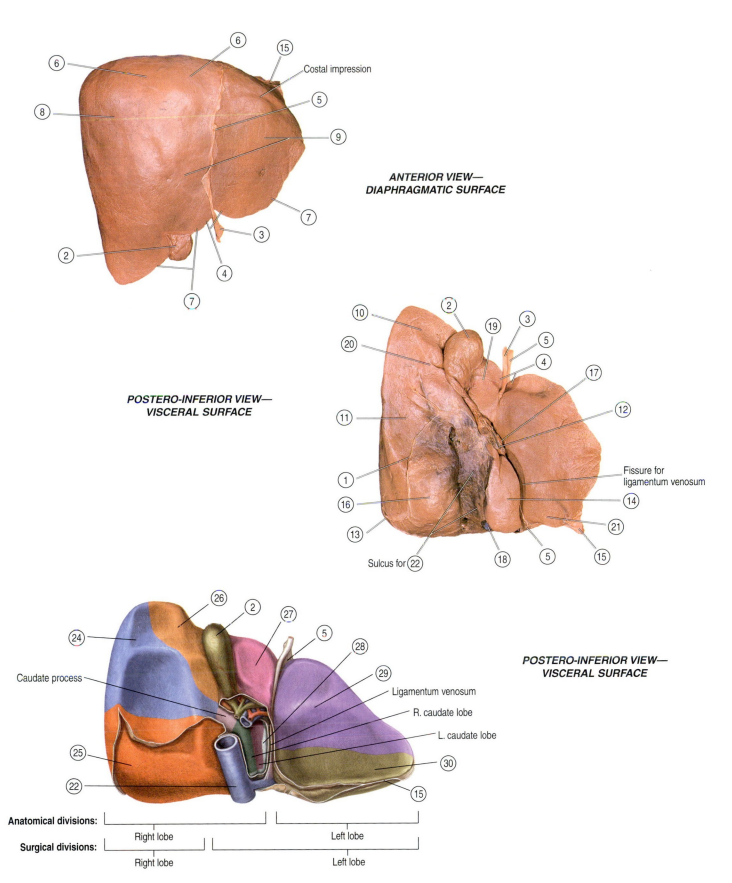

ANTERIOR VIEW—
DIAPHRAGMATIC SURFACE

Costal impression

POSTERO-INFERIOR VIEW—
VISCERAL SURFACE

Fissure for
ligamentum venosum

Sulcus for (22)

POSTERO-INFERIOR VIEW—
VISCERAL SURFACE

Caudate process

Ligamentum venosum

R. caudate lobe

L. caudate lobe

Anatomical divisions:

Right lobe

Left lobe

Surgical divisions:

Right lobe

Left lobe

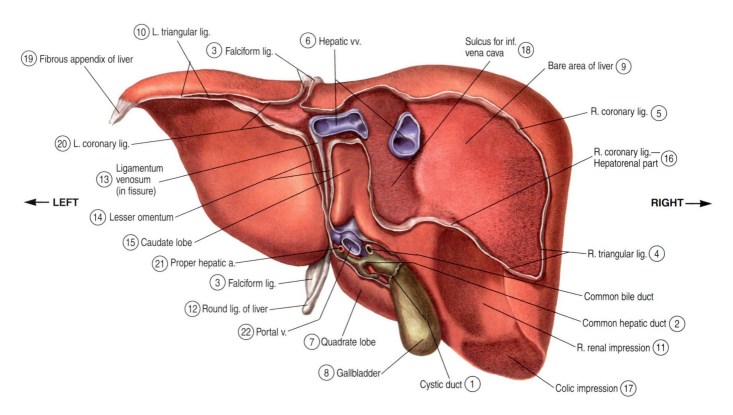

10 L. triangular lig.
19 Fibrous appendix of liver
3 Falciform lig.
6 Hepatic vv.
Sulcus for inf. vena cava 18
Bare area of liver 9
R. coronary lig. 5
20 L. coronary lig.
13 Ligamentum venosum (in fissure)
R. coronary lig.— 16 Hepatorenal part
← LEFT
RIGHT →
14 Lesser omentum
15 Caudate lobe
21 Proper hepatic a.
R. triangular lig. 4
3 Falciform lig.
Common bile duct
12 Round lig. of liver
Common hepatic duct 2
22 Portal v.
R. renal impression 11
7 Quadrate lobe
8 Gallbladder
Cystic duct 1
Colic impression 17

POSTERIOR VIEWS—VISCERO-DIAPHRAGMATIC SURFACE

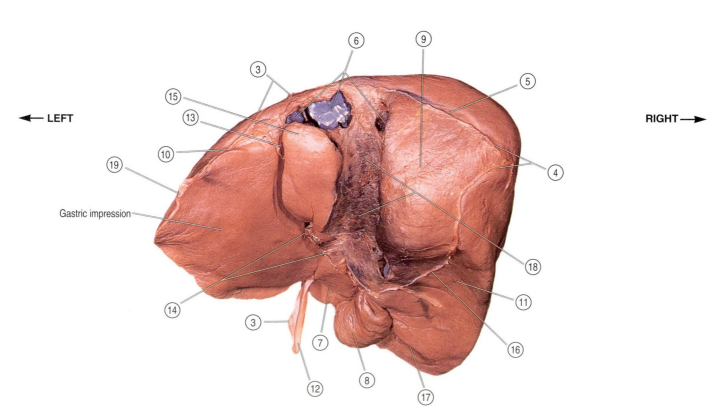

6
9
3
5
15
13
← LEFT
RIGHT →
10
4
19
Gastric impression
18
14
11
3
16
7
12
8
17

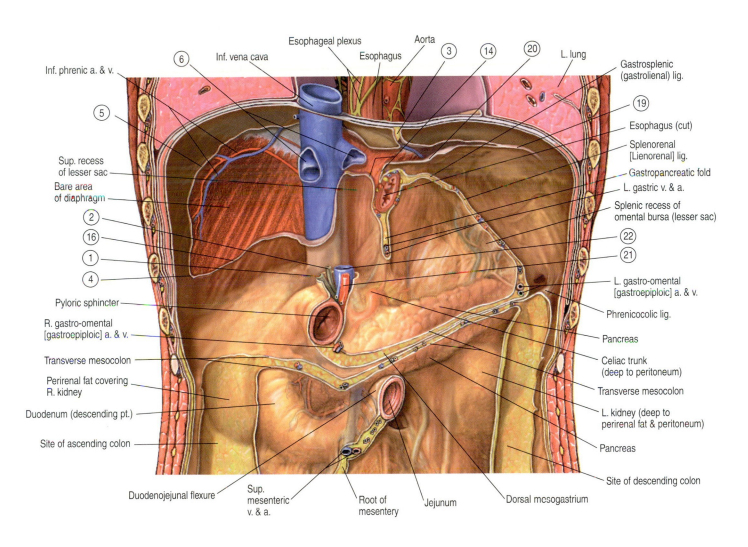

Esophageal plexus

Inf. vena cava

Esophagus

Aorta

③

⑭

⑳

L. lung

Gastrosplenic (gastrolienal) lig.

Inf. phrenic a. & v.

⑥

⑤

⑲

Esophagus (cut)

Sup. recess of lesser sac

Splenorenal [Lienorenal] lig.

Bare area of diaphragm

Gastropancreatic fold

L. gastric v. & a.

②

⑯

Splenic recess of omental bursa (lesser sac)

①

④

㉒

㉑

Pyloric sphincter

L. gastro-omental [gastroepiploic] a. & v.

R. gastro-omental [gastroepiploic] a. & v.

Phrenicocolic lig.

Transverse mesocolon

Pancreas

Perirenal fat covering R. kidney

Celiac trunk (deep to peritoneum)

Duodenum (descending pt.)

Transverse mesocolon

Site of ascending colon

L. kidney (deep to perirenal fat & peritoneum)

Pancreas

Site of descending colon

Duodenojejunal flexure

Sup. mesenteric v. & a.

Root of mesentery

Jejunum

Dorsal mesogastrium

ANTERIOR VIEW—POSTERIOR ABDOMINAL WALL

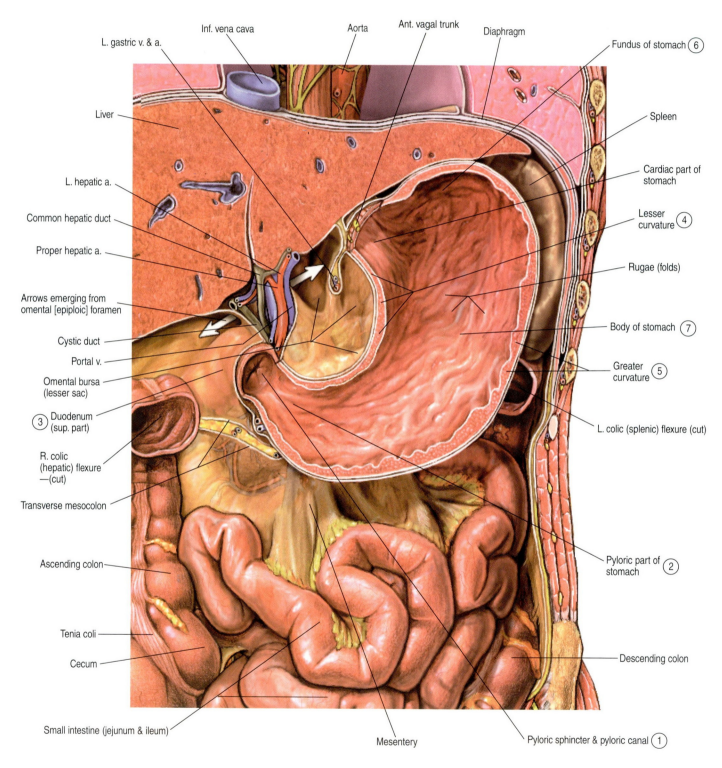

Inf. vena cava

Aorta

Ant. vagal trunk

Diaphragm

L. gastric v. & a.

Fundus of stomach ⑥

Liver

Spleen

Cardiac part of stomach

L. hepatic a.

Lesser curvature ④

Common hepatic duct

Proper hepatic a.

Rugae (folds)

Arrows emerging from omental [epiploic] foramen

Cystic duct

Body of stomach ⑦

Portal v.

Omental bursa (lesser sac)

Greater curvature ⑤

③ Duodenum (sup. part)

L. colic (splenic) flexure (cut)

R. colic (hepatic) flexure —(cut)

Transverse mesocolon

Ascending colon

Pyloric part of stomach ②

Tenia coli

Cecum

Descending colon

Small intestine (jejunum & ileum)

Mesentery

Pyloric sphincter & pyloric canal ①

ANTERIOR VIEW

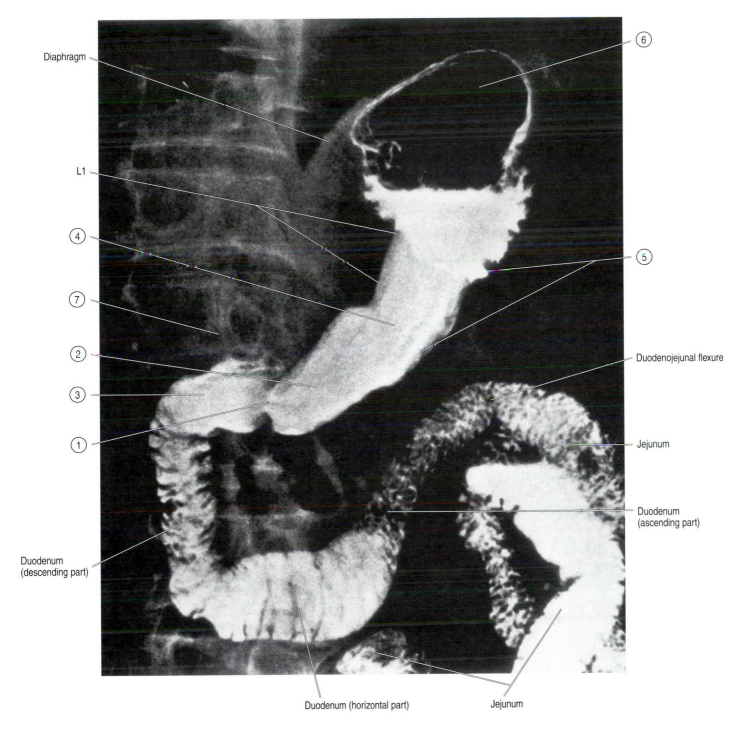

Diaphragm

L1

④

⑦

②

③

①

Duodenum
(descending part)

⑥

⑤

Duodenojejunal flexure

Jejunum

Duodenum
(ascending part)

Duodenum (horizontal part)

Jejunum

RADIOGRAPH OF UPPER G.I. TRACT FOLLOWING BARIUM SWALLOW

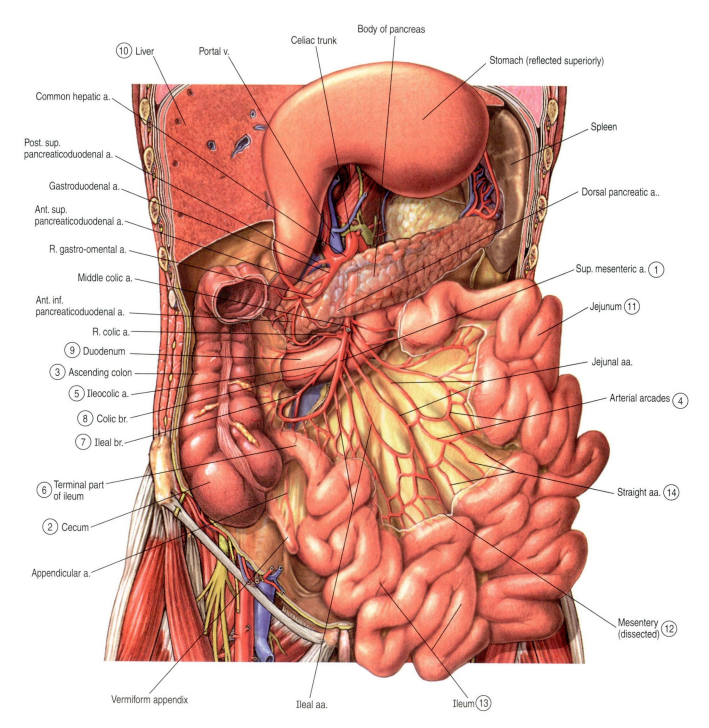

10 Liver

Portal v.

Celiac trunk

Body of pancreas

Stomach (reflected superiorly)

Common hepatic a.

Post. sup. pancreaticoduodenal a.

Gastroduodenal a.

Ant. sup. pancreaticoduodenal a.

R. gastro-omental a.

Middle colic a.

Ant. inf. pancreaticoduodenal a.

R. colic a.

9 Duodenum

3 Ascending colon

5 Ileocolic a.

8 Colic br.

7 Ileal br.

6 Terminal part of ileum

2 Cecum

Appendicular a.

Vermiform appendix

Ileal aa.

Ileum 13

Spleen

Dorsal pancreatic a..

Sup. mesenteric a. 1

Jejunum 11

Jejunal aa.

Arterial arcades 4

Straight aa. 14

Mesentery 12 (dissected)

ANTERIOR VIEW—STOMACH REFLECTED SUPERIORLY

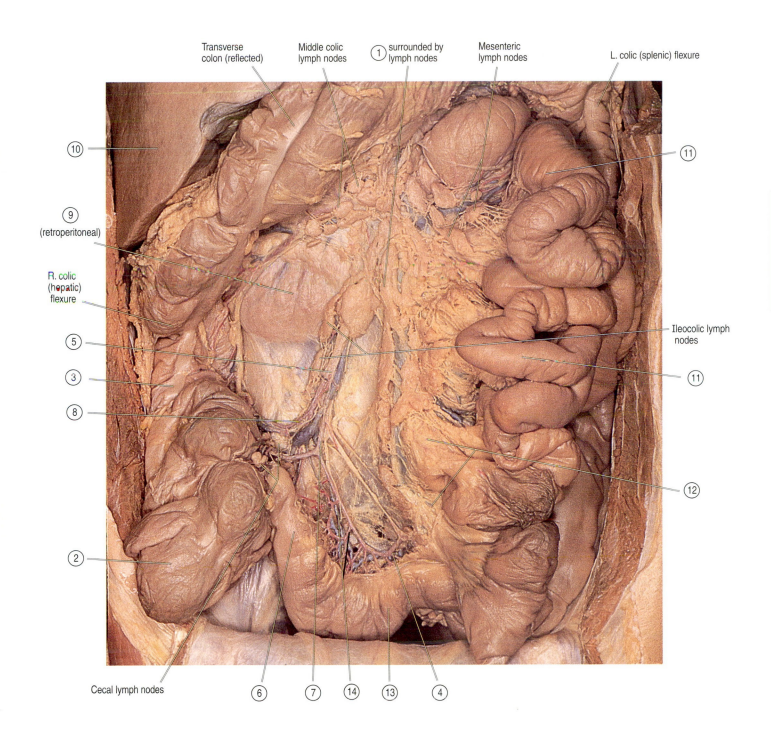

Transverse colon (reflected)

Middle colic lymph nodes

1 surrounded by lymph nodes

Mesenteric lymph nodes

L. colic (splenic) flexure

10

9 (retroperitoneal)

R. colic (hepatic) flexure

5

3

8

2

Cecal lymph nodes

6

7

14

13

4

11

Ileocolic lymph nodes

11

12

ANTERIOR VIEW—TRANSVERSE COLON REFLECTED SUPERIORLY

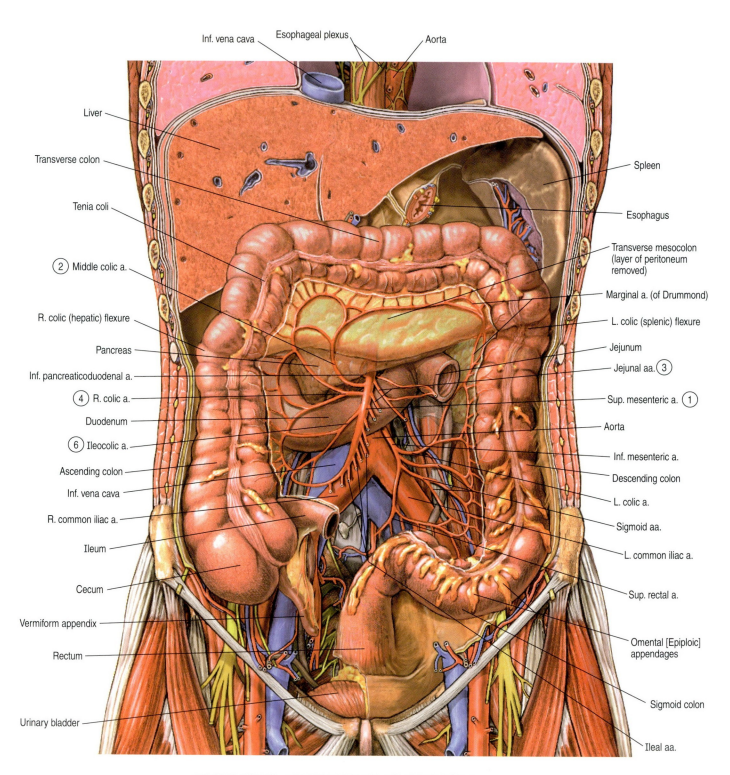

Inf. vena cava
Esophageal plexus
Aorta
Liver
Transverse colon
Tenia coli
② Middle colic a.
R. colic (hepatic) flexure
Pancreas
Inf. pancreaticoduodenal a.
④ R. colic a.
Duodenum
⑥ Ileocolic a.
Ascending colon
Inf. vena cava
R. common iliac a.
Ileum
Cecum
Vermiform appendix
Rectum
Urinary bladder

Spleen
Esophagus
Transverse mesocolon (layer of peritoneum removed)
Marginal a. (of Drummond)
L. colic (splenic) flexure
Jejunum
Jejunal aa. ③
Sup. mesenteric a. ①
Aorta
Inf. mesenteric a.
Descending colon
L. colic a.
Sigmoid aa.
L. common iliac a.
Sup. rectal a.
Omental [Epiploic] appendages
Sigmoid colon
Ileal aa.

**ANTERIOR VIEW—TRANSVERSE COLON REFLECTED SUPERIORLY
& THE MESENTERY PROPER REMOVED**

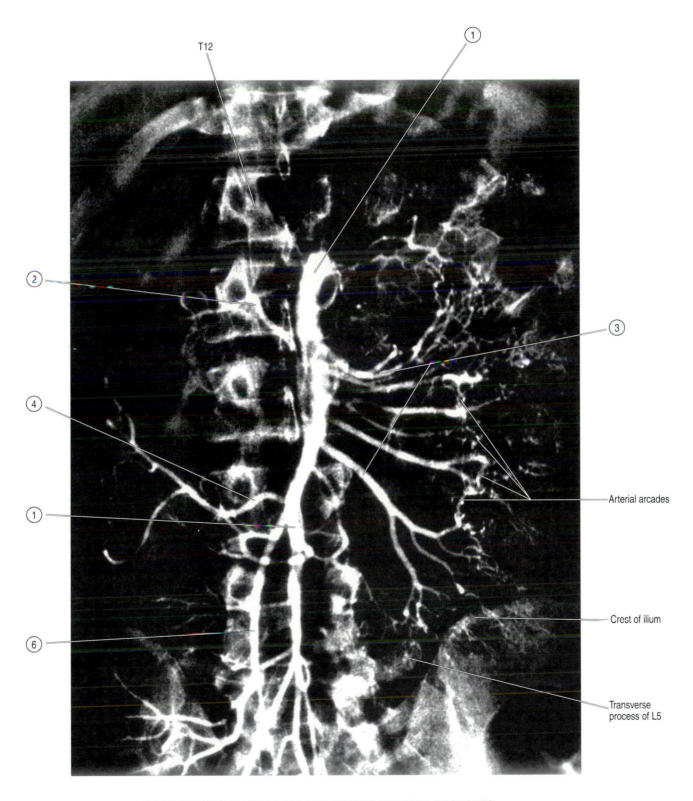

T12

① ② ③ ④ ① ⑥

Arterial arcades

Crest of ilium

Transverse process of L5

ARTERIOGRAPH OF SUPERIOR MESENTERIC ARTERY & BRANCHES

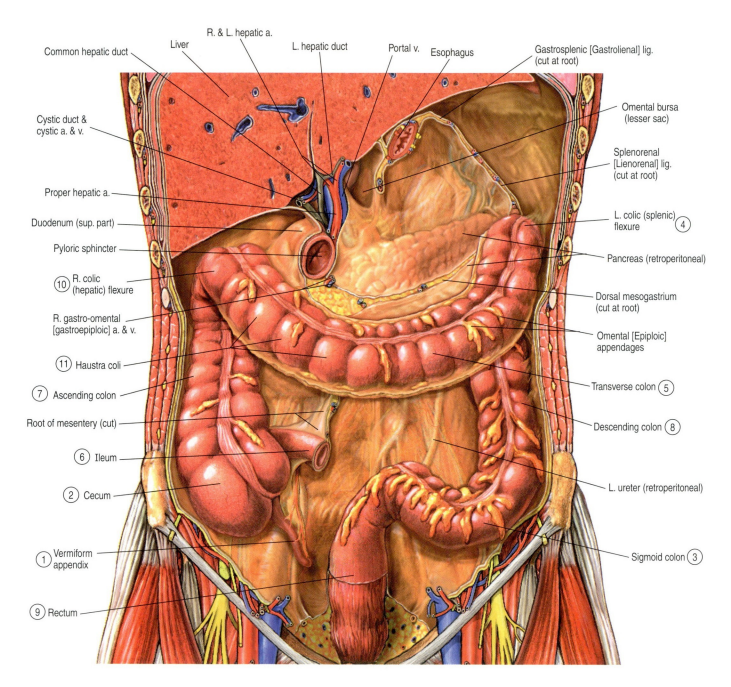

Common hepatic duct

R. & L. hepatic a.

Liver

L. hepatic duct

Portal v.

Esophagus

Gastrosplenic [Gastrolienal] lig. (cut at root)

Cystic duct & cystic a. & v.

Omental bursa (lesser sac)

Splenorenal [Lienorenal] lig. (cut at root)

Proper hepatic a.

L. colic (splenic) flexure ④

Duodenum (sup. part)

Pyloric sphincter

Pancreas (retroperitoneal)

⑩ R. colic (hepatic) flexure

Dorsal mesogastrium (cut at root)

R. gastro-omental [gastroepiploic] a. & v.

Omental [Epiploic] appendages

⑪ Haustra coli

Transverse colon ⑤

⑦ Ascending colon

Descending colon ⑧

Root of mesentery (cut)

⑥ Ileum

② Cecum

L. ureter (retroperitoneal)

① Vermiform appendix

Sigmoid colon ③

⑨ Rectum

ANTERIOR VIEW—SMALL INTESTINES REMOVED

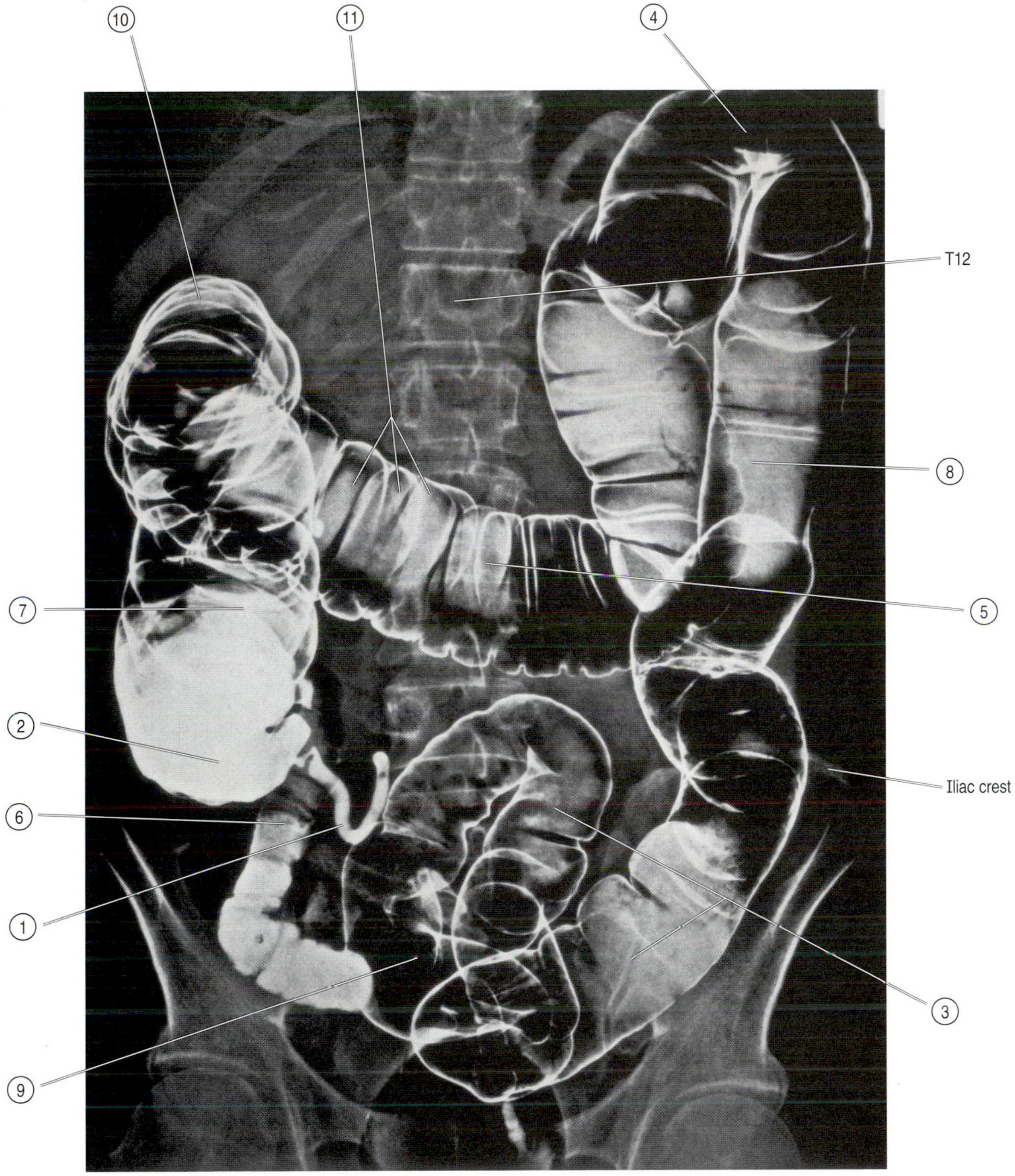
10
11
4
T12
8
5
7
2
Iliac crest
6
1
3
9

DOUBLE CONTRAST (AIR & BARIUM) RADIOGRAPH OF LARGE INTESTINE

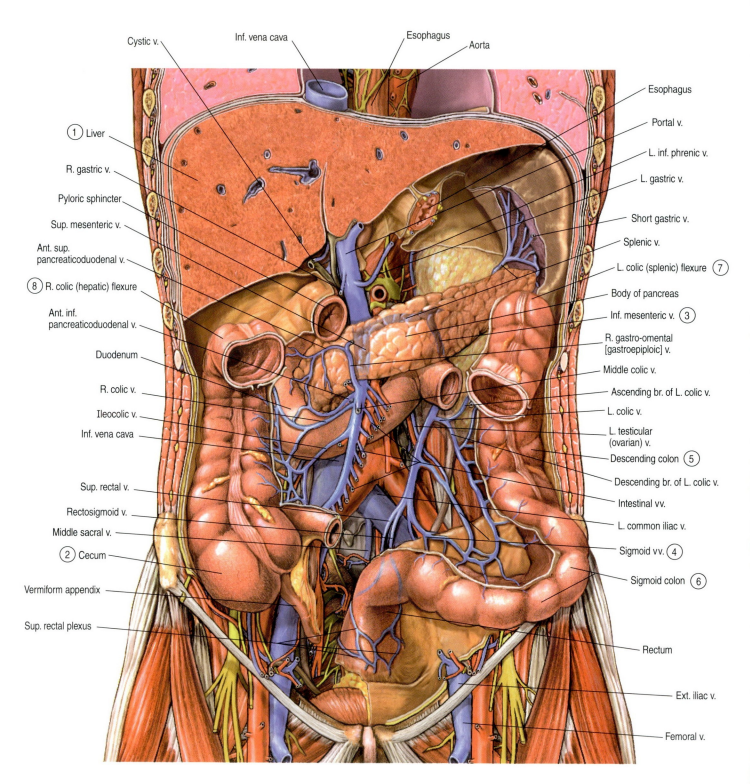

Cystic v.

Inf. vena cava

Esophagus

Aorta

1 Liver

R. gastric v.

Pyloric sphincter

Sup. mesenteric v.

Ant. sup. pancreaticoduodenal v.

8 R. colic (hepatic) flexure

Ant. inf. pancreaticoduodenal v.

Duodenum

R. colic v.

Ileocolic v.

Inf. vena cava

Sup. rectal v.

Rectosigmoid v.

Middle sacral v.

2 Cecum

Vermiform appendix

Sup. rectal plexus

Esophagus

Portal v.

L. inf. phrenic v.

L. gastric v.

Short gastric v.

Splenic v.

L. colic (splenic) flexure 7

Body of pancreas

Inf. mesenteric v. 3

R. gastro-omental [gastroepiploic] v.

Middle colic v.

Ascending br. of L. colic v.

L. colic v.

L. testicular (ovarian) v.

Descending colon 5

Descending br. of L. colic v.

Intestinal vv.

L. common iliac v.

Sigmoid vv. 4

Sigmoid colon 6

Rectum

Ext. iliac v.

Femoral v.

ANTERIOR VIEW

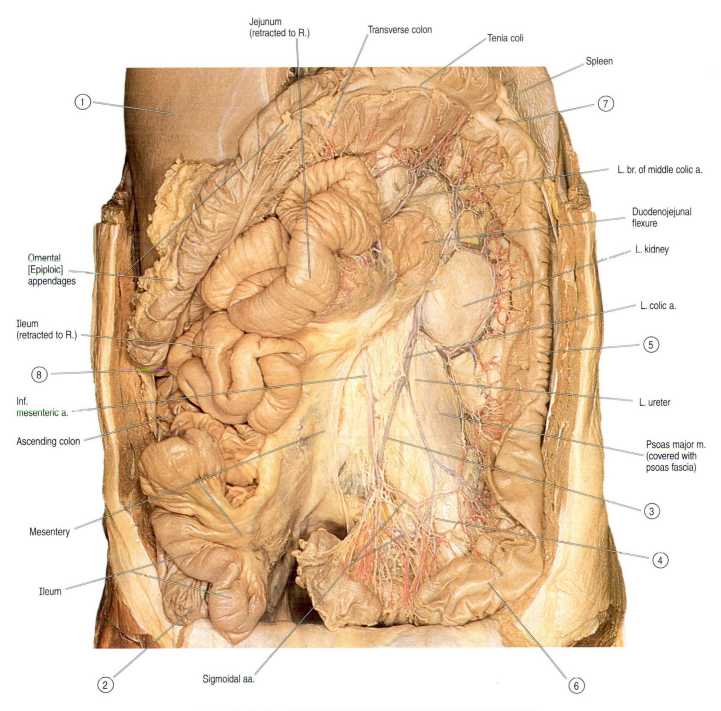

Jejunum
(retracted to R.)

Transverse colon

Tenia coli

Spleen

1

7

L. br. of middle colic a.

Duodenojejunal
flexure

L. kidney

Omental
[Epiploic]
appendages

L. colic a.

Ileum
(retracted to R.)

5

8

L. ureter

Inf.
mesenteric a.

Psoas major m.
(covered with
psoas fascia)

Ascending colon

3

Mesentery

4

Ileum

Sigmoidal aa.

2

6

ANTERIOR VIEW—TRANSVERSE COLON REFLECTED SUPERIORLY

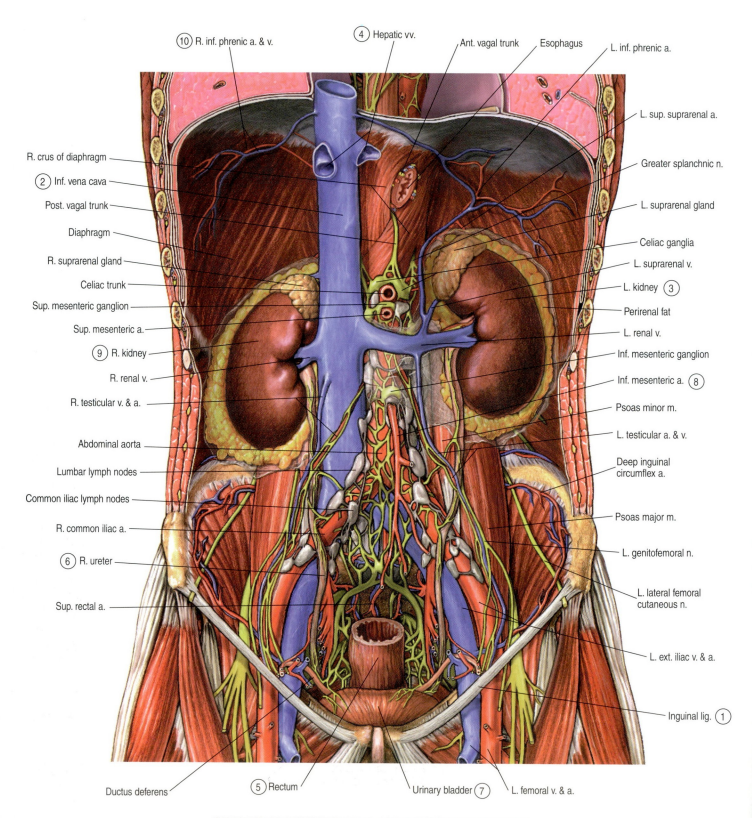

10 R. inf. phrenic a. & v.

4 Hepatic vv.

Ant. vagal trunk

Esophagus

L. inf. phrenic a.

L. sup. suprarenal a.

Greater splanchnic n.

L. suprarenal gland

Celiac ganglia

L. suprarenal v.

L. kidney 3

Perirenal fat

L. renal v.

Inf. mesenteric ganglion

Inf. mesenteric a. 8

Psoas minor m.

L. testicular a. & v.

Deep inguinal circumflex a.

Psoas major m.

L. genitofemoral n.

L. lateral femoral cutaneous n.

L. ext. iliac v. & a.

Inguinal lig. 1

R. crus of diaphragm

2 Inf. vena cava

Post. vagal trunk

Diaphragm

R. suprarenal gland

Celiac trunk

Sup. mesenteric ganglion

Sup. mesenteric a.

9 R. kidney

R. renal v.

R. testicular v. & a.

Abdominal aorta

Lumbar lymph nodes

Common iliac lymph nodes

R. common iliac a.

6 R. ureter

Sup. rectal a.

Ductus deferens

5 Rectum

Urinary bladder 7

L. femoral v. & a.

ANTERIOR VIEW WITH VISCERA AND PERITONEUM REMOVED

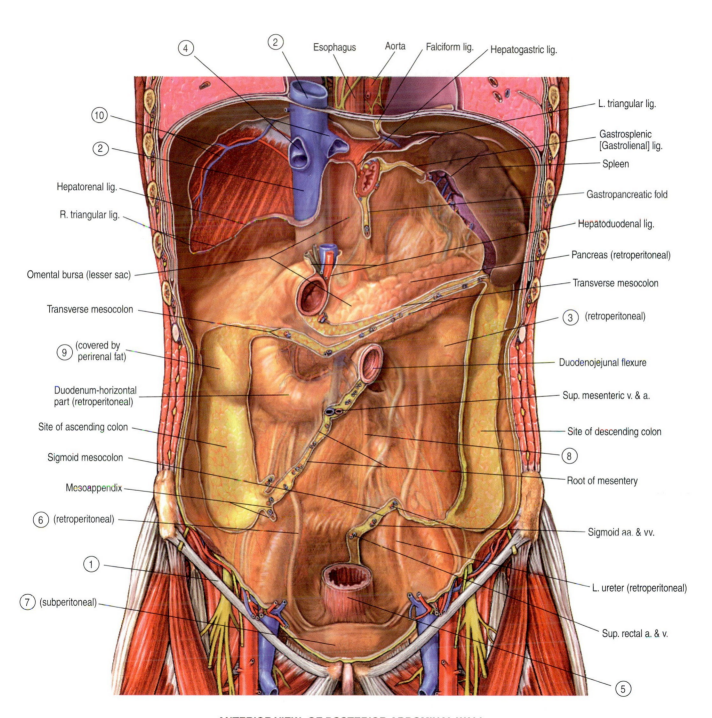

Esophagus Aorta Falciform lig. Hepatogastric lig.

4 2

10

2

Hepatorenal lig.

R. triangular lig.

Omental bursa (lesser sac)

Transverse mesocolon

9 (covered by perirenal fat)

Duodenum-horizontal part (retroperitoneal)

Site of ascending colon

Sigmoid mesocolon

Mesoappendix

6 (retroperitoneal)

1

7 (subperitoneal)

L. triangular lig.

Gastrosplenic [Gastrolienal] lig.

Spleen

Gastropancreatic fold

Hepatoduodenal lig.

Pancreas (retroperitoneal)

Transverse mesocolon

3 (retroperitoneal)

Duodenojejunal flexure

Sup. mesenteric v. & a.

Site of descending colon

8

Root of mesentery

Sigmoid aa. & vv.

L. ureter (retroperitoneal)

Sup. rectal a. & v.

5

**ANTERIOR VIEW OF POSTERIOR ABDOMINAL WALL
SHOWING PERITONEAL COVERINGS AND MESENTERY ORIGINS**

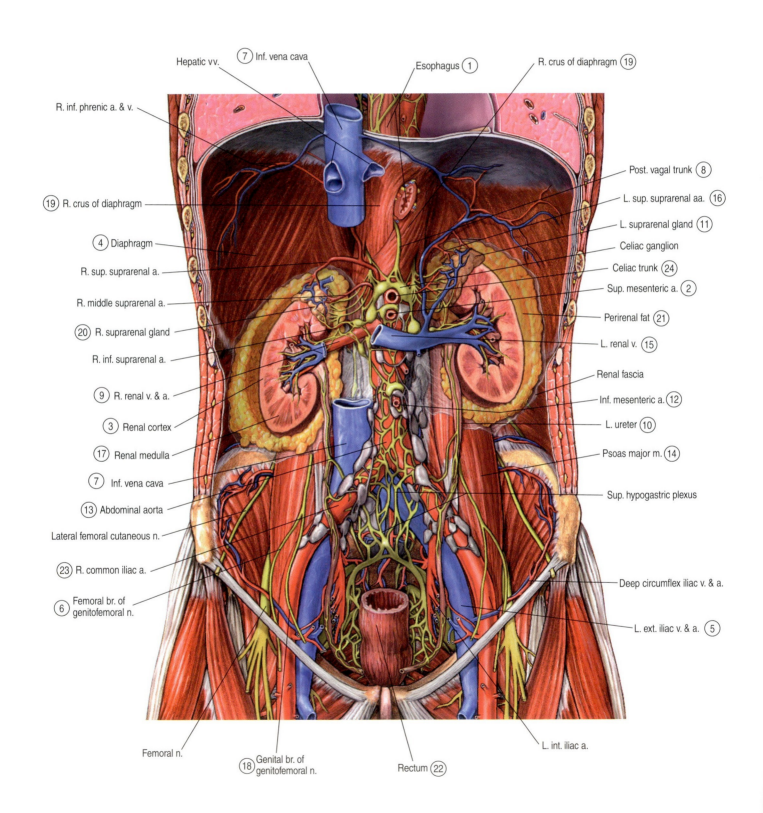

Hepatic vv.

⑦ Inf. vena cava

Esophagus ①

R. crus of diaphragm ⑲

R. inf. phrenic a. & v.

⑲ R. crus of diaphragm

④ Diaphragm

R. sup. suprarenal a.

R. middle suprarenal a.

⑳ R. suprarenal gland

R. inf. suprarenal a.

⑨ R. renal v. & a.

③ Renal cortex

⑰ Renal medulla

⑦ Inf. vena cava

⑬ Abdominal aorta

Lateral femoral cutaneous n.

㉓ R. common iliac a.

⑥ Femoral br. of genitofemoral n.

Post. vagal trunk ⑧

L. sup. suprarenal aa. ⑯

L. suprarenal gland ⑪

Celiac ganglion

Celiac trunk ㉔

Sup. mesenteric a. ②

Perirenal fat ㉑

L. renal v. ⑮

Renal fascia

Inf. mesenteric a. ⑫

L. ureter ⑩

Psoas major m. ⑭

Sup. hypogastric plexus

Deep circumflex iliac v. & a.

L. ext. iliac v. & a. ⑤

Femoral n.

⑱ Genital br. of genitofemoral n.

Rectum ㉒

L. int. iliac a.

ANTERIOR VIEW

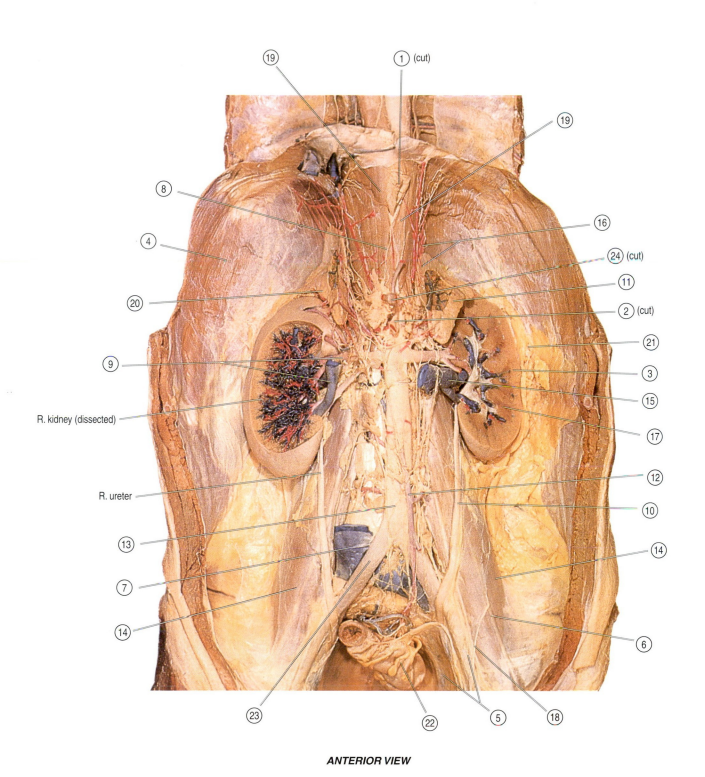

⑲   ① (cut)
⑲
⑧
④   ⑯
                                              ㉔ (cut)
⑳   ⑪
                                              ② (cut)
                                              ㉑
⑨   ③
R. kidney (dissected)   ⑮
                                              ⑰
R. ureter   ⑫
                                              ⑩
⑬   ⑭
⑦   ⑥
⑭
㉓   ㉒   ⑤   ⑱

ANTERIOR VIEW

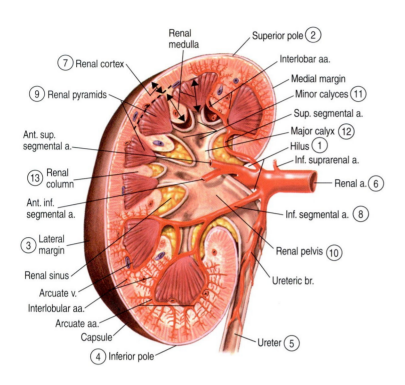

Renal medulla

⑦ Renal cortex

⑨ Renal pyramids

Ant. sup. segmental a.

⑬ Renal column

Ant. inf. segmental a.

③ Lateral margin

Renal sinus

Arcuate v.

Interlobular aa.

Arcuate aa.

Capsule

④ Inferior pole

Superior pole ②

Interlobar aa.

Medial margin

Minor calyces ⑪

Sup. segmental a.

Major calyx ⑫

Hilus ①

Inf. suprarenal a.

Renal a. ⑥

Inf. segmental a. ⑧

Renal pelvis ⑩

Ureteric br.

Ureter ⑤

POSTERIOR VIEWS OF CORONALLY SECTIONED L. KIDNEY

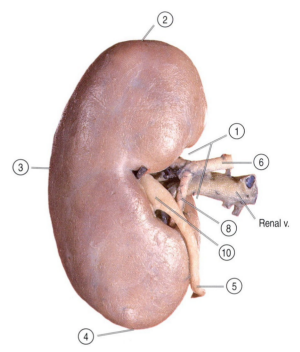

Renal v.

POSTERIOR SURFACE OF LEFT KIDNEY

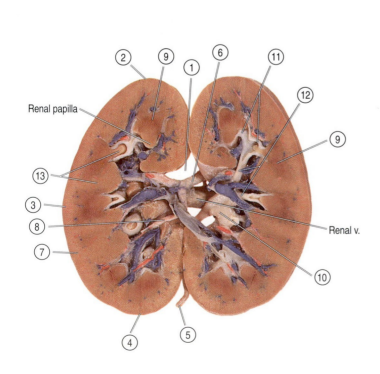

Renal papilla

Renal v.

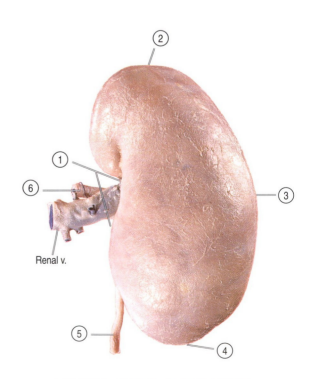

Renal v.

ANTERIOR SURFACE OF LEFT KIDNEY

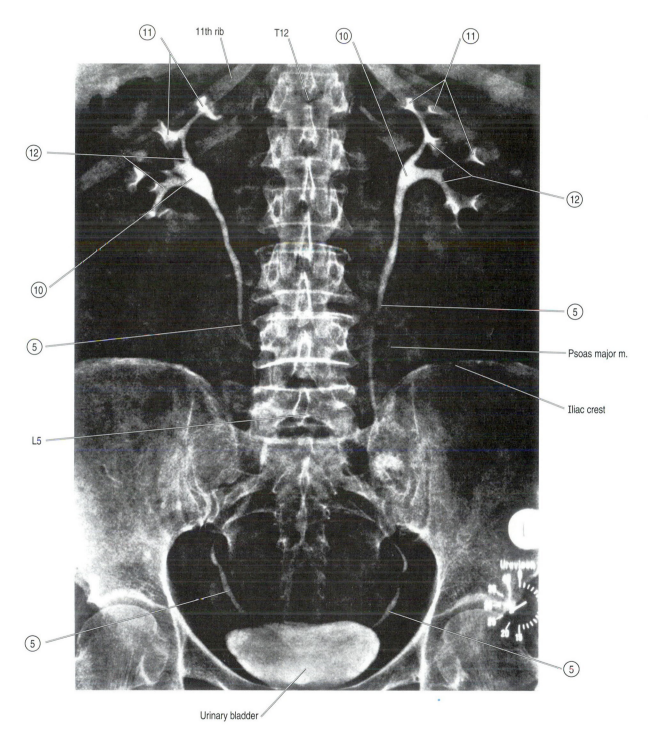

INTRAVENOUS UROGRAM

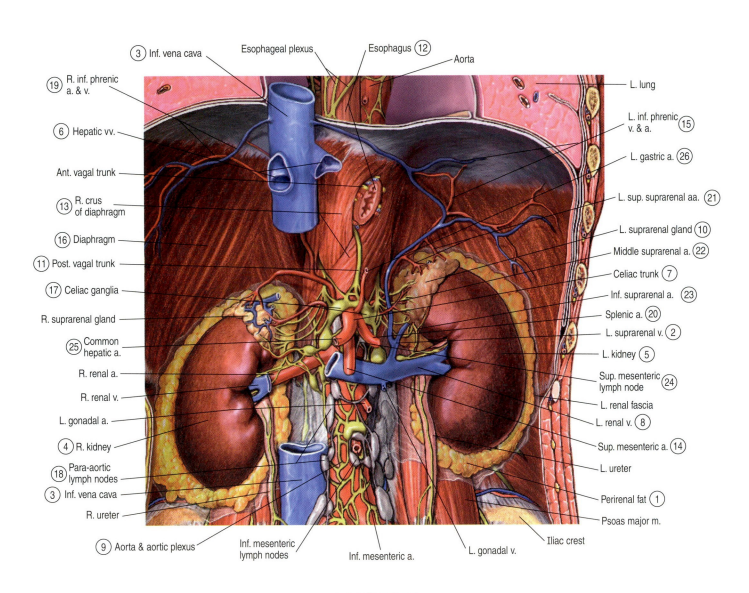

③ Inf. vena cava — Esophageal plexus — Esophagus ⑫ — Aorta

⑲ R. inf. phrenic a. & v.

⑥ Hepatic vv.

Ant. vagal trunk

⑬ R. crus of diaphragm

⑯ Diaphragm

⑪ Post. vagal trunk

⑰ Celiac ganglia

R. suprarenal gland

⑮ Common hepatic a.

R. renal a.

R. renal v.

L. gonadal a.

④ R. kidney

⑱ Para-aortic lymph nodes

③ Inf. vena cava

R. ureter

⑨ Aorta & aortic plexus — Inf. mesenteric lymph nodes — Inf. mesenteric a. — L. gonadal v.

L. lung

L. inf. phrenic v. & a. ⑮

L. gastric a. ㉖

L. sup. suprarenal aa. ㉑

L. suprarenal gland ⑩

Middle suprarenal a. ㉒

Celiac trunk ⑦

Inf. suprarenal a. ㉓

Splenic a. ⑳

L. suprarenal v. ②

L. kidney ⑤

Sup. mesenteric lymph node ㉔

L. renal fascia

L. renal v. ⑧

Sup. mesenteric a. ⑭

L. ureter

Perirenal fat ①

Psoas major m.

Iliac crest

ANTERIOR VIEW

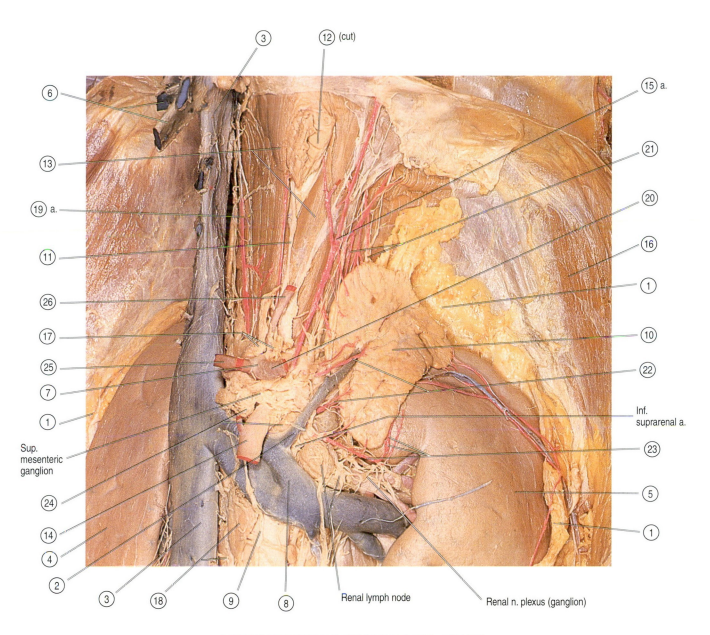

③ ⑫ (cut)
⑥
⑬ ⑮ a.
⑲ a. ㉑
⑪ ⑳
㉖ ⑯
⑰ ①
㉕ ⑩
⑦ ㉒
①
Inf.
suprarenal a.
Sup.
mesenteric
ganglion ㉓
㉔ ⑤
⑭ ①
④
② ③ ⑱ ⑨ ⑧ Renal lymph node Renal n. plexus (ganglion)

ANTERIOR VIEW OF SUPERIOR POLE OF L. KIDNEY

Pelvis and Perineum

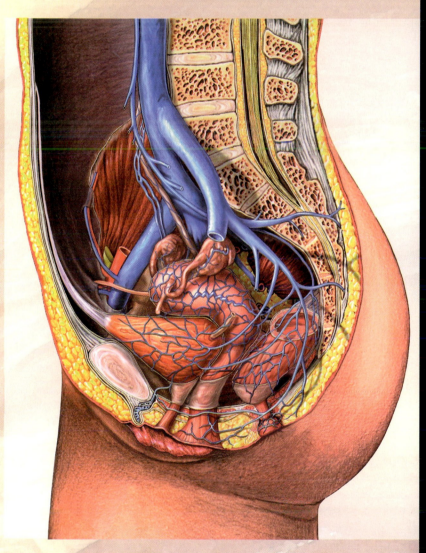

Chapter **4**

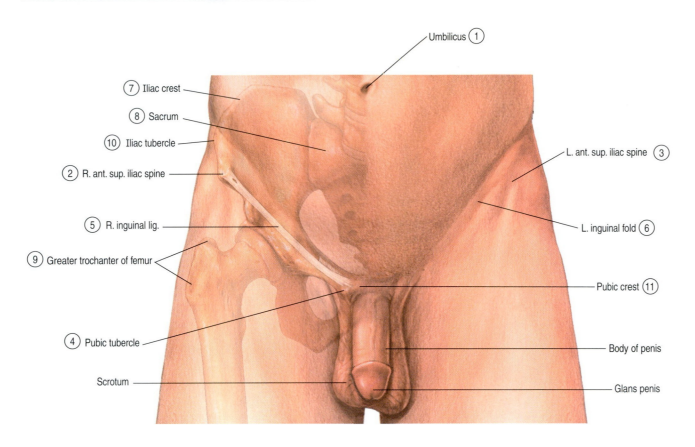

Umbilicus (1)

(7) Iliac crest

(8) Sacrum

(10) Iliac tubercle

(2) R. ant. sup. iliac spine

(5) R. inguinal lig.

(9) Greater trochanter of femur

(4) Pubic tubercle

Scrotum

L. ant. sup. iliac spine (3)

L. inguinal fold (6)

Pubic crest (11)

Body of penis

Glans penis

ANTERIOR VIEW

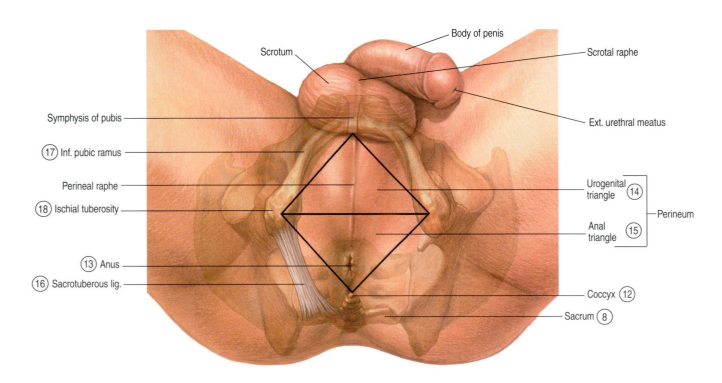

Body of penis

Scrotum

Scrotal raphe

Symphysis of pubis

(17) Inf. pubic ramus

Perineal raphe

(18) Ischial tuberosity

(13) Anus

(16) Sacrotuberous lig.

Ext. urethral meatus

Urogenital triangle (14)

Anal triangle (15)

Perineum

Coccyx (12)

Sacrum (8)

LITHOTOMY VIEW

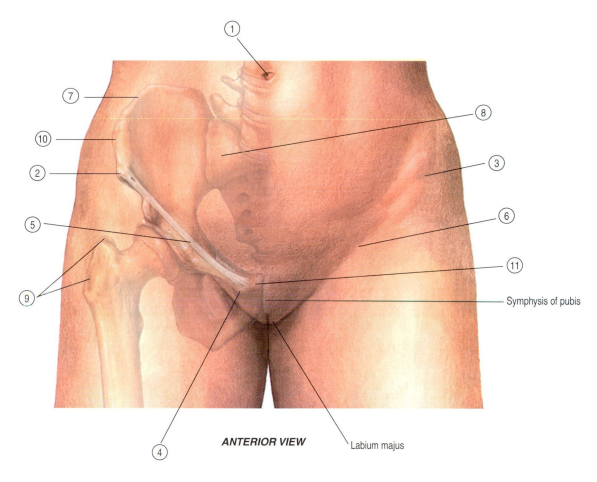

1

7

10

2

5

9

8

3

6

11

Symphysis of pubis

Labium majus

4

ANTERIOR VIEW

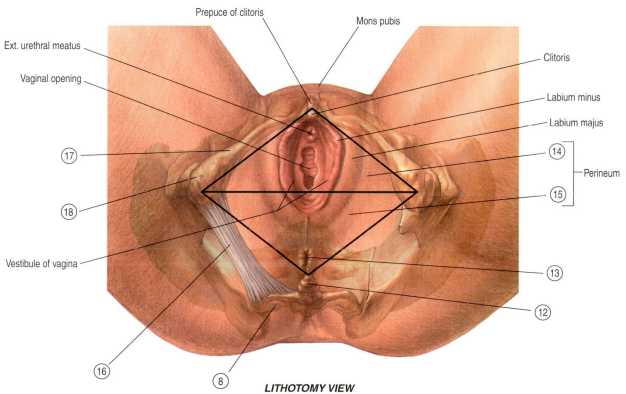

Prepuce of clitoris

Mons pubis

Ext. urethral meatus

Clitoris

Vaginal opening

Labium minus

Labium majus

17

14

Perineum

18

15

Vestibule of vagina

13

16

8

12

LITHOTOMY VIEW

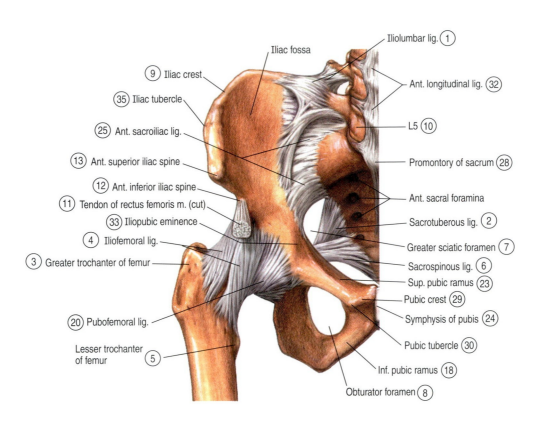

Iliolumbar lig. (1)

(9) Iliac crest

Iliac fossa

Ant. longitudinal lig. (32)

(35) Iliac tubercle

(25) Ant. sacroiliac lig.

L5 (10)

(13) Ant. superior iliac spine

Promontory of sacrum (28)

(12) Ant. inferior iliac spine

(11) Tendon of rectus femoris m. (cut)

Ant. sacral foramina

(33) Iliopubic eminence

Sacrotuberous lig. (2)

(4) Iliofemoral lig.

Greater sciatic foramen (7)

(3) Greater trochanter of femur

Sacrospinous lig. (6)

Sup. pubic ramus (23)

Pubic crest (29)

(20) Pubofemoral lig.

Symphysis of pubis (24)

Lesser trochanter
of femur (5)

Pubic tubercle (30)

Inf. pubic ramus (18)

Obturator foramen (8)

ANTERIOR VIEW

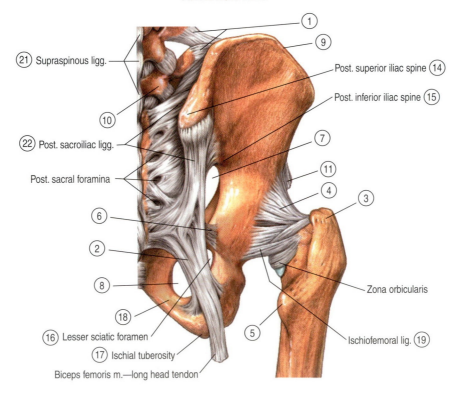

(1)

(9)

(21) Supraspinous ligg.

Post. superior iliac spine (14)

Post. inferior iliac spine (15)

(10)

(22) Post. sacroiliac ligg.

(7)

Post. sacral foramina

(11)

(4)

(6)

(3)

(2)

(8)

Zona orbicularis

(18)

(16) Lesser sciatic foramen

(5)

(17) Ischial tuberosity

Ischiofemoral lig. (19)

Biceps femoris m.—long head tendon

POSTERIOR VIEW

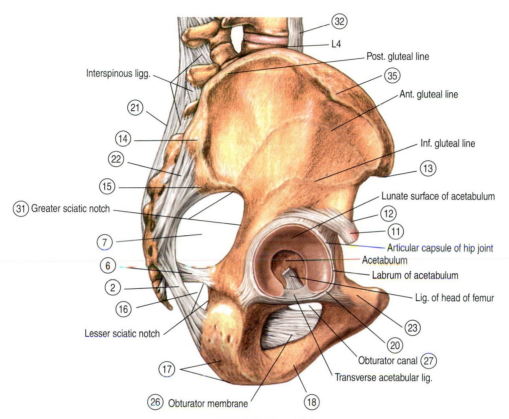

32

L4

Post. gluteal line

35

Ant. gluteal line

Interspinous ligg.

Inf. gluteal line

21

13

14

Lunate surface of acetabulum

22

12

15

11

31 Greater sciatic notch

Articular capsule of hip joint

7

Acetabulum

6

Labrum of acetabulum

2

Lig. of head of femur

16

23

Lesser sciatic notch

20

Obturator canal 27

17

Transverse acetabular lig.

26 Obturator membrane

18

RIGHT LATERAL VIEW

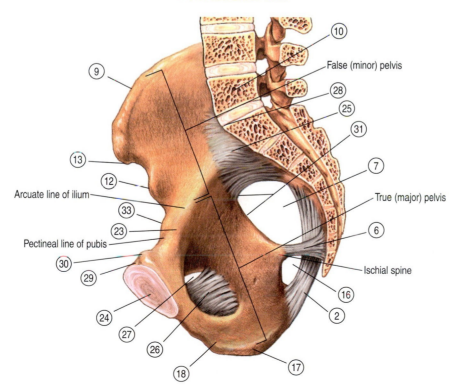

10

9

False (minor) pelvis

28

25

13

31

12

7

Arcuate line of ilium

True (major) pelvis

33

23

6

Pectineal line of pubis

30

Ischial spine

29

16

24

2

27

26

18

17

RIGHT SIDE OF HEMISECTED PELVIS—MEDIAL VIEW

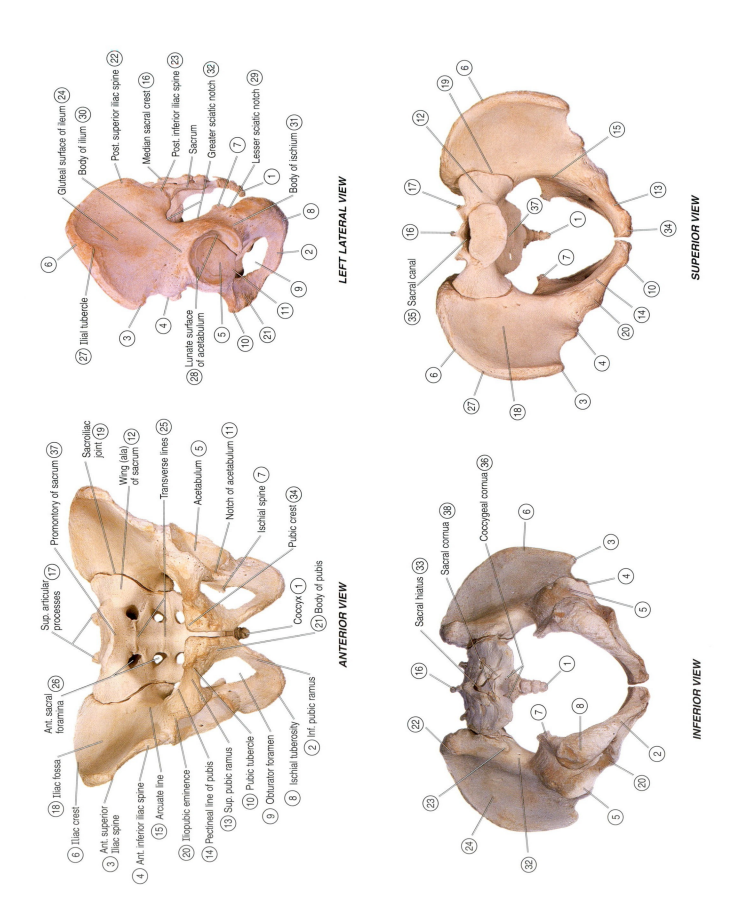

LEFT LATERAL VIEW

Post. superior iliac spine (22)
Gluteal surface of ileum (24)
Body of ilium (30)
Median sacral crest (16)
Post. inferior iliac spine (23)
Sacrum
Greater sciatic notch (32)
(7)
Lesser sciatic notch (29)
Body of ischium (31)
(6)
(27) Ilial tubercle
(3)
(4)
Lunate surface of acetabulum
(28)
(5)
(10)
(21)
(11)
(9)
(2)
(8)
(1)

ANTERIOR VIEW

Promontory of sacrum (37)
Sacroiliac joint (19)
Wing (ala) of sacrum (12)
Transverse lines (25)
Acetabulum (5)
Notch of acetabulum (11)
Ischial spine (7)
Pubic crest (34)
Body of pubis (21)
Coccyx (1)
Sup. articular processes (17)
Ant. sacral foramina (26)
(18) Iliac fossa
(6) Iliac crest
(3) Ant. superior Iliac spine
(4) Ant. inferior iliac spine
(15) Arcuate line
(20) Iliopubic eminence
(14) Pectineal line of pubis
(13) Sup. pubic ramus
(10) Pubic tubercle
(9) Obturator foramen
(8) Ischial tuberosity
(2) Inf. pubic ramus

SUPERIOR VIEW

(19)
(6)
(12)
(15)
(17)
(37)
(13)
(16)
(1)
(34)
(7)
(10)
(14)
(20)
(4)
(3)
(18)
(27)
(6)
(35) Sacral canal

INFERIOR VIEW

Sacral hiatus (33)
Sacral cornua (38)
Coccygeal cornua (36)
(6)
(3)
(4)
(5)
(16)
(1)
(22)
(7)
(8)
(23)
(20)
(2)
(24)
(32)
(5)

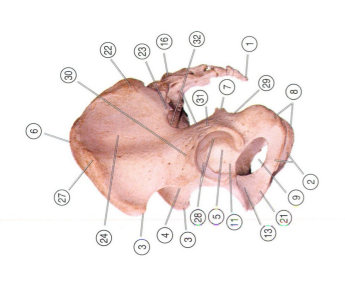

LEFT LATERAL VIEW

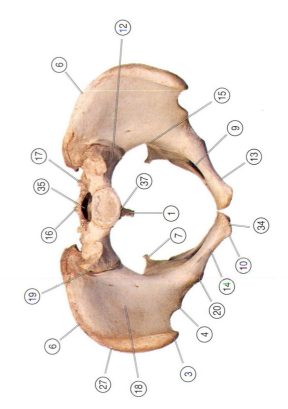

SUPERIOR VIEW

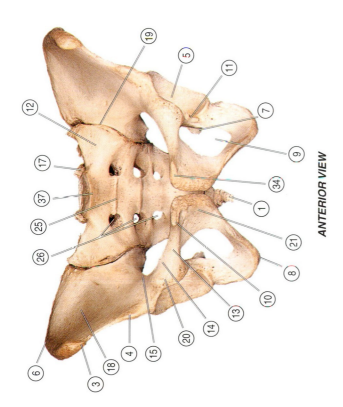

ANTERIOR VIEW

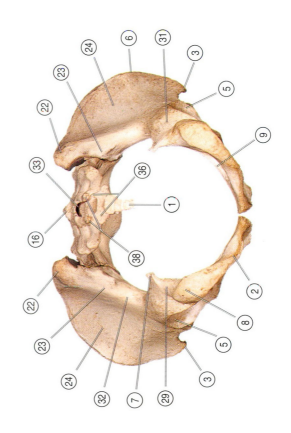

INFERIOR VIEW

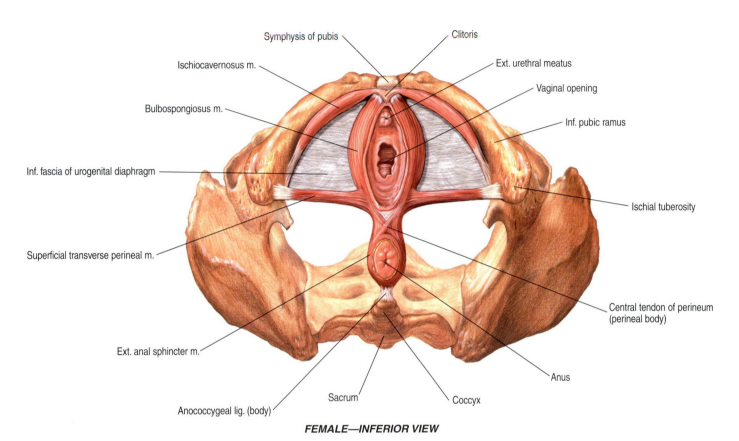

Symphysis of pubis

Clitoris

Ischiocavernosus m.

Ext. urethral meatus

Bulbospongiosus m.

Vaginal opening

Inf. pubic ramus

Inf. fascia of urogenital diaphragm

Ischial tuberosity

Superficial transverse perineal m.

Central tendon of perineum (perineal body)

Ext. anal sphincter m.

Anus

Anococcygeal lig. (body)

Sacrum

Coccyx

FEMALE—INFERIOR VIEW

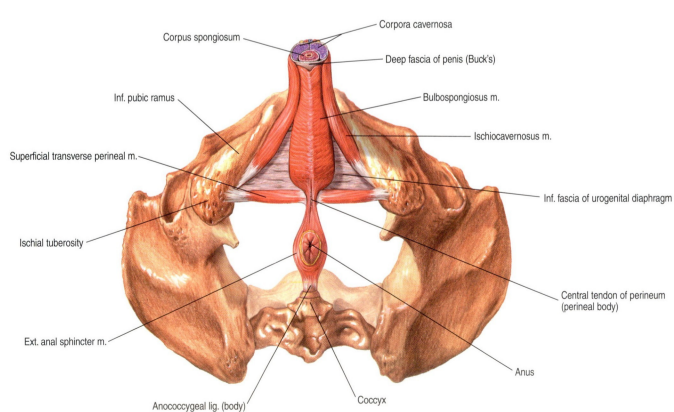

Corpora cavernosa

Corpus spongiosum

Deep fascia of penis (Buck's)

Inf. pubic ramus

Bulbospongiosus m.

Ischiocavernosus m.

Superficial transverse perineal m.

Inf. fascia of urogenital diaphragm

Ischial tuberosity

Central tendon of perineum (perineal body)

Ext. anal sphincter m.

Anus

Anococcygeal lig. (body)

Coccyx

MALE—INFERIOR VIEW

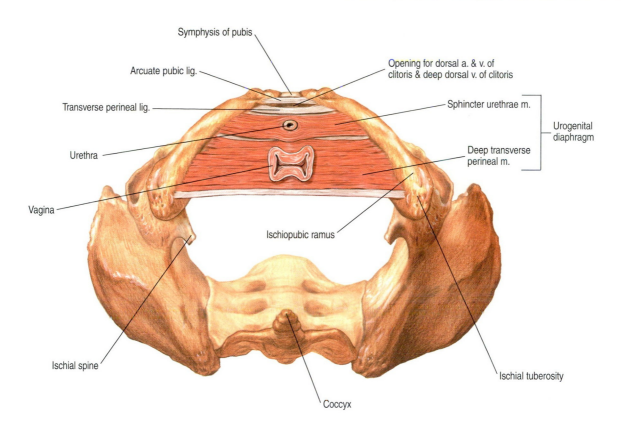

Symphysis of pubis

Arcuate pubic lig.

Transverse perineal lig.

Urethra

Vagina

Ischial spine

Opening for dorsal a. & v. of clitoris & deep dorsal v. of clitoris

Sphincter urethrae m.

Urogenital diaphragm

Deep transverse perineal m.

Ischiopubic ramus

Ischial tuberosity

Coccyx

FEMALE—INFERIOR VIEW

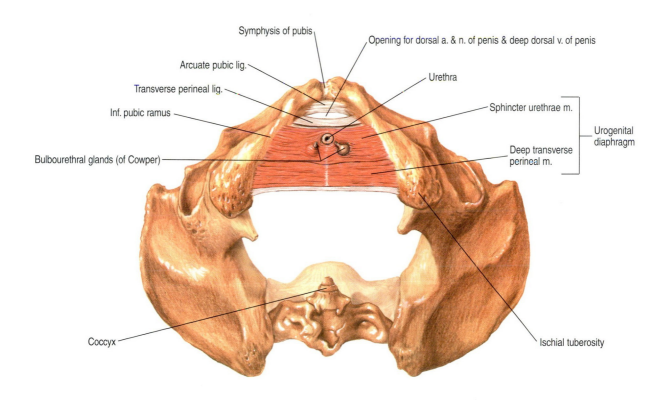

Symphysis of pubis

Arcuate pubic lig.

Transverse perineal lig.

Inf. pubic ramus

Bulbourethral glands (of Cowper)

Coccyx

Opening for dorsal a. & n. of penis & deep dorsal v. of penis

Urethra

Sphincter urethrae m.

Urogenital diaphragm

Deep transverse perineal m.

Ischial tuberosity

MALE—INFERIOR VIEW

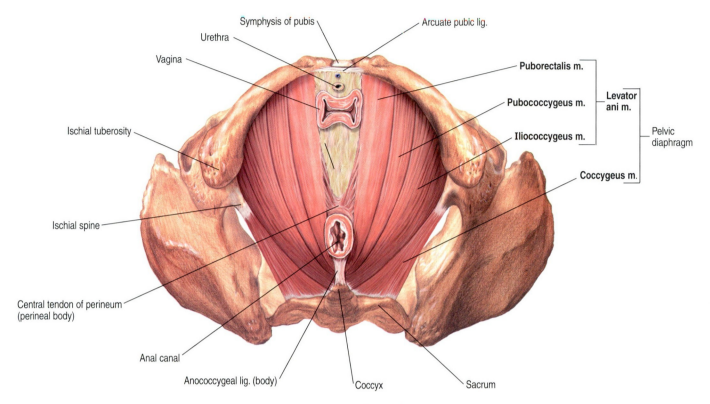

Symphysis of pubis

Urethra

Vagina

Arcuate pubic lig.

Puborectalis m.

Pubococcygeus m.

Iliococcygeus m.

Levator ani m.

Pelvic diaphragm

Coccygeus m.

Ischial tuberosity

Ischial spine

Central tendon of perineum (perineal body)

Anal canal

Anococcygeal lig. (body)

Coccyx

Sacrum

FEMALE—INFERIOR VIEW

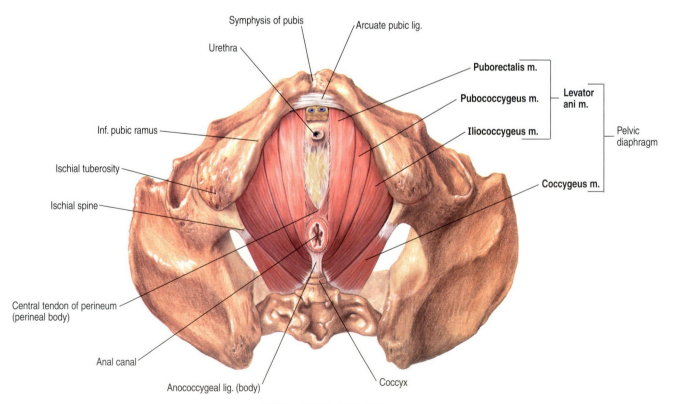

Symphysis of pubis

Urethra

Arcuate pubic lig.

Puborectalis m.

Pubococcygeus m.

Iliococcygeus m.

Levator ani m.

Pelvic diaphragm

Coccygeus m.

Inf. pubic ramus

Ischial tuberosity

Ischial spine

Central tendon of perineum (perineal body)

Anal canal

Anococcygeal lig. (body)

Coccyx

MALE—INFERIOR VIEW

Muscle	Superior or Lateral Attachment	Inferior or Medial Attachment	Innervation	Action(s)
Ischiocavernosus	Int. surface of ischial ramus & tuberosity laterally	Sides & ventrum of crus of penis in ♂ or clitoris medially in ♀	Perineal brr. of pudendal n. (S2–4)	Maintains erection of penis or clitoris
Bulbospongiosus	Dorsum of clitoris in ♀; inf. fascia of urogenital diaphragm, sides & dorsum of penile bulb in ♂	Perineal body, inf. fascia of urogenital diaphragm & median raphe of penile bulb in ♂	Perineal brr. of pudendal n. (S2–4)	Compresses vaginal orifice & erection of clitoris in ♀; compresses urethra, assist in erection & ejaculation in ♂
Superficial transverse perineal	Int. surface of ischial tuberosity laterally	Perineal body (central perineal tendon) medially	Perineal brr. of pudendal n. (S2–4)	Supports pelvic viscera
Ext. anal sphincter	Anococcygeal lig. to coccyx & int. anal sphincter m. superiorly	Perineal body anteriorly & skin superficially	Inf. rectal n. (S2–3) and perineal br. of S4 spinal n.	Compresses anus
Sphincter urethrae	Inf. pubic ramus laterally	Perineal body posteriorly & fibers from opposite side medially	Perineal brr. of pudendal n. (S2–4)	Compresses urethra in ♂ & ♀ & vagina in ♀
Deep transverse perineal	Ischial ramus laterally	Perineal body medially	Perineal brr. of pudendal n. (S2–4)	Supports pelvic viscera

FEMALE PERINEUM & MUSCLES— LEFT LATERAL VIEW

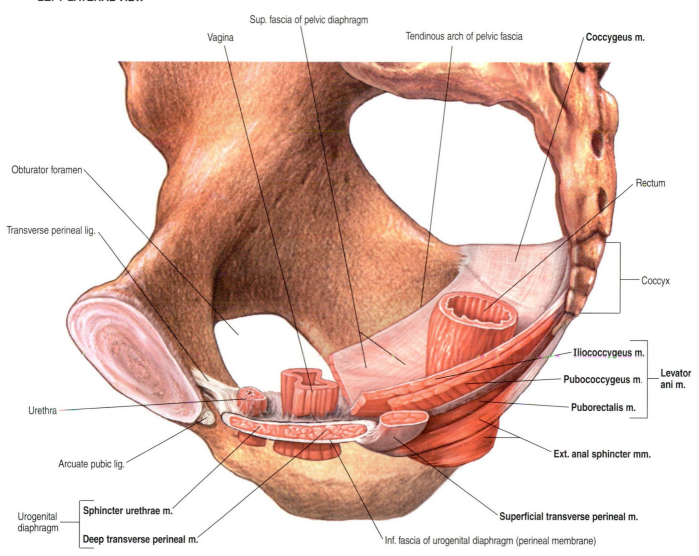

Sup. fascia of pelvic diaphragm

Vagina

Tendinous arch of pelvic fascia

Coccygeus m.

Obturator foramen

Rectum

Transverse perineal lig.

Coccyx

Iliococcygeus m.

Pubococcygeus m.

Puborectalis m.

Levator ani m.

Urethra

Ext. anal sphincter mm.

Arcuate pubic lig.

Urogenital diaphragm

Sphincter urethrae m.

Deep transverse perineal m.

Superficial transverse perineal m.

Inf. fascia of urogenital diaphragm (perineal membrane)

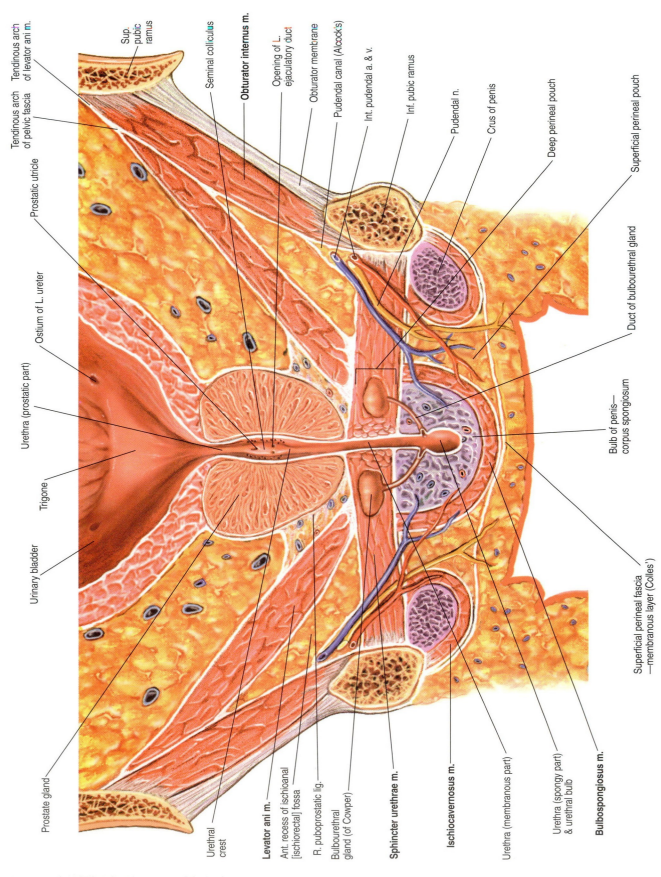

Tendinous arch of levator ani m.

Sup. pubic ramus

Seminal colliculus

Obturator internus m.

Opening of L. ejaculatory duct

Obturator membrane

Pudendal canal (Alcock's)

Int. pudendal a. & v.

Inf. pubic ramus

Pudendal n.

Crus of penis

Deep perineal pouch

Superficial perineal pouch

Tendinous arch of pelvic fascia

Prostatic utricle

Ostium of L. ureter

Urethra (prostatic part)

Trigone

Urinary bladder

Prostate gland

Urethral crest

Levator ani m.

Ant. recess of ischioanal [ischiorectal] fossa

R. puboprostatic lig.

Bulbourethral gland (of Cowper)

Sphincter urethrae m.

Ischiocavernosus m.

Urethra (membranous part)

Urethra (spongy part) & urethral bulb

Bulbospongiosus m.

Superficial perineal fascia —membranous layer (Colles')

Bulb of penis— corpus spongiosum

Duct of bulbourethral gland

MALE CORONAL SECTION—ANTERIOR VIEW

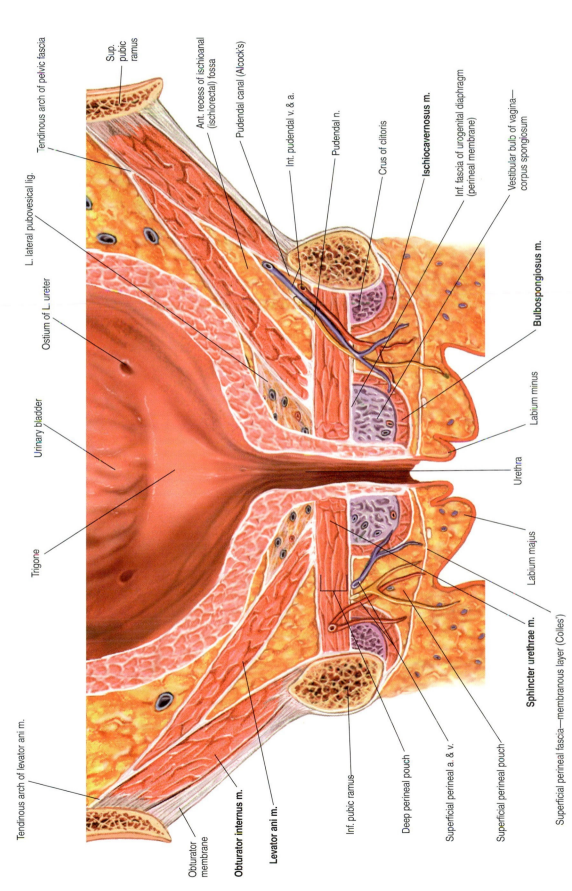

Sup. pubic ramus

Tendinous arch of pelvic fascia

Ant. recess of ischioanal (ischiorectal) fossa

Pudendal canal (Alcock's)

Int. pudendal v. & a.

Pudendal n.

Crus of clitoris

Ischiocavernosus m.

Inf. fascia of urogenital diaphragm (perineal membrane)

Vestibular bulb of vagina—corpus spongiosum

Bulbospongiosus m.

Labium minus

Urethra

Labium majus

Sphincter urethrae m.

Superficial perineal fascia—membranous layer (Colles')

Superficial perineal pouch

Superficial perineal a. & v.

Deep perineal pouch

Inf. pubic ramus

Levator ani m.

Obturator internus m.

Obturator membrane

Tendinous arch of levator ani m.

Trigone

Urinary bladder

Ostium of L. ureter

L. lateral pubovesical lig.

FEMALE CORONAL SECTION—ANTERIOR VIEW

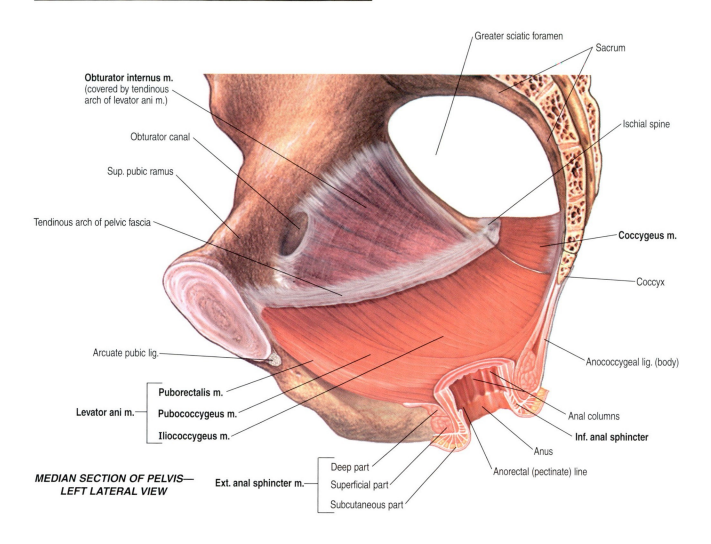

Greater sciatic foramen

Sacrum

Ischial spine

Obturator internus m.
(covered by tendinous
arch of levator ani m.)

Obturator canal

Sup. pubic ramus

Tendinous arch of pelvic fascia

Coccygeus m.

Coccyx

Arcuate pubic lig.

Anococcygeal lig. (body)

Puborectalis m.

Levator ani m. — Pubococcygeus m.

Iliococcygeus m.

Anal columns

Inf. anal sphincter

Anus

Anorectal (pectinate) line

Deep part

**MEDIAN SECTION OF PELVIS—
LEFT LATERAL VIEW**

Ext. anal sphincter m. — Superficial part

Subcutaneous part

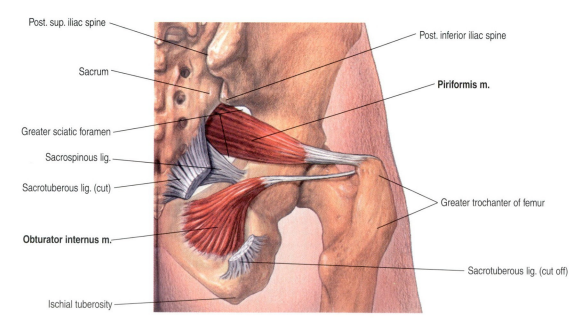

Post. sup. iliac spine

Post. inferior iliac spine

Sacrum

Piriformis m.

Greater sciatic foramen

Sacrospinous lig.

Sacrotuberous lig. (cut)

Greater trochanter of femur

Obturator internus m.

Sacrotuberous lig. (cut off)

Ischial tuberosity

RIGHT GLUTEAL REGION—POSTERIOR VIEW

Muscles of the Pelvic Diaphragm

Muscle	Superior or Lateral Attachment	Inferior or Medial Attachment	Innervation	Action(s)
Puborectalis	Body of pubis anteriorly	Fibers of opposite side post. to rectum	Inf. rectal n. (S2, 3) & perineal brr. of S3, 4 spinal n.	Maintains anorectal flexure by drawing anal canal anteriorly
Pubococcygeus	Body of pubis and obturator fascia anteriorly	Coccyx & anococcygeal lig. posteriorly	Inf. rectal n. (S2, 3) & perineal brr. of S3, 4 spinal n.	Supports pelvic viscera
Iliococcygeus	Ischial spine & tendinous arch of pelvic fascia laterally	Coccyx & anococcygeal lig. posteriorly	Inf. rectal n. (S2, 3) & perineal brr. of S3, 4 spinal n.	Supports pelvic viscera
Coccygeus	Ischial spine & sacrospinous lig. laterally	Coccyx & S5 vertebra medially	Brr. of S3–5 spinal nn.	Supports pelvic viscera

Muscles of the Pelvic Walls

Muscle	Superior or Medial Attachment	Inferior or Lateral Attachment	Innervation	Action(s)
Obturator internus	Pelvic surfaces of ilium & ischium; obturator membrane	Greater trochanter of femur	N. to obturator internus (L5–S2)	Rotates thigh laterally
Piriformis	Pelvic surface of 2nd–4th sacral segments; sup. margin of greater sciatic notch, & sacrotuberous lig.		Ventral rami of S1 & S2	Rotates thigh laterally

MEDIAN VIEW—RIGHT SIDE OF MEDIAL SECTION

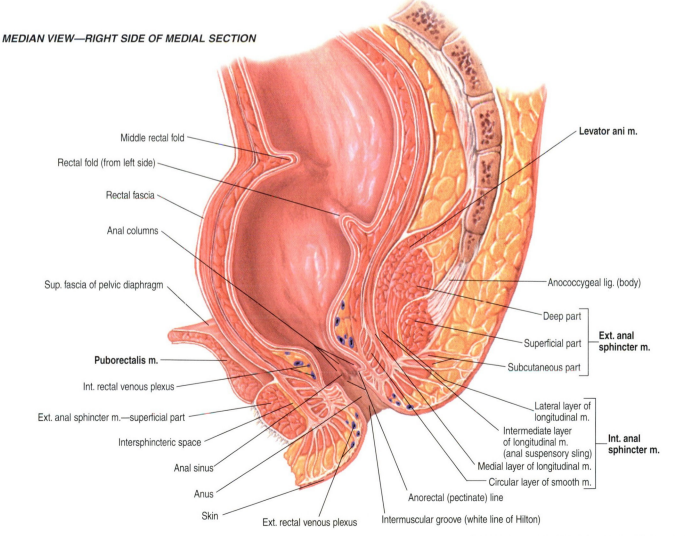

Middle rectal fold

Rectal fold (from left side)

Rectal fascia

Anal columns

Sup. fascia of pelvic diaphragm

Puborectalis m.

Int. rectal venous plexus

Ext. anal sphincter m.—superficial part

Intersphincteric space

Anal sinus

Anus

Skin

Ext. rectal venous plexus

Anorectal (pectinate) line

Intermuscular groove (white line of Hilton)

Circular layer of smooth m.

Medial layer of longitudinal m.

Intermediate layer of longitudinal m. (anal suspensory sling)

Lateral layer of longitudinal m.

Subcutaneous part

Superficial part

Deep part

Anococcygeal lig. (body)

Levator ani m.

Ext. anal sphincter m.

Int. anal sphincter m.

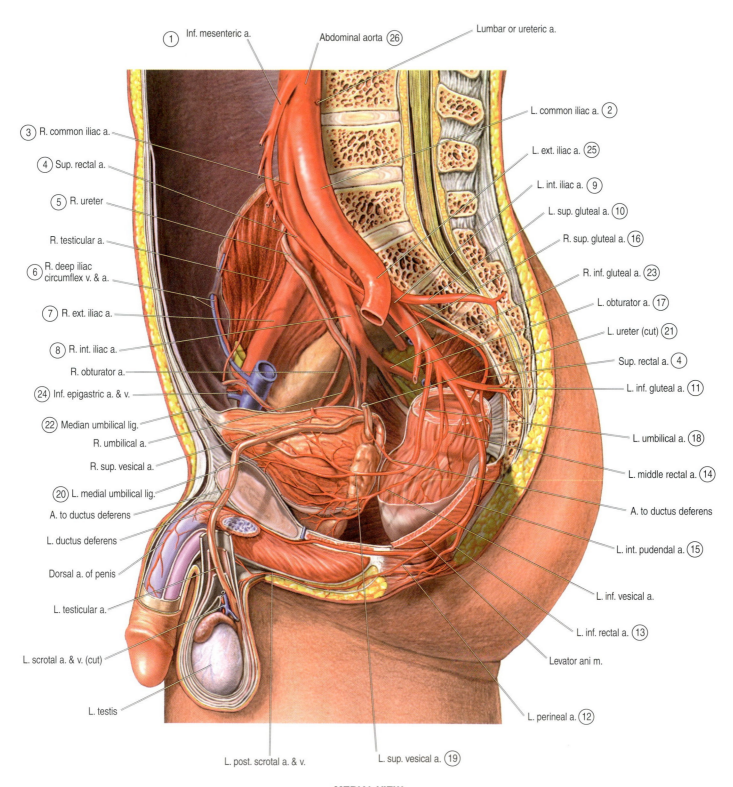

① Inf. mesenteric a.

Abdominal aorta ㉖

Lumbar or ureteric a.

③ R. common iliac a.

④ Sup. rectal a.

⑤ R. ureter

R. testicular a.

⑥ R. deep iliac circumflex v. & a.

⑦ R. ext. iliac a.

⑧ R. int. iliac a.

R. obturator a.

㉔ Inf. epigastric a. & v.

㉒ Median umbilical lig.

R. umbilical a.

R. sup. vesical a.

⑳ L. medial umbilical lig.

A. to ductus deferens

L. ductus deferens

Dorsal a. of penis

L. testicular a.

L. scrotal a. & v. (cut)

L. testis

L. common iliac a. ②

L. ext. iliac a. ㉕

L. int. iliac a. ⑨

L. sup. gluteal a. ⑩

R. sup. gluteal a. ⑯

R. inf. gluteal a. ㉓

L. obturator a. ⑰

L. ureter (cut) ㉑

Sup. rectal a. ④

L. inf. gluteal a. ⑪

L. umbilical a. ⑱

L. middle rectal a. ⑭

A. to ductus deferens

L. int. pudendal a. ⑮

L. inf. vesical a.

L. inf. rectal a. ⑬

Levator ani m.

L. perineal a. ⑫

L. post. scrotal a. & v.

L. sup. vesical a. ⑲

MEDIAL VIEW

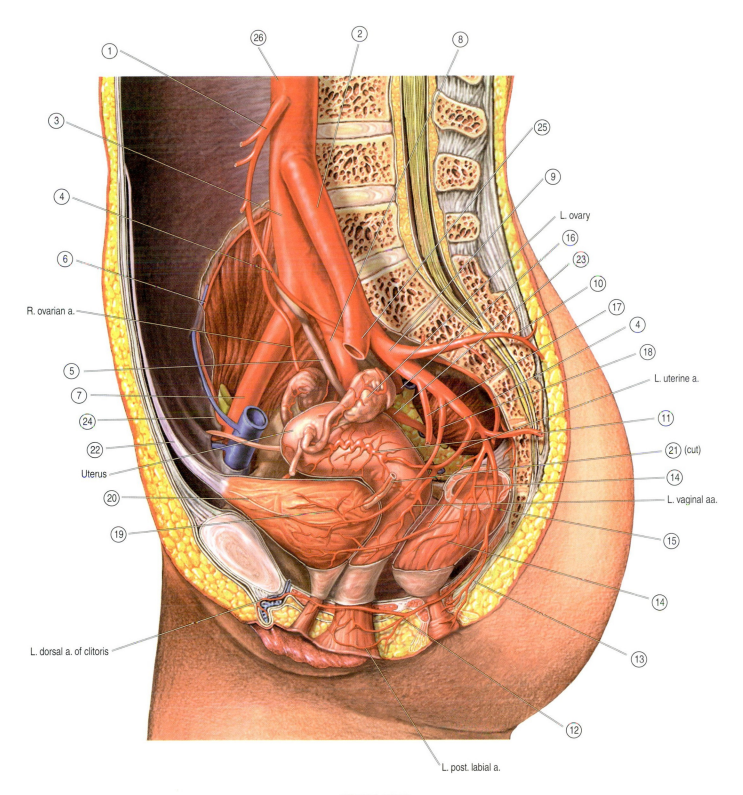

R. ovarian a.

L. ovary

L. uterine a.

L. vaginal aa.

Uterus

L. dorsal a. of clitoris

L. post. labial a.

MEDIAL VIEW

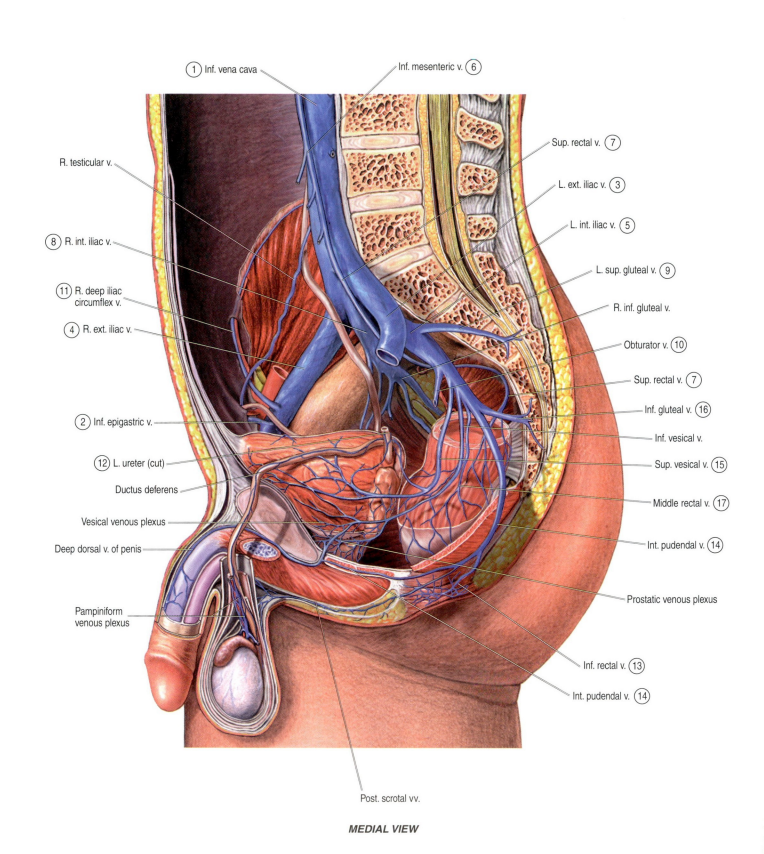

① Inf. vena cava

Inf. mesenteric v. ⑥

R. testicular v.

Sup. rectal v. ⑦

L. ext. iliac v. ③

L. int. iliac v. ⑤

⑧ R. int. iliac v.

L. sup. gluteal v. ⑨

⑪ R. deep iliac circumflex v.

R. inf. gluteal v.

④ R. ext. iliac v.

Obturator v. ⑩

Sup. rectal v. ⑦

② Inf. epigastric v.

Inf. gluteal v. ⑯

Inf. vesical v.

⑫ L. ureter (cut)

Sup. vesical v. ⑮

Ductus deferens

Middle rectal v. ⑰

Vesical venous plexus

Int. pudendal v. ⑭

Deep dorsal v. of penis

Prostatic venous plexus

Pampiniform venous plexus

Inf. rectal v. ⑬

Int. pudendal v. ⑭

Post. scrotal vv.

MEDIAL VIEW

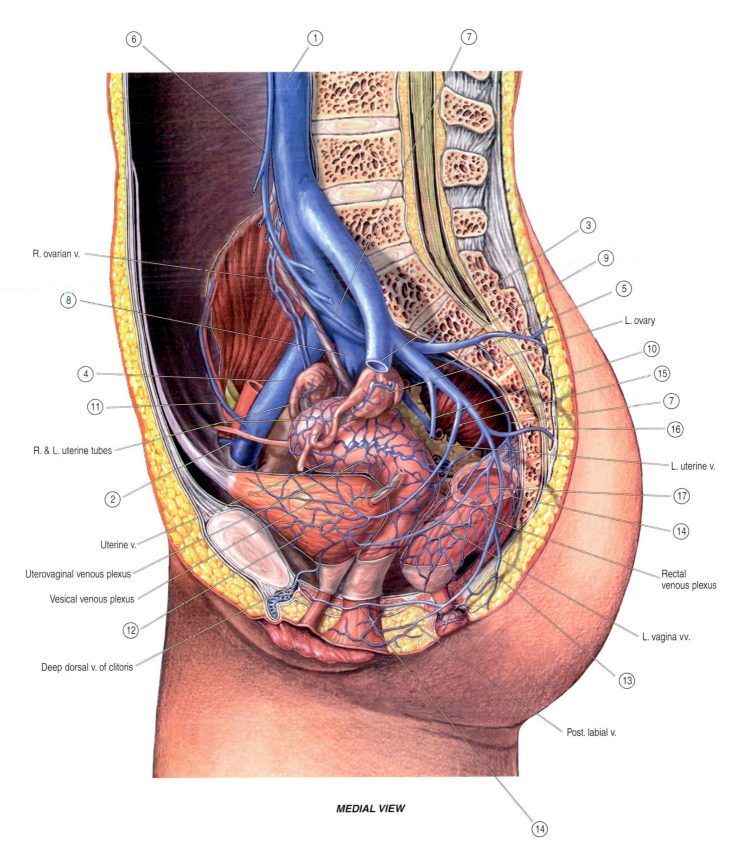

R. ovarian v.

L. ovary

R. & L. uterine tubes

L. uterine v.

Uterine v.

Rectal venous plexus

Uterovaginal venous plexus

Vesical venous plexus

L. vagina vv.

Deep dorsal v. of clitoris

Post. labial v.

MEDIAL VIEW

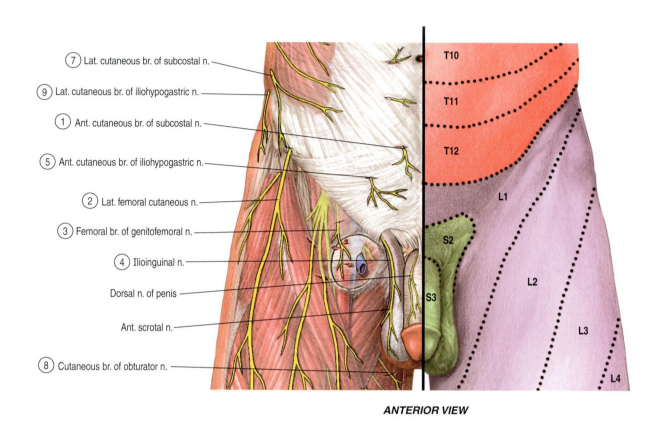

7 Lat. cutaneous br. of subcostal n.

9 Lat. cutaneous br. of iliohypogastric n.

1 Ant. cutaneous br. of subcostal n.

5 Ant. cutaneous br. of iliohypogastric n.

2 Lat. femoral cutaneous n.

3 Femoral br. of genitofemoral n.

4 Ilioinguinal n.

Dorsal n. of penis

Ant. scrotal n.

8 Cutaneous br. of obturator n.

T10
T11
T12
L1
S2
L2
S3
L3
L4

ANTERIOR VIEW

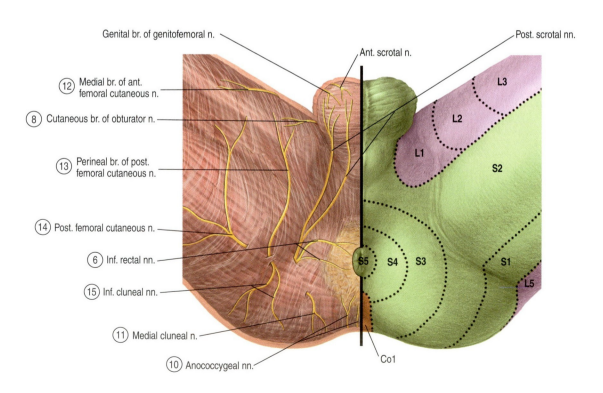

Genital br. of genitofemoral n.

Ant. scrotal n.

Post. scrotal nn.

12 Medial br. of ant. femoral cutaneous n.

8 Cutaneous br. of obturator n.

13 Perineal br. of post. femoral cutaneous n.

14 Post. femoral cutaneous n.

6 Inf. rectal nn.

15 Inf. cluneal nn.

11 Medial cluneal n.

10 Anococcygeal nn.

Co1

L3
L2
L1
S2
S5 S4 S3
S1
L5

LITHOTOMY VIEW

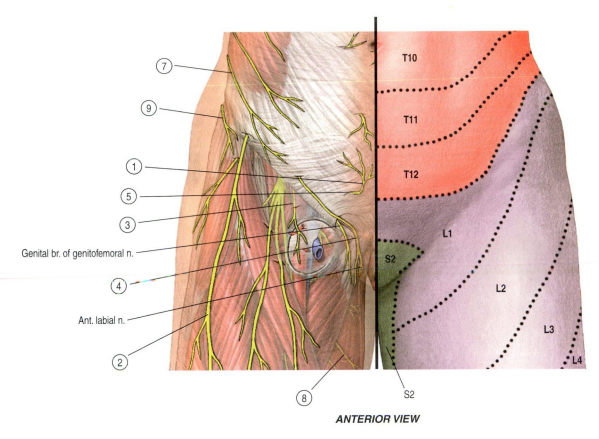

Genital br. of genitofemoral n.

Ant. labial n.

ANTERIOR VIEW

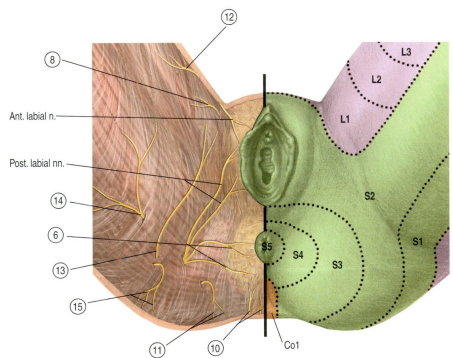

Ant. labial n.

Post. labial nn.

LITHOTOMY VIEW

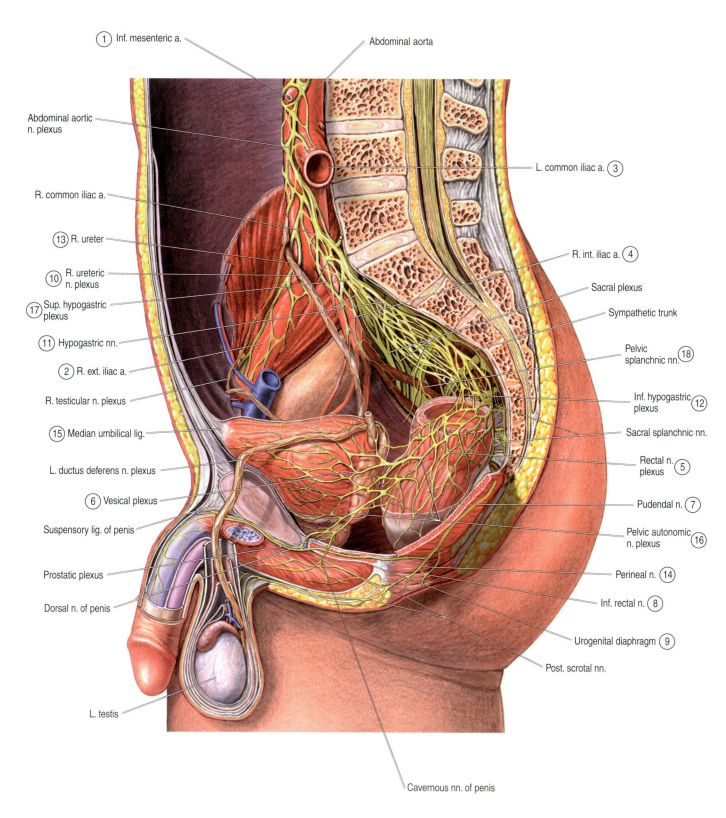

①　Inf. mesenteric a.

Abdominal aorta

Abdominal aortic
n. plexus

L. common iliac a. ③

R. common iliac a.

⑬　R. ureter

R. int. iliac a. ④

⑩　R. ureteric
n. plexus

Sacral plexus

⑰　Sup. hypogastric
plexus

Sympathetic trunk

⑪　Hypogastric nn.

Pelvic
splanchnic nn. ⑱

②　R. ext. iliac a.

R. testicular n. plexus

Inf. hypogastric
plexus ⑫

⑮　Median umbilical lig.

Sacral splanchnic nn.

L. ductus deferens n. plexus

Rectal n. ⑤
plexus

⑥　Vesical plexus

Pudendal n. ⑦

Suspensory lig. of penis

Pelvic autonomic ⑯
n. plexus

Prostatic plexus

Perineal n. ⑭

Dorsal n. of penis

Inf. rectal n. ⑧

Urogenital diaphragm ⑨

Post. scrotal nn.

L. testis

Cavernous nn. of penis

MEDIAL VIEW

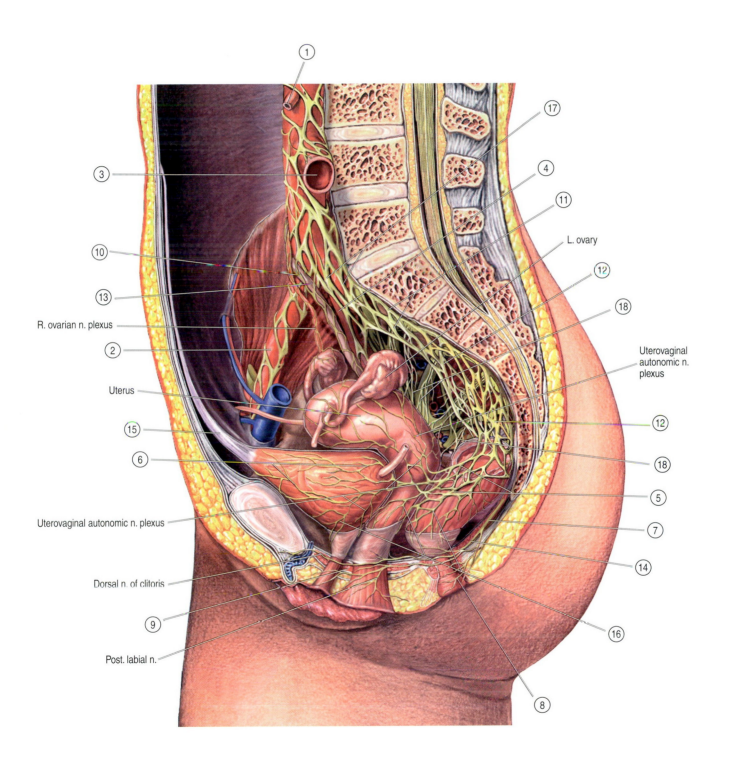

R. ovarian n. plexus

Uterus

Uterovaginal autonomic n. plexus

Dorsal n. of clitoris

Post. labial n.

L. ovary

Uterovaginal autonomic n. plexus

MEDIAL VIEW

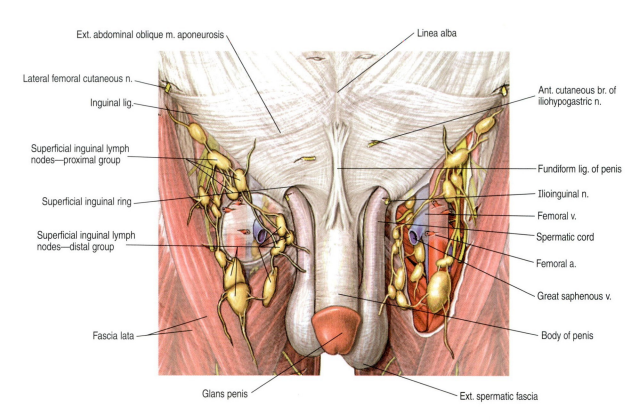

Ext. abdominal oblique m. aponeurosis

Linea alba

Lateral femoral cutaneous n.

Inguinal lig.

Ant. cutaneous br. of iliohypogastric n.

Superficial inguinal lymph nodes—proximal group

Fundiform lig. of penis

Superficial inguinal ring

Ilioinguinal n.

Femoral v.

Superficial inguinal lymph nodes—distal group

Spermatic cord

Femoral a.

Great saphenous v.

Fascia lata

Body of penis

Glans penis

Ext. spermatic fascia

MALE ANTERIOR VIEW

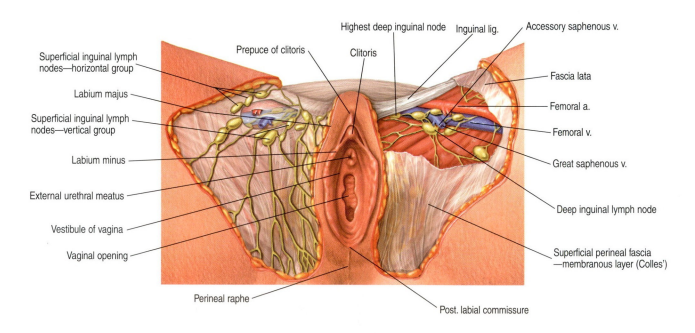

Highest deep inguinal node

Inguinal lig.

Accessory saphenous v.

Prepuce of clitoris

Clitoris

Superficial inguinal lymph nodes—horizontal group

Fascia lata

Labium majus

Femoral a.

Superficial inguinal lymph nodes—vertical group

Femoral v.

Labium minus

Great saphenous v.

External urethral meatus

Deep inguinal lymph node

Vestibule of vagina

Vaginal opening

Superficial perineal fascia —membranous layer (Colles')

Perineal raphe

Post. labial commissure

FEMALE LITHOTOMY VIEW

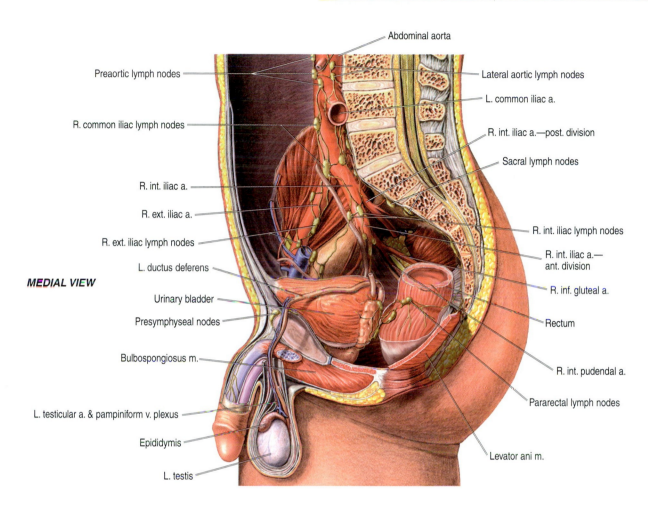

Abdominal aorta

Preaortic lymph nodes

Lateral aortic lymph nodes

R. common iliac lymph nodes

L. common iliac a.

R. int. iliac a.—post. division

Sacral lymph nodes

R. int. iliac a.

R. ext. iliac a.

R. ext. iliac lymph nodes

R. int. iliac lymph nodes

R. int. iliac a.— ant. division

L. ductus deferens

R. inf. gluteal a.

MEDIAL VIEW

Urinary bladder

Rectum

Presymphyseal nodes

Bulbospongiosus m.

R. int. pudendal a.

Pararectal lymph nodes

L. testicular a. & pampiniform v. plexus

Epididymis

Levator ani m.

L. testis

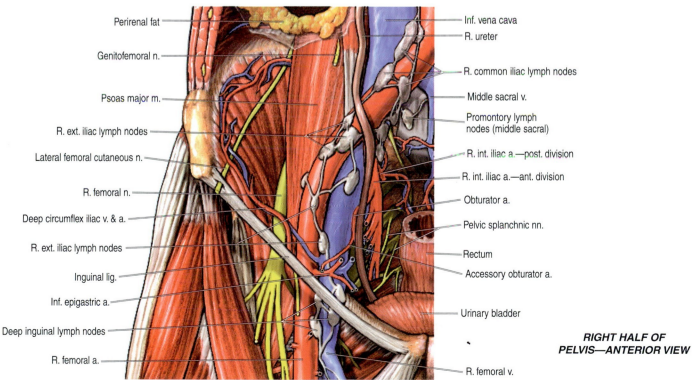

Perirenal fat

Inf. vena cava

R. ureter

Genitofemoral n.

R. common iliac lymph nodes

Psoas major m.

Middle sacral v.

Promontory lymph nodes (middle sacral)

R. ext. iliac lymph nodes

R. int. iliac a.—post. division

Lateral femoral cutaneous n.

R. int. iliac a.—ant. division

R. femoral n.

Obturator a.

Deep circumflex iliac v. & a.

Pelvic splanchnic nn.

R. ext. iliac lymph nodes

Rectum

Inguinal lig.

Accessory obturator a.

Inf. epigastric a.

Deep inguinal lymph nodes

Urinary bladder

R. femoral a.

RIGHT HALF OF PELVIS—ANTERIOR VIEW

R. femoral v.

♀ = **Characteristic Female Structures**

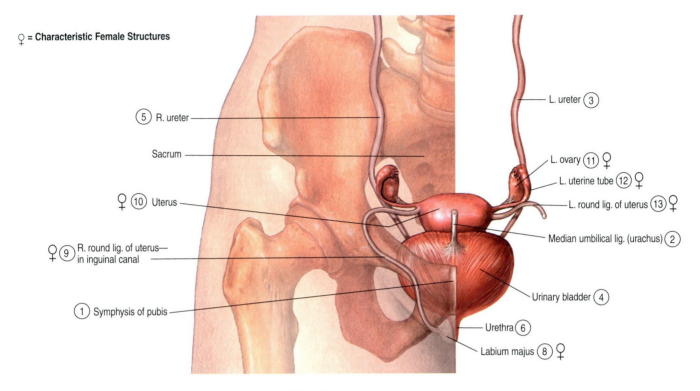

⑤ R. ureter

Sacrum

♀ ⑩ Uterus

♀ ⑨ R. round lig. of uterus— in inguinal canal

① Symphysis of pubis

L. ureter ③

L. ovary ⑪ ♀

L. uterine tube ⑫ ♀

L. round lig. of uterus ⑬ ♀

Median umbilical lig. (urachus) ②

Urinary bladder ④

Urethra ⑥

Labium majus ⑧ ♀

ANTERIOR VIEW

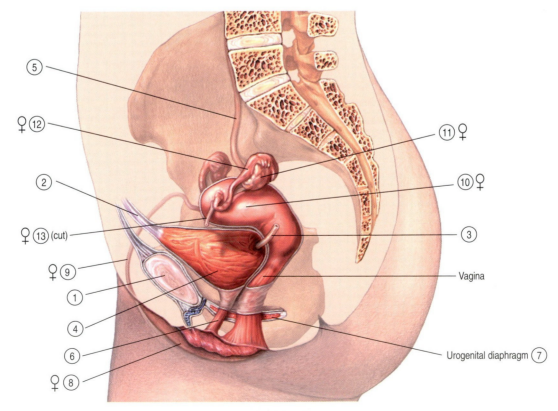

⑤

♀ ⑫

②

♀ ⑬ (cut)

♀ ⑨

①

④

⑥

♀ ⑧

⑪ ♀

⑩ ♀

③

Vagina

Urogenital diaphragm ⑦

MEDIAL VIEW

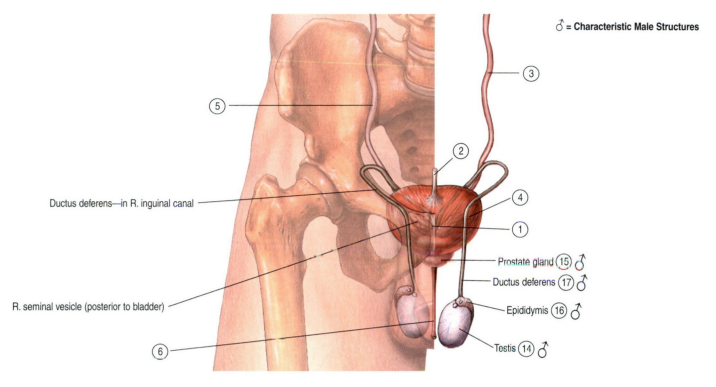

♂ = Characteristic Male Structures

Ductus deferens—in R. inguinal canal

R. seminal vesicle (posterior to bladder)

Prostate gland ⑮ ♂
Ductus deferens ⑰ ♂
Epididymis ⑯ ♂
Testis ⑭ ♂

ANTERIOR VIEW

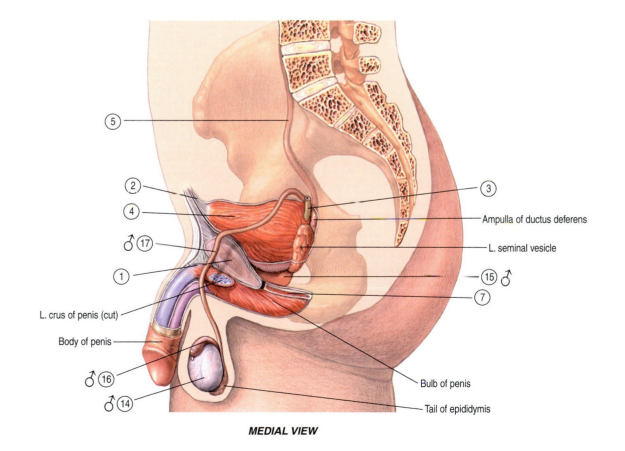

Ampulla of ductus deferens

L. seminal vesicle

⑮ ♂

⑦

L. crus of penis (cut)

Body of penis

♂ ⑯

♂ ⑭

Bulb of penis

Tail of epididymis

MEDIAL VIEW

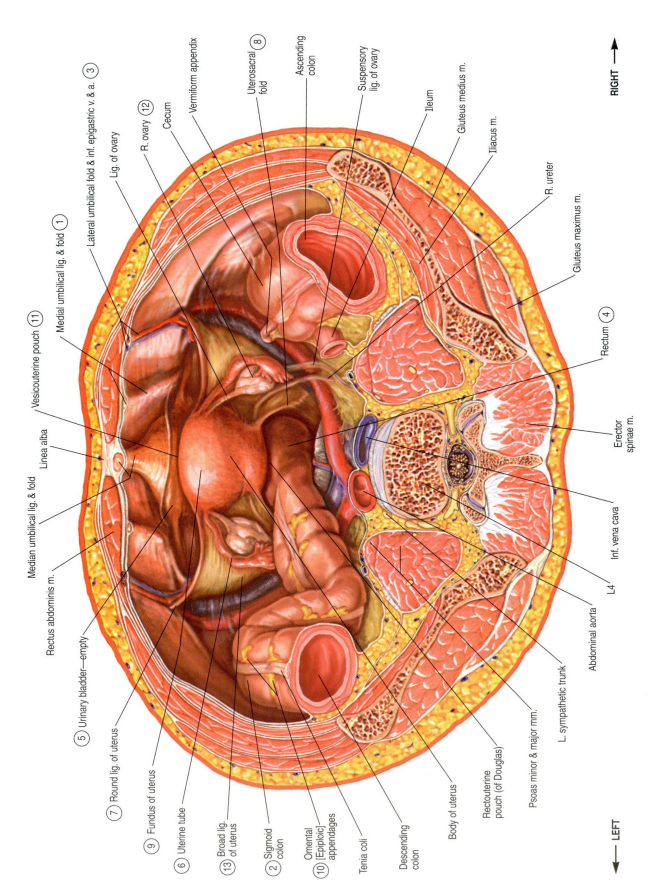

Vesicouterine pouch (11)

Medial umbilical lig. & fold (1)

Lateral umbilical fold & inf. epigastric v. & a. (3)

Lig. of ovary

R. ovary (12)

Cecum

Vermiform appendix

Uterosacral fold (8)

Ascending colon

Suspensory lig. of ovary

Ileum

Gluteus medius m.

Iliacus m.

R. ureter

Gluteus maximus m.

Rectum (4)

Erector spinae m.

Inf. vena cava

L4

Abdominal aorta

L. sympathetic trunk

Psoas minor & major mm.

Rectouterine pouch (of Douglas)

Body of uterus

Descending colon

Tenia coli

Omental [Epiploic] appendages (10)

Sigmoid colon (2)

Broad lig. of uterus (13)

Uterine tube (6)

Fundus of uterus (9)

Round lig. of uterus (7)

Urinary bladder—empty (5)

Rectus abdominis m.

Median umbilical lig. & fold

Linea alba

TRANSVERSE SECTION AT L4—SUPERIOR VIEW

RIGHT →

← LEFT

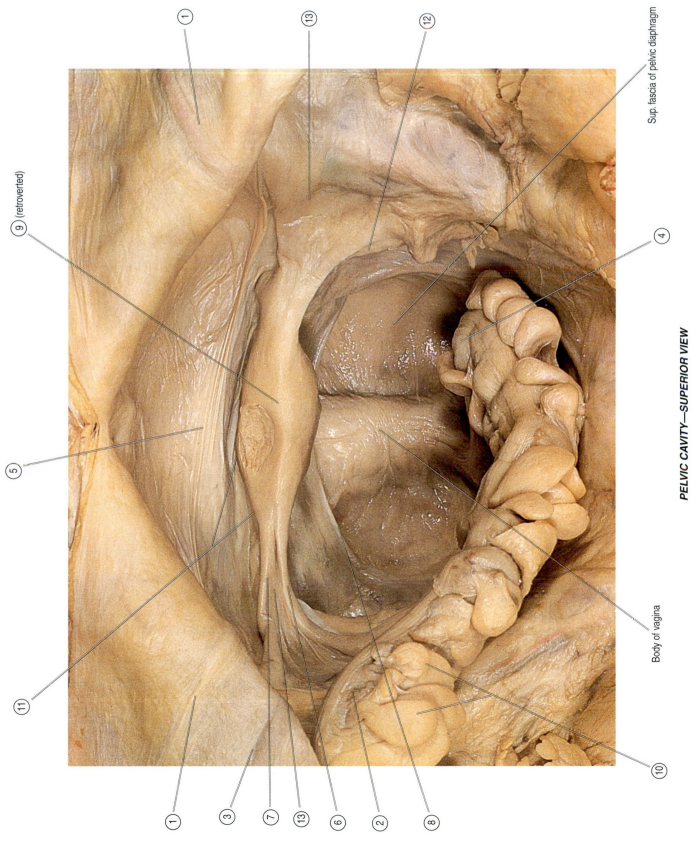

Sup. fascia of pelvic diaphragm

PELVIC CAVITY—SUPERIOR VIEW

9 (retroverted)

Body of vagina

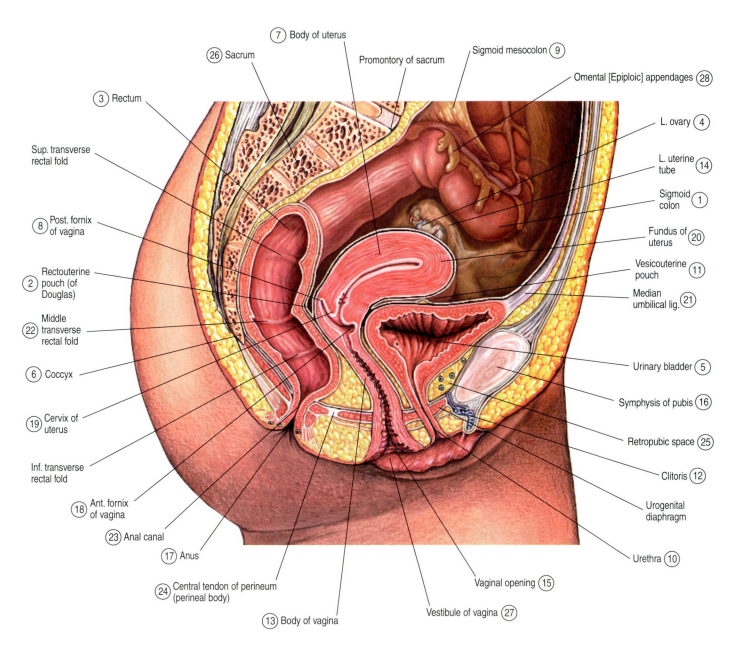

⑦ Body of uterus

㉖ Sacrum

Promontory of sacrum

Sigmoid mesocolon ⑨

Omental [Epiploic] appendages ㉘

③ Rectum

Sup. transverse rectal fold

L. ovary ④

L. uterine tube ⑭

⑧ Post. fornix of vagina

Sigmoid colon ①

Fundus of uterus ⑳

② Rectouterine pouch (of Douglas)

Vesicouterine pouch ⑪

㉒ Middle transverse rectal fold

Median umbilical lig. ㉑

⑥ Coccyx

Urinary bladder ⑤

⑲ Cervix of uterus

Symphysis of pubis ⑯

Inf. transverse rectal fold

Retropubic space ㉕

⑱ Ant. fornix of vagina

Clitoris ⑫

㉓ Anal canal

Urogenital diaphragm

⑰ Anus

Urethra ⑩

㉔ Central tendon of perineum (perineal body)

Vaginal opening ⑮

⑬ Body of vagina

Vestibule of vagina ㉗

MEDIAN SECTION—RIGHT LATERAL VIEW

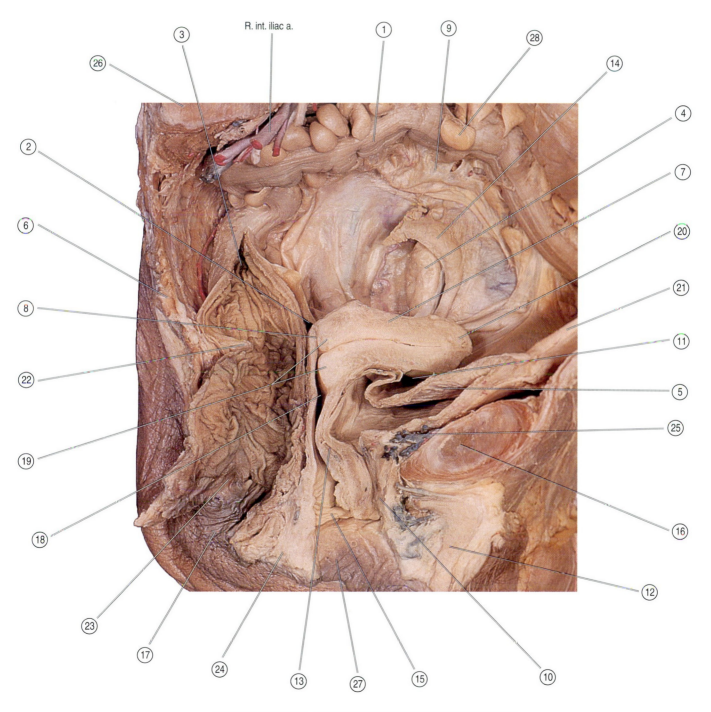

R. int. iliac a.

MEDIAN SECTION—RIGHT LATERAL VIEW OF LEFT PELVIS

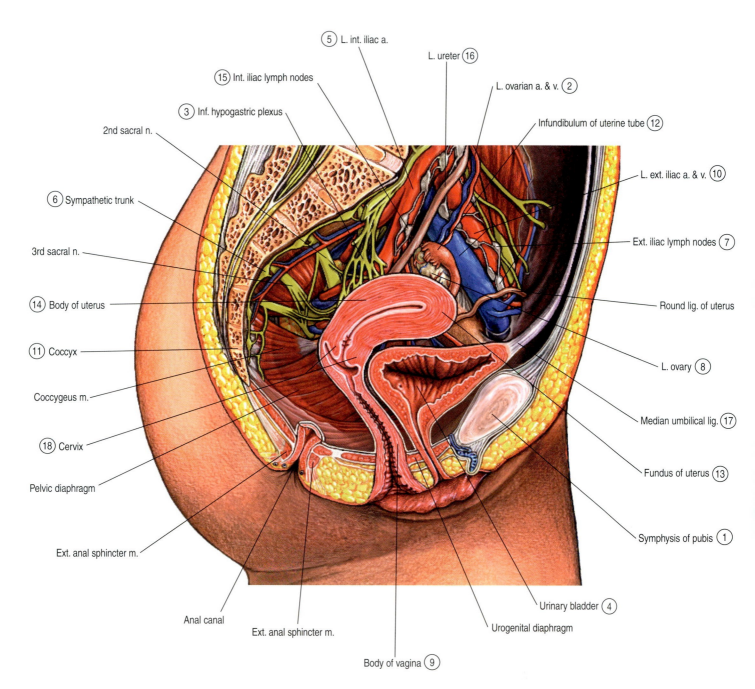

5 L. int. iliac a.

L. ureter 16

15 Int. iliac lymph nodes

L. ovarian a. & v. 2

3 Inf. hypogastric plexus

Infundibulum of uterine tube 12

2nd sacral n.

6 Sympathetic trunk

L. ext. iliac a. & v. 10

3rd sacral n.

Ext. iliac lymph nodes 7

14 Body of uterus

Round lig. of uterus

11 Coccyx

L. ovary 8

Coccygeus m.

Median umbilical lig. 17

18 Cervix

Fundus of uterus 13

Pelvic diaphragm

Symphysis of pubis 1

Ext. anal sphincter m.

Urinary bladder 4

Anal canal

Urogenital diaphragm

Ext. anal sphincter m.

Body of vagina 9

MEDIAN SECTION—RIGHT LATERAL VIEW

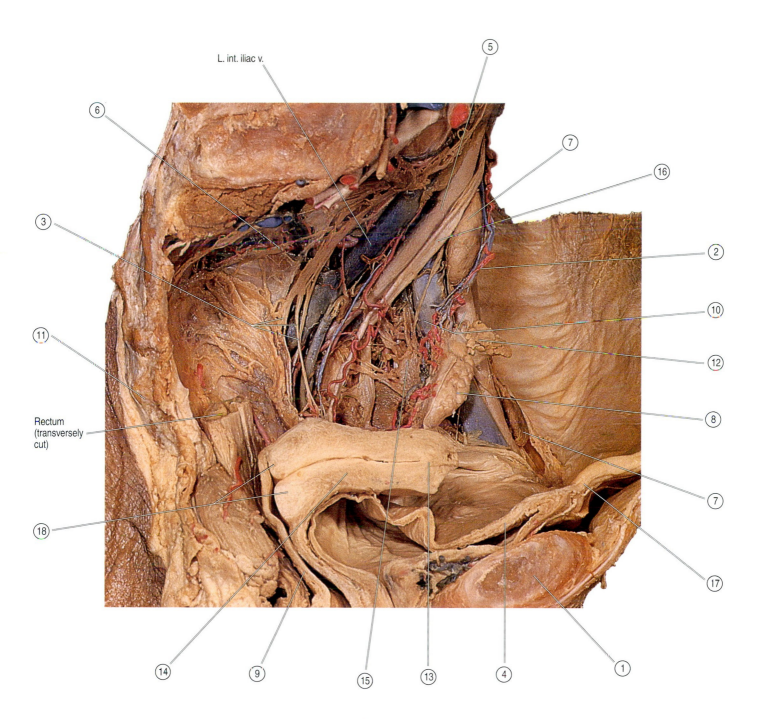

L. int. iliac v.

Rectum
(transversely
cut)

LEFT HALF OF HEMISECTED PELVIS—MEDIAL VIEW

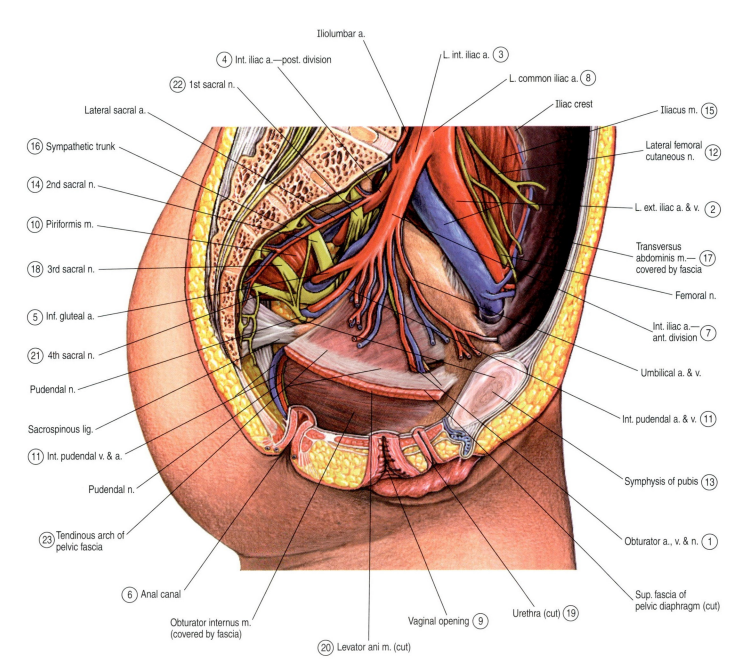

Iliolumbar a.

④ Int. iliac a.—post. division

L. int. iliac a. ③

㉒ 1st sacral n.

L. common iliac a. ⑧

Iliac crest

Lateral sacral a.

Iliacus m. ⑮

⑯ Sympathetic trunk

Lateral femoral cutaneous n. ⑫

⑭ 2nd sacral n.

⑩ Piriformis m.

L. ext. iliac a. & v. ②

⑱ 3rd sacral n.

Transversus abdominis m.— ⑰ covered by fascia

⑤ Inf. gluteal a.

Femoral n.

Int. iliac a.— ⑦ ant. division

㉑ 4th sacral n.

Pudendal n.

Umbilical a. & v.

Sacrospinous lig.

Int. pudendal a. & v. ⑪

⑪ Int. pudendal v. & a.

Pudendal n.

Symphysis of pubis ⑬

㉓ Tendinous arch of pelvic fascia

Obturator a., v. & n. ①

⑥ Anal canal

Sup. fascia of pelvic diaphragm (cut)

Obturator internus m. (covered by fascia)

Vaginal opening ⑨

Urethra (cut) ⑲

㉒ Levator ani m. (cut)

MEDIAN SECTION—RIGHT LATERAL VIEW

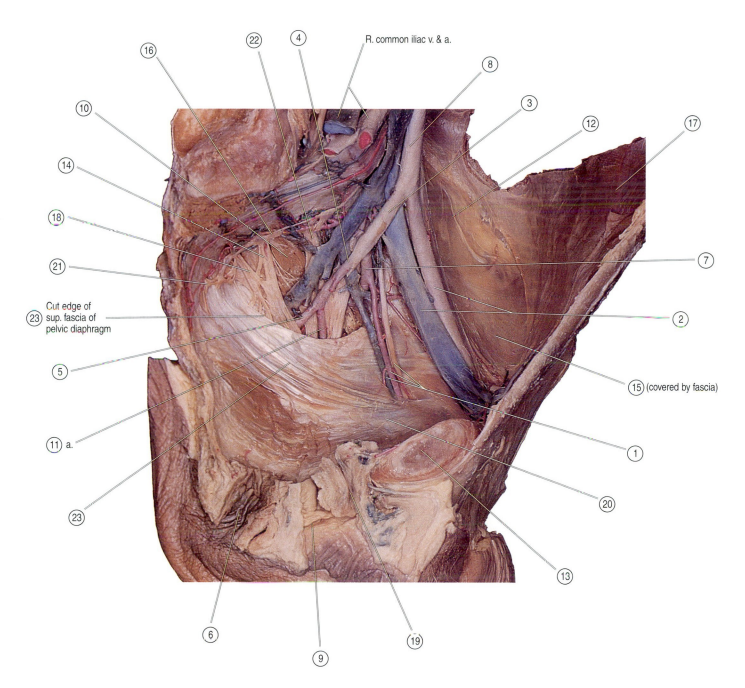

R. common iliac v. & a.

Cut edge of
sup. fascia of
pelvic diaphragm

(15) (covered by fascia)

(11) a.

MEDIAN SECTION—RIGHT LATERAL VIEW

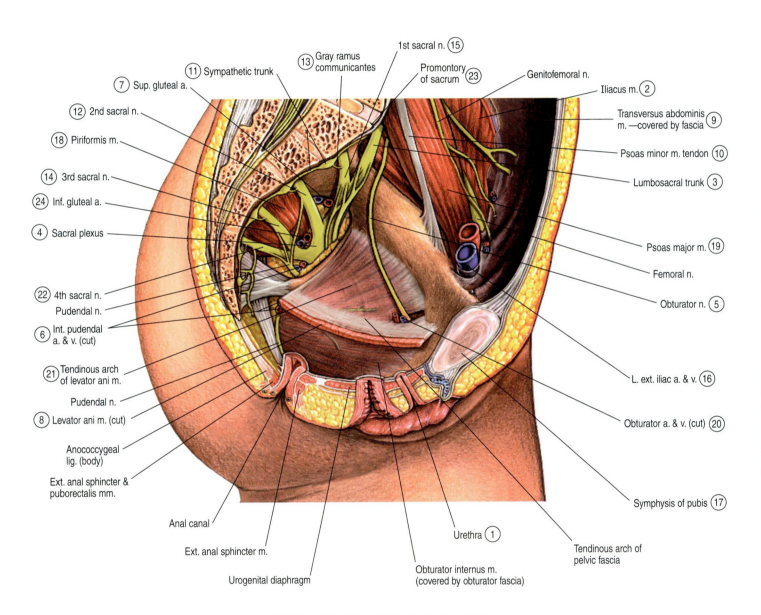

1st sacral n. (15)

(13) Gray ramus communicantes

Promontory of sacrum (23)

Genitofemoral n.

(11) Sympathetic trunk

(7) Sup. gluteal a.

Iliacus m. (2)

(12) 2nd sacral n.

Transversus abdominis m. —covered by fascia (9)

(18) Piriformis m.

Psoas minor m. tendon (10)

(14) 3rd sacral n.

Lumbosacral trunk (3)

(24) Inf. gluteal a.

(4) Sacral plexus

Psoas major m. (19)

Femoral n.

(22) 4th sacral n.

Obturator n. (5)

Pudendal n.

(6) Int. pudendal a. & v. (cut)

(21) Tendinous arch of levator ani m.

L. ext. iliac a. & v. (16)

Pudendal n.

(8) Levator ani m. (cut)

Obturator a. & v. (cut) (20)

Anococcygeal lig. (body)

Ext. anal sphincter & puborectalis mm.

Symphysis of pubis (17)

Anal canal

Ext. anal sphincter m.

Urethra (1)

Tendinous arch of pelvic fascia

Urogenital diaphragm

Obturator internus m. (covered by obturator fascia)

MEDIAN SECTION—RIGHT LATERAL VIEW

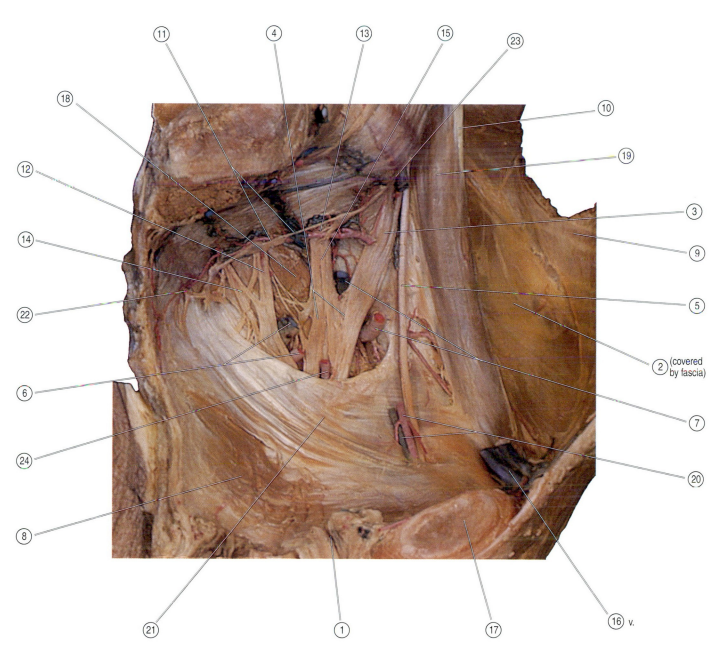

MEDIAN SECTION—RIGHT LATERAL VIEW

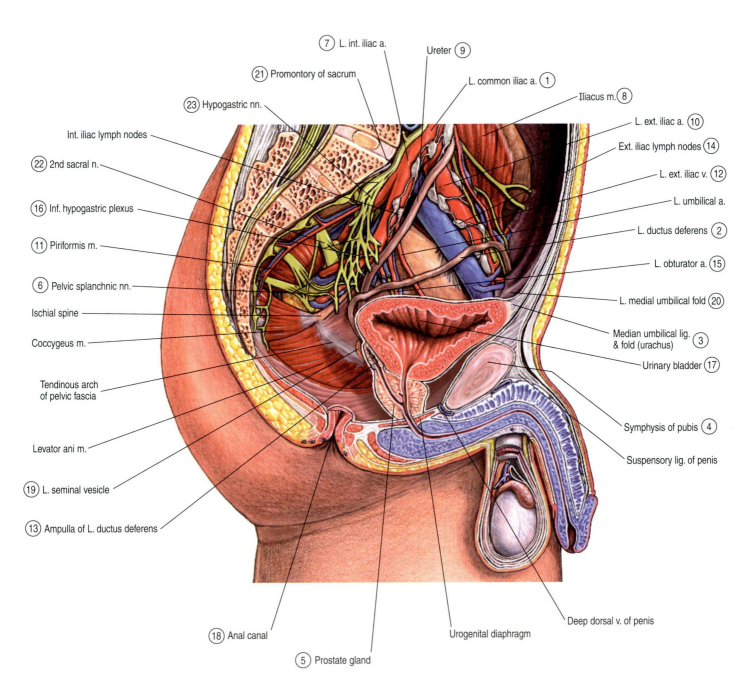

⑦ L. int. iliac a.

Ureter ⑨

㉑ Promontory of sacrum

L. common iliac a. ①

㉓ Hypogastric nn.

Iliacus m. ⑧

Int. iliac lymph nodes

L. ext. iliac a. ⑩

Ext. iliac lymph nodes ⑭

㉒ 2nd sacral n.

L. ext. iliac v. ⑫

⑯ Inf. hypogastric plexus

L. umbilical a.

L. ductus deferens ②

⑪ Piriformis m.

L. obturator a. ⑮

⑥ Pelvic splanchnic nn.

L. medial umbilical fold ⑳

Ischial spine

Median umbilical lig. & fold (urachus) ③

Coccygeus m.

Urinary bladder ⑰

Tendinous arch of pelvic fascia

Levator ani m.

Symphysis of pubis ④

⑲ L. seminal vesicle

Suspensory lig. of penis

⑬ Ampulla of L. ductus deferens

Deep dorsal v. of penis

⑱ Anal canal

Urogenital diaphragm

⑤ Prostate gland

MEDIAN SECTION—RIGHT LATERAL VIEW

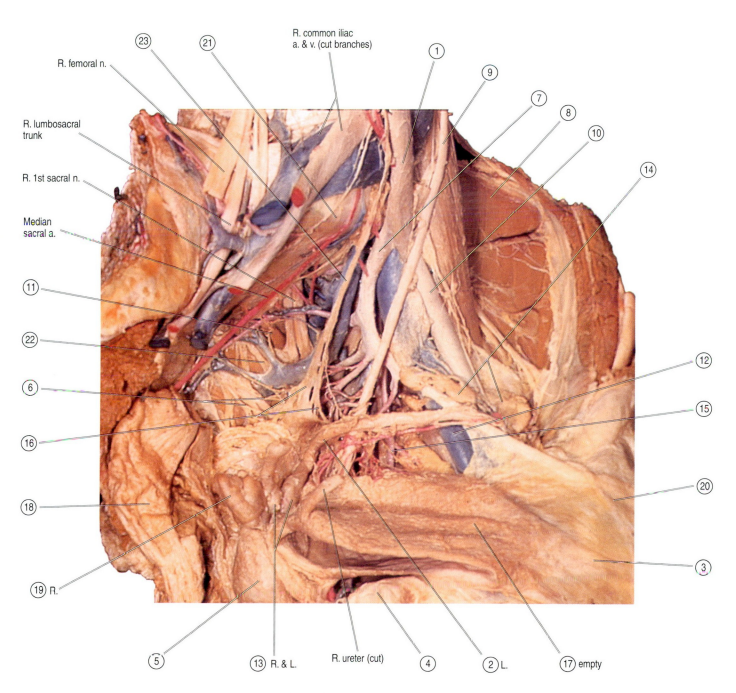

R. common iliac
a. & v. (cut branches)

R. femoral n.

R. lumbosacral
trunk

R. 1st sacral n.

Median
sacral a.

R.

R. & L.

R. ureter (cut)

L.

empty

**LEFT HALF OF HEMISECTED PELVIS WITH
BLADDER PULLED ANTERIORLY—MEDIAL VIEW**

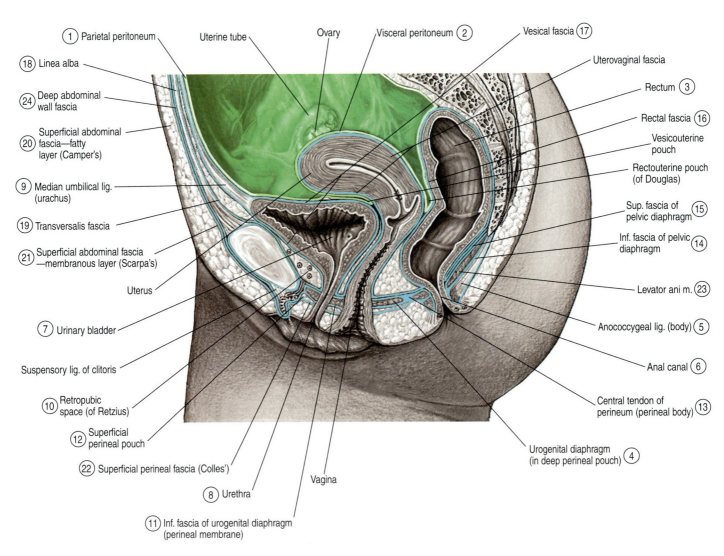

① Parietal peritoneum

Uterine tube

Ovary

Visceral peritoneum ②

Vesical fascia ⑰

⑱ Linea alba

Uterovaginal fascia

㉔ Deep abdominal wall fascia

Rectum ③

⑳ Superficial abdominal fascia—fatty layer (Camper's)

Rectal fascia ⑯

Vesicouterine pouch

⑨ Median umbilical lig. (urachus)

Rectouterine pouch (of Douglas)

⑲ Transversalis fascia

Sup. fascia of pelvic diaphragm ⑮

㉑ Superficial abdominal fascia —membranous layer (Scarpa's)

Inf. fascia of pelvic diaphragm ⑭

Uterus

Levator ani m. ㉓

⑦ Urinary bladder

Anococcygeal lig. (body) ⑤

Suspensory lig. of clitoris

Anal canal ⑥

⑩ Retropubic space (of Retzius)

Central tendon of perineum (perineal body) ⑬

⑫ Superficial perineal pouch

Urogenital diaphragm (in deep perineal pouch) ④

㉒ Superficial perineal fascia (Colles')

Vagina

⑧ Urethra

⑪ Inf. fascia of urogenital diaphragm (perineal membrane)

MEDIAN SECTION—LEFT LATERAL VIEW

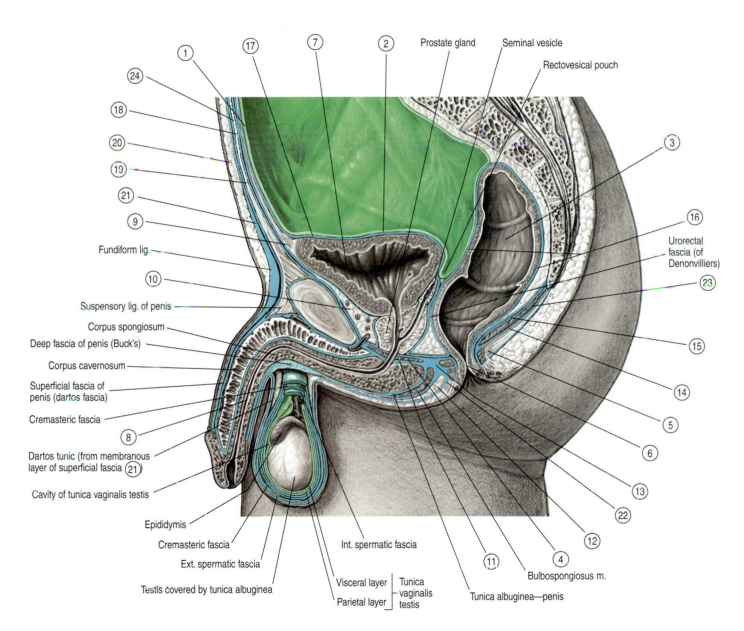

Prostate gland

Seminal vesicle

Rectovesical pouch

Fundiform lig.

Suspensory lig. of penis

Corpus spongiosum

Deep fascia of penis (Buck's)

Corpus cavernosum

Superficial fascia of penis (dartos fascia)

Cremasteric fascia

Dartos tunic (from membranous layer of superficial fascia (21))

Cavity of tunica vaginalis testis

Epididymis

Cremasteric fascia

Ext. spermatic fascia

Testis covered by tunica albuginea

Int. spermatic fascia

Visceral layer | Tunica
Parietal layer | vaginalis testis

Tunica albuginea—penis

Bulbospongiosus m.

Urorectal fascia (of Denonvilliers)

MEDIAN SECTION—LEFT LATERAL VIEW

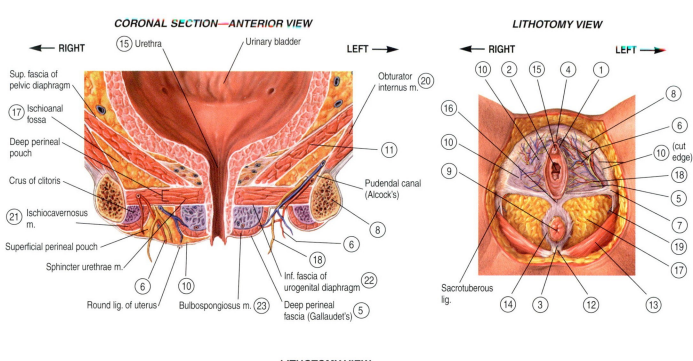

CORONAL SECTION—ANTERIOR VIEW

← RIGHT   LEFT →

- (15) Urethra
- Urinary bladder
- Sup. fascia of pelvic diaphragm
- (17) Ischioanal fossa
- Deep perineal pouch
- Crus of clitoris
- (21) Ischiocavernosus m.
- Superficial perineal pouch
- Sphincter urethrae m.
- (6)
- (10)
- Round lig. of uterus
- Bulbospongiosus m. (23)
- Obturator internus m. (20)
- (11)
- Pudendal canal (Alcock's)
- (8)
- (6)
- (18)
- Inf. fascia of urogenital diaphragm (22)
- Deep perineal fascia (Gallaudet's) (5)

LITHOTOMY VIEW

← RIGHT   LEFT →

- (10) (2) (15) (4) (1)
- (16)
- (10)
- (9)
- (8)
- (6)
- (10) (cut edge)
- (18)
- (5)
- (7)
- (19)
- (17)
- Sacrotuberous lig.
- (14) (3) (12) (13)

LITHOTOMY VIEW

← RIGHT   LEFT →

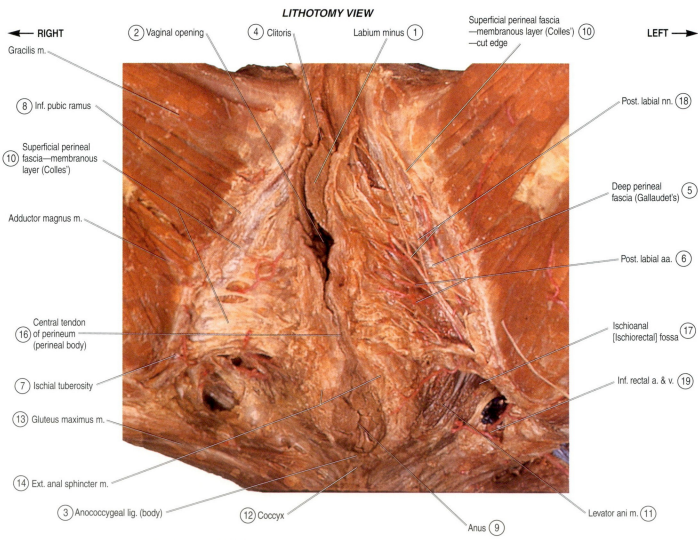

- (2) Vaginal opening
- (4) Clitoris
- Labium minus (1)
- Superficial perineal fascia —membranous layer (Colles') (10) —cut edge
- Gracilis m.
- (8) Inf. pubic ramus
- (10) Superficial perineal fascia—membranous layer (Colles')
- Adductor magnus m.
- (16) Central tendon of perineum (perineal body)
- (7) Ischial tuberosity
- (13) Gluteus maximus m.
- (14) Ext. anal sphincter m.
- (3) Anococcygeal lig. (body)
- (12) Coccyx
- Anus (9)
- Post. labial nn. (18)
- Deep perineal fascia (Gallaudet's) (5)
- Post. labial aa. (6)
- Ischioanal [Ischiorectal] fossa (17)
- Inf. rectal a. & v. (19)
- Levator ani m. (11)

LITHOTOMY VIEW

← **RIGHT**   **LEFT** →

Ext. spermatic fascia over testis & spermatic cord

24

25

10

7

Sacrotuberous lig.

17

14

13

3

12

9

16

CORONAL SECTION—ANTERIOR VIEW

← **RIGHT**   **LEFT** →

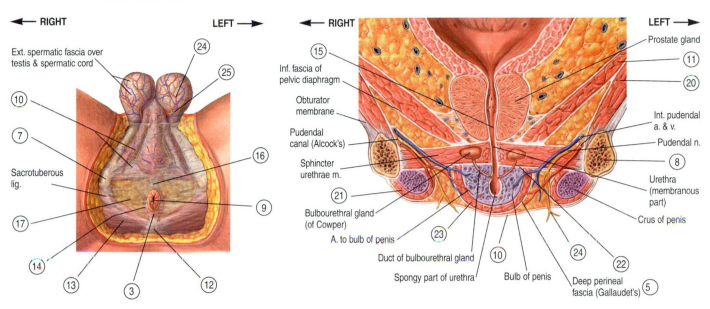

15

Inf. fascia of pelvic diaphragm

Obturator membrane

Pudendal canal (Alcock's)

Sphincter urethrae m.

21

Bulbourethral gland (of Cowper)

A. to bulb of penis

23

Duct of bulbourethral gland

Spongy part of urethra

Bulb of penis

10

Prostate gland

11

20

Int. pudendal a. & v.

Pudendal n.

8

Urethra (membranous part)

Crus of penis

Deep perineal fascia (Gallaudet's) 5

24

22

LITHOTOMY VIEW

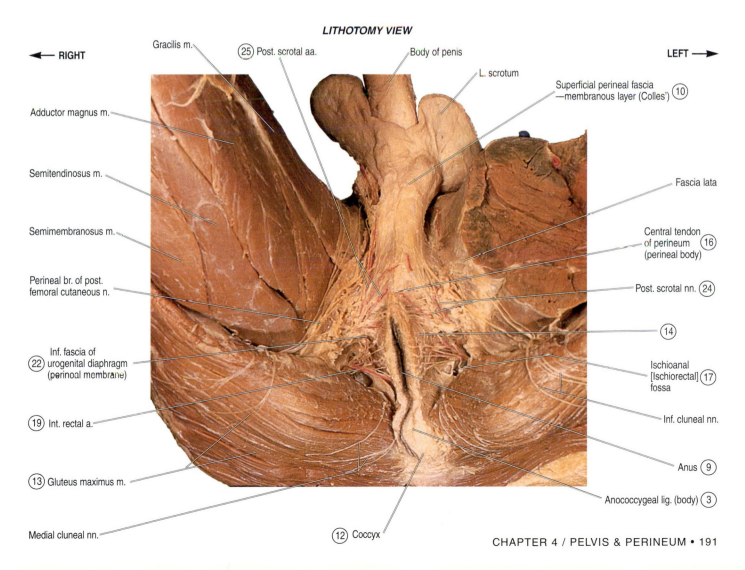

← **RIGHT**   **LEFT** →

Gracilis m.

25 Post. scrotal aa.

Body of penis

L. scrotum

Superficial perineal fascia —membranous layer (Colles') 10

Adductor magnus m.

Semitendinosus m.

Semimembranosus m.

Perineal br. of post. femoral cutaneous n.

Inf. fascia of
22 urogenital diaphragm (perineal membrane)

19 Int. rectal a.

13 Gluteus maximus m.

Medial cluneal nn.

12 Coccyx

Fascia lata

Central tendon of perineum (perineal body) 16

Post. scrotal nn. 24

14

Ischioanal [Ischiorectal] 17 fossa

Inf. cluneal nn.

Anus 9

Anococcygeal lig. (body) 3

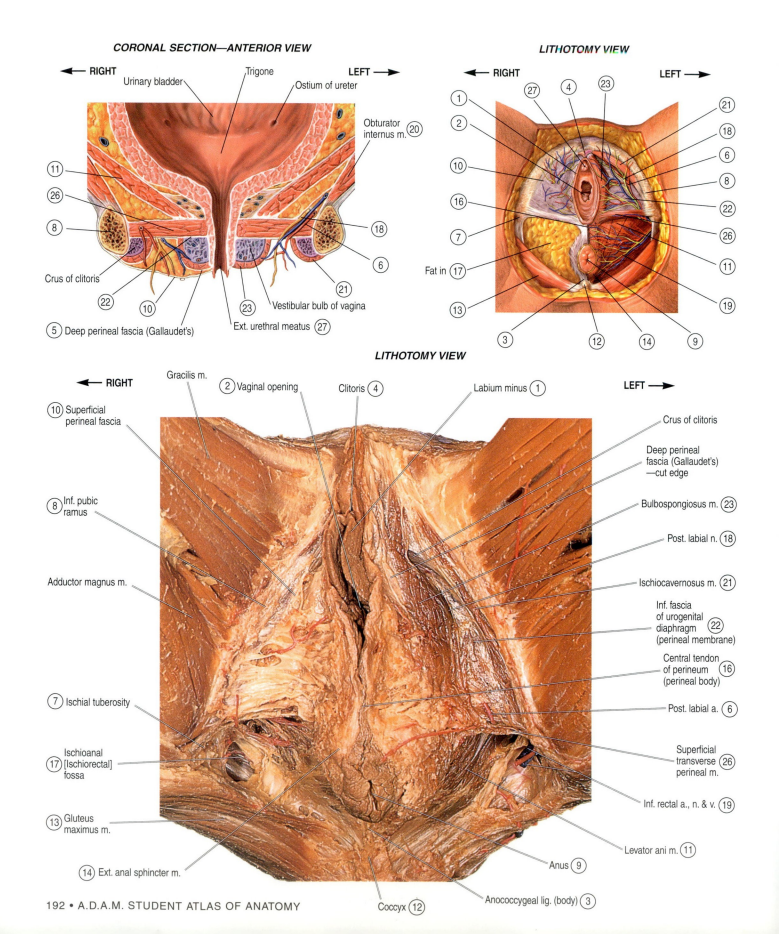

CORONAL SECTION—ANTERIOR VIEW

← RIGHT   LEFT →

- Urinary bladder
- Trigone
- Ostium of ureter
- Obturator internus m. (20)
- (11)
- (26)
- (8)
- (18)
- (6)
- Crus of clitoris
- (22)
- (10)
- (23)
- Vestibular bulb of vagina
- (21)
- (5) Deep perineal fascia (Gallaudet's)
- Ext. urethral meatus (27)

LITHOTOMY VIEW

← RIGHT   LEFT →

- (1)
- (27) (4) (23)
- (2)
- (21)
- (18)
- (10)
- (6)
- (16)
- (8)
- (7)
- (22)
- Fat in (17)
- (26)
- (11)
- (13)
- (19)
- (3)
- (12) (14) (9)

LITHOTOMY VIEW

← RIGHT   LEFT →

- Gracilis m.
- (2) Vaginal opening
- Clitoris (4)
- Labium minus (1)
- (10) Superficial perineal fascia
- Crus of clitoris
- Deep perineal fascia (Gallaudet's) —cut edge
- (8) Inf. pubic ramus
- Bulbospongiosus m. (23)
- Post. labial n. (18)
- Adductor magnus m.
- Ischiocavernosus m. (21)
- Inf. fascia of urogenital diaphragm (22) (perineal membrane)
- Central tendon of perineum (16) (perineal body)
- (7) Ischial tuberosity
- Post. labial a. (6)
- (17) Ischioanal [Ischiorectal] fossa
- Superficial transverse (26) perineal m.
- Inf. rectal a., n. & v. (19)
- (13) Gluteus maximus m.
- Levator ani m. (11)
- (14) Ext. anal sphincter m.
- Anus (9)
- Coccyx (12)
- Anococcygeal lig. (body) (3)

LITHOTOMY VIEW

← RIGHT   LEFT →

L. spermatic cord (cut)

CORONAL SECTION—ANTERIOR VIEW

← LEFT   RIGHT →

Prostate gland   Urinary bladder   Lateral puboprostatic lig.   Obturator internus m. (20)

(11)

(22)

(30)

(32) Perineal n.

(15) Urethra   (23)   Corpus spongiosum (28)

(31)

(8)

(21)

LITHOTOMY VIEW

← RIGHT   LEFT →

Body of penis   L. scrotum

(5) Deep perineal fascia (Gallaudet's)

(23) Bulbospongiosus m.

(21) Ischiocavernosus m.

Femoral a. & v.

Adductor longus m.

(30) Crus of penis

(26) Superficial transverse perineal m.

(7) Ischial tuberosity

(17) Ischioanal [Ischiorectal] fossa

(13) Gluteus maximus m.

(9) Anus   (12) Coccyx   (3) Anococcygeal lig. (body)

Corpus spongiosum (28)

Superficial perineal fascia (10)

Inf. pubic ramus (8)

Obturator externus m.

N. to bulbospongiosus m.

Perineal a. (29)

Pudendal n. (31)

Central tendon of perineum (perineal body)

Ext. anal sphincter m. (14)

Inf. rectal a., n. & v. (19)

Levator ani m. (11)

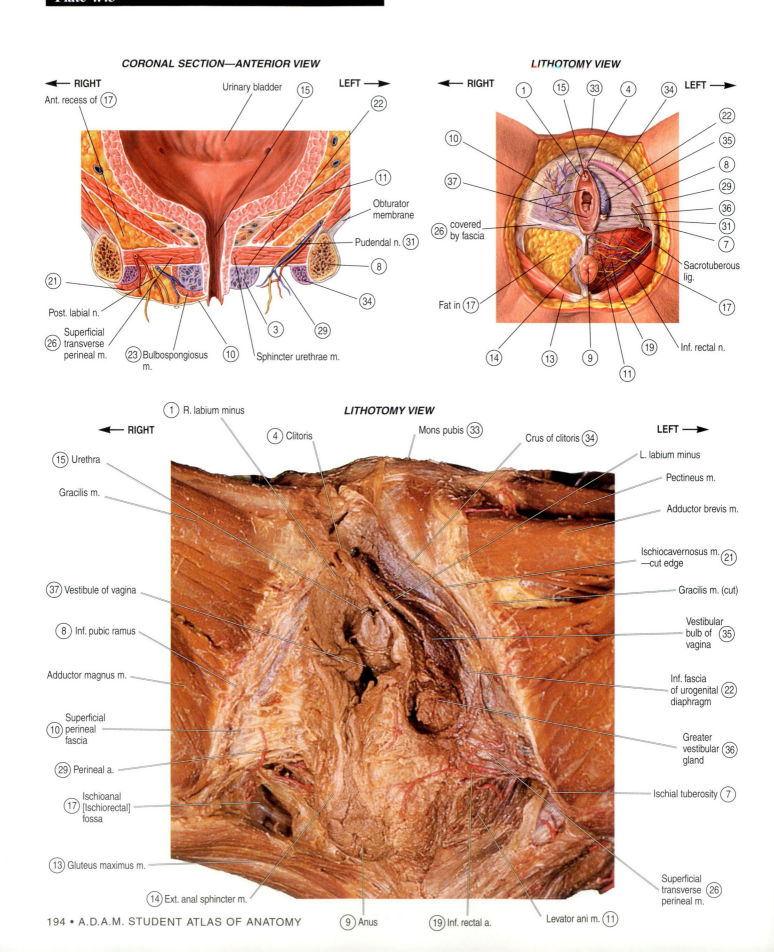

CORONAL SECTION—ANTERIOR VIEW

← RIGHT   Urinary bladder (15)   LEFT →

Ant. recess of (17)
(22)
(11)
Obturator membrane
Pudendal n. (31)
(8)
(34)
(21)
Post. labial n.
(26) Superficial transverse perineal m.
(23) Bulbospongiosus m.
(10)
(3)
(29)
Sphincter urethrae m.

LITHOTOMY VIEW

← RIGHT   (1) (15) (33) (4) (34)   LEFT →
(10)
(37)
(26) covered by fascia
Fat in (17)
(22)
(35)
(8)
(29)
(36)
(31)
(7)
Sacrotuberous lig.
(17)
(14) (13) (9)
(19) Inf. rectal n.
(11)

LITHOTOMY VIEW

(1) R. labium minus
(4) Clitoris
Mons pubis (33)
Crus of clitoris (34)

← RIGHT   LEFT →

(15) Urethra
Gracilis m.
(37) Vestibule of vagina
(8) Inf. pubic ramus
Adductor magnus m.
(10) Superficial perineal fascia
(29) Perineal a.
(17) Ischioanal [Ischiorectal] fossa
(13) Gluteus maximus m.
(14) Ext. anal sphincter m.
(9) Anus

L. labium minus
Pectineus m.
Adductor brevis m.
Ischiocavernosus m. (21) —cut edge
Gracilis m. (cut)
Vestibular bulb of (35) vagina
Inf. fascia (22) of urogenital diaphragm
Greater vestibular (36) gland
Ischial tuberosity (7)
Superficial transverse (26) perineal m.
(19) Inf. rectal a.
Levator ani m. (11)

LITHOTOMY VIEW

← **RIGHT**   **LEFT** →

(15)

Deep fascia of penis   Corpus cavernosum

(28)

Spermatic cord (cut)

(23)

(30)

(21)

(28)

(8)

(22)

(31)

(7)

(11)

(19)

(38)

(9)

(14)

CORONAL SECTION—ANTERIOR VIEW

← **RIGHT**   **LEFT** →

Urinary bladder

Prostate gland   Urogenital diaphragm

(11)

(11)

(31)

Ant. recess of (17)

(8)

(30)

(29)

(21)

Urethra (15)

(24) Post. scrotal n.

(22)

(23)

(28)

Post. scrotal a. (25)

Bulbourethral gland (of Cowper)

LITHOTOMY VIEW

← **RIGHT**   **LEFT** →

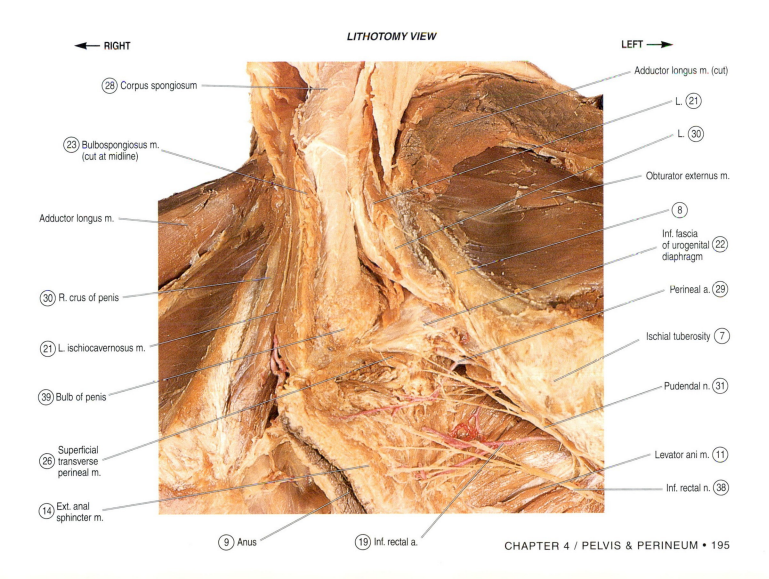

(28) Corpus spongiosum

Adductor longus m. (cut)

(23) Bulbospongiosus m. (cut at midline)

L. (21)

L. (30)

Adductor longus m.

Obturator externus m.

(8)

Inf. fascia of urogenital (22) diaphragm

(30) R. crus of penis

Perineal a. (29)

(21) L. ischiocavernosus m.

Ischial tuberosity (7)

(39) Bulb of penis

Pudendal n. (31)

(26) Superficial transverse perineal m.

Levator ani m. (11)

(14) Ext. anal sphincter m.

Inf. rectal n. (38)

(9) Anus

(19) Inf. rectal a.

CORONAL SECTION—ANTERIOR VIEW

← RIGHT   LEFT →

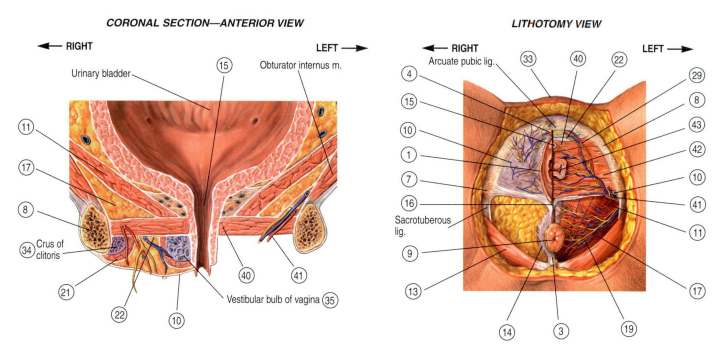

Urinary bladder
⑮
Obturator internus m.
⑪
⑰
⑧
㉞ Crus of clitoris
㉑
㉒
⑩
④⓪
④①
Vestibular bulb of vagina ㉟

LITHOTOMY VIEW

← RIGHT   LEFT →

Arcuate pubic lig.
④
⑮
⑩
①
⑦
⑯
Sacrotuberous lig.
⑨
⑬
㉝ ④⓪ ㉒
㉙
⑧
④③
④②
⑩
④①
⑪
⑰
⑭ ③ ⑲

LITHOTOMY VIEW

← RIGHT   LEFT →

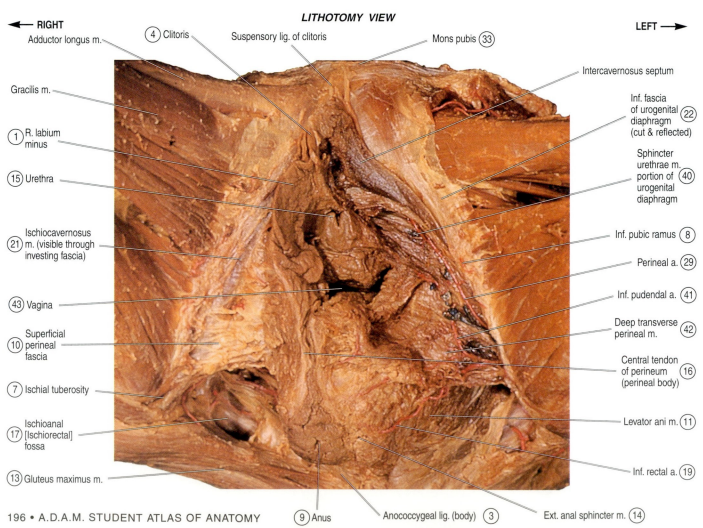

Adductor longus m.
④ Clitoris
Suspensory lig. of clitoris
Mons pubis ㉝

Gracilis m.
Intercavernosus septum

① R. labium minus
Inf. fascia of urogenital diaphragm (cut & reflected) ㉒

⑮ Urethra
Sphincter urethrae m. portion of urogenital diaphragm ④⓪

㉑ Ischiocavernosus m. (visible through investing fascia)
Inf. pubic ramus ⑧

④③ Vagina
Perineal a. ㉙

⑩ Superficial perineal fascia
Inf. pudendal a. ④①

⑦ Ischial tuberosity
Deep transverse perineal m. ④②

⑰ Ischioanal [Ischiorectal] fossa
Central tendon of perineum (perineal body) ⑯

⑬ Gluteus maximus m.
Levator ani m. ⑪

Inf. rectal a. ⑲

⑨ Anus
Anococcygeal lig. (body) ③
Ext. anal sphincter m. ⑭

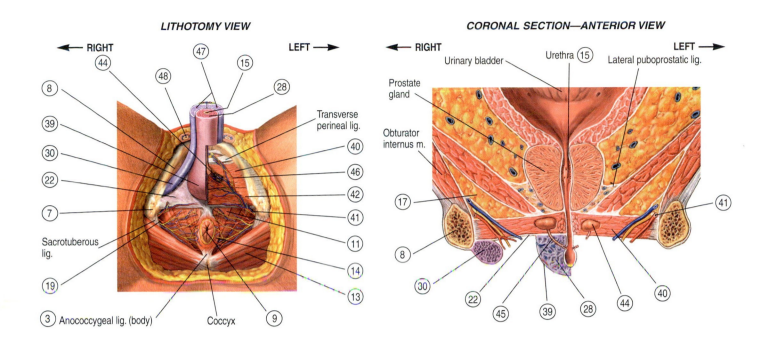

LITHOTOMY VIEW

← RIGHT   LEFT →

(44) (47) (48) (15) (28)
(8)
(39)
(30)
(22)
(7)

Transverse perineal lig. (40)
(46)
(42)
(41)
(11)
(14)
(13)

Sacrotuberous lig.

(19)

(3) Anococcygeal lig. (body)   Coccyx   (9)

CORONAL SECTION—ANTERIOR VIEW

← RIGHT   LEFT →

Urinary bladder   Urethra (15)   Lateral puboprostatic lig.

Prostate gland

Obturator internus m.

(17)

(8)

(30)   (22)   (45)   (39)   (28)   (44)   (40)   (41)

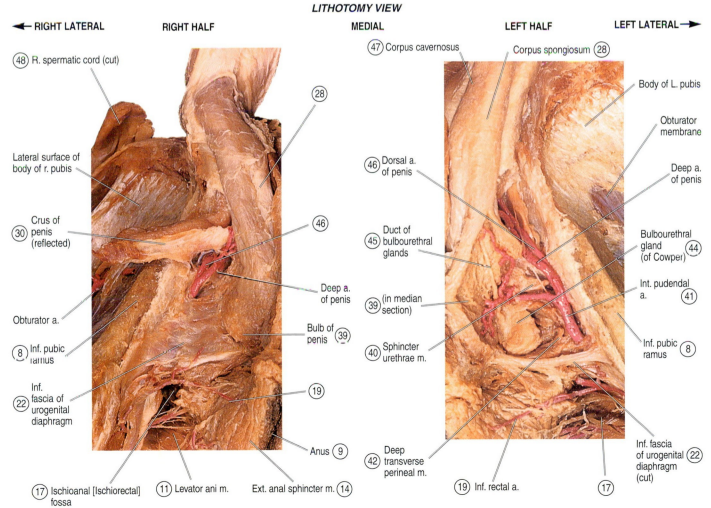

LITHOTOMY VIEW

← RIGHT LATERAL   RIGHT HALF   MEDIAL   LEFT HALF   LEFT LATERAL →

(48) R. spermatic cord (cut)

(47) Corpus cavernosus   Corpus spongiosum (28)

Body of L. pubis

(28)

Lateral surface of body of r. pubis

Obturator membrane

(46) Dorsal a. of penis

Deep a. of penis

Crus of
(30) penis (reflected)

(46)

Duct of
(45) bulbourethral glands

Bulbourethral gland (44) (of Cowper)

Deep a. of penis

Obturator a.

(39) (in median section)

Int. pudendal a. (41)

(8) Inf. pubic ramus

Bulb of penis (39)

(40) Sphincter urethrae m.

Inf. pubic ramus (8)

Inf.
(22) fascia of urogenital diaphragm

(19)

Anus (9)

(42) Deep transverse perineal m.

Inf. fascia of urogenital (22) diaphragm (cut)

(17) Ischioanal [Ischiorectal] fossa   (11) Levator ani m.   Ext. anal sphincter m. (14)

(19) Inf. rectal a.   (17)

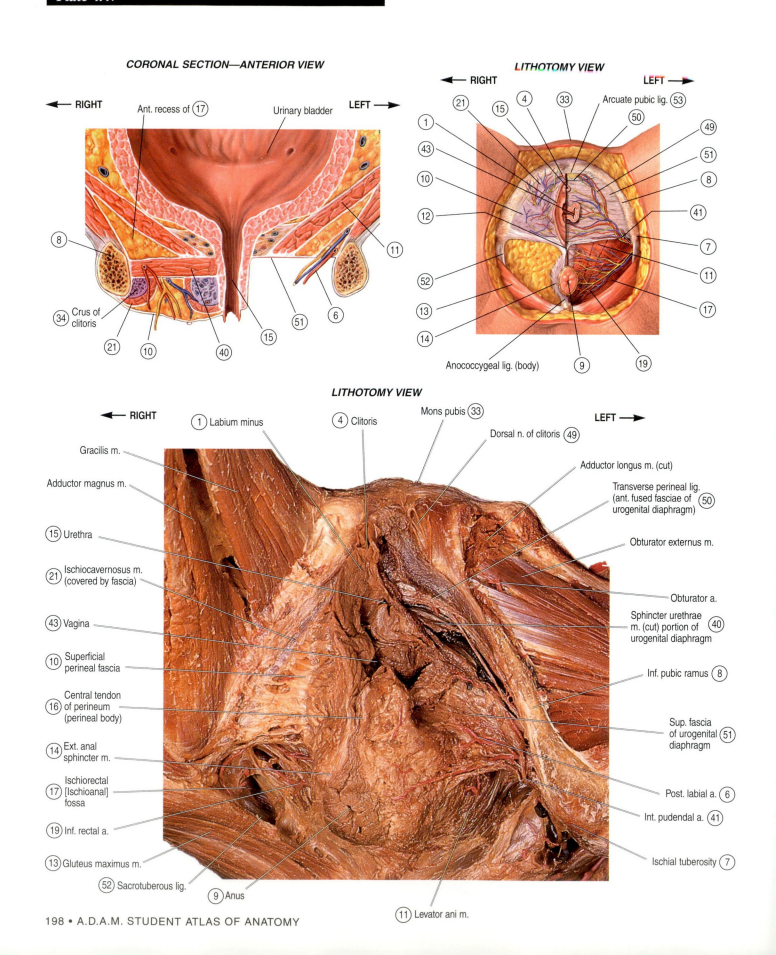

CORONAL SECTION—ANTERIOR VIEW

← RIGHT

Ant. recess of ⑰

Urinary bladder

LEFT →

⑧

③④ Crus of clitoris

㉑ ⑩ ㊵ ⑮ ⑥ ⑪

LITHOTOMY VIEW

← RIGHT   LEFT →

㉑ ⑮ ④ ㉝   Arcuate pubic lig. ㊿ ㊼

⑤⓪ ㊾ ㊿ ⑤① ⑧ ㊶ ⑦ ⑪ ⑰

① ㊸ ⑩ ⑫ ㊼ ⑤② ⑬ ⑭

Anococcygeal lig. (body)   ⑨   ⑲

LITHOTOMY VIEW

← RIGHT

① Labium minus   ④ Clitoris   Mons pubis ㉝   Dorsal n. of clitoris ㊾   LEFT →

Gracilis m.

Adductor magnus m.

⑮ Urethra

㉑ Ischiocavernosus m. (covered by fascia)

㊸ Vagina

⑩ Superficial perineal fascia

⑯ Central tendon of perineum (perineal body)

⑭ Ext. anal sphincter m.

⑰ Ischiorectal [Ischioanal] fossa

⑲ Inf. rectal a.

⑬ Gluteus maximus m.

⑤② Sacrotuberous lig.

⑨ Anus

Adductor longus m. (cut)

Transverse perineal lig. (ant. fused fasciae of urogenital diaphragm) ㊿

Obturator externus m.

Obturator a.

Sphincter urethrae m. (cut) portion of urogenital diaphragm ㊵

Inf. pubic ramus ⑧

Sup. fascia of urogenital ⑤① diaphragm

Post. labial a. ⑥

Int. pudendal a. ㊶

Ischial tuberosity ⑦

⑪ Levator ani m.

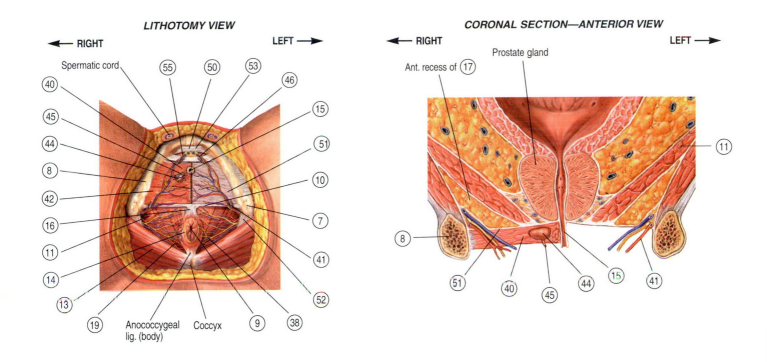

LITHOTOMY VIEW

◄── RIGHT   LEFT ──►

Spermatic cord   55   50   53   46
40
45
44
8
42
16
11
14
13
19   Anococcygeal lig. (body)   Coccyx   9   38
15
51
10
7
41
52

CORONAL SECTION—ANTERIOR VIEW

◄── RIGHT   LEFT ──►

Ant. recess of 17   Prostate gland
8
51   40   45   44   15   41
11

LITHOTOMY VIEWS

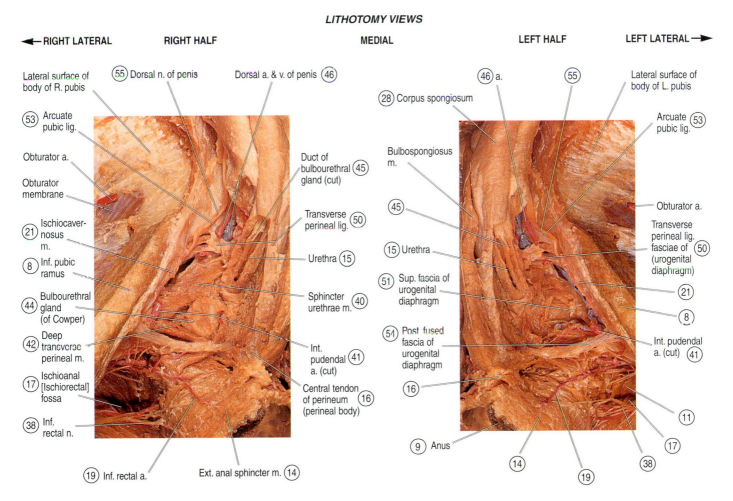

◄── RIGHT LATERAL   RIGHT HALF   MEDIAL   LEFT HALF   LEFT LATERAL ──►

Lateral surface of body of R. pubis
55 Dorsal n. of penis   Dorsal a. & v. of penis 46
53 Arcuate pubic lig.
Obturator a.
Obturator membrane
21 Ischiocaver-nosus m.
8 Inf. pubic ramus
44 Bulbourethral gland (of Cowper)
42 Deep transverse perineal m.
17 Ischioanal [Ischiorectal] fossa
38 Inf. rectal n.
19 Inf. rectal a.
Ext. anal sphincter m. 14

Duct of bulbourethral gland (cut) 45
Transverse perineal lig. 50
Urethra 15
Sphincter urethrae m. 40
Int. pudendal a. (cut) 41
Central tendon of perineum (perineal body) 16

46 a.   55
28 Corpus spongiosum
Bulbospongiosus m.
45
15 Urethra
51 Sup. fascia of urogenital diaphragm
54 Post. fused fascia of urogenital diaphragm
16
9 Anus
14   19   38

Lateral surface of body of L. pubis
Arcuate pubic lig. 53
Obturator a.
Transverse perineal lig. 50 fasciae of (urogenital diaphragm)
21
8
Int. pudendal a. (cut) 41
11
17

CORONAL SECTION—ANTERIOR VIEW

← RIGHT   LEFT →

Sup. fascia of pelvic diaphragm
Obturator internus m.
Urinary bladder

Inf. fascia of pelvic diaphragm

Ant. recess of (17)

LITHOTOMY VIEW

← RIGHT   LEFT →

Arcuate pubic lig.

Fat in (17)

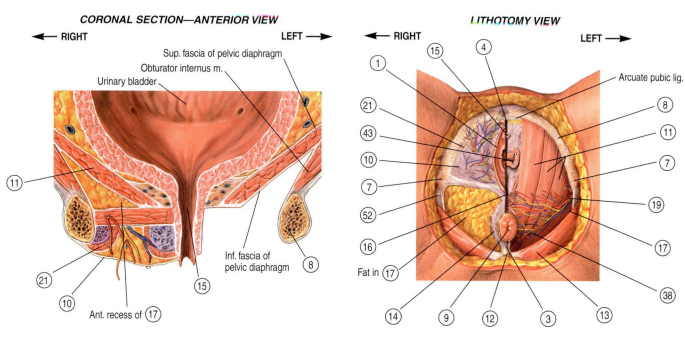

LITHOTOMY VIEW

← RIGHT   LEFT →

(1) Labium minus
(4) Clitoris
Sup. pubic ramus
Femoral v.
Obturator externus m.

(15) Urethra

Int. pudendal v.

(21) Ischiocavernosus m.—covered by fascia

Inf. pubic ramus (8)

(43) Vagina

Deep a. of clitoris

(10) Superficial perineal fascia

Inf. rectal a. (19)

Inf. rectal n. (38)

(16) Central tendon of perineum (perineal body)

Ischial tuberosity (7)

Sacrotuberous lig. (52)

(17) Ischioanal [Ischiorectal] fossa

Levator ani m. (11)

Ext. anal sphincter m. (14)

(13) Gluteus maximus m.
(9) Anus
(12) Coccyx
Anococcygeal lig. (body) (3)

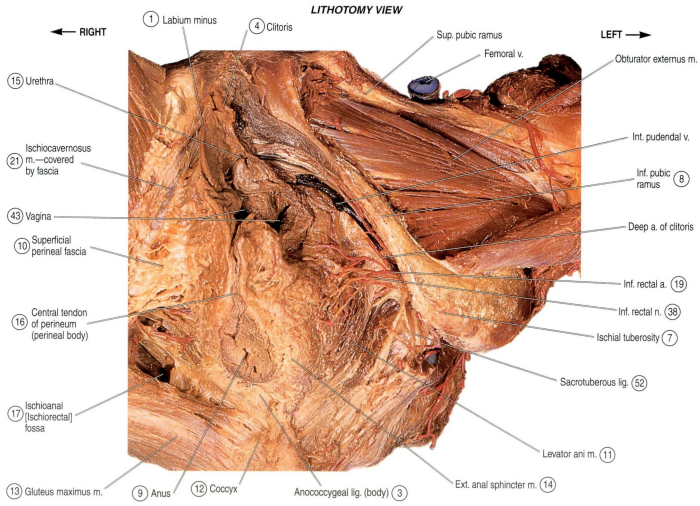

LITHOTOMY VIEW

← RIGHT   LEFT →

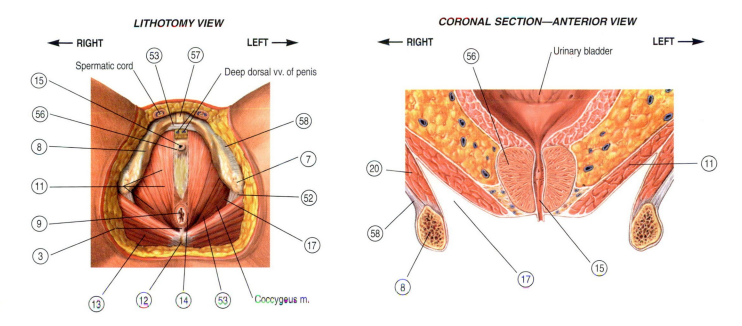

(53) (57)

Spermatic cord

(15)

Deep dorsal vv. of penis

(56)

(8)

(58)

(7)

(11)

(52)

(9)

(17)

(3)

(13) (12) (14) (53)   Coccygeus m.

CORONAL SECTION—ANTERIOR VIEW

← RIGHT   LEFT →

(56)   Urinary bladder

(20)

(11)

(58)

(8)

(17)

(15)

LITHOTOMY VIEW

← RIGHT   LEFT →

(15) Urethra   Puboprostatic m.   (57) Pubic symphysis   Arcuate pubic lig. (53)   Obturator membrane (58)

(56) Prostate gland   Obturator canal

(11) Levator ani m.   Puborectalis m. part of (11)

Inf. pubic ramus (8)

Obturator internus m. fascia

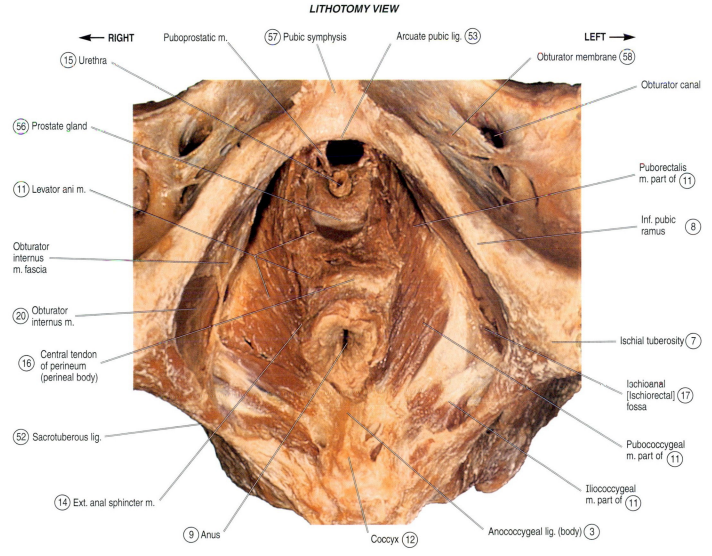

(20) Obturator internus m.

Ischial tuberosity (7)

(16) Central tendon of perineum (perineal body)

Ischioanal [Ischiorectal] (17) fossa

(52) Sacrotuberous lig.

Pubococcygeal m. part of (11)

(14) Ext. anal sphincter m.

Iliococcygeal m. part of (11)

(9) Anus   Coccyx (12)   Anococcygeal lig. (body) (3)

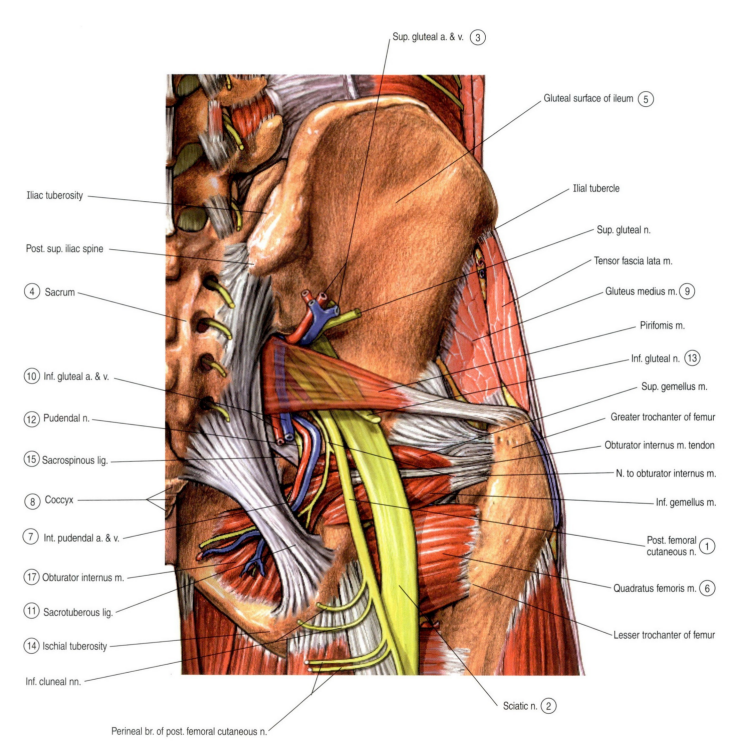

Sup. gluteal a. & v. ③

Gluteal surface of ileum ⑤

Iliac tuberosity

Ilial tubercle

Post. sup. iliac spine

Sup. gluteal n.

Tensor fascia lata m.

④ Sacrum

Gluteus medius m. ⑨

Pirifomis m.

⑩ Inf. gluteal a. & v.

Inf. gluteal n. ⑬

⑫ Pudendal n.

Sup. gemellus m.

Greater trochanter of femur

⑮ Sacrospinous lig.

Obturator internus m. tendon

N. to obturator internus m.

⑧ Coccyx

Inf. gemellus m.

⑦ Int. pudendal a. & v.

Post. femoral cutaneous n. ①

⑰ Obturator internus m.

Quadratus femoris m. ⑥

⑪ Sacrotuberous lig.

Lesser trochanter of femur

⑭ Ischial tuberosity

Inf. cluneal nn.

Sciatic n. ②

Perineal br. of post. femoral cutaneous n.

GLUTEAL REGION—POSTERIOR VIEW

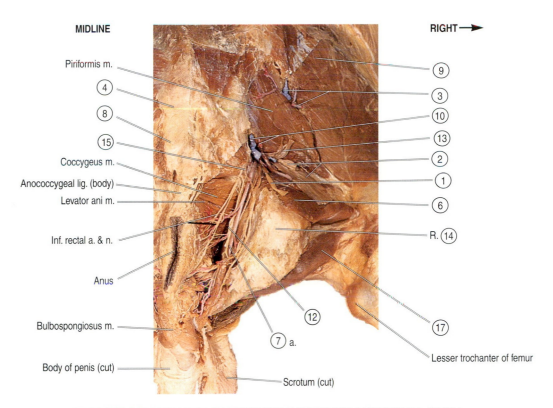

MIDLINE

RIGHT →

Piriformis m.

④

⑧

⑮

Coccygeus m.

Anococcygeal lig. (body)

Levator ani m.

Inf. rectal a. & n.

Anus

Bulbospongiosus m.

Body of penis (cut)

⑨

③

⑩

⑬

②

①

⑥

R. ⑭

⑰

⑫

⑦ a.

Lesser trochanter of femur

Scrotum (cut)

INFERIOR OBLIQUE VIEW OF RIGHT MALE PERINEUM & PUDENDAL CANAL

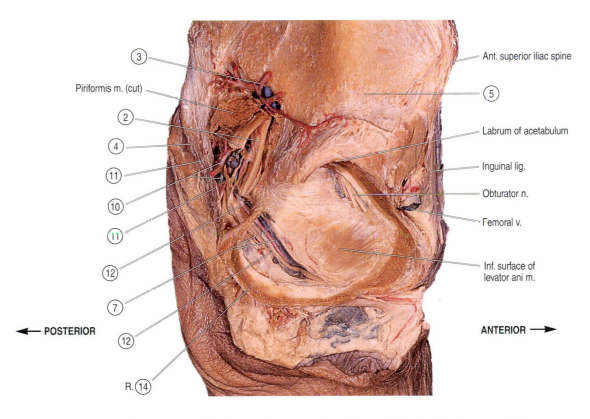

③

Piriformis m. (cut)

②

④

⑪

⑩

⑪

⑫

⑦

⑫

Ant. superior iliac spine

⑤

Labrum of acetabulum

Inguinal lig.

Obturator n.

Femoral v.

Inf. surface of
levator ani m.

← POSTERIOR

ANTERIOR →

R. ⑭

DISSECTION OF FEMALE PERINEUM FROM LATERAL APPROACH (ACETABULUM REMOVED)

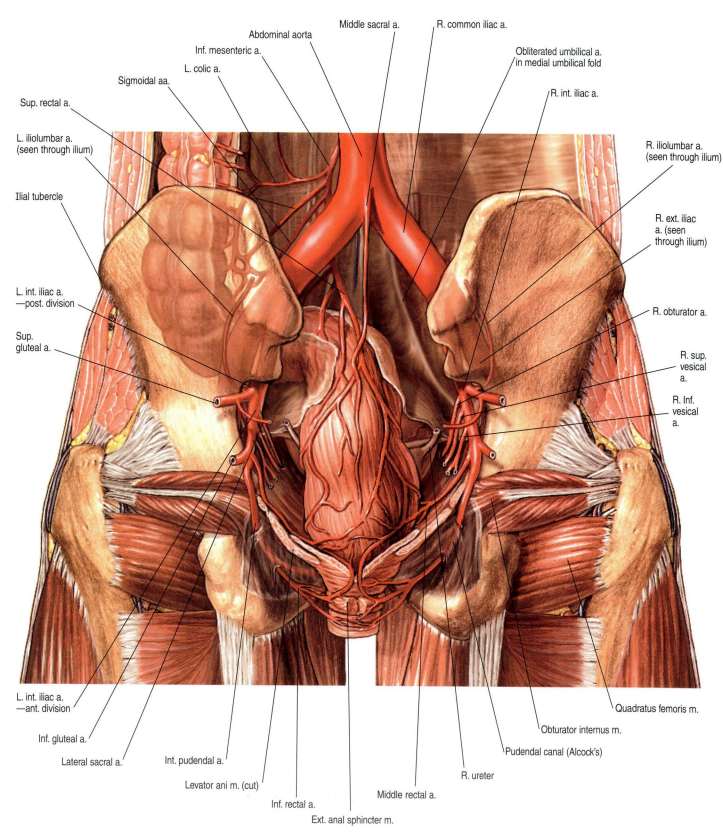

Middle sacral a.

R. common iliac a.

Abdominal aorta

Inf. mesenteric a.

Obliterated umbilical a. in medial umbilical fold

L. colic a.

Sigmoidal aa.

R. int. iliac a.

Sup. rectal a.

L. iliolumbar a. (seen through ilium)

R. iliolumbar a. (seen through ilium)

Ilial tubercle

R. ext. iliac a. (seen through ilium)

L. int. iliac a. —post. division

R. obturator a.

Sup. gluteal a.

R. sup. vesical a.

R. Inf. vesical a.

L. int. iliac a. —ant. division

Quadratus femoris m.

Inf. gluteal a.

Obturator internus m.

Lateral sacral a.

Pudendal canal (Alcock's)

Int. pudendal a.

R. ureter

Levator ani m. (cut)

Middle rectal a.

Inf. rectal a.

Ext. anal sphincter m.

POSTERIOR VIEW WITH SACRUM REMOVED

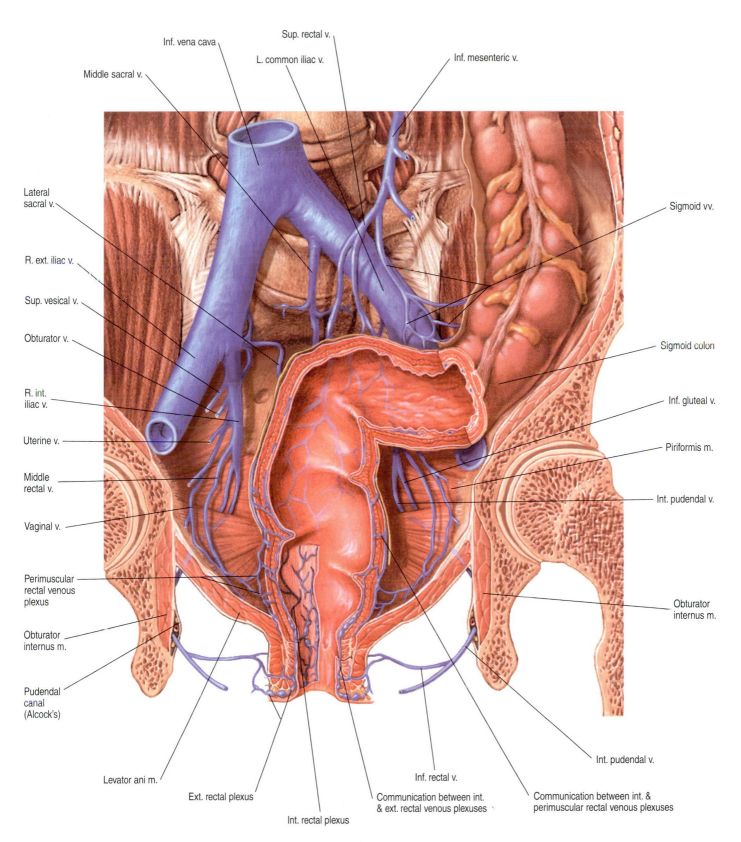

Inf. vena cava

Sup. rectal v.

Middle sacral v.

L. common iliac v.

Inf. mesenteric v.

Lateral sacral v.

Sigmoid vv.

R. ext. iliac v.

Sup. vesical v.

Obturator v.

Sigmoid colon

R. int. iliac v.

Inf. gluteal v.

Uterine v.

Piriformis m.

Middle rectal v.

Int. pudendal v.

Vaginal v.

Perimuscular rectal venous plexus

Obturator internus m.

Obturator internus m.

Pudendal canal (Alcock's)

Int. pudendal v.

Levator ani m.

Ext. rectal plexus

Inf. rectal v.

Communication between int. & ext. rectal venous plexuses

Communication between int. & perimuscular rectal venous plexuses

Int. rectal plexus

CORONAL SECTION—ANTERIOR VIEW

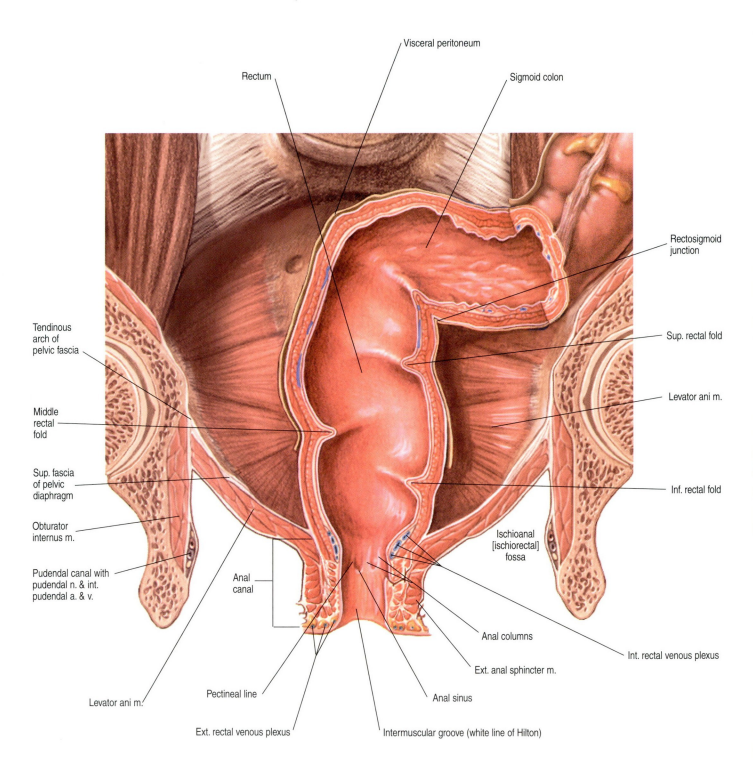

Visceral peritoneum

Rectum

Sigmoid colon

Rectosigmoid junction

Tendinous arch of pelvic fascia

Sup. rectal fold

Middle rectal fold

Levator ani m.

Sup. fascia of pelvic diaphragm

Inf. rectal fold

Obturator internus m.

Pudendal canal with pudendal n. & int. pudendal a. & v.

Ischioanal [ischiorectal] fossa

Anal canal

Anal columns

Int. rectal venous plexus

Levator ani m.

Pectineal line

Ext. anal sphincter m.

Ext. rectal venous plexus

Anal sinus

Intermuscular groove (white line of Hilton)

CORONAL SECTION—ANTERIOR VIEW

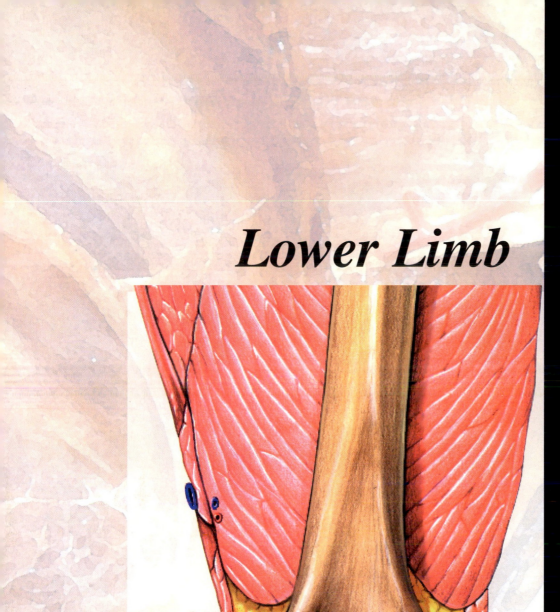

Lower Limb

Chapter **5**

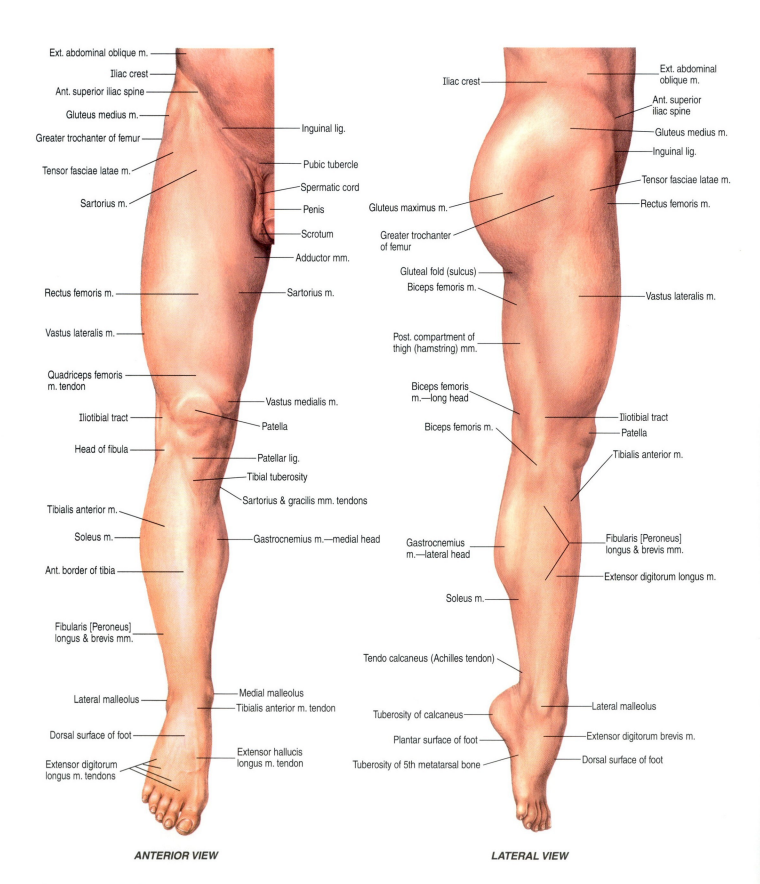

Ext. abdominal oblique m.
Iliac crest
Ant. superior iliac spine
Gluteus medius m.
Greater trochanter of femur
Tensor fasciae latae m.
Sartorius m.
Rectus femoris m.
Vastus lateralis m.
Quadriceps femoris m. tendon
Iliotibial tract
Head of fibula
Tibialis anterior m.
Soleus m.
Ant. border of tibia
Fibularis [Peroneus] longus & brevis mm.
Lateral malleolus
Dorsal surface of foot
Extensor digitorum longus m. tendons

Inguinal lig.
Pubic tubercle
Spermatic cord
Penis
Scrotum
Adductor mm.
Sartorius m.
Vastus medialis m.
Patella
Patellar lig.
Tibial tuberosity
Sartorius & gracilis mm. tendons
Gastrocnemius m.—medial head
Medial malleolus
Tibialis anterior m. tendon
Extensor hallucis longus m. tendon

ANTERIOR VIEW

Iliac crest
Gluteus maximus m.
Greater trochanter of femur
Gluteal fold (sulcus)
Biceps femoris m.
Post. compartment of thigh (hamstring) mm.
Biceps femoris m.—long head
Biceps femoris m.
Gastrocnemius m.—lateral head
Soleus m.
Tendo calcaneus (Achilles tendon)
Tuberosity of calcaneus
Plantar surface of foot
Tuberosity of 5th metatarsal bone

Ext. abdominal oblique m.
Ant. superior iliac spine
Gluteus medius m.
Inguinal lig.
Tensor fasciae latae m.
Rectus femoris m.
Vastus lateralis m.
Iliotibial tract
Patella
Tibialis anterior m.
Fibularis [Peroneus] longus & brevis mm.
Extensor digitorum longus m.
Lateral malleolus
Extensor digitorum brevis m.
Dorsal surface of foot

LATERAL VIEW

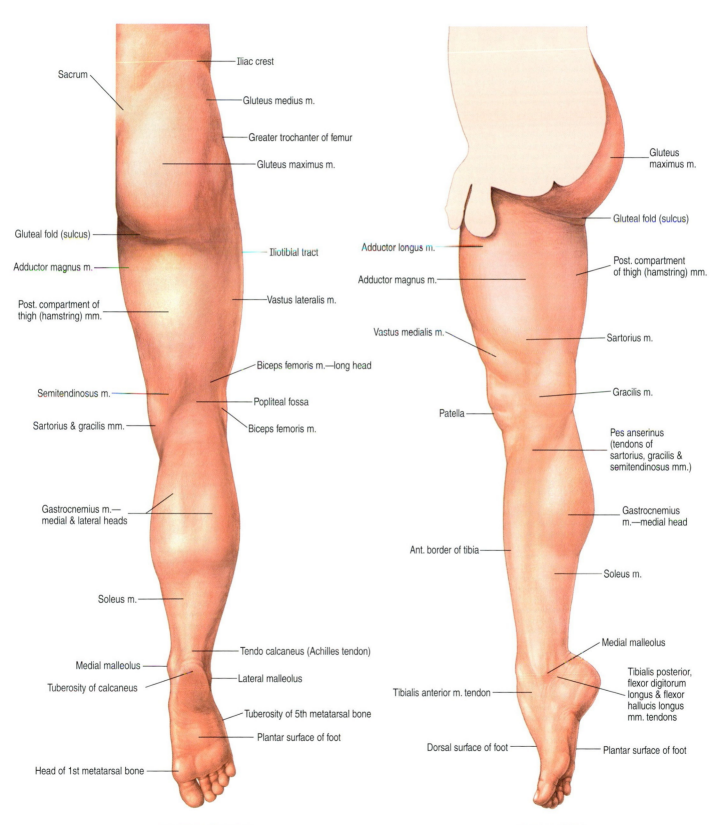

Iliac crest

Sacrum

Gluteus medius m.

Greater trochanter of femur

Gluteus maximus m.

Gluteal fold (sulcus)

Adductor magnus m.

Iliotibial tract

Post. compartment of thigh (hamstring) mm.

Vastus lateralis m.

Biceps femoris m.—long head

Semitendinosus m.

Popliteal fossa

Sartorius & gracilis mm.

Biceps femoris m.

Gastrocnemius m.—medial & lateral heads

Soleus m.

Tendo calcaneus (Achilles tendon)

Medial malleolus

Lateral malleolus

Tuberosity of calcaneus

Tuberosity of 5th metatarsal bone

Plantar surface of foot

Head of 1st metatarsal bone

Gluteus maximus m.

Gluteal fold (sulcus)

Adductor longus m.

Post. compartment of thigh (hamstring) mm.

Adductor magnus m.

Vastus medialis m.

Sartorius m.

Gracilis m.

Patella

Pes anserinus (tendons of sartorius, gracilis & semitendinosus mm.)

Gastrocnemius m.—medial head

Ant. border of tibia

Soleus m.

Medial malleolus

Tibialis posterior, flexor digitorum longus & flexor hallucis longus mm. tendons

Tibialis anterior m. tendon

Dorsal surface of foot

Plantar surface of foot

POSTERIOR VIEW

MEDIAL VIEW

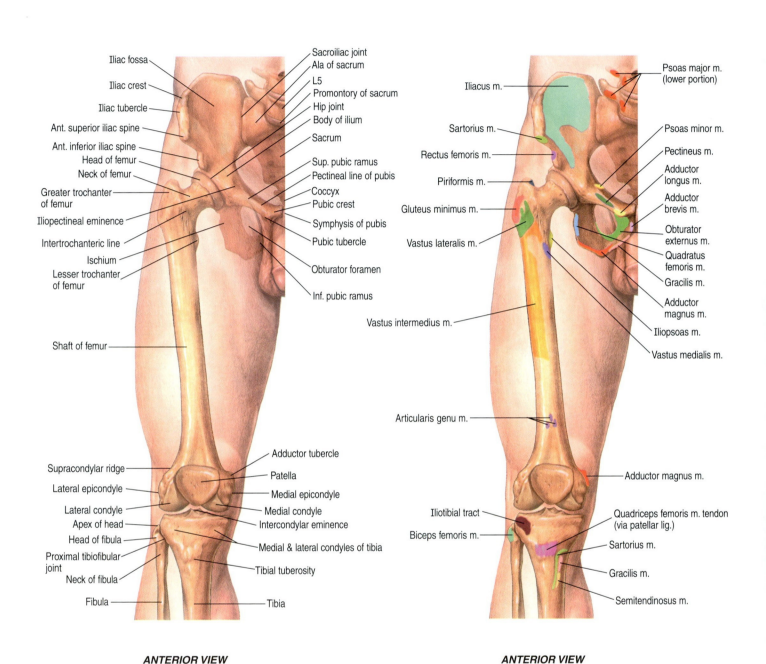

Iliac fossa
Iliac crest
Iliac tubercle
Ant. superior iliac spine
Ant. inferior iliac spine
Head of femur
Neck of femur
Greater trochanter of femur
Iliopectineal eminence
Intertrochanteric line
Ischium
Lesser trochanter of femur
Shaft of femur
Supracondylar ridge
Lateral epicondyle
Lateral condyle
Apex of head
Head of fibula
Proximal tibiofibular joint
Neck of fibula
Fibula

Sacroiliac joint
Ala of sacrum
L5
Promontory of sacrum
Hip joint
Body of ilium
Sacrum
Sup. pubic ramus
Pectineal line of pubis
Coccyx
Pubic crest
Symphysis of pubis
Pubic tubercle
Obturator foramen
Inf. pubic ramus
Adductor tubercle
Patella
Medial epicondyle
Medial condyle
Intercondylar eminence
Medial & lateral condyles of tibia
Tibial tuberosity
Tibia

ANTERIOR VIEW

Iliacus m.
Sartorius m.
Rectus femoris m.
Piriformis m.
Gluteus minimus m.
Vastus lateralis m.
Vastus intermedius m.
Articularis genu m.
Iliotibial tract
Biceps femoris m.

Psoas major m. (lower portion)
Psoas minor m.
Pectineus m.
Adductor longus m.
Adductor brevis m.
Obturator externus m.
Quadratus femoris m.
Gracilis m.
Adductor magnus m.
Iliopsoas m.
Vastus medialis m.
Adductor magnus m.
Quadriceps femoris m. tendon (via patellar lig.)
Sartorius m.
Gracilis m.
Semitendinosus m.

ANTERIOR VIEW

- Gluteus minimus
- Vastus lateralis
- Vastus medialis
- Iliopsoas
- Vastus intermedius
- Obturator externus

- Adductor longus
- Iliotibial tract
- Piriformis
- Articularis genu
- Patellar ligament
- Sartorius

- Gracilis
- Adductor brevis
- Quadratus femoris
- Biceps femoris
- Semitendinosus
- Iliacus

- Psoas major
- Rectus femoris
- Psoas minor
- Adductor magnus
- Pectineus

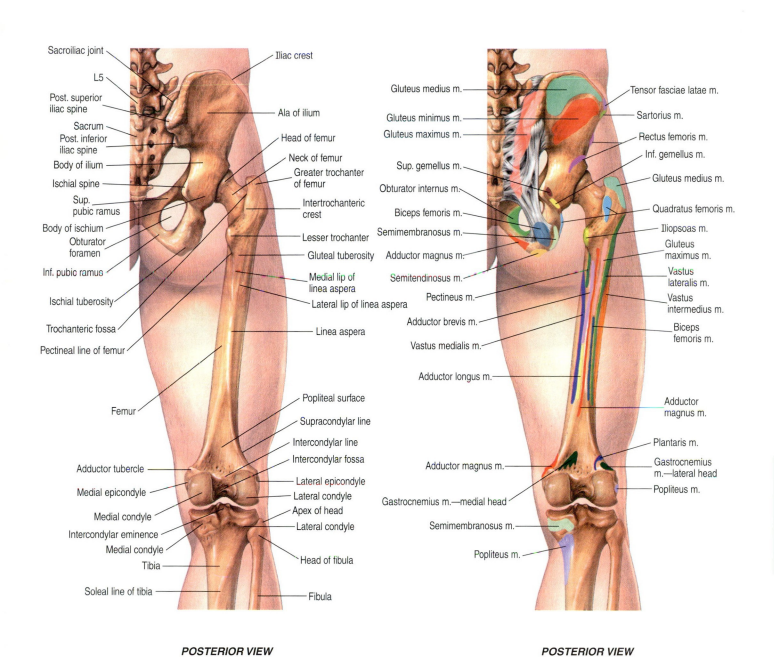

Sacroiliac joint
Iliac crest
L5
Post. superior iliac spine
Ala of ilium
Sacrum
Post. inferior iliac spine
Head of femur
Body of ilium
Neck of femur
Greater trochanter of femur
Ischial spine
Sup. pubic ramus
Intertrochanteric crest
Body of ischium
Lesser trochanter
Obturator foramen
Gluteal tuberosity
Inf. pubic ramus
Medial lip of linea aspera
Ischial tuberosity
Lateral lip of linea aspera
Trochanteric fossa
Pectineal line of femur
Linea aspera
Femur
Popliteal surface
Supracondylar line
Intercondylar line
Intercondylar fossa
Adductor tubercle
Lateral epicondyle
Medial epicondyle
Lateral condyle
Medial condyle
Apex of head
Intercondylar eminence
Lateral condyle
Medial condyle
Tibia
Head of fibula
Soleal line of tibia
Fibula

POSTERIOR VIEW

Gluteus medius m.
Tensor fasciae latae m.
Gluteus minimus m.
Sartorius m.
Gluteus maximus m.
Rectus femoris m.
Inf. gemellus m.
Sup. gemellus m.
Gluteus medius m.
Obturator internus m.
Quadratus femoris m.
Biceps femoris m.
Iliopsoas m.
Semimembranosus m.
Gluteus maximus m.
Adductor magnus m.
Vastus lateralis m.
Semitendinosus m.
Vastus intermedius m.
Pectineus m.
Adductor brevis m.
Biceps femoris m.
Vastus medialis m.
Adductor longus m.
Adductor magnus m.
Plantaris m.
Adductor magnus m.
Gastrocnemius m.—lateral head
Popliteus m.
Gastrocnemius m.—medial head
Semimembranosus m.
Popliteus m.

POSTERIOR VIEW

- Sartorius
- Rectus femoris
- Tensor fasciae latae
- Gluteus medius
- Gluteus minimus
- Obturator internus
- Semimembranosus
- Popliteus
- Adductor magnus
- Gluteus maximus
- Quadratus femoris
- Inferior gemellus
- Superior gemellus
- Semitendinosus
- Biceps femoris
- Gastrocnemius
- Iliopsoas
- Pectineus
- Vastus medialis
- Adductor brevis
- Adductor longus
- Vastus lateralis
- Vastus intermedius
- Plantaris

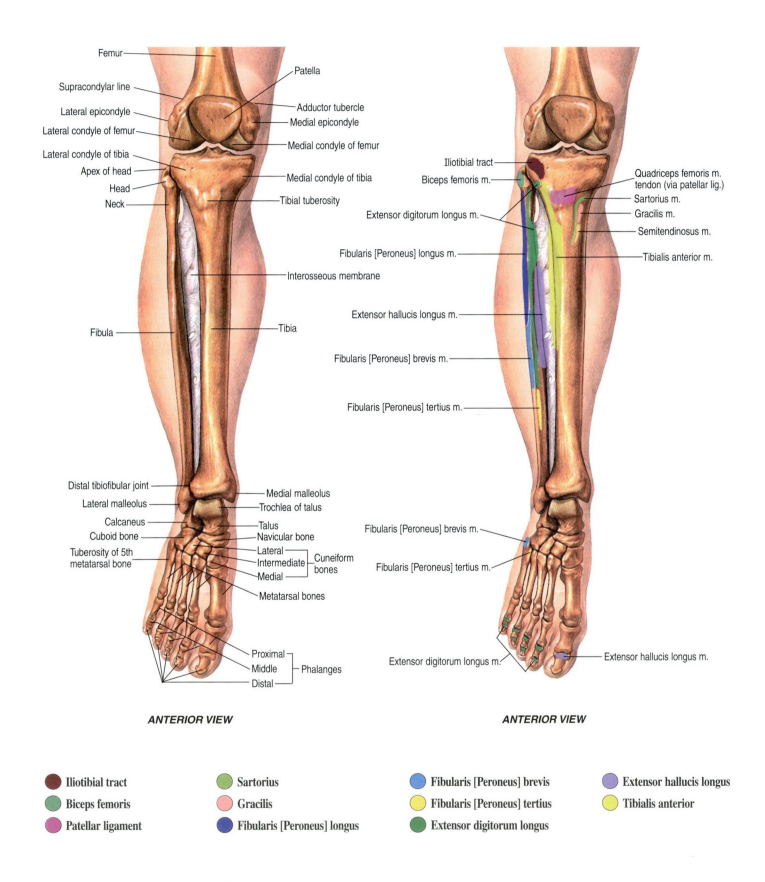

Femur

Supracondylar line

Lateral epicondyle

Lateral condyle of femur

Lateral condyle of tibia

Apex of head

Head

Neck

Fibula

Distal tibiofibular joint

Lateral malleolus

Calcaneus

Cuboid bone

Tuberosity of 5th metatarsal bone

Patella

Adductor tubercle

Medial epicondyle

Medial condyle of femur

Medial condyle of tibia

Tibial tuberosity

Interosseous membrane

Tibia

Medial malleolus

Trochlea of talus

Talus

Navicular bone

Lateral
Intermediate — Cuneiform bones
Medial

Metatarsal bones

Proximal
Middle — Phalanges
Distal

ANTERIOR VIEW

Iliotibial tract

Biceps femoris m.

Extensor digitorum longus m.

Fibularis [Peroneus] longus m.

Extensor hallucis longus m.

Fibularis [Peroneus] brevis m.

Fibularis [Peroneus] tertius m.

Fibularis [Peroneus] brevis m.

Fibularis [Peroneus] tertius m.

Extensor digitorum longus m.

Quadriceps femoris m. tendon (via patellar lig.)

Sartorius m.

Gracilis m.

Semitendinosus m.

Tibialis anterior m.

Extensor hallucis longus m.

ANTERIOR VIEW

Iliotibial tract

Biceps femoris

Patellar ligament

Sartorius

Gracilis

Fibularis [Peroneus] longus

Fibularis [Peroneus] brevis

Fibularis [Peroneus] tertius

Extensor digitorum longus

Extensor hallucis longus

Tibialis anterior

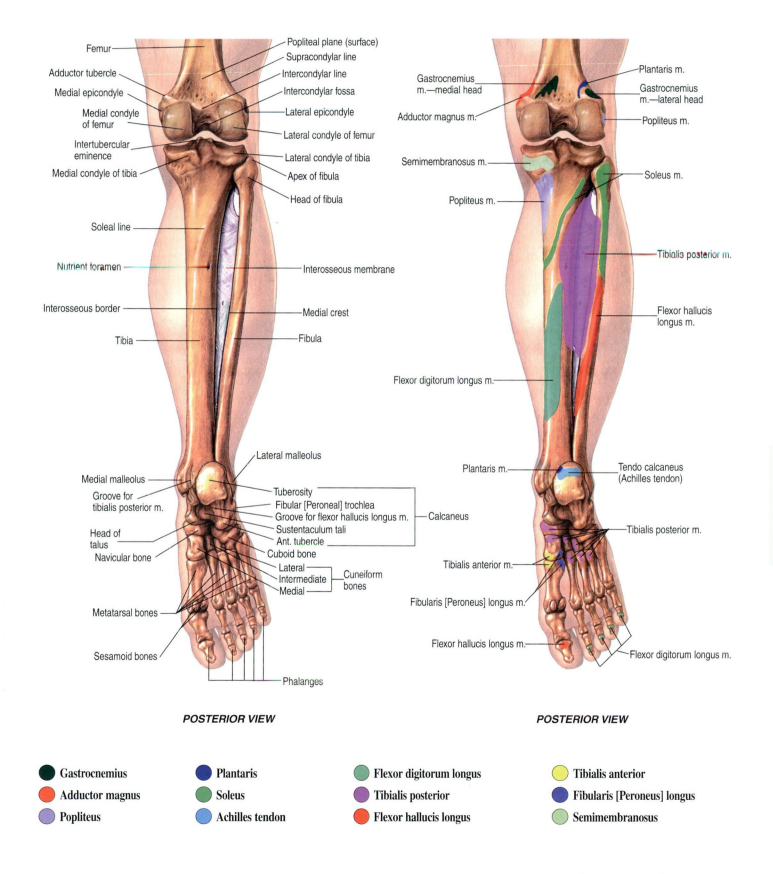

Femur
Popliteal plane (surface)
Supracondylar line
Adductor tubercle
Intercondylar line
Medial epicondyle
Intercondylar fossa
Medial condyle of femur
Lateral epicondyle
Lateral condyle of femur
Intertubercular eminence
Lateral condyle of tibia
Medial condyle of tibia
Apex of fibula
Head of fibula
Soleal line
Nutrient foramen
Interosseous membrane
Interosseous border
Medial crest
Tibia
Fibula

Lateral malleolus
Medial malleolus
Tuberosity
Groove for tibialis posterior m.
Fibular [Peroneal] trochlea
Groove for flexor hallucis longus m.
Calcaneus
Head of talus
Sustentaculum tali
Ant. tubercle
Navicular bone
Cuboid bone
Metatarsal bones
Lateral
Intermediate
Cuneiform bones
Medial
Sesamoid bones
Phalanges

Gastrocnemius m.—medial head
Plantaris m.
Gastrocnemius m.—lateral head
Adductor magnus m.
Popliteus m.
Semimembranosus m.
Soleus m.
Popliteus m.
Tibialis posterior m.
Flexor hallucis longus m.
Flexor digitorum longus m.
Plantaris m.
Tendo calcaneus (Achilles tendon)
Calcaneus
Tibialis posterior m.
Tibialis anterior m.
Fibularis [Peroneus] longus m.
Flexor hallucis longus m.
Flexor digitorum longus m.

POSTERIOR VIEW

POSTERIOR VIEW

● **Gastrocnemius**   ● **Plantaris**   ● **Flexor digitorum longus**   ● **Tibialis anterior**

● **Adductor magnus**   ● **Soleus**   ● **Tibialis posterior**   ● **Fibularis [Peroneus] longus**

● **Popliteus**   ● **Achilles tendon**   ● **Flexor hallucis longus**   ● **Semimembranosus**

Anterior Thigh Muscles
Table 5.1

Muscle	Proximal Attachment	Distal Attachment	Innervation	Main Actions
Iliopsoas Psoas major	Sides of T12 to L5 vertebral bodies, intervertebral discs between them & transverse processes of L1–L5	Lesser trochanter of femur	Ventral rami of lumbar nn. (**L1**, **L2** & L3)[a]	Act conjointly in flexing thigh at hip joint and in stabilizing this joint.
Psoas minor	Sides of T12 & L1 vertebrae & intervertebral disc	Pectineal line, iliopectineal eminence via iliopectineal arch lig.	Ventral rami of lumbar nn. (L1 & L2)	
Iliacus	Iliac crest, iliac fossa, ala of sacrum, ant. sacroiliac ligg. & capsule of hip joint	Tendon of psoas major & body of femur, inf. to lesser trochanter	Femoral n. (**L2** & L3)	
Tensor fasciae latae	Ant. sup. iliac spine & ant. part of ext. lip of iliac crest	Anterolateral aspect of lateral tibial condyle via iliotibial tract	Sup. gluteal n. (L4 & L5)	Abducts, medially rotates, and flexes thigh; helps to keep knee extended
Sartorius	Ant. sup. iliac spine & sup. part of notch inf. to it	Sup. part of medial surface of tibia	Femoral n. (L2 & L3)	Flexes, abducts & laterally rotates thigh at hip joint & flexes leg at knee joint
Quadriceps femoris Rectus femoris	Ant. inf. iliac spine & groove sup. to acetabulum			
Vastus lateralis	Greater trochanter & lateral lip of linea aspera of femur	Base of patella & via patellar lig. to tibial tuberosity	Femoral n. (L2, **L3** & **L4**)	Extend leg at knee joint; rectus femoris also helps iliopsoas to flex thigh
Vastus medialis	Intertrochanteric line & medial lip of linea aspera of femur			
Vastus intermedius	Ant. & lateral surfaces of shaft of femur			

[a]In this and subsequent tables, the numbers indicate the spinal cord segmental innervation of the nerves. For example, **L1**, **L2**, and L3 indicate that the nerves supplying the psoas major muscle are derived from the first three lumbar segments of the spinal cord; the boldface (**L1**, **L2**) indicates the main segmental innervation. Damage to one or more of these spinal cord segments or to the motor nerve roots arising from them results in paralysis of the muscles concerned.

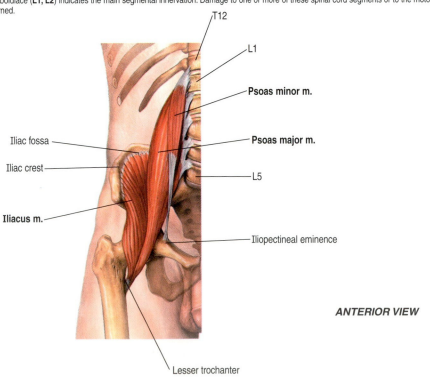

ANTERIOR VIEW

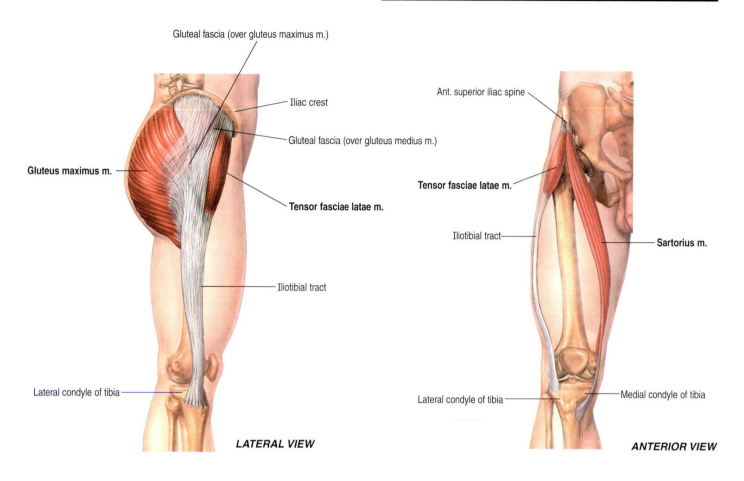

Gluteal fascia (over gluteus maximus m.)

Iliac crest

Gluteal fascia (over gluteus medius m.)

Gluteus maximus m.

Tensor fasciae latae m.

Iliotibial tract

Lateral condyle of tibia

LATERAL VIEW

Ant. superior iliac spine

Tensor fasciae latae m.

Iliotibial tract

Sartorius m.

Lateral condyle of tibia

Medial condyle of tibia

ANTERIOR VIEW

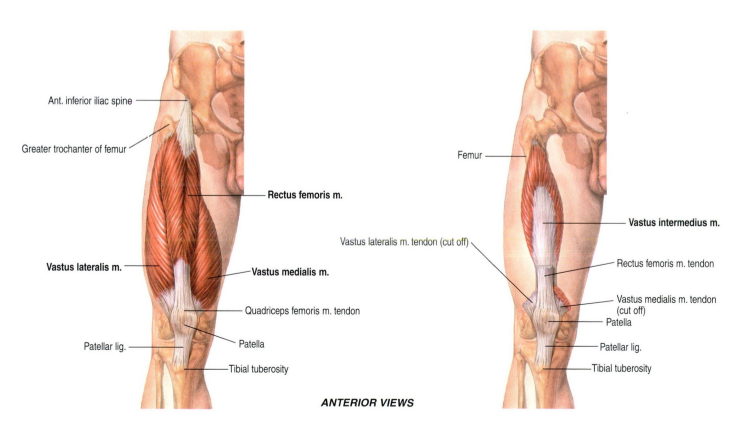

Ant. inferior iliac spine

Greater trochanter of femur

Rectus femoris m.

Vastus lateralis m.

Vastus medialis m.

Quadriceps femoris m. tendon

Patellar lig.

Patella

Tibial tuberosity

Femur

Vastus intermedius m.

Vastus lateralis m. tendon (cut off)

Rectus femoris m. tendon

Vastus medialis m. tendon (cut off)

Patella

Patellar lig.

Tibial tuberosity

ANTERIOR VIEWS

Gluteal & Posterior Thigh Muscles
Table 5.2

Gluteal Muscle	Proximal Attachment	Distal Attachment	Innervation	Main Actions
Gluteus maximus	Ext. surface of ala of ilium, including iliac crest, dorsal surface of sacrum & coccyx, and sacrotuberous lig.	Most fibers end in iliotibial tract which inserts into lateral condyle of tibia; some fibers insert on gluteal tuberosity of femur	Inf. gluteal n. (L5, **S1** & **S2**)	Extends thigh & assists in its lat. rotation; also assists in raising trunk from flexed position
Gluteus medius	Ext. surface of ilium between ant. & post. gluteal lines	Lateral surface of greater trochanter of femur	Sup. gluteal n. (**L5** & S1)	Abduct & medially rotate thigh; steady pelvis
Gluteus minimus	Ext. surface of ilium between ant. & inf. gluteal lines	Ant. surface of greater trochanter of femur		
Piriformis	Ant. surface of sacrum between S2 & S4	Superior border of greater trochanter of femur	Brr. from ventral rami of **S1** & S2	Laterally rotate extended thigh & abduct flexed thigh
Obturator internus	Pelvic surface of obturator membrane & surrounding bones	Trochanteric fossa[a]	N. to obturator internus (L5 & **S1**)	
Gemelli, superior & inferior	*Sup.:* ischial spine *Inf.:* ischial tuberosity		*Sup. gemellus,* same nerve supply as obturator internus *Inf. gemellus,* same nerve supply as quadratus femoris	
Quadratus femoris	Lateral border of ischial tuberosity	Quadrate tubercle on intertrochanteric crest of femur & inf. to it	N. to quadratus femoris (L5 & S1)	Laterally rotates thigh[b]

[a]The gemelli muscles blend with the tendon of the obturator internus muscle as it attaches to the trochanteric fossa.
[b]There are six lateral rotators of the thigh: piriformis, obturator internus, gemelli (superior and inferior), quadratus femoris, and obturator externus. These muscles also stabilize the hip joint.

Post. Thigh Muscle	Proximal Attachment	Distal Attachment	Innervation	Main Actions
Semitendinosus	Ischial tuberosity	Medial surface of sup. part of tibia	Tibial division of sciatic n. (**L5, S1** & S2)	Extend thigh; flex leg and rotate it medially; when thigh & leg are flexed, they can extend trunk
Semimembranous		Post. part of medial condyle of tibia		
Biceps femoris	*Long head:* Ischial tuberosity *Short head:* Lateral lip of distal half of linea aspera & lateral supracondylar line	Lateral side of head of fibular	*Long head:* Tibial division of sciatic n. (L5, **S1** & S2) *Short head:* Common fibular (peroneal) division of sciatic n. (L5, **S1** & S2)	Flexes leg & rotates it laterally; extends thigh (*e.g.,* when starting to walk)

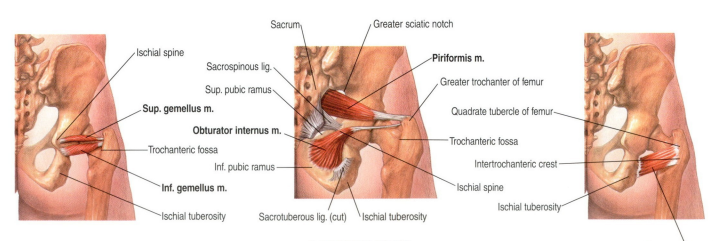

POSTERIOR VIEWS

POSTERIOR VIEW

LATERAL VIEWS

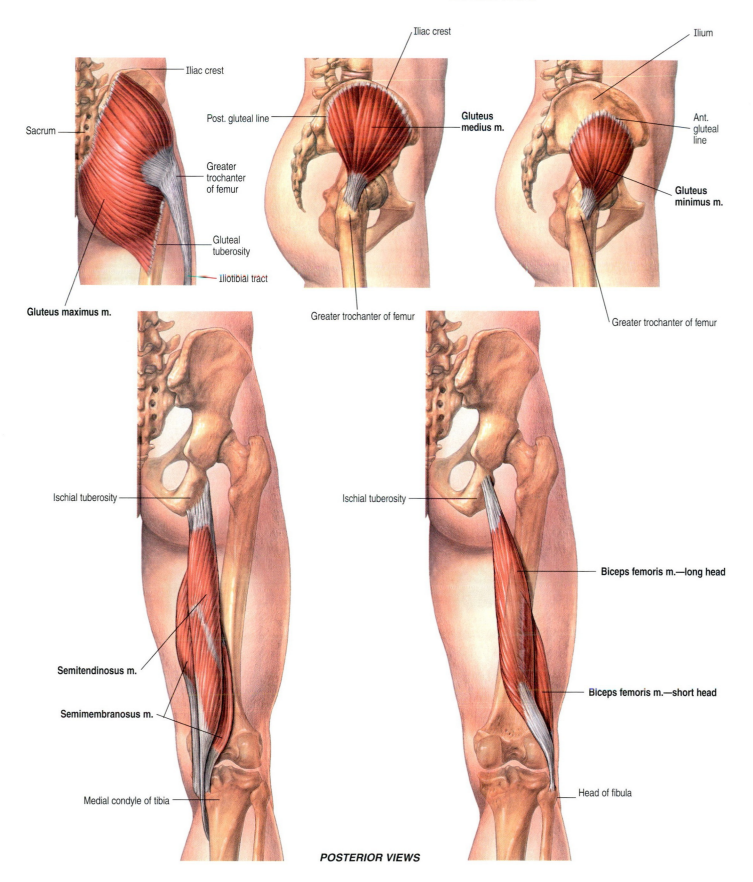

Iliac crest

Ilium

Iliac crest

Post. gluteal line

**Gluteus
medius m.**

Ant.
gluteal
line

Sacrum

Greater
trochanter
of femur

**Gluteus
minimus m.**

Gluteal
tuberosity

Iliotibial tract

Gluteus maximus m.

Greater trochanter of femur

Greater trochanter of femur

Ischial tuberosity

Ischial tuberosity

Biceps femoris m.—long head

Semitendinosus m.

Semimembranosus m.

Biceps femoris m.—short head

Medial condyle of tibia

Head of fibula

POSTERIOR VIEWS

Medial Thigh Muscles
Table 5.3

Muscle[a]	Proximal Attachment	Distal Attachment	Innervation	Main Actions
Pectineus	Pecten pubis	Pectineal line of femur	Femoral nerve (**L2** & L3) & br. from obturator n. (L2, L3)	Adducts; flexes & laterally rotates thigh
Adductor longus	Body of pubis, inf. to pubic crest	Middle third of linea aspera of femur	Obturator n. ant. br. (L2, **L3** & L4)	Adducts thigh
Adductor brevis	Body & inf. ramus of pubis	Pectineal line & proximal part of linea aspera of femur	Obturator n. (L2, **L3** & L4)	Adducts thigh & to some extent flexes it
Adductor magnus	Inf. ramus of pubis, ramus of ischium (adductor part) & ischial tuberosity	Gluteal tuberosity, linea aspera med., supracondylar line (adductor part) & adductor tubercle of femur (hamstring part)	*Adductor part,* obturator n. (L2, **L3** & L4) *Hamstring part,* tibial portion of sciatic n. (**L4**)	Adducts thigh; its adductor part also flexes thigh & its hamstring part extends it
Gracilis	Body & inf. ramus of pubis	Sup. part of med. surface of tibia	Obturator n. (**L2**, L3 & L4)	Adducts thigh, flexes leg & helps to rotate it medially
Obturator externus	Margins of obturator foramen & ext. surface of obturator membrane	Trochanteric fossa of femur	Obturator n. (L3 & **L4**)	Laterally rotates thigh

[a]Collectively, the first five muscles listed are known as the *adductors of the thigh*, but their actions are more complex than this, *e.g.,* they act as *fixors of the hip* during flexion of the knee joint and are active during walking.

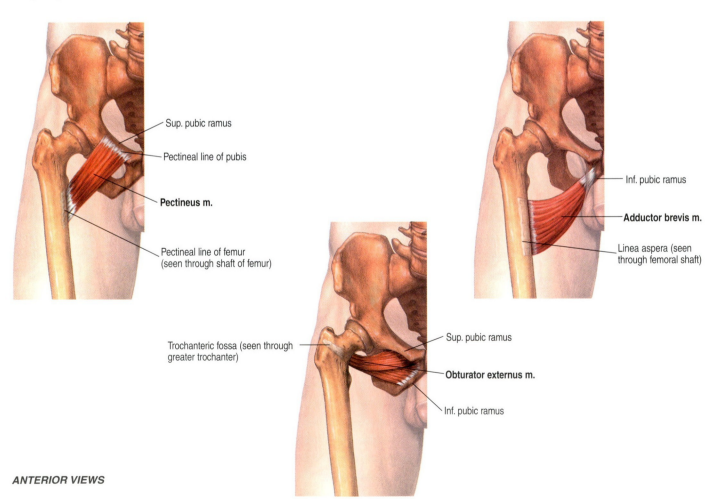

Sup. pubic ramus

Pectineal line of pubis

Pectineus m.

Pectineal line of femur (seen through shaft of femur)

Inf. pubic ramus

Adductor brevis m.

Linea aspera (seen through femoral shaft)

Trochanteric fossa (seen through greater trochanter)

Sup. pubic ramus

Obturator externus m.

Inf. pubic ramus

ANTERIOR VIEWS

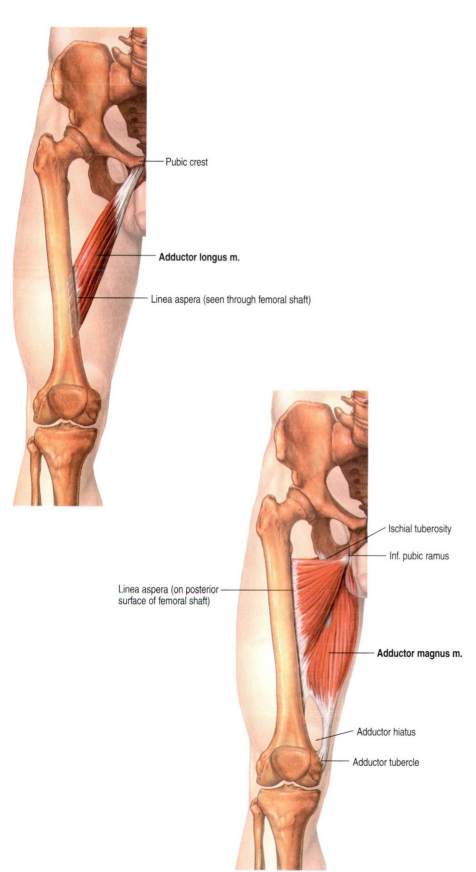

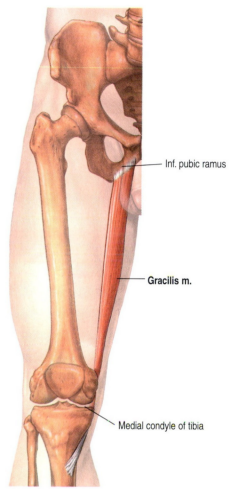

Pubic crest

Adductor longus m.

Linea aspera (seen through femoral shaft)

Inf. pubic ramus

Gracilis m.

Medial condyle of tibia

Ischial tuberosity

Inf. pubic ramus

Linea aspera (on posterior surface of femoral shaft)

Adductor magnus m.

Adductor hiatus

Adductor tubercle

ANTERIOR VIEWS

Anterior Muscle	Proximal Attachment	Distal Attachment	Innervation	Main Actions
Tibialis anterior	Lateral condyle & sup. half of lateral surface of tibia	Medial & inf. surfaces of medial cuneiform bone & base of 1st metatarsal bone	Deep fibular [peroneal] n. (**L4** & L5)	Dorsiflexes & inverts foot
Extensor hallucis longus	Middle part of ant. surface of fibula & interosseous membrane	Dorsal aspect of base of distal phalanx of 1st digit (hallux)		Extends 1st digit & dorsiflexes foot
Extensor digitorum longus	Lateral condyle of tibia, sup. 3/4 of ant. surface of fibula & interosseous membrane	Middle & distal phalanges of lateral 4 digits	Deep fibular [peroneal] n. (L5 & S1)	Extends lateral 4 digits dorsiflexes foot
Fibularis [Peroneus] tertius	Inferior third of ant. surface of fibula & interosseous membrane	Dorsum of base of 5th metatarsal bone		Dorsiflexes foot & aids in eversion of it

Lateral Muscle[a]	Proximal Attachment	Distal Attachment	Innervation	Main Actions
Fibularis [Peroneus] longus	Head & sup. 2/3 of lateral surface of fibula	Base of metatarsal 1st bone & medial cuneiform bone	Superficial fibular (peroneal) n. (**L5**, **S1** & S2)	Everts & plantar flexes foot
Fibularis [Peroneus] brevis	Inf. 2/3 of lateral surface of fibula	Dorsal surface of tuberosity of 5th metatarsal bone		Everts foot & weakly plantarflexes foot

[a]The fibularis [peroneus] longus and brevis were named because their proximal attachment is to the fibula. *Peroneus* is the Greek word for the Latin term *fibula* and was formerly used to describe these muscles.

ANTERIOR VIEWS

Lateral condyle of tibia

Tibialis anterior m.

Medial cuneiform bone

Base of 1st metatarsal bone

Lateral condyle of tibia

Head of fibula

Interosseous membrane

Extensor digitorum longus m.

Fibularis [Peroneus] tertius m. tendon

Extensor digitorum longus m. tendons

Extensor expansions

Distal phalanges

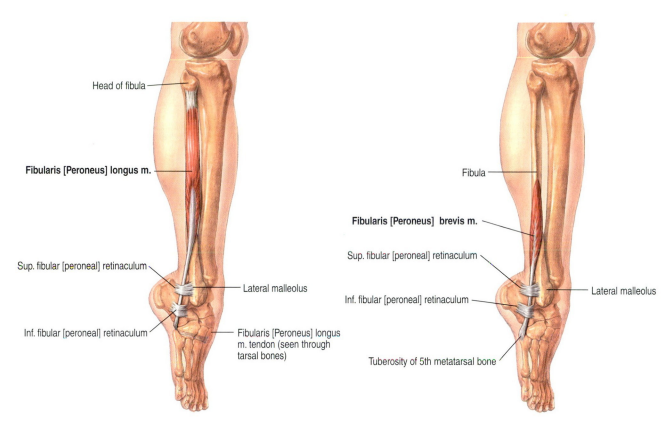

Head of fibula

Fibularis [Peroneus] longus m.

Sup. fibular [peroneal] retinaculum

Lateral malleolus

Inf. fibular [peroneal] retinaculum

Fibularis [Peroneus] longus m. tendon (seen through tarsal bones)

Fibula

Fibularis [Peroneus] brevis m.

Sup. fibular [peroneal] retinaculum

Inf. fibular [peroneal] retinaculum

Lateral malleolus

Tuberosity of 5th metatarsal bone

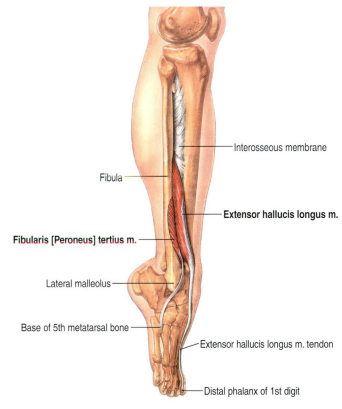

Interosseous membrane

Fibula

Extensor hallucis longus m.

Fibularis [Peroneus] tertius m.

Lateral malleolus

Base of 5th metatarsal bone

Extensor hallucis longus m. tendon

Distal phalanx of 1st digit

LATERAL VIEWS

Posterior Leg Muscles
Table 5.5

Superficial Muscle	Proximal Attachment	Distal Attachment	Innervation	Main Actions
Gastrocnemius	*Lateral head:* Lateral aspect of lateral condyle of femur *Medial head:* Popliteal surface of femur, sup. to medial condyle	Post. surface of tuberosity of calcaneus via tendo calcaneus	Tibial n. (L5, S1 & **S2**)	Plantarflexes foot, raises heel during walking & flexes knee joint
Soleus	Post. aspect of head of fibula, sup. 4th of post. surface of fibula, soleal line & medial border of tibia			Plantarflexes foot
Plantaris	Inf. end of lat. supracondylar line of femur & oblique popliteal lig.	Medial side of tendo calcaneus		Weakly assists gastrocnemius in plantarflexing foot & flexing knee joint

Deep Muscle	Proximal Attachment	Distal Attachment	Innervation	Main Actions
Popliteus	Lateral epicondyle of femur & lateral meniscus	Post. surface of tibia, sup. to soleal line	Tibial n. (**L4, L5** & S1)	Weakly flexes knee & unlocks it
Flexor hallucis longus	Inf. 2/3 of post. surface of fibula & inf. part of interosseous membrane	Base of distal phalanx of 1st digit (hallux)	Tibial n. (**S2**–S3)	Flexes 1st digit at all joints and plantarflexes foot
Flexor digitorum longus	Medial part of post. surface of tibia, inf. to soleal line & by a broad aponeurosis to fibula	Bases of distal phalanges of lateral 4 digits		Flexes 4 digits & plantarflexes foot
Tibialis posterior	Interosseous membrane, post. surface of tibia inf. to soleal line & post. surface of fibula	Tuberosity of navicular, cuneiform & cuboid bones, & bases of 2nd, 3rd & 4th metatarsal bones	Tibial n. (L4–L5)	Plantarflexes & inverts foot

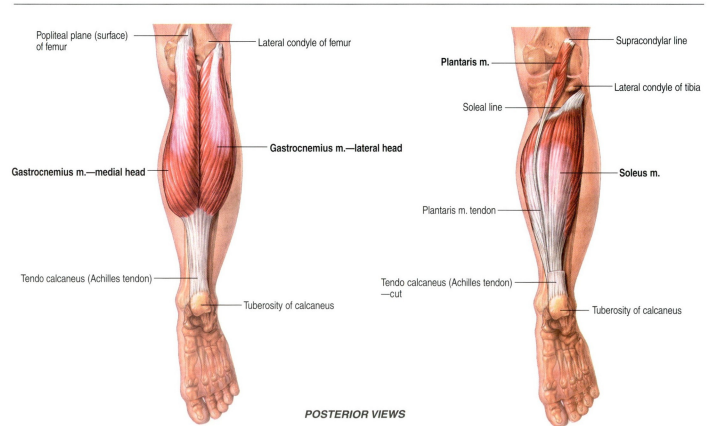

Popliteal plane (surface) of femur — Lateral condyle of femur — Gastrocnemius m.—lateral head — **Gastrocnemius m.—medial head** — Tendo calcaneus (Achilles tendon) — Tuberosity of calcaneus

Plantaris m. — Supracondylar line — Soleal line — Lateral condyle of tibia — **Soleus m.** — Plantaris m. tendon — Tendo calcaneus (Achilles tendon)—cut — Tuberosity of calcaneus

POSTERIOR VIEWS

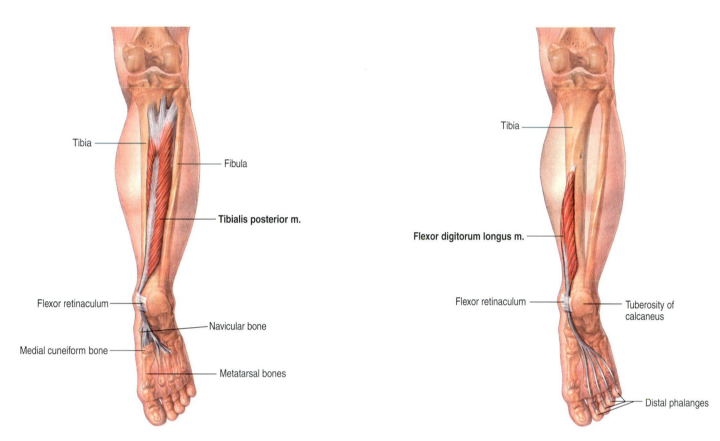

Tibia

Fibula

Tibialis posterior m.

Flexor retinaculum

Navicular bone

Medial cuneiform bone

Metatarsal bones

Tibia

Flexor digitorum longus m.

Flexor retinaculum

Tuberosity of calcaneus

Distal phalanges

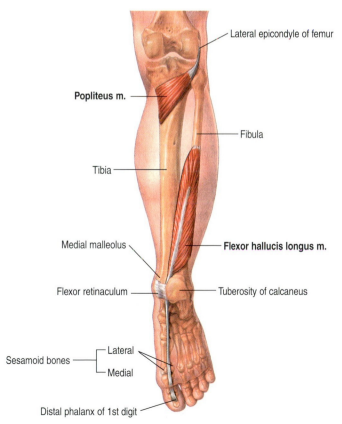

Lateral epicondyle of femur

Popliteus m.

Fibula

Tibia

Medial malleolus

Flexor hallucis longus m.

Flexor retinaculum

Tuberosity of calcaneus

Sesamoid bones — Lateral
— Medial

Distal phalanx of 1st digit

POSTERIOR VIEWS

Intrinsic Foot Muscles
Table 5.6

Muscle	Proximal Attachment	Distal Attachment	Innervation	Main Actions
FIRST LAYER[a]				
Abductor hallucis	Medial process of tuber calcanei, flexor retinaculum & plantar aponeurosis	Medial side of base of proximal phalanx & medial sesamoid bone of 1st digit (hallux)	Medial plantar n. (S2 & **S3**)	Abducts & flexes 1st digit
Flexor digitorum brevis	Medial process of tuber calcanei, plantar aponeurosis & intermuscular septa	Both sides of middle phalanges of lateral 4 digits		Flexes lateral 4 digits (toes)
Abductor digiti minimi	Medial & lateral processes of tuber calcanei, plantar aponeurosis & intermuscular septa	Lateral side of base of proximal phalanx of 5th digit (little toe)	Lateral plantar n. (S2 & **S3**)	Abducts & flexes 5th digit
SECOND LAYER				
Quadratus plantae	Medial surface & lateral margin of plantar surface of calcaneus	Posterolateral margin of tendon of flexor digitorum longus	Lateral plantar n. (S2 & **S3**)	Assists flexor digitorum longus in flexing lateral 4 digits
Lumbricalis	Tendons of flexor digitorum longus	Medial sides of bases of proximal phalanges of lateral 4 digits & extensor expansions of tendons of extensor digitorum longus	*Medial one:* medial plantar n. (S2 & **S3**) *Lateral three:* lateral plantar n. (S2 & **S3**)	Flex proximal phalanges & extend middle & distal phalanges of lateral 4 digits
THIRD LAYER				
Flexor hallucis brevis	Plantar surfaces of cuboid & lateral cuneiform bones	Both sides of base of proximal phalanx of 1st digit	Medial plantar n. (S2 & **S3**)	Flexes proximal phalanx of 1st digit (hallux)
Adductor hallucis	*Oblique head:* Bases of metatarsal bones 2–4 *Transverse head:* Plantar ligg. of metatarsophalangeal joints 2–5	*Tendons of both heads* attached to lateral side of base of proximal phalanx & lat. sesamoid bone of 1st digit (hallux)	Deep br. of lateral plantar n. (S2 & **S3**)	Adducts 1st digit; assists in maintaining transverse arch of foot
Flexor digiti minimi brevis	Base of 5th metatarsal bone	Base of proximal phalanx of 5th digit	Superficial br. of lateral plantar n. (S2 & **S3**)	Flexes proximal phalanx of 5th digit, thereby assisting with its flexion
FOURTH LAYER				
Plantar interossei (3 muscles)	Bases & medial sides of metatarsal bones 3–5	Medial sides of bases of proximal phalanges of digits 3–5	Lateral plantar n. (S2 & **S3**)	Adduct digits (2–4) & flex metatarsophalangeal joints
Dorsal interossei (4 muscles)	Adjacent side of metatarsal bones 1–5	*1st:* medial side of proximal phalanx of 2nd digit *2nd–4th:* lateral sides of digits 2–4		Abduct digits (2–4) & flex metatarsorphalangeal joints

[a]In spite of the individual actions ascribed to them, the primary function of the first layer of intrinsic muscles of the foot is to provide dynamic support of the longitudinal arch of the foot (i.e., resisting forces tending to spread or flatten it).

Dorsal interossei mm.

Metatarsal bones

Extensor expansions

DORSAL SURFACE VIEW

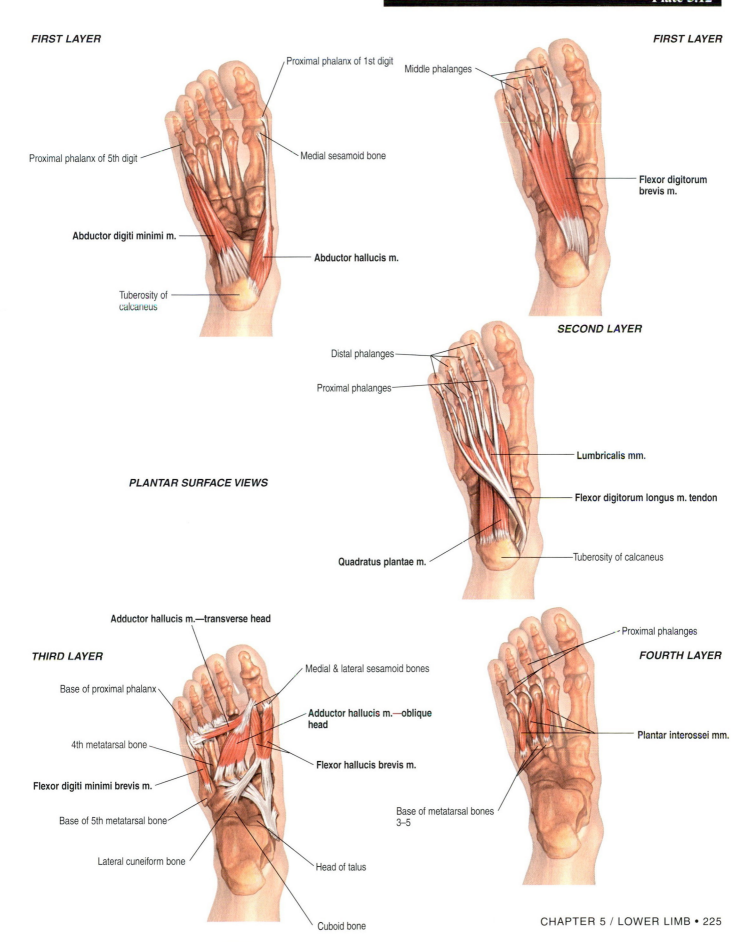

FIRST LAYER

Proximal phalanx of 1st digit

Proximal phalanx of 5th digit

Medial sesamoid bone

Abductor digiti minimi m.

Abductor hallucis m.

Tuberosity of calcaneus

FIRST LAYER

Middle phalanges

Flexor digitorum brevis m.

SECOND LAYER

Distal phalanges

Proximal phalanges

Lumbricalis mm.

Flexor digitorum longus m. tendon

Quadratus plantae m.

Tuberosity of calcaneus

PLANTAR SURFACE VIEWS

THIRD LAYER

Adductor hallucis m.—transverse head

Base of proximal phalanx

4th metatarsal bone

Flexor digiti minimi brevis m.

Base of 5th metatarsal bone

Lateral cuneiform bone

Medial & lateral sesamoid bones

Adductor hallucis m.—oblique head

Flexor hallucis brevis m.

Head of talus

Cuboid bone

FOURTH LAYER

Proximal phalanges

Plantar interossei mm.

Base of metatarsal bones 3–5

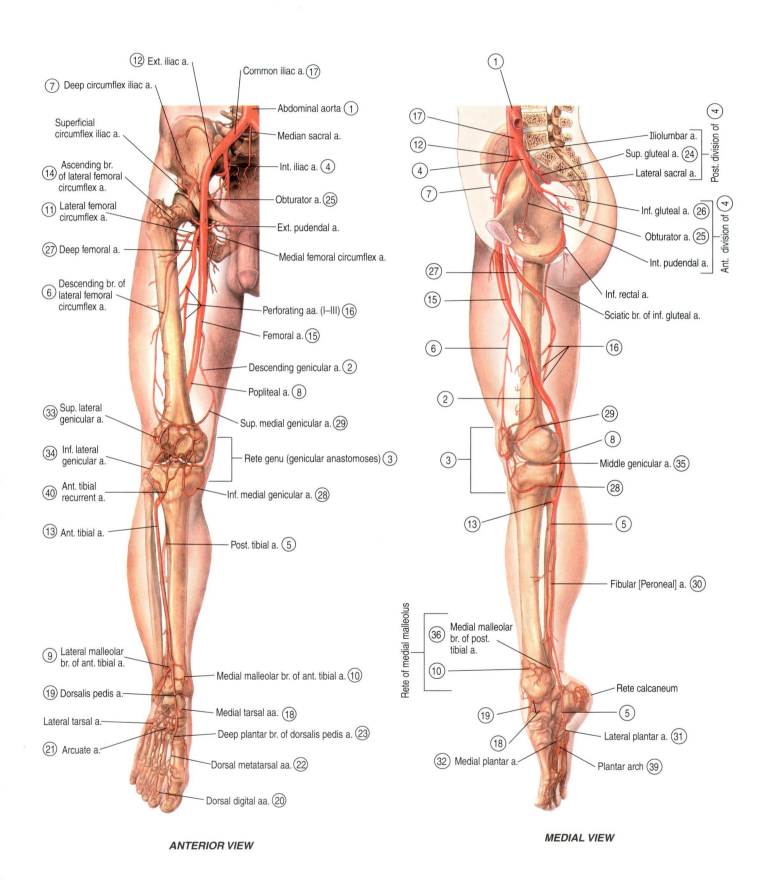

12 Ext. iliac a.

7 Deep circumflex iliac a.

Common iliac a. 17

Superficial circumflex iliac a.

Abdominal aorta 1

Median sacral a.

14 Ascending br. of lateral femoral circumflex a.

Int. iliac a. 4

11 Lateral femoral circumflex a.

Obturator a. 25

27 Deep femoral a.

Ext. pudendal a.

6 Descending br. of lateral femoral circumflex a.

Medial femoral circumflex a.

Perforating aa. (I–III) 16

Femoral a. 15

Descending genicular a. 2

Popliteal a. 8

33 Sup. lateral genicular a.

Sup. medial genicular a. 29

34 Inf. lateral genicular a.

Rete genu (genicular anastomoses) 3

40 Ant. tibial recurrent a.

Inf. medial genicular a. 28

13 Ant. tibial a.

Post. tibial a. 5

9 Lateral malleolar br. of ant. tibial a.

19 Dorsalis pedis a.

Medial malleolar br. of ant. tibial a. 10

Lateral tarsal a.

Medial tarsal aa. 18

21 Arcuate a.

Deep plantar br. of dorsalis pedis a. 23

Dorsal metatarsal aa. 22

Dorsal digital aa. 20

ANTERIOR VIEW

1

17

12

4

7

Iliolumbar a.

Sup. gluteal a. 24

Lateral sacral a.

Post. division of 4

Inf. gluteal a. 26

Obturator a. 25

Int. pudendal a.

Ant. division of 4

27

15

Inf. rectal a.

Sciatic br. of inf. gluteal a.

6

16

2

29

3

8

Middle genicular a. 35

13

28

5

Fibular [Peroneal] a. 30

Rete of medial malleolus

36 Medial malleolar br. of post. tibial a.

10

Rete calcaneum

19

5

18

Lateral plantar a. 31

32 Medial plantar a.

Plantar arch 39

MEDIAL VIEW

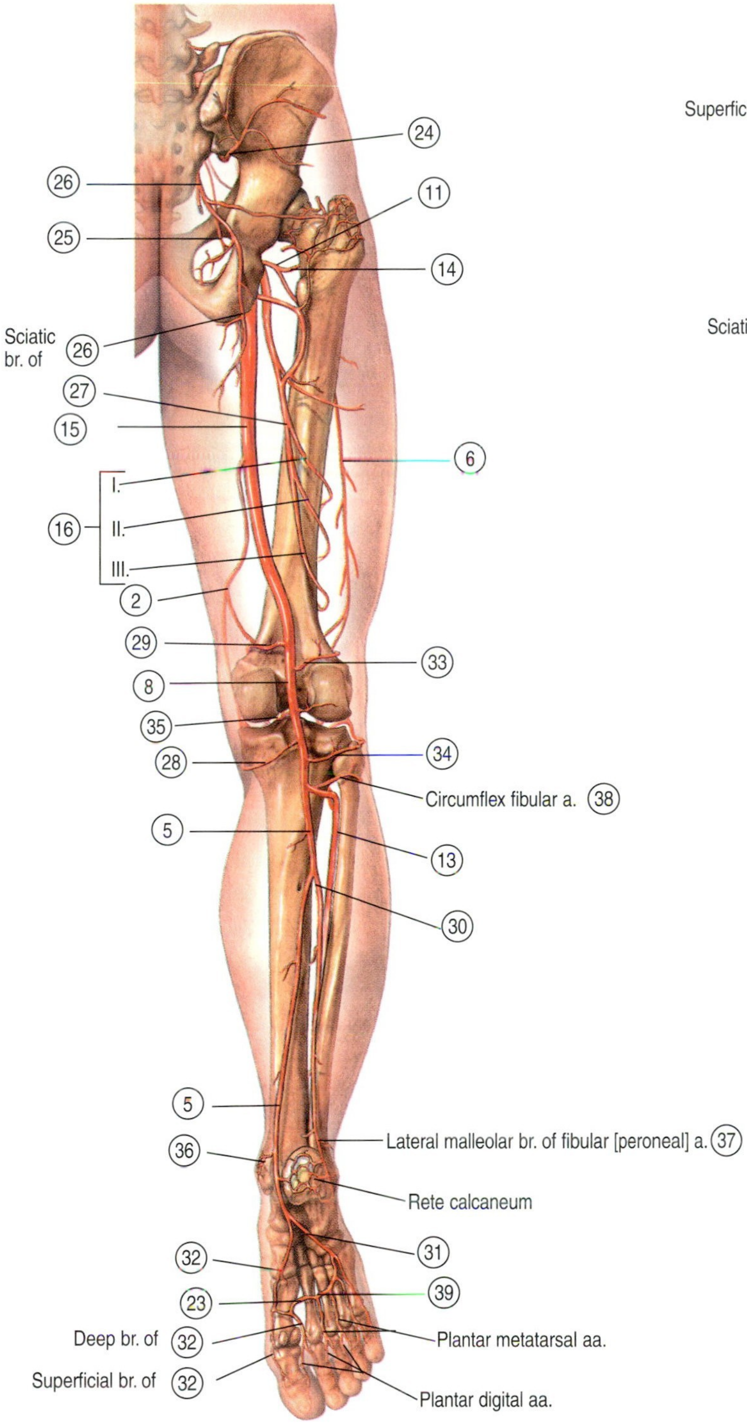

(24)
(26)
(11)
(25)
(14)
Sciatic br. of (26)
(27)
(15)
(6)
I.
(16) II.
III.
(2)
(29)
(33)
(8)
(35)
(34)
(28)
Circumflex fibular a. (38)
(5)
(13)
(30)
(5)
Lateral malleolar br. of fibular [peroneal] a. (37)
(36)
Rete calcaneum
(32)
(31)
(23)
(39)
Deep br. of (32)
Plantar metatarsal aa.
Superficial br. of (32)
Plantar digital aa.

POSTERIOR VIEW

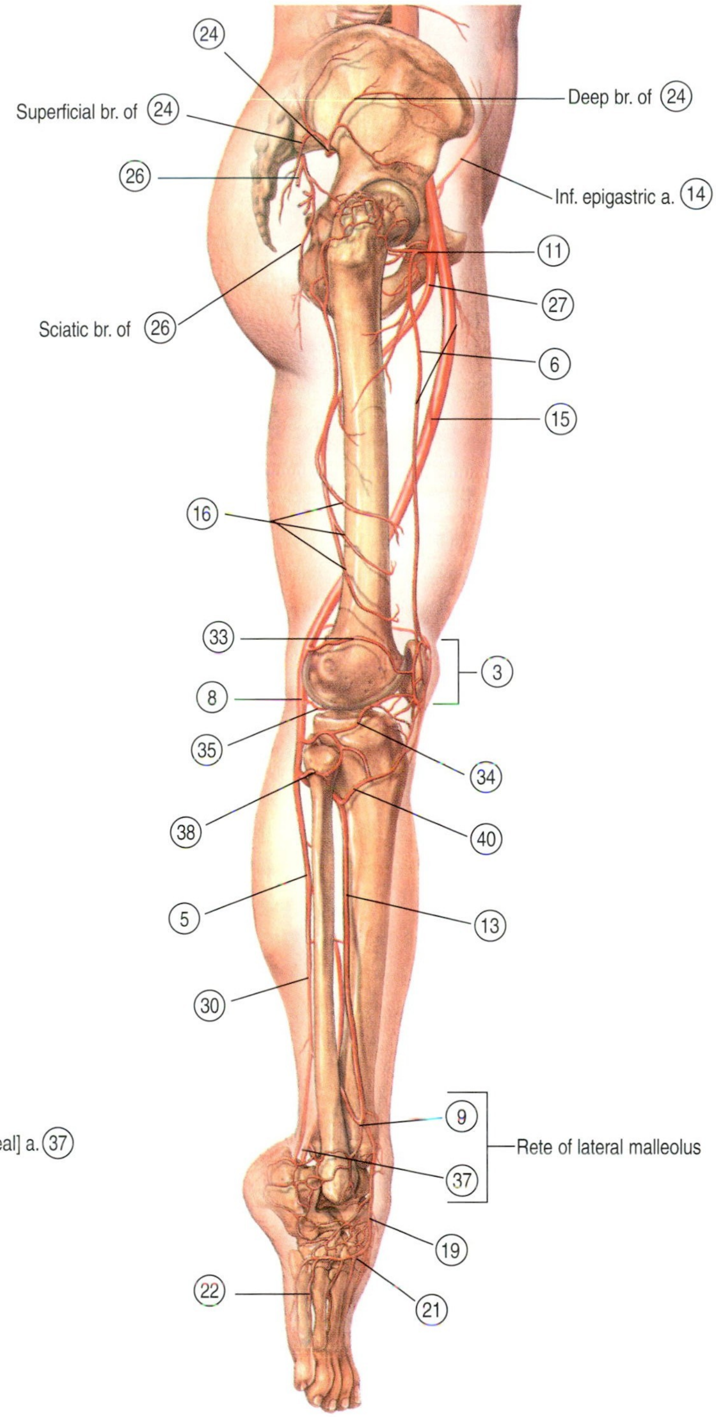

(24)
Deep br. of (24)
Superficial br. of (24)
(26)
Inf. epigastric a. (14)
(11)
(27)
Sciatic br. of (26)
(6)
(15)
(16)
(33)
(3)
(8)
(35)
(34)
(38)
(40)
(5)
(13)
(30)
(9)
Rete of lateral malleolus
(37)
(19)
(22)
(21)

LATERAL VIEW

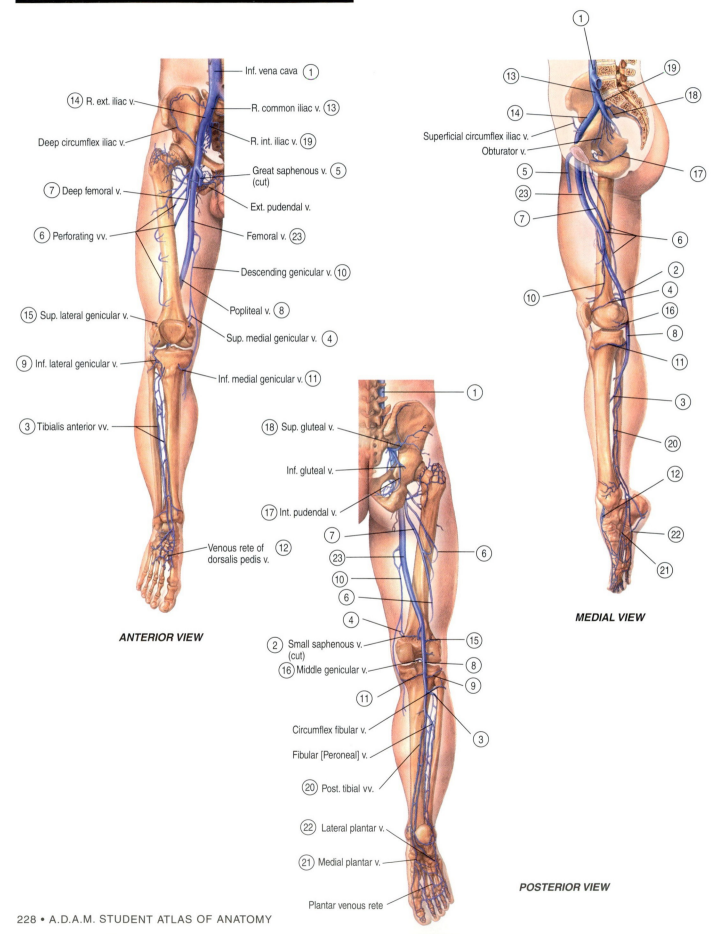

Inf. vena cava (1)

(14) R. ext. iliac v.

R. common iliac v. (13)

Deep circumflex iliac v.

R. int. iliac v. (19)

(7) Deep femoral v.

Great saphenous v. (5)
(cut)

Ext. pudendal v.

(6) Perforating vv.

Femoral v. (23)

Descending genicular v. (10)

(15) Sup. lateral genicular v.

Popliteal v. (8)

Sup. medial genicular v. (4)

(9) Inf. lateral genicular v.

Inf. medial genicular v. (11)

(3) Tibialis anterior vv.

Venous rete of (12)
dorsalis pedis v.

ANTERIOR VIEW

Superficial circumflex iliac v.

Obturator v.

(13)

(14)

(19)

(18)

(5)

(23)

(7)

(17)

(6)

(2)

(4)

(16)

(8)

(11)

(10)

(3)

(20)

(12)

(22)

(21)

MEDIAL VIEW

(1)

(18) Sup. gluteal v.

Inf. gluteal v.

(17) Int. pudendal v.

(7)

(23)

(10)

(6)

(6)

(4)

(2) Small saphenous v.
(cut)

(16) Middle genicular v.

(15)

(8)

(9)

(11)

(3)

Circumflex fibular v.

Fibular [Peroneal] v.

(20) Post. tibial vv.

(22) Lateral plantar v.

(21) Medial plantar v.

Plantar venous rete

POSTERIOR VIEW

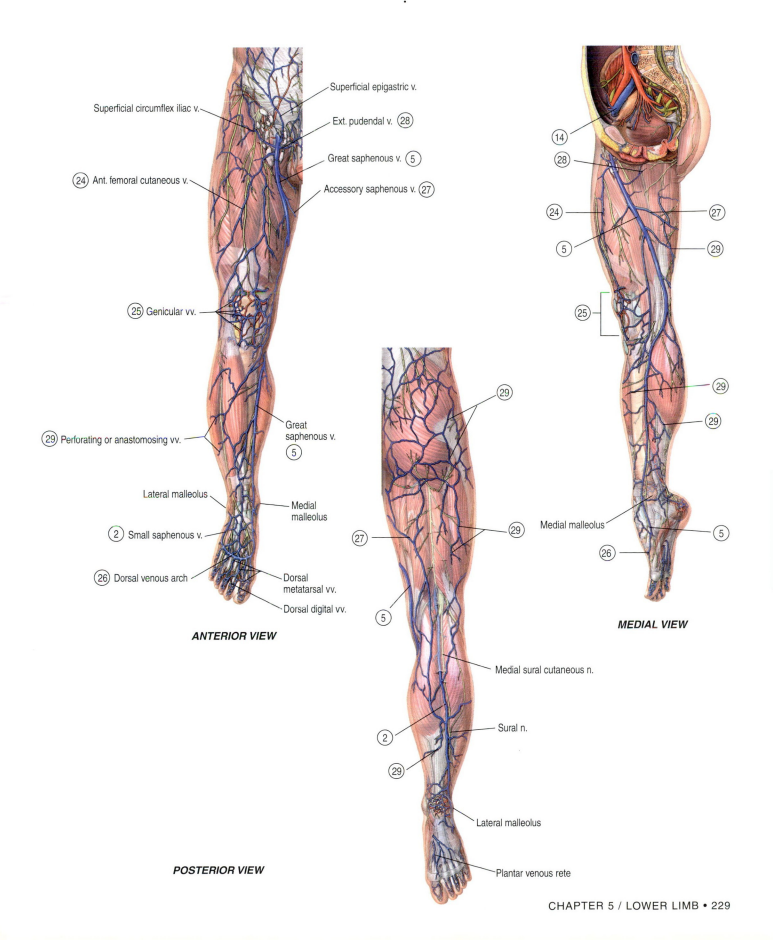

Superficial epigastric v.

Superficial circumflex iliac v.

Ext. pudendal v. (28)

Great saphenous v. (5)

(24) Ant. femoral cutaneous v.

Accessory saphenous v. (27)

(14)

(28)

(24) (27)

(5) (29)

(25) Genicular vv.

(25)

(29)

(29) Perforating or anastomosing vv.

Great saphenous v. (5)

(29)

Lateral malleolus

Medial malleolus

(2) Small saphenous v.

Medial malleolus

(5)

(26) Dorsal venous arch

Dorsal metatarsal vv.

(26)

Dorsal digital vv.

ANTERIOR VIEW

MEDIAL VIEW

(29)

(27)

(29)

(5)

Medial sural cutaneous n.

(2) Sural n.

(29)

Lateral malleolus

POSTERIOR VIEW

Plantar venous rete

Dermatomes & Cutaneous Nerves of Lower Limb
Plate 5.17

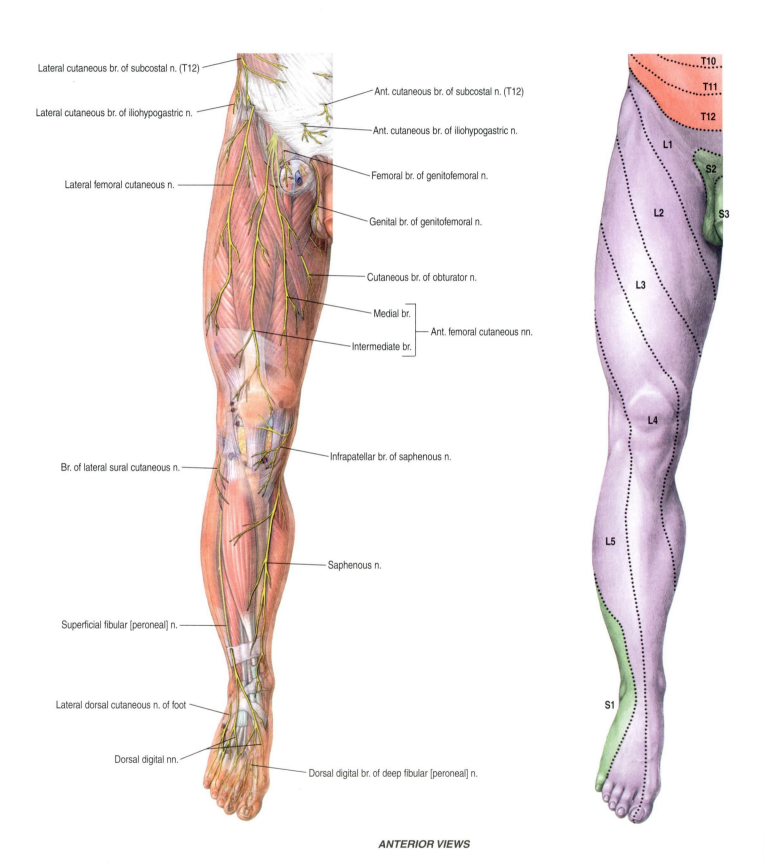

Lateral cutaneous br. of subcostal n. (T12)

Lateral cutaneous br. of iliohypogastric n.

Lateral femoral cutaneous n.

Ant. cutaneous br. of subcostal n. (T12)

Ant. cutaneous br. of iliohypogastric n.

Femoral br. of genitofemoral n.

Genital br. of genitofemoral n.

Cutaneous br. of obturator n.

Medial br.

Intermediate br.

Ant. femoral cutaneous nn.

Infrapatellar br. of saphenous n.

Br. of lateral sural cutaneous n.

Saphenous n.

Superficial fibular [peroneal] n.

Lateral dorsal cutaneous n. of foot

Dorsal digital nn.

Dorsal digital br. of deep fibular [peroneal] n.

T10
T11
T12
L1
S2
S3
L2
L3
L4
L5
S1

ANTERIOR VIEWS

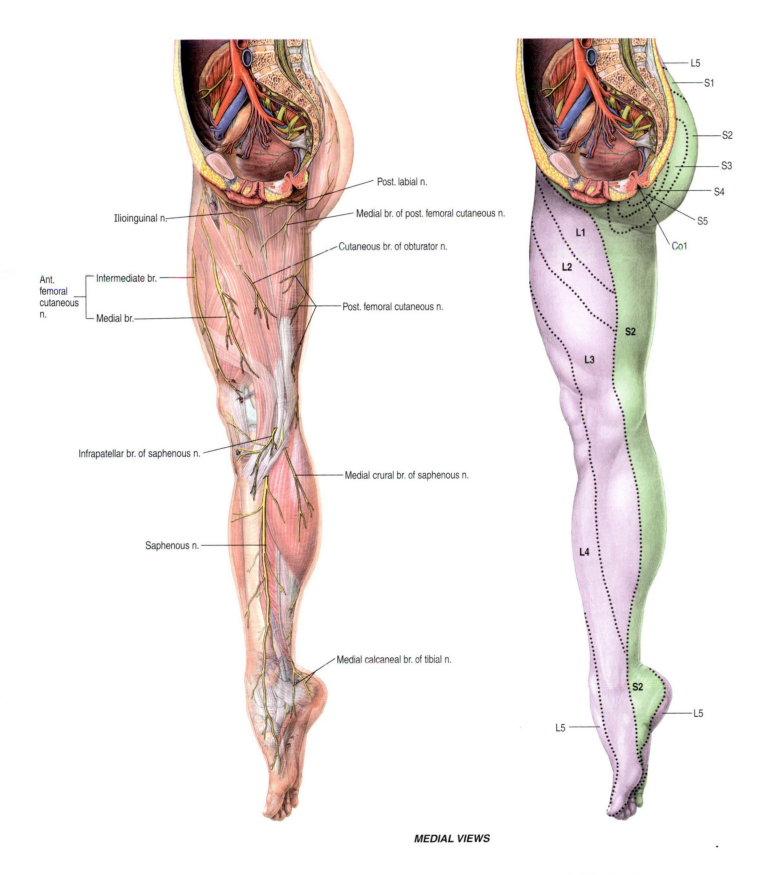

Post. labial n.

Ilioinguinal n.

Medial br. of post. femoral cutaneous n.

Cutaneous br. of obturator n.

Ant. femoral cutaneous n.

Intermediate br.

Medial br.

Post. femoral cutaneous n.

Infrapatellar br. of saphenous n.

Medial crural br. of saphenous n.

Saphenous n.

Medial calcaneal br. of tibial n.

L5
S1
S2
S3
S4
S5
Co1

L1
L2
S2
L3
L4
S2
L5
L5

MEDIAL VIEWS

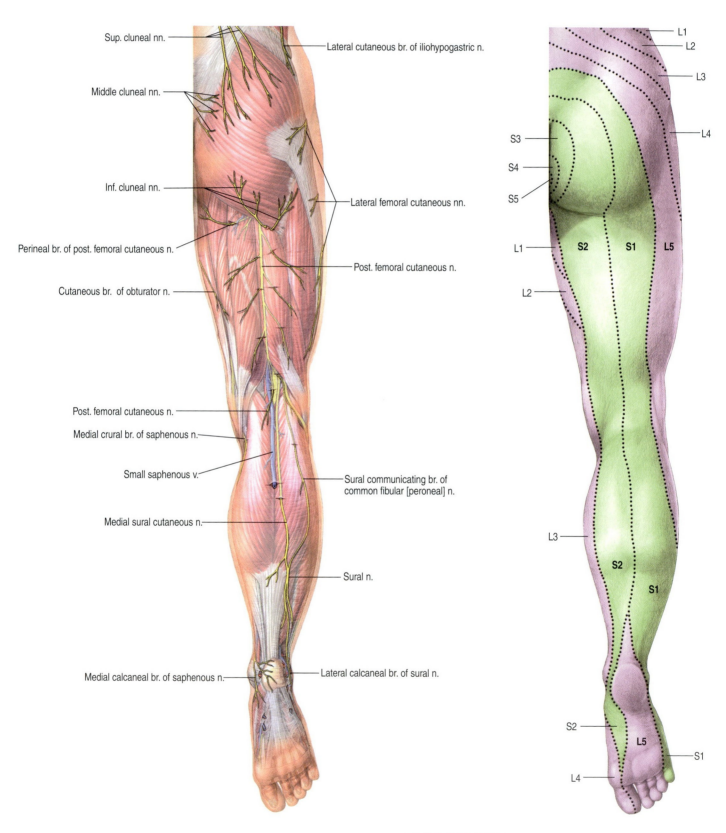

Sup. cluneal nn.

Lateral cutaneous br. of iliohypogastric n.

Middle cluneal nn.

Inf. cluneal nn.

Lateral femoral cutaneous nn.

Perineal br. of post. femoral cutaneous n.

Post. femoral cutaneous n.

Cutaneous br. of obturator n.

Post. femoral cutaneous n.

Medial crural br. of saphenous n.

Small saphenous v.

Sural communicating br. of common fibular [peroneal] n.

Medial sural cutaneous n.

Sural n.

Medial calcaneal br. of saphenous n.

Lateral calcaneal br. of sural n.

L1
L2
L3
L4
S3
S4
S5
L1
S2
S1
L5
L2
L3
S2
S1
S2
L5
L4
S1

POSTERIOR VIEWS

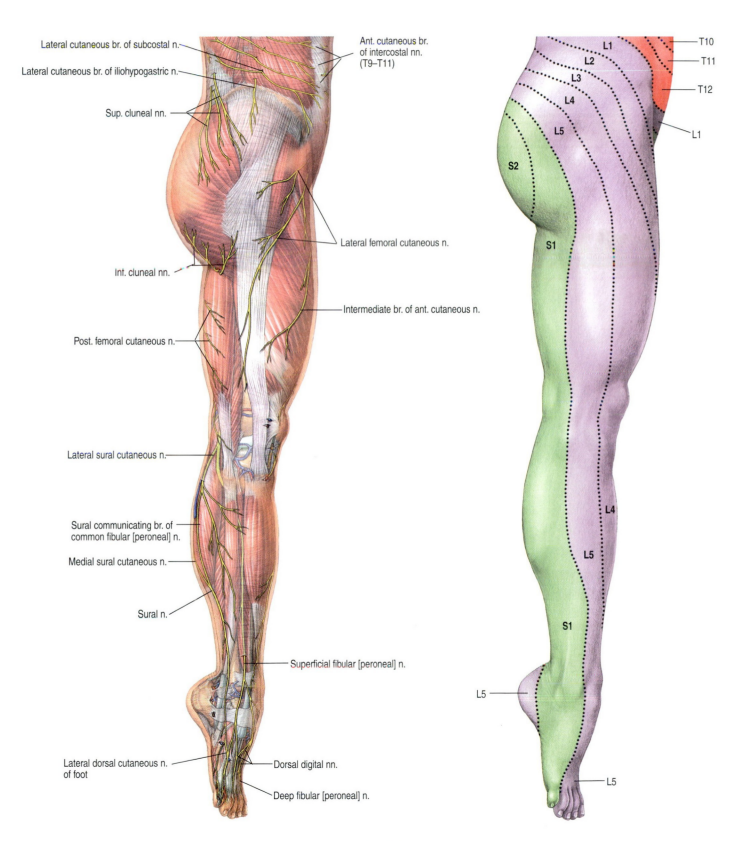

Lateral cutaneous br. of subcostal n.

Lateral cutaneous br. of iliohypogastric n.

Sup. cluneal nn.

Int. cluneal nn.

Post. femoral cutaneous n.

Lateral sural cutaneous n.

Sural communicating br. of common fibular [peroneal] n.

Medial sural cutaneous n.

Sural n.

Lateral dorsal cutaneous n. of foot

Ant. cutaneous br. of intercostal nn. (T9–T11)

Lateral femoral cutaneous n.

Intermediate br. of ant. cutaneous n.

Superficial fibular [peroneal] n.

Dorsal digital nn.

Deep fibular [peroneal] n.

T10

T11

T12

L1

L1

L2

L3

L4

L5

S2

S1

L4

L5

S1

L5

L5

LATERAL VIEWS

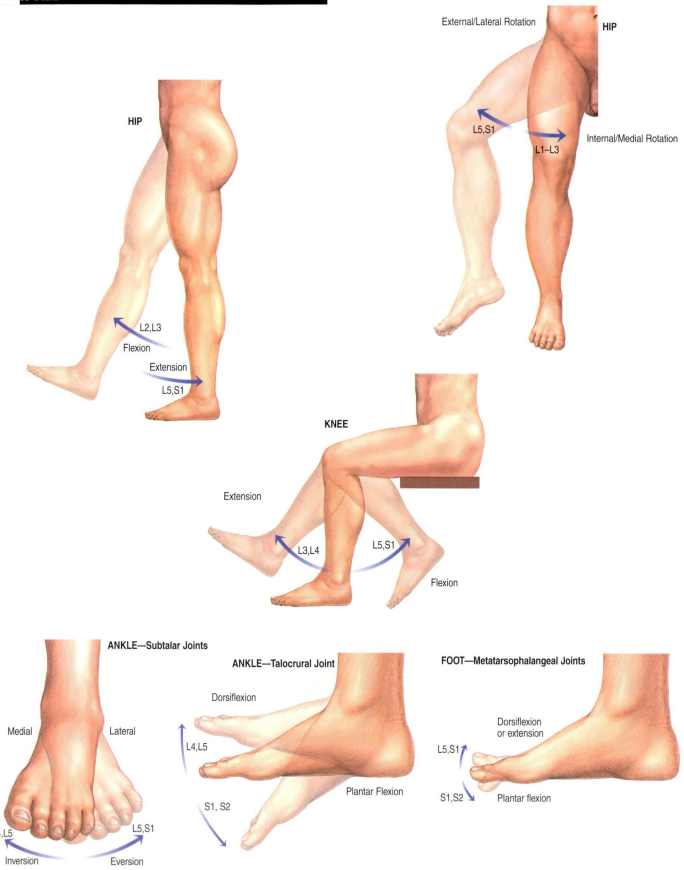

HIP

External/Lateral Rotation

HIP

L5,S1

Internal/Medial Rotation

L1–L3

HIP

L2,L3

Flexion

Extension

L5,S1

KNEE

Extension

L3,L4

L5,S1

Flexion

ANKLE—Subtalar Joints

Medial

Lateral

L4,L5

L5,S1

Inversion

Eversion

ANKLE—Talocrural Joint

Dorsiflexion

L4,L5

S1, S2

Plantar Flexion

FOOT—Metatarsophalangeal Joints

Dorsiflexion or extension

L5,S1

S1,S2

Plantar flexion

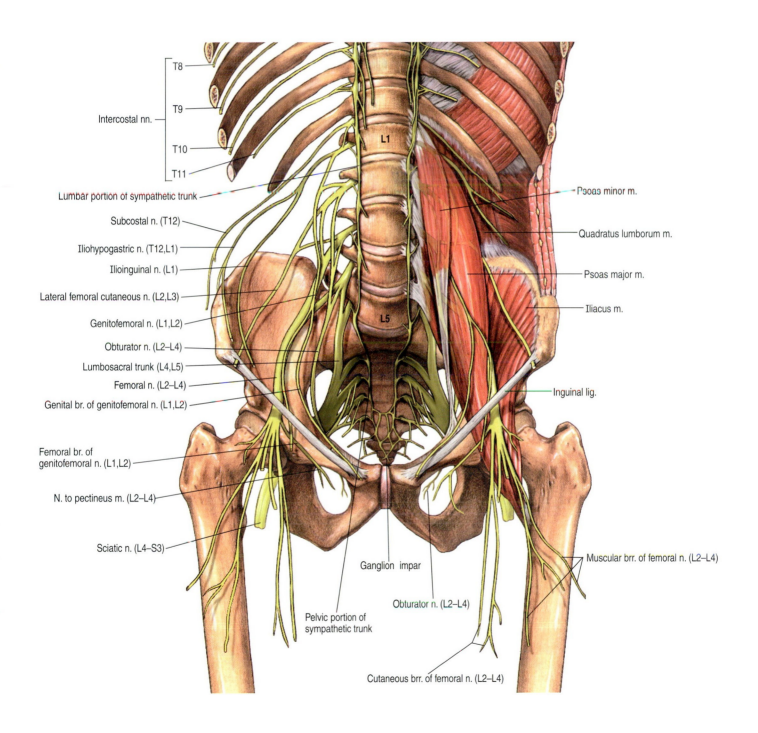

Intercostal nn.

T8
T9
T10
T11

Lumbar portion of sympathetic trunk

Subcostal n. (T12)

Iliohypogastric n. (T12,L1)

Ilioinguinal n. (L1)

Lateral femoral cutaneous n. (L2,L3)

Genitofemoral n. (L1,L2)

Obturator n. (L2–L4)

Lumbosacral trunk (L4,L5)

Femoral n. (L2–L4)

Genital br. of genitofemoral n. (L1,L2)

Femoral br. of genitofemoral n. (L1,L2)

N. to pectineus m. (L2–L4)

Sciatic n. (L4–S3)

L1

L5

Psoas minor m.

Quadratus lumborum m.

Psoas major m.

Iliacus m.

Inguinal lig.

Muscular brr. of femoral n. (L2–L4)

Ganglion impar

Obturator n. (L2–L4)

Pelvic portion of sympathetic trunk

Cutaneous brr. of femoral n. (L2–L4)

ANTERIOR VIEW

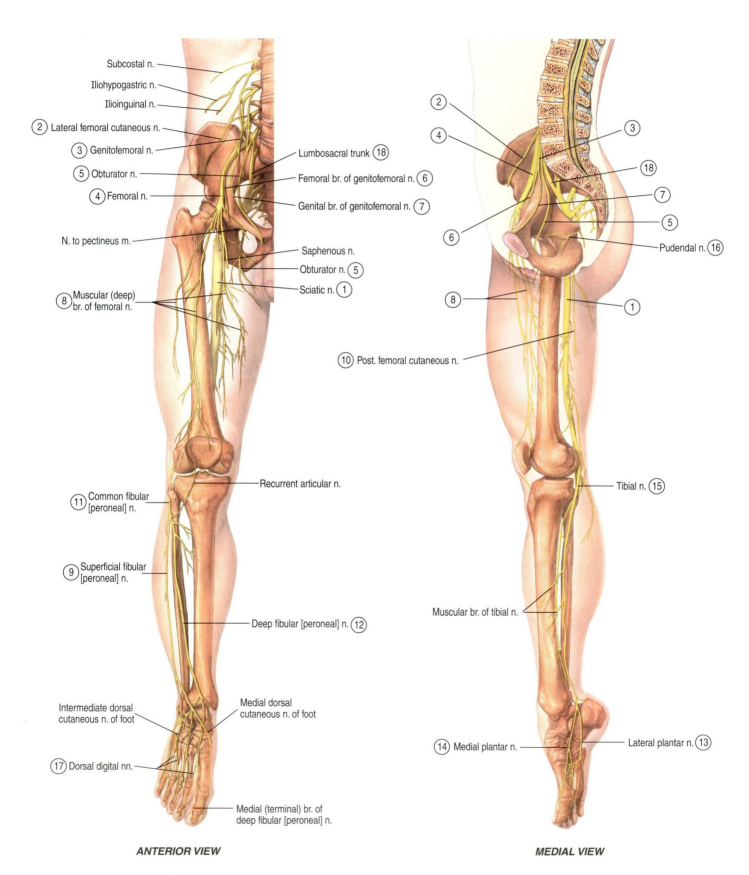

Subcostal n.

Iliohypogastric n.

Ilioinguinal n.

② Lateral femoral cutaneous n.

③ Genitofemoral n.

⑤ Obturator n.

④ Femoral n.

N. to pectineus m.

⑧ Muscular (deep) br. of femoral n.

Lumbosacral trunk ⑱

Femoral br. of genitofemoral n. ⑥

Genital br. of genitofemoral n. ⑦

Saphenous n.

Obturator n. ⑤

Sciatic n. ①

⑩ Post. femoral cutaneous n.

Recurrent articular n.

⑪ Common fibular [peroneal] n.

⑨ Superficial fibular [peroneal] n.

Deep fibular [peroneal] n. ⑫

Intermediate dorsal cutaneous n. of foot

Medial dorsal cutaneous n. of foot

⑰ Dorsal digital nn.

Medial (terminal) br. of deep fibular [peroneal] n.

② ④ ③ ⑱ ⑦ ⑤

⑥

Pudendal n. ⑯

⑧ ①

Tibial n. ⑮

Muscular br. of tibial n.

⑭ Medial plantar n.

Lateral plantar n. ⑬

ANTERIOR VIEW

MEDIAL VIEW

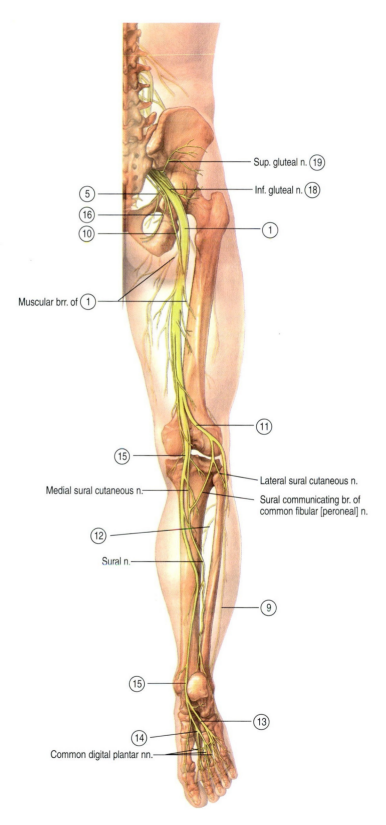

Sup. gluteal n. (19)

Inf. gluteal n. (18)

(5)

(16)

(10)

(1)

Muscular brr. of (1)

(11)

(15)

Lateral sural cutaneous n.

Medial sural cutaneous n.

Sural communicating br. of
common fibular [peroneal] n.

(12)

Sural n.

(9)

(15)

(13)

(14)

Common digital plantar nn.

POSTERIOR VIEW

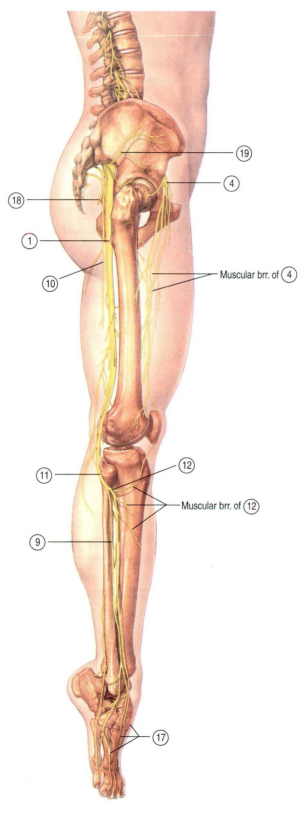

(19)

(4)

(18)

(1)

(10)

Muscular brr. of (4)

(11)

(12)

Muscular brr. of (12)

(9)

(17)

LATERAL VIEW

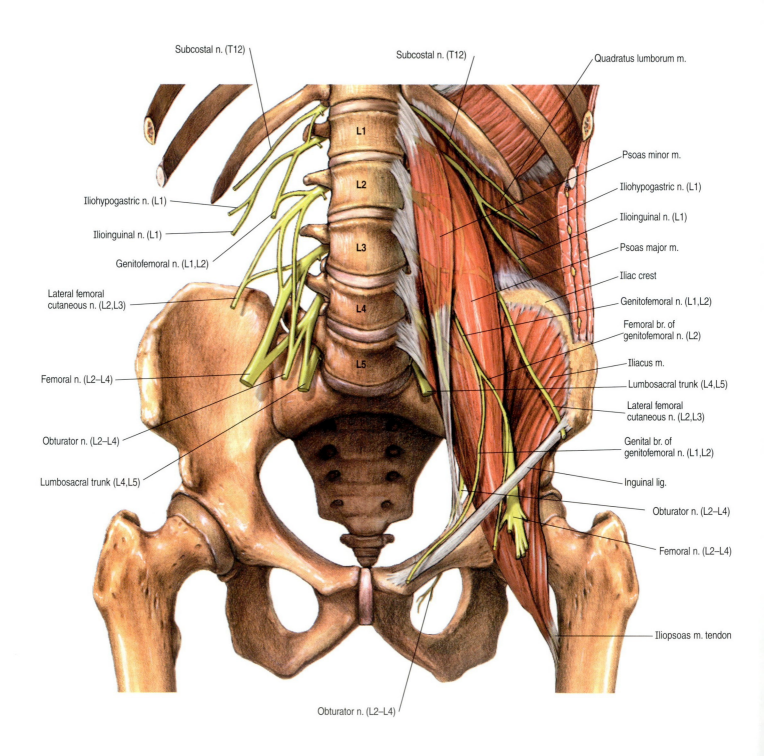

Subcostal n. (T12)

Subcostal n. (T12)

Quadratus lumborum m.

L1

Psoas minor m.

Iliohypogastric n. (L1)

Iliohypogastric n. (L1)

Ilioinguinal n. (L1)

Ilioinguinal n. (L1)

L2

Psoas major m.

Genitofemoral n. (L1,L2)

Iliac crest

L3

Genitofemoral n. (L1,L2)

Lateral femoral cutaneous n. (L2,L3)

Femoral br. of genitofemoral n. (L2)

L4

Iliacus m.

Lumbosacral trunk (L4,L5)

L5

Lateral femoral cutaneous n. (L2,L3)

Femoral n. (L2–L4)

Genital br. of genitofemoral n. (L1,L2)

Inguinal lig.

Obturator n. (L2–L4)

Obturator n. (L2–L4)

Lumbosacral trunk (L4,L5)

Femoral n. (L2–L4)

Iliopsoas m. tendon

Obturator n. (L2–L4)

ANTERIOR VIEW

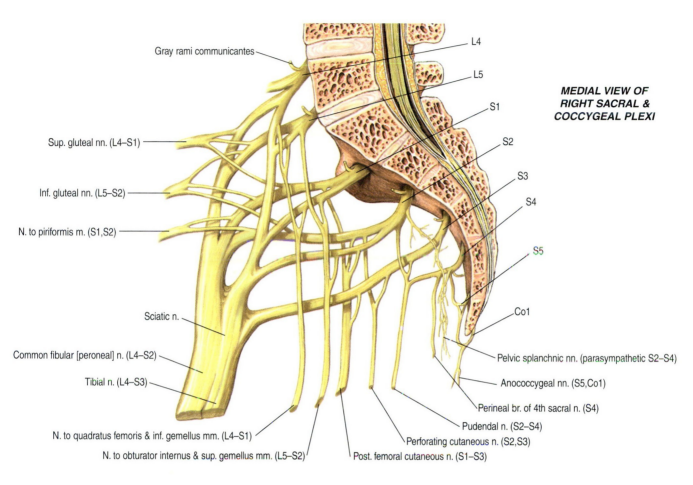

MEDIAL VIEW OF RIGHT SACRAL & COCCYGEAL PLEXI

Gray rami communicantes

L4
L5
S1
S2
S3
S4
S5
Co1

Sup. gluteal nn. (L4–S1)

Inf. gluteal nn. (L5–S2)

N. to piriformis m. (S1,S2)

Sciatic n.

Common fibular [peroneal] n. (L4–S2)

Tibial n. (L4–S3)

N. to quadratus femoris & inf. gemellus mm. (L4–S1)

N. to obturator internus & sup. gemellus mm. (L5–S2)

Post. femoral cutaneous n. (S1–S3)

Perforating cutaneous n. (S2,S3)

Pudendal n. (S2–S4)

Perineal br. of 4th sacral n. (S4)

Anococcygeal nn. (S5,Co1)

Pelvic splanchnic nn. (parasympathetic S2–S4)

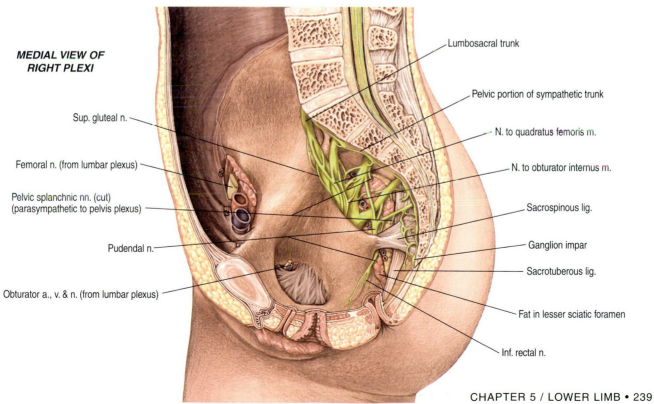

MEDIAL VIEW OF RIGHT PLEXI

Lumbosacral trunk

Pelvic portion of sympathetic trunk

N. to quadratus femoris m.

N. to obturator internus m.

Sacrospinous lig.

Ganglion impar

Sacrotuberous lig.

Fat in lesser sciatic foramen

Inf. rectal n.

Sup. gluteal n.

Femoral n. (from lumbar plexus)

Pelvic splanchnic nn. (cut)
(parasympathetic to pelvis plexus)

Pudendal n.

Obturator a., v. & n. (from lumbar plexus)

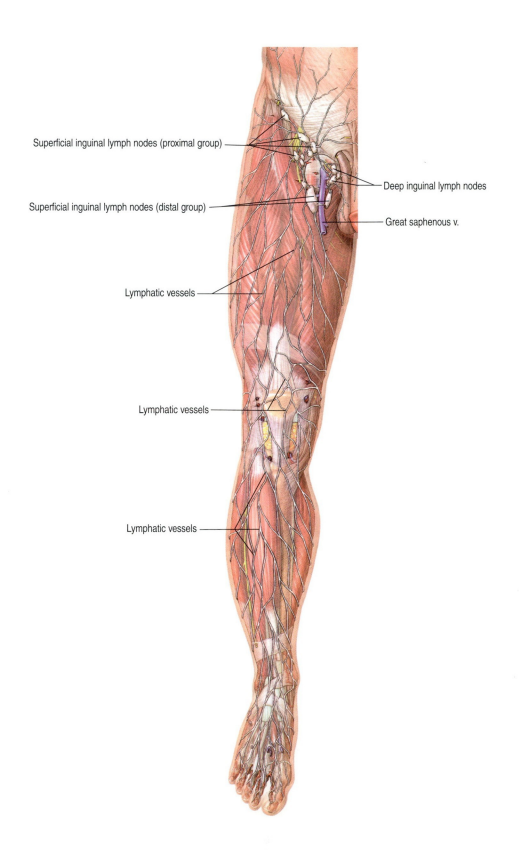

Superficial inguinal lymph nodes (proximal group)

Deep inguinal lymph nodes

Superficial inguinal lymph nodes (distal group)

Great saphenous v.

Lymphatic vessels

Lymphatic vessels

Lymphatic vessels

ANTERIOR VIEW

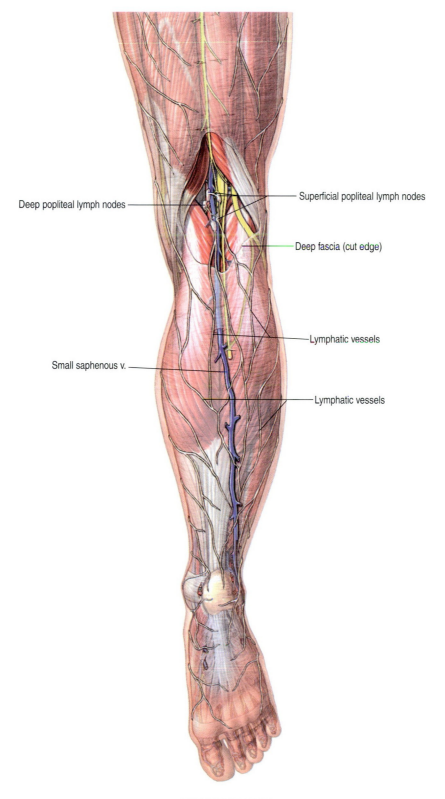

Deep popliteal lymph nodes

Superficial popliteal lymph nodes

Deep fascia (cut edge)

Lymphatic vessels

Small saphenous v.

Lymphatic vessels

POSTERIOR VIEW

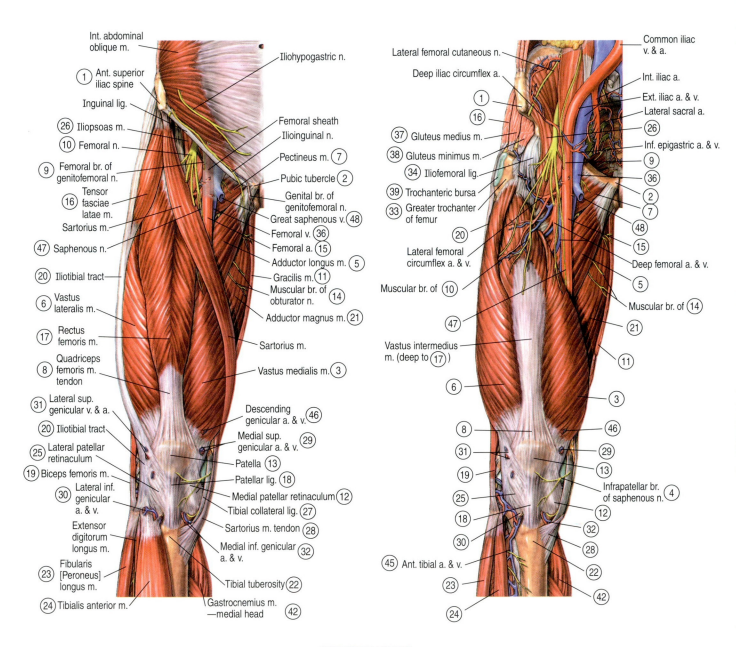

Int. abdominal oblique m.

Iliohypogastric n.

① Ant. superior iliac spine

Inguinal lig.

㉖ Iliopsoas m.

⑩ Femoral n.

⑨ Femoral br. of genitofemoral n.

⑯ Tensor fasciae latae m.

Sartorius m.

㊼ Saphenous n.

⑳ Iliotibial tract

⑥ Vastus lateralis m.

⑰ Rectus femoris m.

⑧ Quadriceps femoris m. tendon

㉛ Lateral sup. genicular v. & a.

⑳ Iliotibial tract

㉕ Lateral patellar retinaculum

⑲ Biceps femoris m.

㉚ Lateral inf. genicular a. & v.

Extensor digitorum longus m.

㉓ Fibularis [Peroneus] longus m.

㉔ Tibialis anterior m.

Femoral sheath

Ilioinguinal n.

Pectineus m. ⑦

Pubic tubercle ②

Genital br. of genitofemoral n.

Great saphenous v. ㊽

Femoral v. ㊱

Femoral a. ⑮

Adductor longus m. ⑤

Gracilis m. ⑪

Muscular br. of obturator n. ⑭

Adductor magnus m. ㉑

Sartorius m.

Vastus medialis m. ③

Descending genicular a. & v. ㊻

Medial sup. genicular a. & v. ㉙

Patella ⑬

Patellar lig. ⑱

Medial patellar retinaculum ⑫

Tibial collateral lig. ㉗

Sartorius m. tendon ㉘

Medial inf. genicular a. & v. ㉜

Tibial tuberosity ㉒

Gastrocnemius m. —medial head ㊷

Lateral femoral cutaneous n.

Deep iliac circumflex a.

①
⑯

㊲ Gluteus medius m.

㊳ Gluteus minimus m.

㉞ Iliofemoral lig.

㊴ Trochanteric bursa

㉝ Greater trochanter of femur

⑳

Lateral femoral circumflex a. & v.

Muscular br. of ⑩

㊼

Vastus intermedius m. (deep to ⑰)

⑥

⑧

㉛

⑲

㉕

⑱

㉚

㊺ Ant. tibial a. & v.

㉓

㉔

Common iliac v. & a.

Int. iliac a.

Ext. iliac a. & v.

Lateral sacral a.

㉖

Inf. epigastric a. & v.

⑨

㊱

②

⑦

㊽

⑮

Deep femoral a. & v.

⑤

Muscular br. of ⑭

㉑

⑪

③

㊻

㉙

⑬

Infrapatellar br. of saphenous n. ④

⑫

㉜

㉘

㉒

㊷

ANTERIOR VIEWS

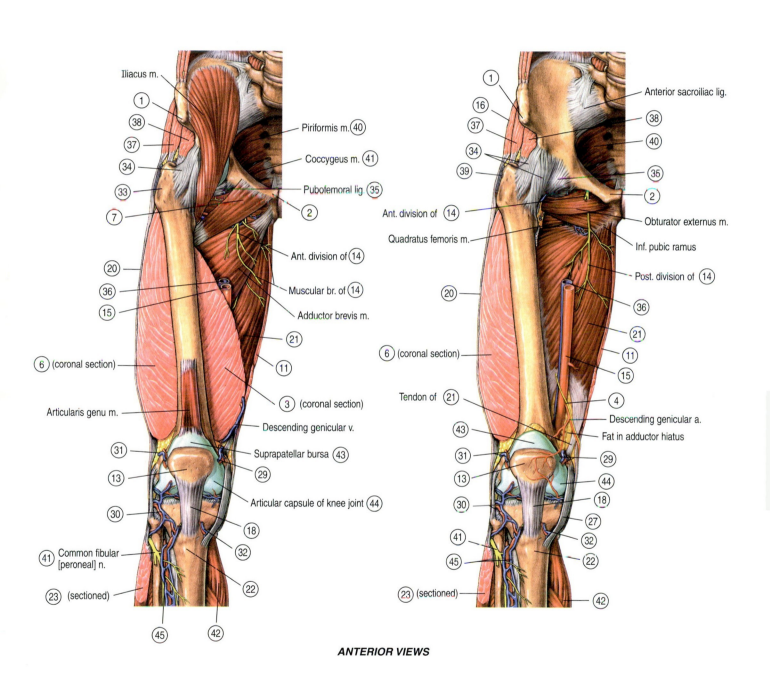

Iliacus m.

Piriformis m. (40)

Coccygeus m. (41)

Pubofemoral lig (35)

Ant. division of (14)

Muscular br. of (14)

Adductor brevis m.

(3) (coronal section)

Descending genicular v.

Suprapatellar bursa (43)

Articular capsule of knee joint (44)

Articularis genu m.

Common fibular [peroneal] n.

(6) (coronal section)

Anterior sacroiliac lig.

Ant. division of (14)

Quadratus femoris m.

Obturator externus m.

Inf. pubic ramus

Post. division of (14)

Tendon of (21)

Descending genicular a.

Fat in adductor hiatus

ANTERIOR VIEWS

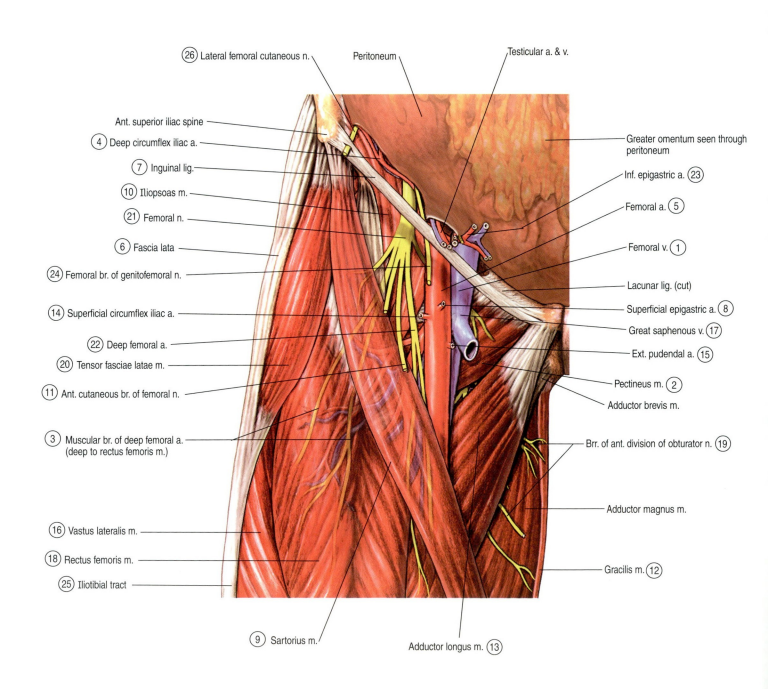

26 Lateral femoral cutaneous n.

Peritoneum

Testicular a. & v.

Ant. superior iliac spine

4 Deep circumflex iliac a.

7 Inguinal lig.

10 Iliopsoas m.

21 Femoral n.

6 Fascia lata

24 Femoral br. of genitofemoral n.

14 Superficial circumflex iliac a.

22 Deep femoral a.

20 Tensor fasciae latae m.

11 Ant. cutaneous br. of femoral n.

3 Muscular br. of deep femoral a. (deep to rectus femoris m.)

16 Vastus lateralis m.

18 Rectus femoris m.

25 Iliotibial tract

9 Sartorius m.

Adductor longus m. 13

Greater omentum seen through peritoneum

Inf. epigastric a. 23

Femoral a. 5

Femoral v. 1

Lacunar lig. (cut)

Superficial epigastric a. 8

Great saphenous v. 17

Ext. pudendal a. 15

Pectineus m. 2

Adductor brevis m.

Brr. of ant. division of obturator n. 19

Adductor magnus m.

Gracilis m. 12

ANTERIOR VIEW OF RIGHT PROXIMAL THIGH

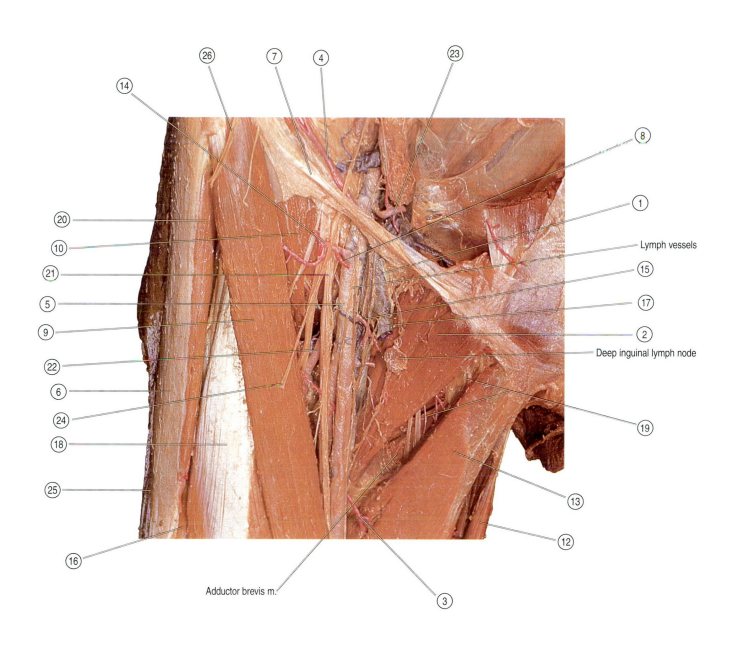

Lymph vessels

Deep inguinal lymph node

Adductor brevis m.

ANTERIOR VIEW OF RIGHT PROXIMAL THIGH

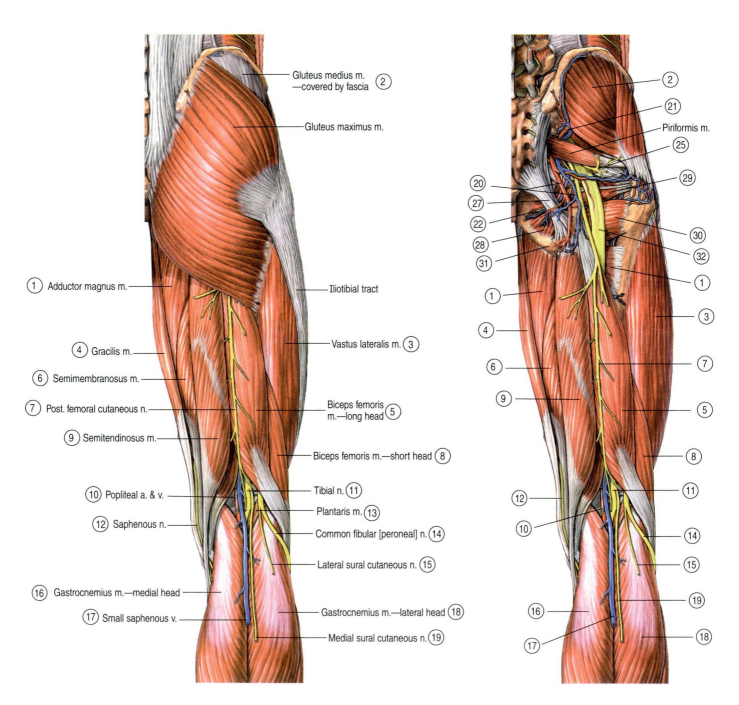

Gluteus medius m. ②
—covered by fascia

Gluteus maximus m.

① Adductor magnus m.

Iliotibial tract

④ Gracilis m.

Vastus lateralis m. ③

⑥ Semimembranosus m.

⑦ Post. femoral cutaneous n.

Biceps femoris
m.—long head ⑤

⑨ Semitendinosus m.

Biceps femoris m.—short head ⑧

⑩ Popliteal a. & v.

Tibial n. ⑪

Plantaris m. ⑬

⑫ Saphenous n.

Common fibular [peroneal] n. ⑭

Lateral sural cutaneous n. ⑮

⑯ Gastrocnemius m.—medial head

⑰ Small saphenous v.

Gastrocnemius m.—lateral head ⑱

Medial sural cutaneous n. ⑲

②

㉑

Piriformis m.

㉕

㉙

⑳

㉗

㉒

㉘

㉛

㉚

㉜

①

③

④

⑦

⑥

⑨

⑤

⑧

⑪

⑫

⑭

⑩

⑮

⑲

⑯

⑰

⑱

POSTERIOR VIEWS

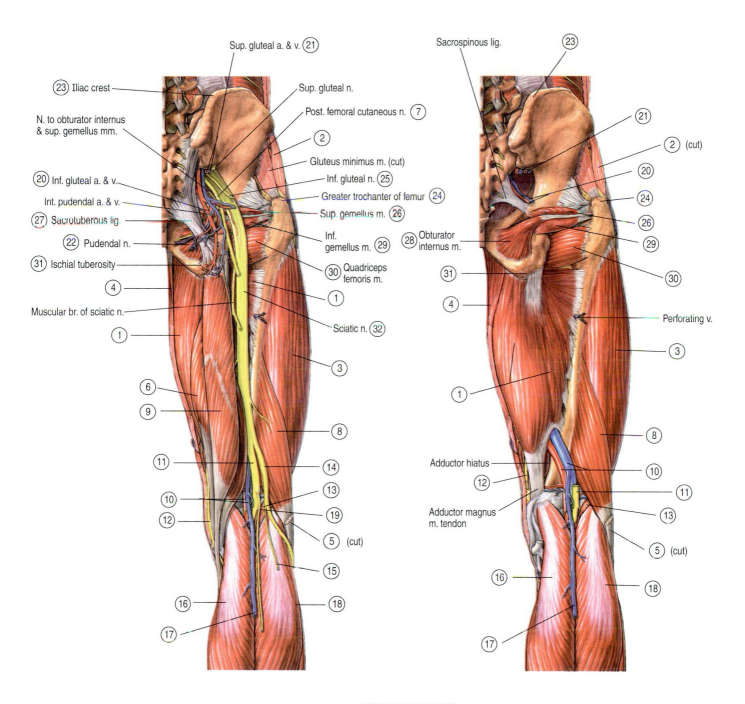

Sup. gluteal a. & v. (21)

(23) Iliac crest

Sup. gluteal n.

Post. femoral cutaneous n. (7)

N. to obturator internus
& sup. gemellus mm.

(2)

Gluteus minimus m. (cut)

(20) Inf. gluteal a. & v.

Inf. gluteal n. (25)

Int. pudendal a. & v.

Greater trochanter of femur (24)

(27) Sacrotuberous lig.

Sup. gemellus m. (26)

(22) Pudendal n.

Inf.
gemellus m. (29)

(31) Ischial tuberosity

(30) Quadriceps
femoris m.

(4)

(1)

Muscular br. of sciatic n.

Sciatic n. (32)

(1)

(3)

(6)

(9)

(8)

(11)

(14)

(10)

(13)

(12)

(19)

(5) (cut)

(15)

(16)

(18)

(17)

Sacrospinous lig.

(23)

(21)

(2) (cut)

(20)

(24)

(28) Obturator
internus m.

(26)

(29)

(31)

(30)

(4)

Perforating v.

(1)

(3)

(8)

Adductor hiatus

(10)

(12)

(11)

Adductor magnus
m. tendon

(13)

(5) (cut)

(16)

(18)

(17)

POSTERIOR VIEWS

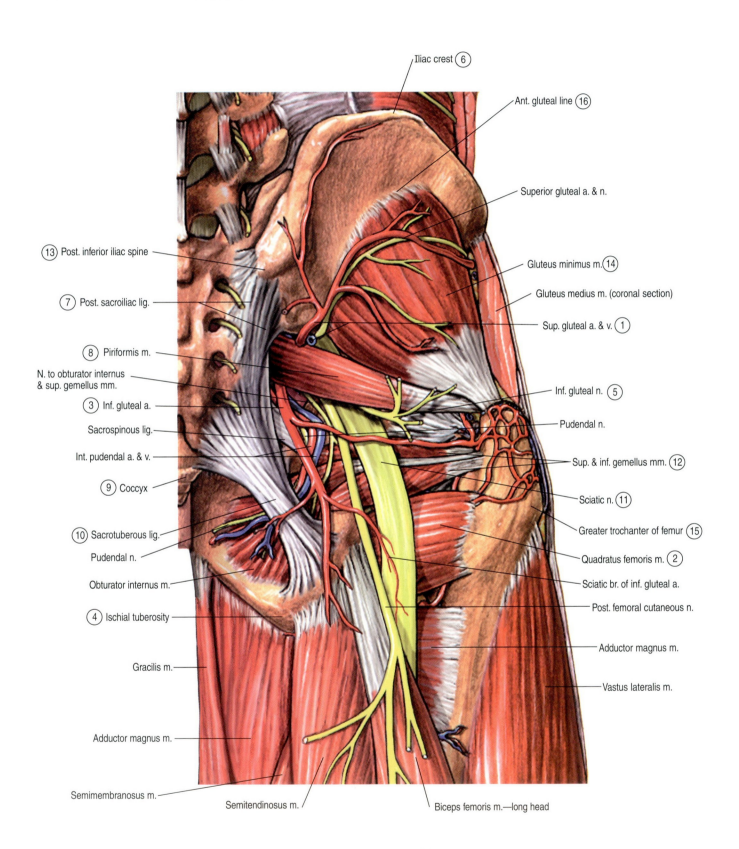

Iliac crest ⑥

Ant. gluteal line ⑯

Superior gluteal a. & n.

⑬ Post. inferior iliac spine

Gluteus minimus m. ⑭

Gluteus medius m. (coronal section)

⑦ Post. sacroiliac lig.

Sup. gluteal a. & v. ①

⑧ Piriformis m.

N. to obturator internus
& sup. gemellus mm.

Inf. gluteal n. ⑤

③ Inf. gluteal a.

Pudendal n.

Sacrospinous lig.

Int. pudendal a. & v.

Sup. & inf. gemellus mm. ⑫

⑨ Coccyx

Sciatic n. ⑪

⑩ Sacrotuberous lig.

Greater trochanter of femur ⑮

Pudendal n.

Quadratus femoris m. ②

Obturator internus m.

Sciatic br. of inf. gluteal a.

④ Ischial tuberosity

Post. femoral cutaneous n.

Gracilis m.

Adductor magnus m.

Vastus lateralis m.

Adductor magnus m.

Semimembranosus m.

Semitendinosus m.

Biceps femoris m.—long head

POSTERIOR VIEW

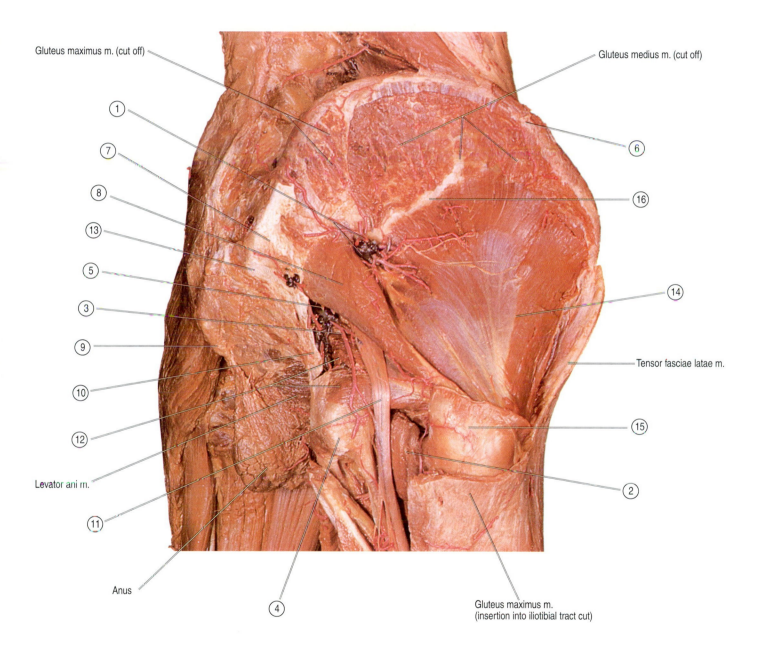

Gluteus maximus m. (cut off)

Gluteus medius m. (cut off)

1

7

8

13

5

3

9

10

12

Levator ani m.

11

Anus

4

6

16

14

Tensor fasciae latae m.

15

2

Gluteus maximus m.
(insertion into iliotibial tract cut)

POSTEROLATERAL VIEW

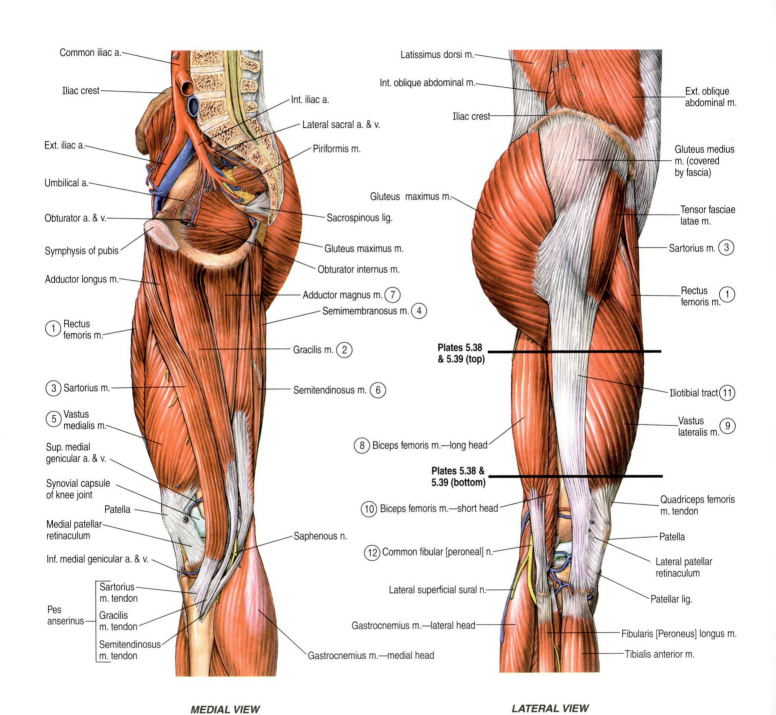

Common iliac a.
Iliac crest
Ext. iliac a.
Umbilical a.
Obturator a. & v.
Symphysis of pubis
Adductor longus m.
1 Rectus femoris m.
3 Sartorius m.
5 Vastus medialis m.
Sup. medial genicular a. & v.
Synovial capsule of knee joint
Patella
Medial patellar retinaculum
Inf. medial genicular a. & v.
Pes anserinus
Sartorius m. tendon
Gracilis m. tendon
Semitendinosus m. tendon

Int. iliac a.
Lateral sacral a. & v.
Piriformis m.
Sacrospinous lig.
Gluteus maximus m.
Obturator internus m.
Adductor magnus m. 7
Semimembranosus m. 4
Gracilis m. 2
Semitendinosus m. 6
Saphenous n.
Gastrocnemius m.—medial head

MEDIAL VIEW

Latissimus dorsi m.
Int. oblique abdominal m.
Iliac crest
Gluteus maximus m.
Plates 5.38 & 5.39 (top)
8 Biceps femoris m.—long head
Plates 5.38 & 5.39 (bottom)
10 Biceps femoris m.—short head
12 Common fibular [peroneal] n.
Lateral superficial sural n.
Gastrocnemius m.—lateral head

Ext. oblique abdominal m.
Gluteus medius m. (covered by fascia)
Tensor fasciae latae m.
Sartorius m. 3
Rectus femoris m. 1
Iliotibial tract 11
Vastus lateralis m. 9
Quadriceps femoris m. tendon
Patella
Lateral patellar retinaculum
Patellar lig.
Fibularis [Peroneus] longus m.
Tibialis anterior m.

LATERAL VIEW

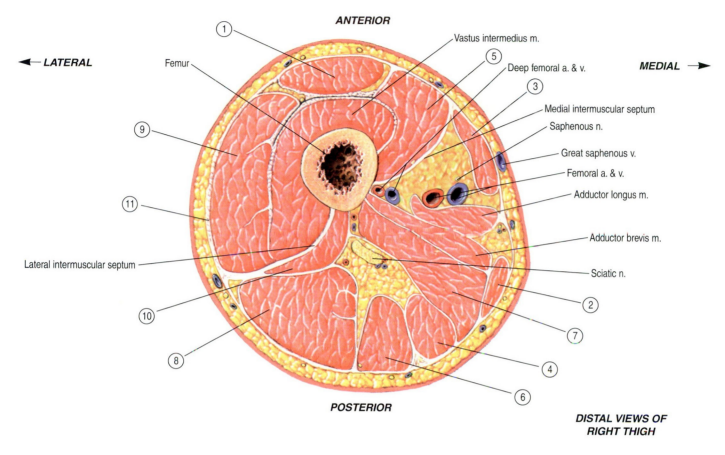

ANTERIOR

1

Vastus intermedius m.

5

Deep femoral a. & v.

3

LATERAL ←   MEDIAL →

Femur

Medial intermuscular septum

9

Saphenous n.

Great saphenous v.

Femoral a. & v.

11

Adductor longus m.

Adductor brevis m.

Lateral intermuscular septum

Sciatic n.

10

2

8

7

4

6

POSTERIOR

DISTAL VIEWS OF
RIGHT THIGH

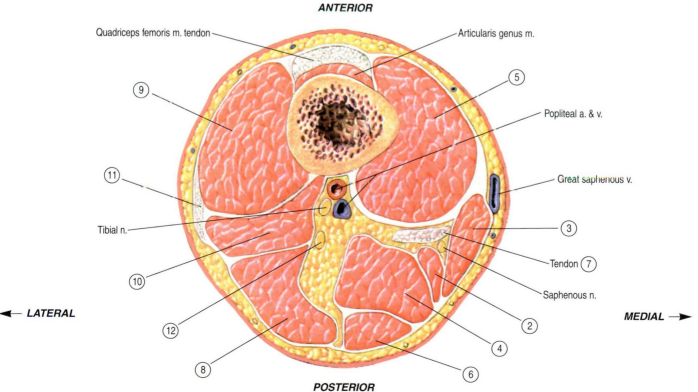

ANTERIOR

Quadriceps femoris m. tendon

Articularis genus m.

9

5

Popliteal a. & v.

11

Great saphenous v.

Tibial n.

3

10

Tendon 7

12

Saphenous n.

8

2

4

6

LATERAL ←   MEDIAL →

POSTERIOR

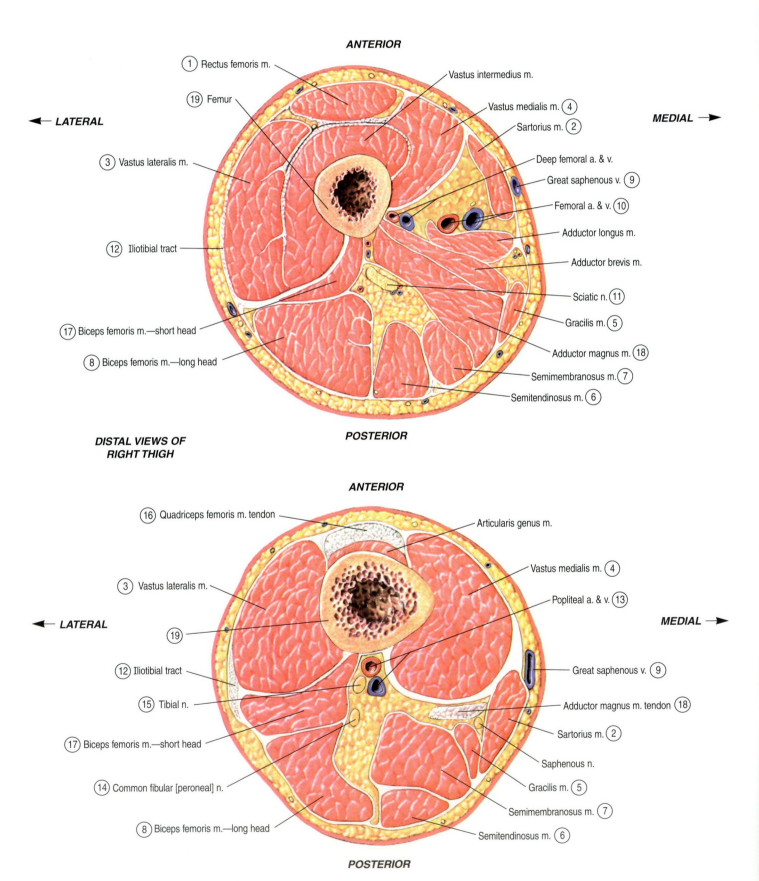

ANTERIOR

① Rectus femoris m.

⑲ Femur

◄ LATERAL

③ Vastus lateralis m.

⑫ Iliotibial tract

⑰ Biceps femoris m.—short head

⑧ Biceps femoris m.—long head

Vastus intermedius m.

Vastus medialis m. ④

Sartorius m. ②

Deep femoral a. & v.

Great saphenous v. ⑨

Femoral a. & v. ⑩

Adductor longus m.

Adductor brevis m.

Sciatic n. ⑪

Gracilis m. ⑤

Adductor magnus m. ⑱

Semimembranosus m. ⑦

Semitendinosus m. ⑥

MEDIAL ►

DISTAL VIEWS OF
RIGHT THIGH

POSTERIOR

ANTERIOR

⑯ Quadriceps femoris m. tendon

③ Vastus lateralis m.

⑲

◄ LATERAL

⑫ Iliotibial tract

⑮ Tibial n.

⑰ Biceps femoris m.—short head

⑭ Common fibular [peroneal] n.

⑧ Biceps femoris m.—long head

Articularis genus m.

Vastus medialis m. ④

Popliteal a. & v. ⑬

Great saphenous v. ⑨

Adductor magnus m. tendon ⑱

Sartorius m. ②

Saphenous n.

Gracilis m. ⑤

Semimembranosus m. ⑦

Semitendinosus m. ⑥

MEDIAL ►

POSTERIOR

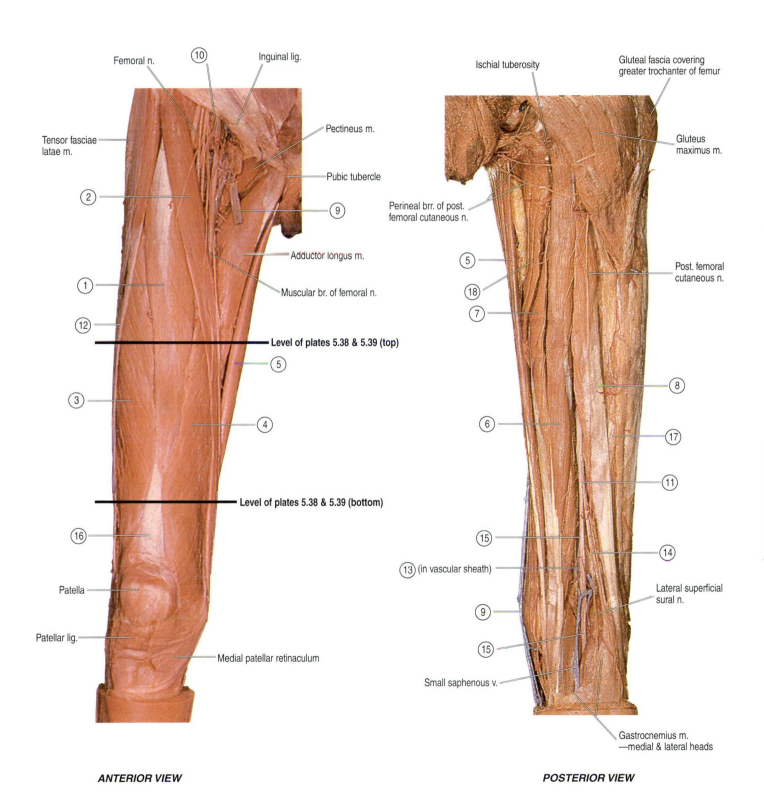

Femoral n.

10

Inguinal lig.

Tensor fasciae latae m.

Pectineus m.

Pubic tubercle

2

9

Adductor longus m.

Muscular br. of femoral n.

1

12

Level of plates 5.38 & 5.39 (top)

5

3

4

Level of plates 5.38 & 5.39 (bottom)

16

Patella

Patellar lig.

Medial patellar retinaculum

ANTERIOR VIEW

Ischial tuberosity

Gluteal fascia covering greater trochanter of femur

Gluteus maximus m.

Perineal brr. of post. femoral cutaneous n.

5

18

Post. femoral cutaneous n.

7

8

6

17

11

15

14

13 (in vascular sheath)

Lateral superficial sural n.

9

15

Small saphenous v.

Gastrocnemius m. —medial & lateral heads

POSTERIOR VIEW

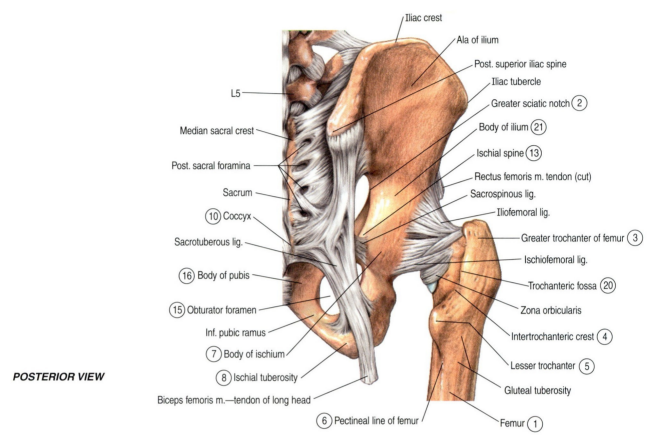

Iliac crest

Ala of ilium

Post. superior iliac spine

Iliac tubercle

Greater sciatic notch ②

Body of ilium ㉑

Ischial spine ⑬

Rectus femoris m. tendon (cut)

Sacrospinous lig.

Iliofemoral lig.

Greater trochanter of femur ③

Ischiofemoral lig.

Trochanteric fossa ⑳

Zona orbicularis

Intertrochanteric crest ④

Lesser trochanter ⑤

Gluteal tuberosity

Femur ①

L5

Median sacral crest

Post. sacral foramina

Sacrum

⑩ Coccyx

Sacrotuberous lig.

⑯ Body of pubis

⑮ Obturator foramen

Inf. pubic ramus

⑦ Body of ischium

⑧ Ischial tuberosity

Biceps femoris m.—tendon of long head

⑥ Pectineal line of femur

POSTERIOR VIEW

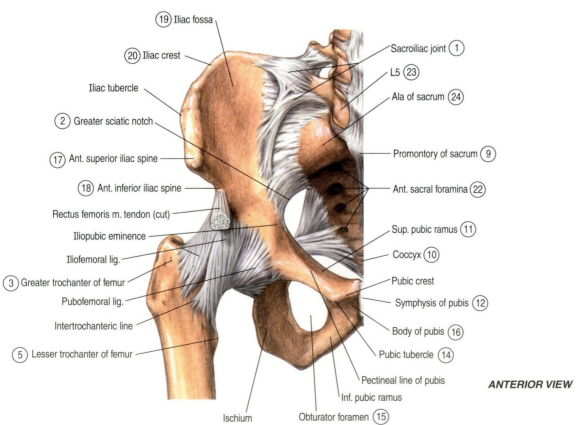

⑲ Iliac fossa

⑳ Iliac crest

Iliac tubercle

② Greater sciatic notch

⑰ Ant. superior iliac spine

⑱ Ant. inferior iliac spine

Rectus femoris m. tendon (cut)

Iliopubic eminence

Iliofemoral lig.

③ Greater trochanter of femur

Pubofemoral lig.

Intertrochanteric line

⑤ Lesser trochanter of femur

Sacroiliac joint ①

L5 ㉓

Ala of sacrum ㉔

Promontory of sacrum ⑨

Ant. sacral foramina ㉒

Sup. pubic ramus ⑪

Coccyx ⑩

Pubic crest

Symphysis of pubis ⑫

Body of pubis ⑯

Pubic tubercle ⑭

Pectineal line of pubis

Inf. pubic ramus

Ischium

Obturator foramen ⑮

ANTERIOR VIEW

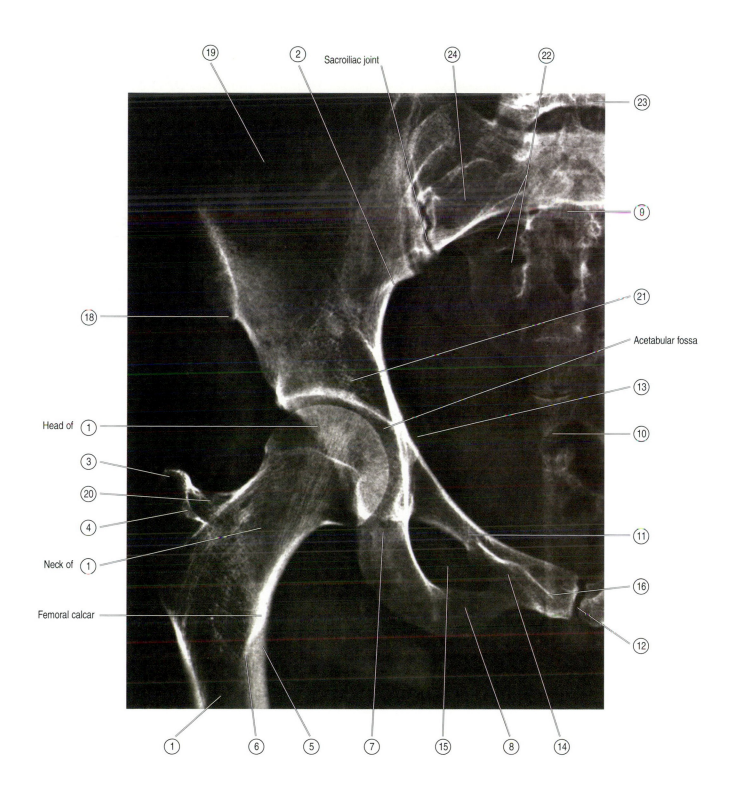

Sacroiliac joint

Acetabular fossa

Head of ①

Neck of ①

Femoral calcar

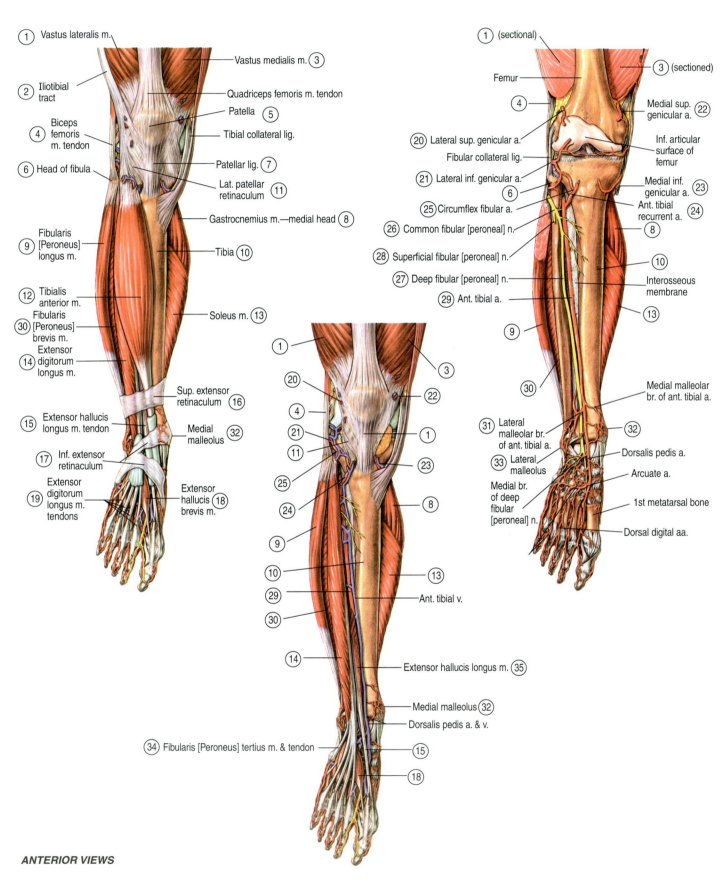

① Vastus lateralis m.
② Iliotibial tract
④ Biceps femoris m. tendon
⑥ Head of fibula
⑨ Fibularis [Peroneus] longus m.
⑫ Tibialis anterior m.
㉚ Fibularis [Peroneus] brevis m.
⑭ Extensor digitorum longus m.
⑮ Extensor hallucis longus m. tendon
⑰ Inf. extensor retinaculum
⑲ Extensor digitorum longus m. tendons

Vastus medialis m. ③
Quadriceps femoris m. tendon
Patella ⑤
Tibial collateral lig.
Patellar lig. ⑦
Lat. patellar retinaculum ⑪
Gastrocnemius m.—medial head ⑧
Tibia ⑩
Soleus m. ⑬
Sup. extensor retinaculum ⑯
Medial malleolus ㉜
Extensor hallucis ⑱ brevis m.

① (sectional)
Femur
④
⑳ Lateral sup. genicular a.
Fibular collateral lig.
㉑ Lateral inf. genicular a.
⑥
㉕ Circumflex fibular a.
㉖ Common fibular [peroneal] n.
㉘ Superficial fibular [peroneal] n.
㉗ Deep fibular [peroneal] n.
㉙ Ant. tibial a.
⑨
㉚

③ (sectioned)
Medial sup. genicular a. ㉒
Inf. articular surface of femur
Medial inf. genicular a. ㉓
Ant. tibial recurrent a. ㉔
⑧
⑩
Interosseous membrane
⑬

㉛ Lateral malleolar br. of ant. tibial a.
㉝ Lateral malleolus
Medial br. of deep fibular [peroneal] n.

Medial malleolar br. of ant. tibial a.
㉜
Dorsalis pedis a.
Arcuate a.
1st metatarsal bone
Dorsal digital aa.

⑳
④
㉑
⑪
㉕
㉔
⑨
⑩
㉙
㉚
⑭

①
㉒
③
㉓
⑧
⑬
Ant. tibial v.
Extensor hallucis longus m. ㉟
Medial malleolus ㉜
Dorsalis pedis a. & v.
㉞ Fibularis [Peroneus] tertius m. & tendon
⑮
⑱

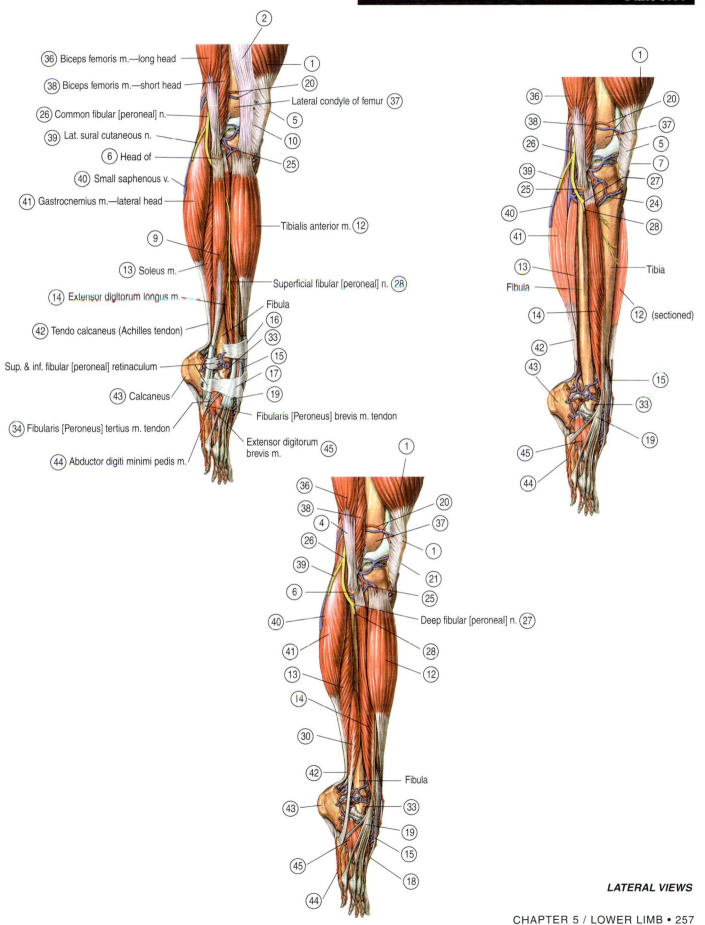

36 Biceps femoris m.—long head
38 Biceps femoris m.—short head
26 Common fibular [peroneal] n.
39 Lat. sural cutaneous n.
6 Head of
40 Small saphenous v.
41 Gastrocnemius m.—lateral head

2
1
20
Lateral condyle of femur 37
5
10
25

9
13 Soleus m.
14 Extensor digitorum longus m.
42 Tendo calcaneus (Achilles tendon)
Sup. & inf. fibular [peroneal] retinaculum
43 Calcaneus
34 Fibularis [Peroneus] tertius m. tendon
44 Abductor digiti minimi pedis m.

Tibialis anterior m. 12
Superficial fibular [peroneal] n. 28
Fibula
16
33
15
17
19
Fibularis [Peroneus] brevis m. tendon
Extensor digitorum brevis m. 45

1
36
38
26
39
25
40
41
13
Fibula
14
42
43
45
44

20
37
5
7
27
24
28
Tibia
12 (sectioned)
15
33
19

36
38
4
26
39
6
40
41
13
14
30
42
43
45
44

1
20
37
1
21
25
Deep fibular [peroneal] n. 27
28
12
Fibula
33
19
15
18

LATERAL VIEWS

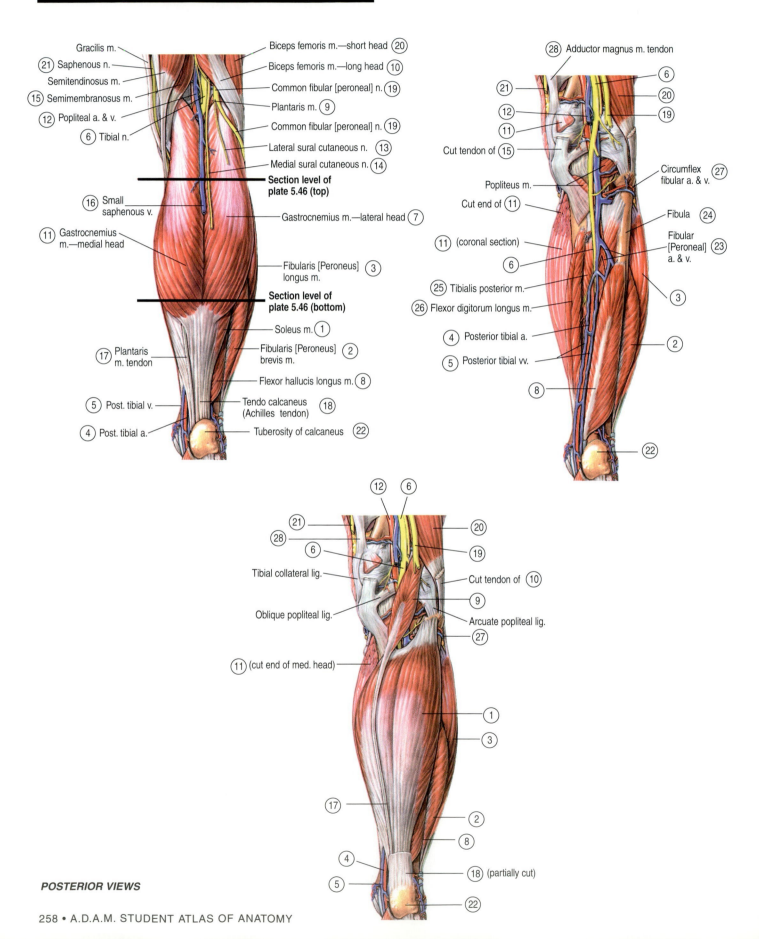

Gracilis m.
(21) Saphenous n.
Semitendinosus m.
(15) Semimembranosus m.
(12) Popliteal a. & v.
(6) Tibial n.

Biceps femoris m.—short head (20)
Biceps femoris m.—long head (10)
Common fibular [peroneal] n. (19)
Plantaris m. (9)
Common fibular [peroneal] n. (19)
Lateral sural cutaneous n. (13)
Medial sural cutaneous n. (14)
Section level of plate 5.46 (top)

(16) Small saphenous v.
Gastrocnemius m.—lateral head (7)

(11) Gastrocnemius m.—medial head
Fibularis [Peroneus] longus m. (3)

Section level of plate 5.46 (bottom)

Soleus m. (1)
(17) Plantaris m. tendon
Fibularis [Peroneus] brevis m. (2)
Flexor hallucis longus m. (8)
(5) Post. tibial v.
Tendo calcaneus (Achilles tendon) (18)
(4) Post. tibial a.
Tuberosity of calcaneus (22)

(28) Adductor magnus m. tendon
(21)
(12)
(11)
Cut tendon of (15)
Popliteus m.
Cut end of (11)
(11) (coronal section)
(6)
(25) Tibialis posterior m.
(26) Flexor digitorum longus m.
(4) Posterior tibial a.
(5) Posterior tibial vv.
(8)

(6)
(20)
(19)
Circumflex fibular a. & v. (27)
Fibula (24)
Fibular [Peroneal] a. & v. (23)
(3)
(2)
(22)

(12) (6)
(21)
(28)
(6)
Tibial collateral lig.
Oblique popliteal lig.
(11) (cut end of med. head)

(20)
(19)
Cut tendon of (10)
(9)
Arcuate popliteal lig.
(27)
(1)
(3)
(17)
(2)
(8)
(4)
(18) (partially cut)
(5)
(22)

POSTERIOR VIEWS

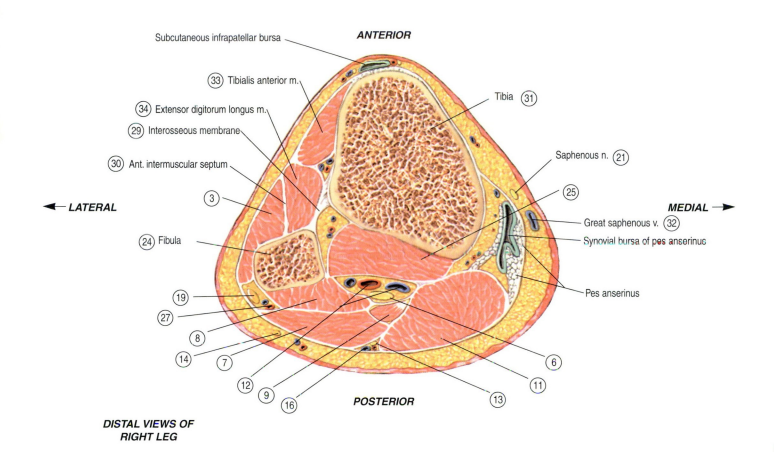

Subcutaneous infrapatellar bursa

ANTERIOR

(33) Tibialis anterior m.

(34) Extensor digitorum longus m.

(29) Interosseous membrane

(30) Ant. intermuscular septum

← **LATERAL**

(3)

(24) Fibula

(19)

(27)

(8)

(14)   (7)

(12)

(9)

(16)

Tibia (31)

Saphenous n. (21)

(25)

MEDIAL →

Great saphenous v. (32)

Synovial bursa of pes anserinus

Pes anserinus

(6)

(11)

(13)

POSTERIOR

**DISTAL VIEWS OF
RIGHT LEG**

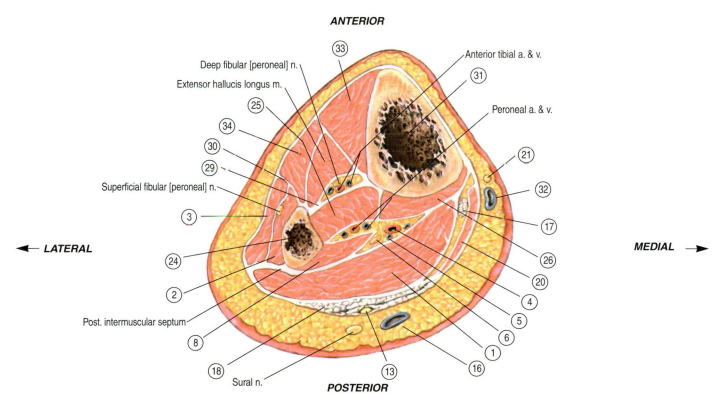

ANTERIOR

(33)

Deep fibular [peroneal] n.

Extensor hallucis longus m.

(25)

(34)

(30)

(29)

Superficial fibular [peroneal] n.

(3)

← **LATERAL**

(24)

(2)

Post. intermuscular septum

(8)

(18)

Sural n.

Anterior tibial a. & v.

(31)

Peroneal a. & v.

(21)

(32)

(17)

MEDIAL →

(26)

(20)

(4)

(5)

(6)

(1)

(16)

(13)

POSTERIOR

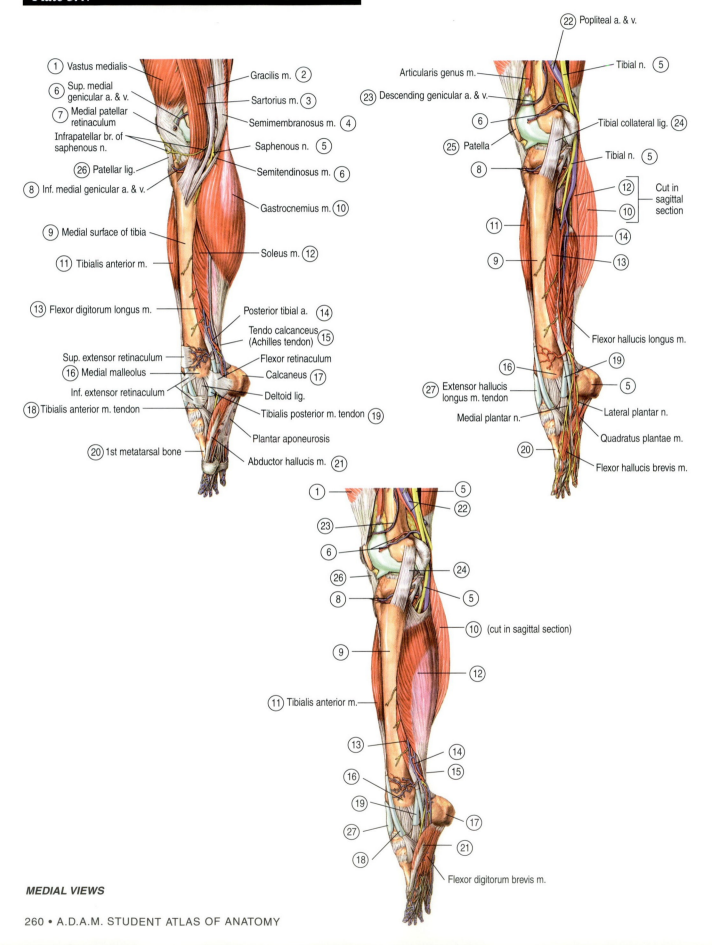

① Vastus medialis
⑥ Sup. medial genicular a. & v.
⑦ Medial patellar retinaculum
Infrapatellar br. of saphenous n.
㉖ Patellar lig.
⑧ Inf. medial genicular a. & v.
⑨ Medial surface of tibia
⑪ Tibialis anterior m.
⑬ Flexor digitorum longus m.
Sup. extensor retinaculum
⑯ Medial malleolus
Inf. extensor retinaculum
⑱ Tibialis anterior m. tendon
⑳ 1st metatarsal bone

Gracilis m. ②
Sartorius m. ③
Semimembranosus m. ④
Saphenous n. ⑤
Semitendinosus m. ⑥
Gastrocnemius m. ⑩
Soleus m. ⑫
Posterior tibial a. ⑭
Tendo calcanceus (Achilles tendon) ⑮
Flexor retinaculum
Calcaneus ⑰
Deltoid lig.
Tibialis posterior m. tendon ⑲
Plantar aponeurosis
Abductor hallucis m. ㉑

㉒ Popliteal a. & v.
Articularis genus m.
㉓ Descending genicular a. & v.
⑥
㉕ Patella
⑧
⑪
⑨

Tibial n. ⑤
Tibial collateral lig. ㉔
Tibial n. ⑤
⑫ ⑩ Cut in sagittal section
⑭
⑬
Flexor hallucis longus m.
⑯ ⑲
㉗ Extensor hallucis longus m. tendon ⑤
Medial plantar n.
⑳
Lateral plantar n.
Quadratus plantae m.
Flexor hallucis brevis m.

①
㉓
⑥
㉖
⑧
⑤ ㉒
⑤
㉔
⑤
⑩ (cut in sagittal section)
⑫
⑪ Tibialis anterior m.
⑨
⑬
⑯
⑲
㉗
⑱
⑭
⑮
⑰
㉑
Flexor digitorum brevis m.

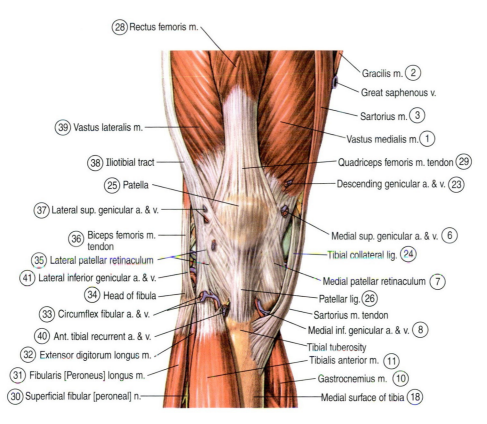

(28) Rectus femoris m.

(39) Vastus lateralis m.

(38) Iliotibial tract

(25) Patella

(37) Lateral sup. genicular a. & v.

(36) Biceps femoris m. tendon

(35) Lateral patellar retinaculum

(41) Lateral inferior genicular a. & v.

(34) Head of fibula

(33) Circumflex fibular a. & v.

(40) Ant. tibial recurrent a. & v.

(32) Extensor digitorum longus m.

(31) Fibularis [Peroneus] longus m.

(30) Superficial fibular [peroneal] n.

Gracilis m. (2)

Great saphenous v.

Sartorius m. (3)

Vastus medialis m. (1)

Quadriceps femoris m. tendon (29)

Descending genicular a. & v. (23)

Medial sup. genicular a. & v. (6)

Tibial collateral lig. (24)

Medial patellar retinaculum (7)

Patellar lig. (26)

Sartorius m. tendon

Medial inf. genicular a. & v. (8)

Tibial tuberosity

Tibialis anterior m. (11)

Gastrocnemius m. (10)

Medial surface of tibia (18)

ANTERIOR VIEW

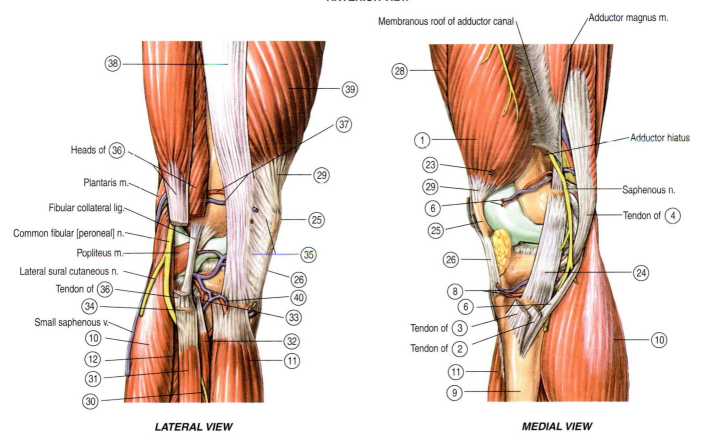

(38)

(39)

(37)

Heads of (36)

Plantaris m.

Fibular collateral lig.

Common fibular [peroneal] n.

Popliteus m.

Lateral sural cutaneous n.

Tendon of (36)

(34)

Small saphenous v.

(10)

(12)

(31)

(30)

(29)

(25)

(35)

(26)

(40)

(33)

(32)

(11)

LATERAL VIEW

Membranous roof of adductor canal

Adductor magnus m.

(28)

(1)

(23)

(29)

(6)

(25)

(26)

(8)

(6)

Tendon of (3)

Tendon of (2)

(11)

(9)

Adductor hiatus

Saphenous n.

Tendon of (4)

(24)

(10)

MEDIAL VIEW

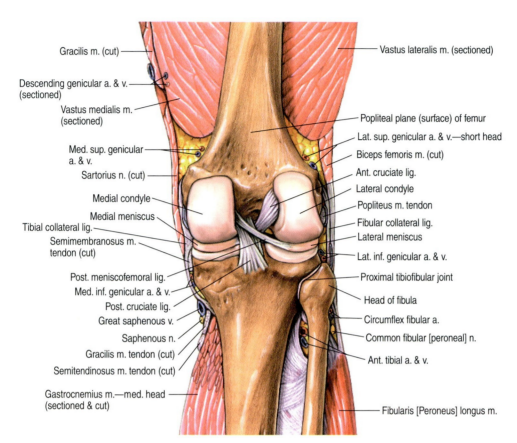

Gracilis m. (cut)

Descending genicular a. & v. (sectioned)

Vastus medialis m. (sectioned)

Med. sup. genicular a. & v.

Sartorius n. (cut)

Medial condyle

Medial meniscus

Tibial collateral lig.

Semimembranosus m. tendon (cut)

Post. meniscofemoral lig.

Med. inf. genicular a. & v.

Post. cruciate lig.

Great saphenous v.

Saphenous n.

Gracilis m. tendon (cut)

Semitendinosus m. tendon (cut)

Gastrocnemius m.—med. head (sectioned & cut)

Vastus lateralis m. (sectioned)

Popliteal plane (surface) of femur

Lat. sup. genicular a. & v.—short head

Biceps femoris m. (cut)

Ant. cruciate lig.

Lateral condyle

Popliteus m. tendon

Fibular collateral lig.

Lateral meniscus

Lat. inf. genicular a. & v.

Proximal tibiofibular joint

Head of fibula

Circumflex fibular a.

Common fibular [peroneal] n.

Ant. tibial a. & v.

Fibularis [Peroneus] longus m.

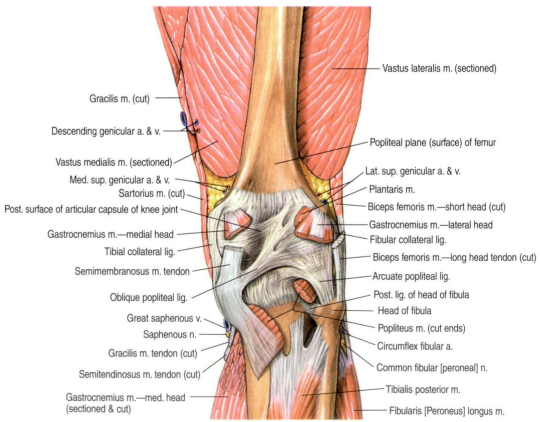

Vastus lateralis m. (sectioned)

Gracilis m. (cut)

Descending genicular a. & v.

Vastus medialis m. (sectioned)

Med. sup. genicular a. & v.

Sartorius m. (cut)

Post. surface of articular capsule of knee joint

Gastrocnemius m.—medial head

Tibial collateral lig.

Semimembranosus m. tendon

Oblique popliteal lig.

Great saphenous v.

Saphenous n.

Gracilis m. tendon (cut)

Semitendinosus m. tendon (cut)

Gastrocnemius m.—med. head (sectioned & cut)

Popliteal plane (surface) of femur

Lat. sup. genicular a. & v.

Plantaris m.

Biceps femoris m.—short head (cut)

Gastrocnemius m.—lateral head

Fibular collateral lig.

Biceps femoris m.—long head tendon (cut)

Arcuate popliteal lig.

Post. lig. of head of fibula

Head of fibula

Popliteus m. (cut ends)

Circumflex fibular a.

Common fibular [peroneal] n.

Tibialis posterior m.

Fibularis [Peroneus] longus m.

POSTERIOR VIEWS

**DISTAL VIEW OF ARTICULAR
SURFACE OF RIGHT FEMUR**

ANTERIOR

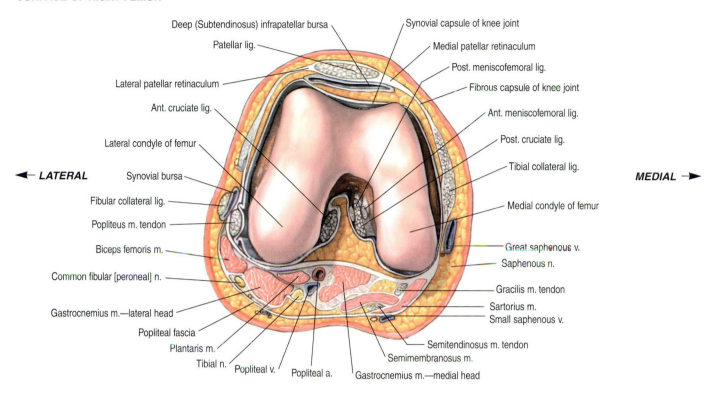

Deep (Subtendinosus) infrapatellar bursa

Patellar lig.

Lateral patellar retinaculum

Ant. cruciate lig.

Lateral condyle of femur

◄ LATERAL

Synovial bursa

Fibular collateral lig.

Popliteus m. tendon

Biceps femoris m.

Common fibular [peroneal] n.

Gastrocnemius m.—lateral head

Popliteal fascia

Plantaris m.

Tibial n.

Popliteal v.

Popliteal a.

Synovial capsule of knee joint

Medial patellar retinaculum

Post. meniscofemoral lig.

Fibrous capsule of knee joint

Ant. meniscofemoral lig.

Post. cruciate lig.

Tibial collateral lig.

MEDIAL ►

Medial condyle of femur

Great saphenous v.

Saphenous n.

Gracilis m. tendon

Sartorius m.

Small saphenous v.

Semitendinosus m. tendon

Semimembranosus m.

Gastrocnemius m.—medial head

**DISTAL VIEW OF ARTICULAR
SURFACE OF RIGHT TIBIA**

POSTERIOR

Popliteal v. & a.

Popliteal fascia

Tibial n.

Plantaris m.

Medial sural cutaneous n.

Gastrocnemius m.—lateral head

Common fibular [peroneal] n.

Post. meniscofemoral lig.

Biceps femoris m.

◄ LATERAL

Popliteus m. tendon

Post. cruciate ligament

Fibular collateral lig.

Lateral meniscus

Ant. meniscofemoral lig.

Sup. articular surface of tibia (lateral condyle)

Infrapatellar fat pad

Patellar lig.

Gastrocnemius m.—medial head

Semimembranosus m.

Small saphenous v.

Semitendinous m. tendon

Sartorius m.

Gracilis m.

Saphenous n.

Great saphenous v.

Sup. articular surface of tibia

Med. meniscus

MEDIAL ►

Tibial collateral lig.

Synovial capsule of knee joint

Intercondylar eminence

Ant. cruciate lig.

Transverse lig. of knee joint

ANTERIOR

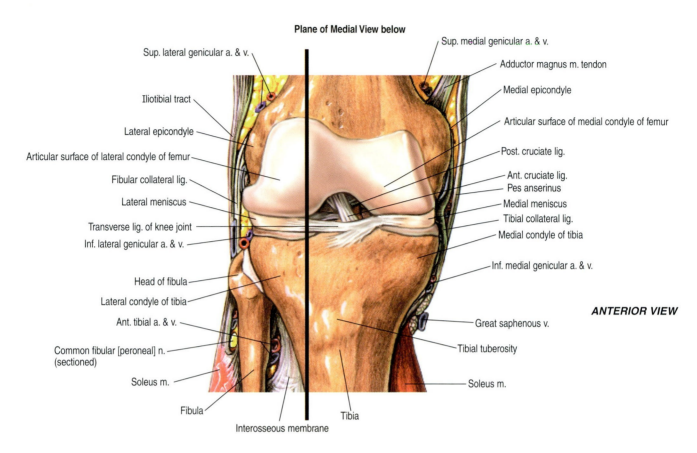

Plane of Medial View below

Sup. lateral genicular a. & v.

Iliotibial tract

Lateral epicondyle

Articular surface of lateral condyle of femur

Fibular collateral lig.

Lateral meniscus

Transverse lig. of knee joint

Inf. lateral genicular a. & v.

Head of fibula

Lateral condyle of tibia

Ant. tibial a. & v.

Common fibular [peroneal] n. (sectioned)

Soleus m.

Fibula

Interosseous membrane

Sup. medial genicular a. & v.

Adductor magnus m. tendon

Medial epicondyle

Articular surface of medial condyle of femur

Post. cruciate lig.

Ant. cruciate lig.
Pes anserinus

Medial meniscus

Tibial collateral lig.

Medial condyle of tibia

Inf. medial genicular a. & v.

Great saphenous v.

Tibial tuberosity

Soleus m.

Tibia

ANTERIOR VIEW

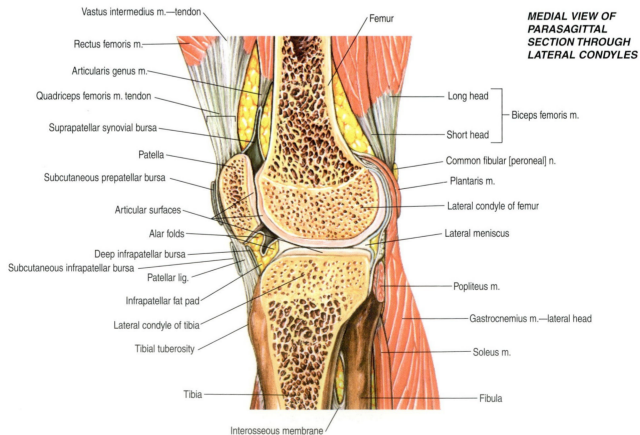

MEDIAL VIEW OF PARASAGITTAL SECTION THROUGH LATERAL CONDYLES

Vastus intermedius m.—tendon

Rectus femoris m.

Articularis genus m.

Quadriceps femoris m. tendon

Suprapatellar synovial bursa

Patella

Subcutaneous prepatellar bursa

Articular surfaces

Alar folds

Deep infrapatellar bursa

Subcutaneous infrapatellar bursa

Patellar lig.

Infrapatellar fat pad

Lateral condyle of tibia

Tibial tuberosity

Tibia

Interosseous membrane

Femur

Long head

Biceps femoris m.

Short head

Common fibular [peroneal] n.

Plantaris m.

Lateral condyle of femur

Lateral meniscus

Popliteus m.

Gastrocnemius m.—lateral head

Soleus m.

Fibula

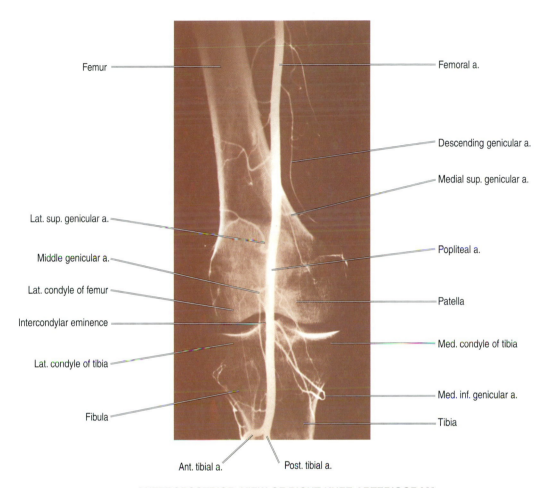

Femur

Femoral a.

Descending genicular a.

Medial sup. genicular a.

Lat. sup. genicular a.

Popliteal a.

Middle genicular a.

Lat. condyle of femur

Patella

Intercondylar eminence

Med. condyle of tibia

Lat. condyle of tibia

Med. inf. genicular a.

Fibula

Tibia

Ant. tibial a.

Post. tibial a.

ANTEROPOSTRIOR VIEW OF RIGHT KNEE ARTERIOGRAM

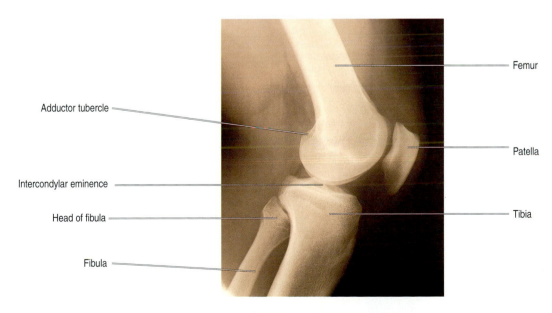

Adductor tubercle

Femur

Patella

Intercondylar eminence

Head of fibula

Tibia

Fibula

LATERAL VIEW OF RIGHT KNEE

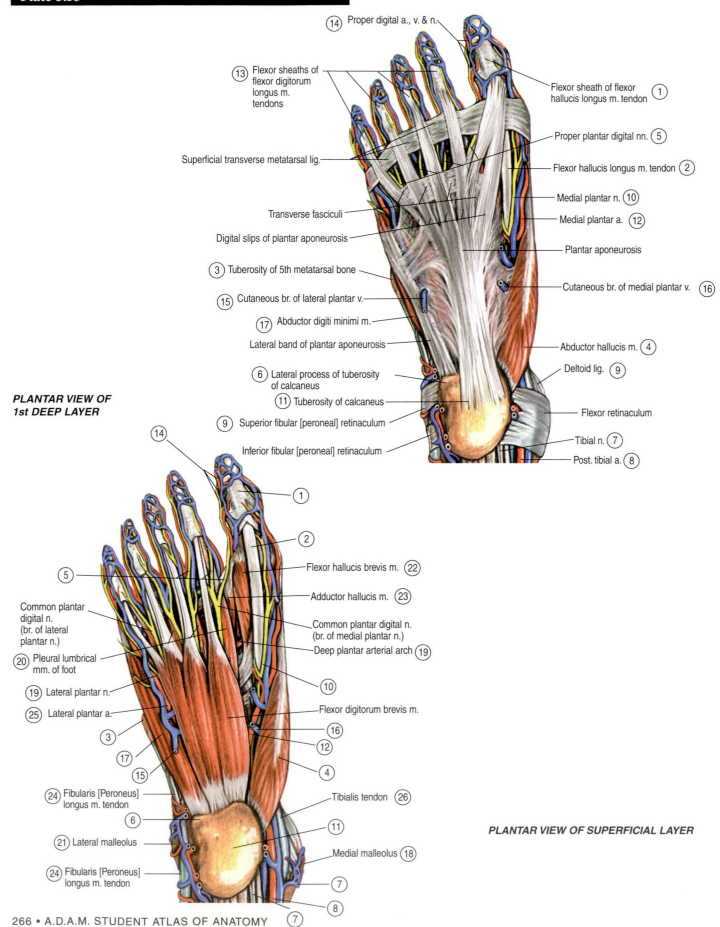

(14) Proper digital a., v. & n.

(13) Flexor sheaths of flexor digitorum longus m. tendons

Flexor sheath of flexor hallucis longus m. tendon (1)

Proper plantar digital nn. (5)

Flexor hallucis longus m. tendon (2)

Medial plantar n. (10)

Medial plantar a. (12)

Superficial transverse metatarsal lig.

Transverse fasciculi

Plantar aponeurosis

Digital slips of plantar aponeurosis

Cutaneous br. of medial plantar v. (16)

(3) Tuberosity of 5th metatarsal bone

(15) Cutaneous br. of lateral plantar v.

(17) Abductor digiti minimi m.

Abductor hallucis m. (4)

Lateral band of plantar aponeurosis

Deltoid lig. (9)

(6) Lateral process of tuberosity of calcaneus

(11) Tuberosity of calcaneus

Flexor retinaculum

(9) Superior fibular [peroneal] retinaculum

Inferior fibular [peroneal] retinaculum

Tibial n. (7)

Post. tibial a. (8)

**PLANTAR VIEW OF
1st DEEP LAYER**

(14)

(1)

(2)

Flexor hallucis brevis m. (22)

(5)

Adductor hallucis m. (23)

Common plantar digital n. (br. of lateral plantar n.)

Common plantar digital n. (br. of medial plantar n.)

Deep plantar arterial arch (19)

(20) Pleural lumbrical mm. of foot

(19) Lateral plantar n.

(10)

(25) Lateral plantar a.

Flexor digitorum brevis m.

(3)

(16)

(17)

(12)

(15)

(4)

(24) Fibularis [Peroneus] longus m. tendon

Tibialis tendon (26)

(6)

PLANTAR VIEW OF SUPERFICIAL LAYER

(21) Lateral malleolus

(11)

Medial malleolus (18)

(24) Fibularis [Peroneus] longus m. tendon

(7)

(8)

(7)

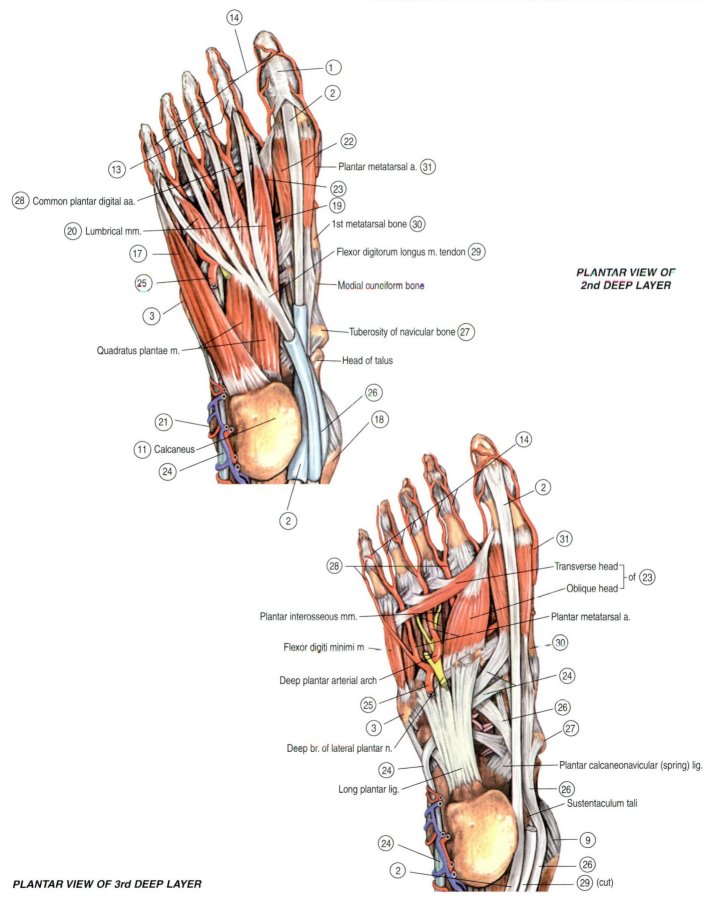

14

1

2

22

Plantar metatarsal a. 31

13

23

19

28 Common plantar digital aa.

20 Lumbrical mm.

1st metatarsal bone 30

17

Flexor digitorum longus m. tendon 29

25

Medial cuneiform bone

3

Tuberosity of navicular bone 27

Quadratus plantae m.

Head of talus

**PLANTAR VIEW OF
2nd DEEP LAYER**

26

21

18

11 Calcaneus

24

2

14

2

31

28

Transverse head ⎤
                ⎬ of 23
Oblique head ⎦

Plantar interosseous mm.

Plantar metatarsal a.

Flexor digiti minimi m.

30

Deep plantar arterial arch

24

25

26

3

27

Deep br. of lateral plantar n.

Plantar calcaneonavicular (spring) lig.

24

26

Long plantar lig.

Sustentaculum tali

9

26

24

2

29 (cut)

PLANTAR VIEW OF 3rd DEEP LAYER

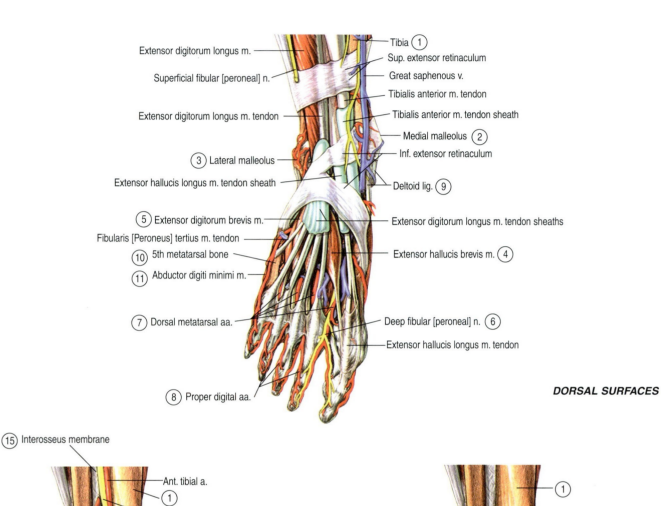

Extensor digitorum longus m.

Superficial fibular [peroneal] n.

Extensor digitorum longus m. tendon

③ Lateral malleolus

Extensor hallucis longus m. tendon sheath

⑤ Extensor digitorum brevis m.

Fibularis [Peroneus] tertius m. tendon

⑩ 5th metatarsal bone

⑪ Abductor digiti minimi m.

⑦ Dorsal metatarsal aa.

⑧ Proper digital aa.

Tibia ①

Sup. extensor retinaculum

Great saphenous v.

Tibialis anterior m. tendon

Tibialis anterior m. tendon sheath

Medial malleolus ②

Inf. extensor retinaculum

Deltoid lig. ⑨

Extensor digitorum longus m. tendon sheaths

Extensor hallucis brevis m. ④

Deep fibular [peroneal] n. ⑥

Extensor hallucis longus m. tendon

DORSAL SURFACES

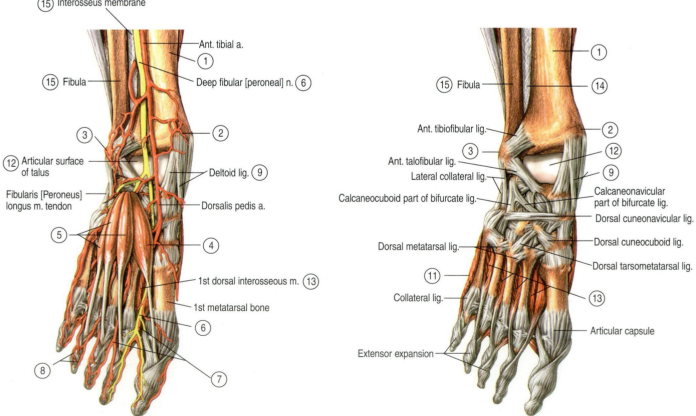

⑮ Interosseus membrane

⑮ Fibula

⑫ Articular surface of talus

Fibularis [Peroneus] longus m. tendon

⑤

⑧

Ant. tibial a.

①

Deep fibular [peroneal] n. ⑥

②

Deltoid lig. ⑨

Dorsalis pedis a.

④

1st dorsal interosseous m. ⑬

1st metatarsal bone

⑥

⑦

⑮ Fibula

①

⑭

Ant. tibiofibular lig.

②

Ant. talofibular lig.

③

⑫

Lateral collateral lig.

⑨

Calcaneocuboid part of bifurcate lig.

Calcaneonavicular part of bifurcate lig.

Dorsal cuneonavicular lig.

Dorsal metatarsal lig.

Dorsal cuneocuboid lig.

Dorsal tarsometatarsal lig.

⑪

Collateral lig.

⑬

Articular capsule

Extensor expansion

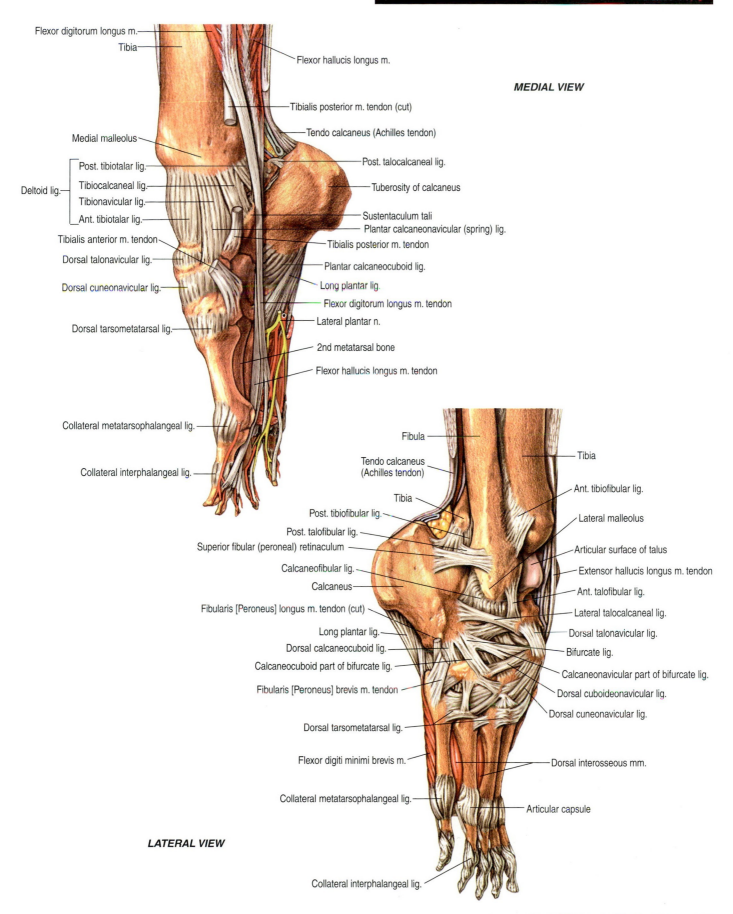

Flexor digitorum longus m.
Tibia
Flexor hallucis longus m.

MEDIAL VIEW

Tibialis posterior m. tendon (cut)
Tendo calcaneus (Achilles tendon)
Medial malleolus
Post. talocalcaneal lig.
Post. tibiotalar lig.
Tibiocalcaneal lig.
Tuberosity of calcaneus
Deltoid lig.
Tibionavicular lig.
Sustentaculum tali
Ant. tibiotalar lig.
Plantar calcaneonavicular (spring) lig.
Tibialis anterior m. tendon
Tibialis posterior m. tendon
Dorsal talonavicular lig.
Plantar calcaneocuboid lig.
Dorsal cuneonavicular lig.
Long plantar lig.
Flexor digitorum longus m. tendon
Lateral plantar n.
Dorsal tarsometatarsal lig.
2nd metatarsal bone
Flexor hallucis longus m. tendon

Collateral metatarsophalangeal lig.

Fibula
Tibia
Tendo calcaneus
(Achilles tendon)
Ant. tibiofibular lig.
Collateral interphalangeal lig.
Tibia
Post. tibiofibular lig.
Lateral malleolus
Post. talofibular lig.
Superior fibular (peroneal) retinaculum
Articular surface of talus
Calcaneofibular lig.
Extensor hallucis longus m. tendon
Calcaneus
Ant. talofibular lig.
Fibularis [Peroneus] longus m. tendon (cut)
Lateral talocalcaneal lig.
Long plantar lig.
Dorsal talonavicular lig.
Dorsal calcaneocuboid lig.
Bifurcate lig.
Calcaneocuboid part of bifurcate lig.
Calcaneonavicular part of bifurcate lig.
Fibularis [Peroneus] brevis m. tendon
Dorsal cuboideonavicular lig.
Dorsal cuneonavicular lig.
Dorsal tarsometatarsal lig.
Flexor digiti minimi brevis m.
Dorsal interosseous mm.
Collateral metatarsophalangeal lig.
Articular capsule

LATERAL VIEW

Collateral interphalangeal lig.

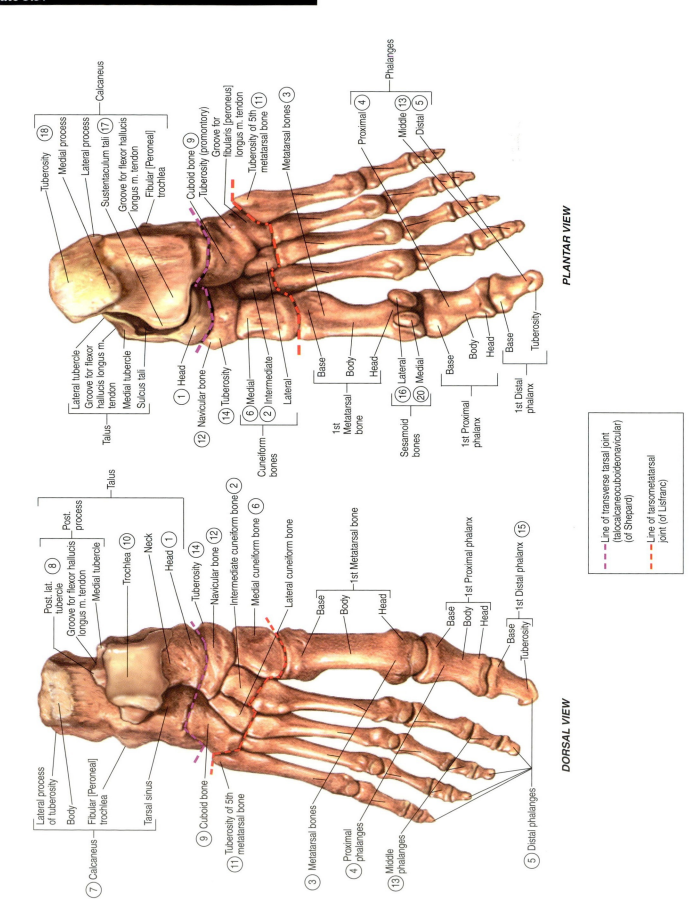

PLANTAR VIEW

Tuberosity (18)
Medial process
Lateral process
Calcaneus
Sustentaculum tali (17)
Groove for flexor hallucis longus m. tendon
Fibular [Peroneal] trochlea
Cuboid bone (9)
Tuberosity (promontory)
Groove for fibularis [peroneus] longus m. tendon
Tuberosity of 5th metatarsal bone (11)
Metatarsal bones (3)
Phalanges
Proximal (4)
Middle (13)
Distal (5)

Lateral tubercle
Groove for flexor hallucis longus m. tendon
Medial tubercle
Sulcus tali
Talus

(1) Head
(12) Navicular bone
(14) Tuberosity
Cuneiform bones
(6) Medial
(2) Intermediate
Lateral

Base
1st Metatarsal bone
Body
Head
Sesamoid bones
(16) Lateral
(20) Medial
Base
1st Proximal phalanx
Body
Head
Base
1st Distal phalanx
Tuberosity

DORSAL VIEW

Post. lat. tubercle (8)
Groove for flexor hallucis longus m. tendon
Medial tubercle
Post. process
Talus

Trochlea (10)
Neck
Head (1)
Tuberosity (14)
Navicular bone (12)
Intermediate cuneiform bone (2)
Medial cuneiform bone (6)
Lateral cuneiform bone

Lateral process of tuberosity
Body
Fibular [Peroneal] trochlea
Tarsal sinus
Calcaneus (7)

Cuboid bone (9)
Tuberosity of 5th metatarsal bone (11)

Base
Body
1st Metatarsal bone
Head
Base
Body
Head
1st Proximal phalanx
Base
Tuberosity
1st Distal phalanx (15)

Metatarsal bones (3)
Proximal phalanges (4)
Middle phalanges (13)
Distal phalanges (5)

- - - Line of transverse tarsal joint (talocalcaneocuboideonavicular) (of Shepard)
- - - Line of tarsometatarsal joint (of Lisfranc)

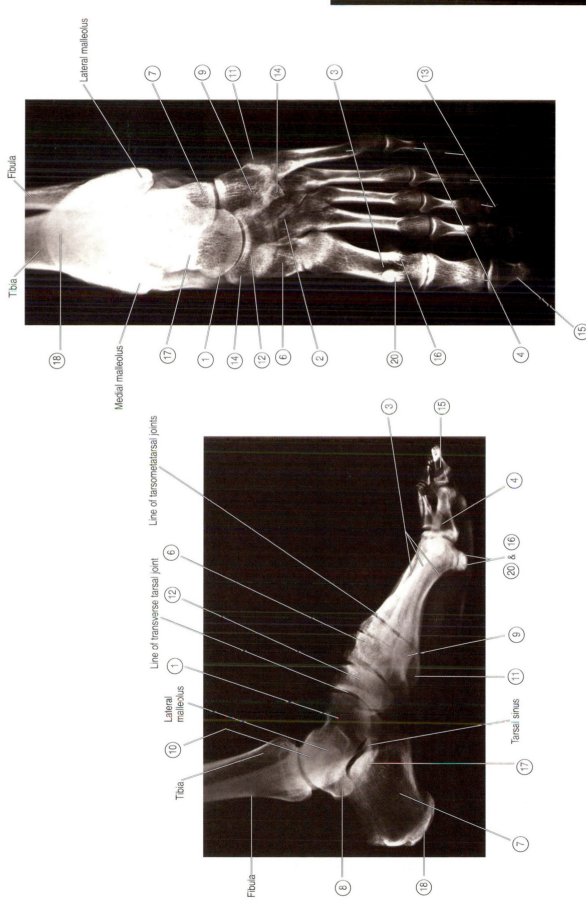

Lateral malleolus

Fibula

Tibia

Medial malleolus

ANTEROPOSTERIOR VIEW

Line of tarsometatarsal joints

Line of transverse tarsal joint

Lateral malleolus

Tibia

Fibula

Tarsal sinus

LATERAL VIEW

Upper Limb

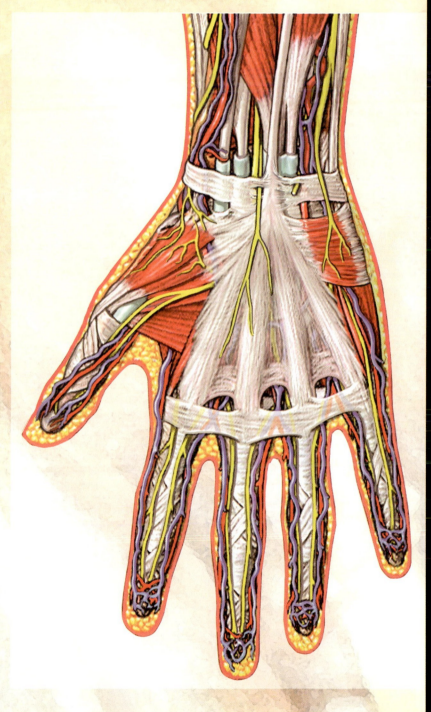

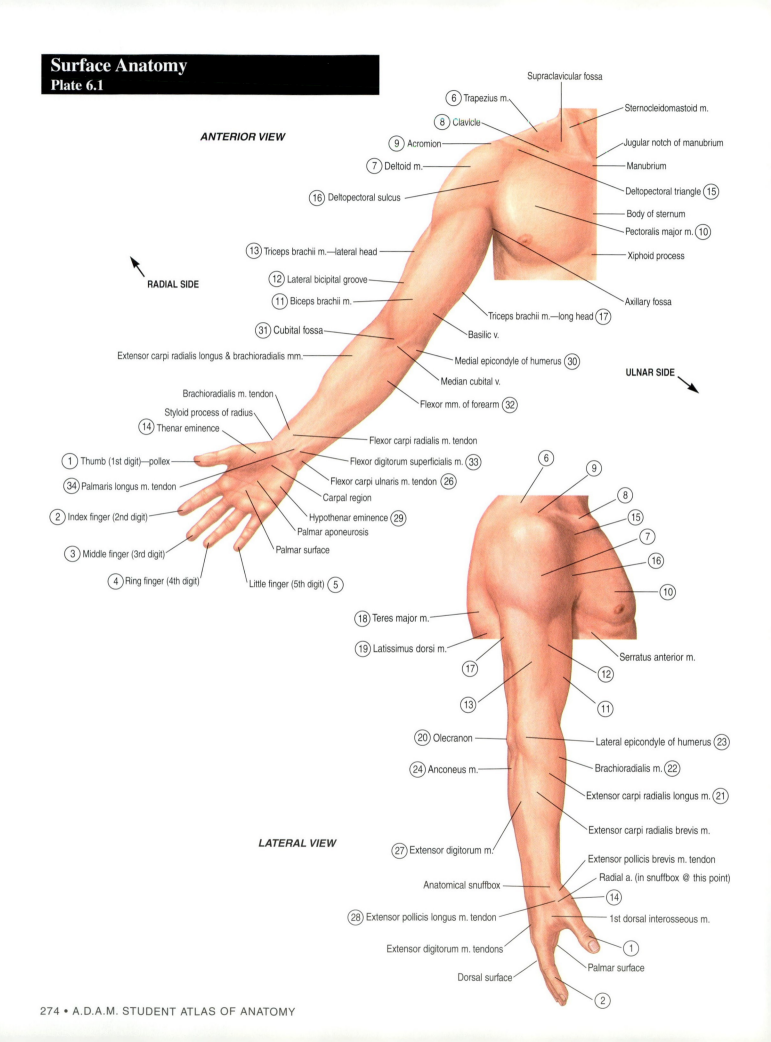

ANTERIOR VIEW

RADIAL SIDE

ULNAR SIDE

Supraclavicular fossa

⑥ Trapezius m.

⑧ Clavicle

⑨ Acromion

⑦ Deltoid m.

⑯ Deltopectoral sulcus

⑬ Triceps brachii m.—lateral head

⑫ Lateral bicipital groove

⑪ Biceps brachii m.

③① Cubital fossa

Extensor carpi radialis longus & brachioradialis mm.

Brachioradialis m. tendon

Styloid process of radius

⑭ Thenar eminence

① Thumb (1st digit)—pollex

③④ Palmaris longus m. tendon

② Index finger (2nd digit)

③ Middle finger (3rd digit)

④ Ring finger (4th digit)

Sternocleidomastoid m.

Jugular notch of manubrium

Manubrium

Deltopectoral triangle ⑮

Body of sternum

Pectoralis major m. ⑩

Xiphoid process

Axillary fossa

Triceps brachii m.—long head ⑰

Basilic v.

Medial epicondyle of humerus ㉚

Median cubital v.

Flexor mm. of forearm ㉜

Flexor carpi radialis m. tendon

Flexor digitorum superficialis m. ㉝

Flexor carpi ulnaris m. tendon ㉖

Carpal region

Hypothenar eminence ㉙

Palmar aponeurosis

Palmar surface

Little finger (5th digit) ⑤

⑥

⑨

⑧

⑮

⑦

⑯

⑩

⑱ Teres major m.

⑲ Latissimus dorsi m.

⑰

⑬

Serratus anterior m.

⑫

⑪

㉚ Olecranon

㉔ Anconeus m.

Lateral epicondyle of humerus ㉓

Brachioradialis m. ㉒

Extensor carpi radialis longus m. ㉑

Extensor carpi radialis brevis m.

LATERAL VIEW

㉗ Extensor digitorum m.

Anatomical snuffbox

㉘ Extensor pollicis longus m. tendon

Extensor digitorum m. tendons

Dorsal surface

Extensor pollicis brevis m. tendon

Radial a. (in snuffbox @ this point)

⑭

1st dorsal interosseous m.

①

Palmar surface

②

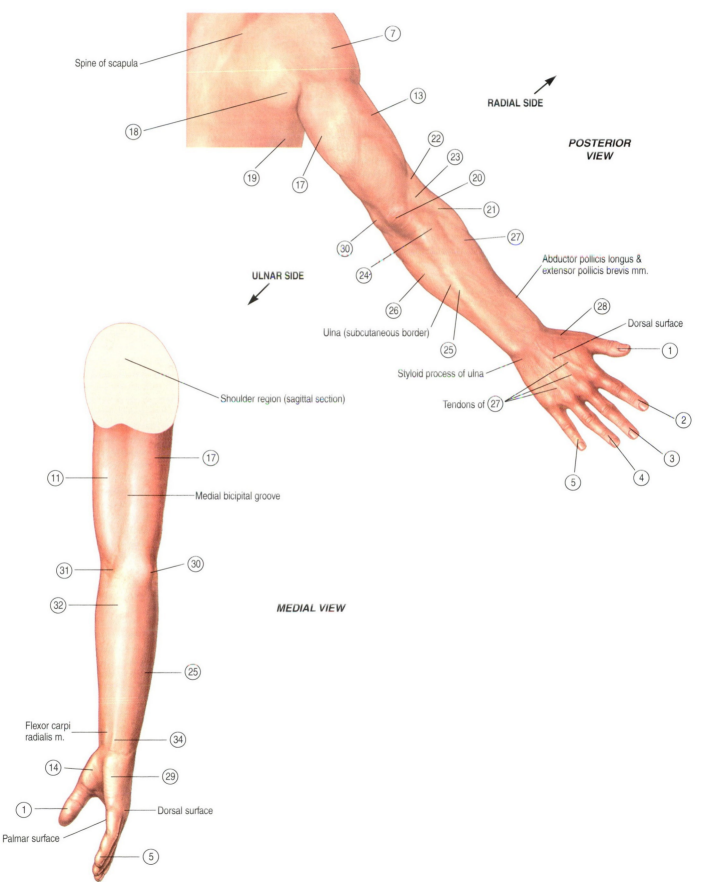

Spine of scapula

⑦

⑬

RADIAL SIDE

⑱

⑲   ⑰

⑳

㉒

㉓

㉑

POSTERIOR VIEW

⑰

ULNAR SIDE

㉚

㉗

Abductor pollicis longus & extensor pollicis brevis mm.

㉔

㉘

Dorsal surface

㉖

Ulna (subcutaneous border)

㉕

①

Styloid process of ulna

②

Tendons of ㉗

③

Shoulder region (sagittal section)

⑤   ④

⑪   ⑰

Medial bicipital groove

㉛   ㉚

㉜

MEDIAL VIEW

㉕

Flexor carpi radialis m.

㉞

⑭

㉙

①   Dorsal surface

Palmar surface

⑤

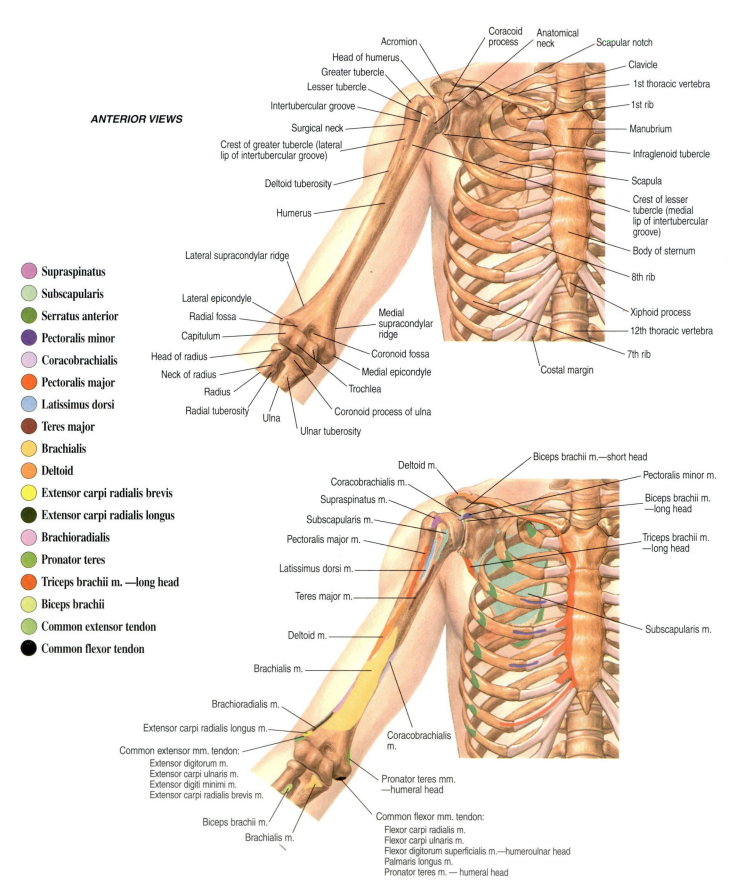

ANTERIOR VIEWS

Coracoid process
Anatomical neck
Acromion
Scapular notch
Head of humerus
Clavicle
Greater tubercle
1st thoracic vertebra
Lesser tubercle
1st rib
Intertubercular groove
Manubrium
Surgical neck
Infraglenoid tubercle
Crest of greater tubercle (lateral lip of intertubercular groove)
Scapula
Deltoid tuberosity
Crest of lesser tubercle (medial lip of intertubercular groove)
Humerus
Body of sternum
8th rib
Lateral supracondylar ridge
Xiphoid process
Lateral epicondyle
Medial supracondylar ridge
12th thoracic vertebra
Radial fossa
7th rib
Capitulum
Coronoid fossa
Head of radius
Medial epicondyle
Costal margin
Neck of radius
Trochlea
Radius
Coronoid process of ulna
Radial tuberosity
Ulna
Ulnar tuberosity

Supraspinatus
Subscapularis
Serratus anterior
Pectoralis minor
Coracobrachialis
Pectoralis major
Latissimus dorsi
Teres major
Brachialis
Deltoid
Extensor carpi radialis brevis
Extensor carpi radialis longus
Brachioradialis
Pronator teres
Triceps brachii m. —long head
Biceps brachii
Common extensor tendon
Common flexor tendon

Deltoid m.
Biceps brachii m.—short head
Coracobrachialis m.
Pectoralis minor m.
Supraspinatus m.
Biceps brachii m. —long head
Subscapularis m.
Pectoralis major m.
Triceps brachii m. —long head
Latissimus dorsi m.
Teres major m.
Subscapularis m.
Deltoid m.
Brachialis m.
Brachioradialis m.
Extensor carpi radialis longus m.
Coracobrachialis m.
Common extensor mm. tendon:
  Extensor digitorum m.
  Extensor carpi ulnaris m.
  Extensor digiti minimi m.
  Extensor carpi radialis brevis m.
Pronator teres mm. —humeral head
Biceps brachii m.
Brachialis m.
Common flexor mm. tendon:
  Flexor carpi radialis m.
  Flexor carpi ulnaris m.
  Flexor digitorum superficialis m.—humeroulnar head
  Palmaris longus m.
  Pronator teres m. — humeral head

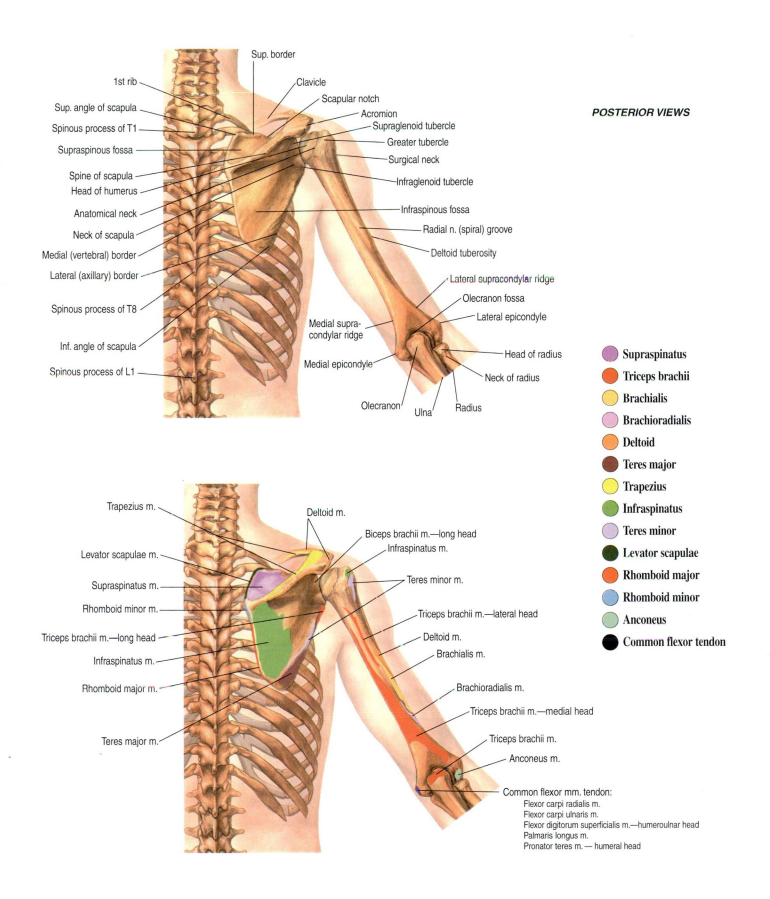

POSTERIOR VIEWS

Sup. border
1st rib
Clavicle
Scapular notch
Sup. angle of scapula
Acromion
Spinous process of T1
Supraglenoid tubercle
Supraspinous fossa
Greater tubercle
Surgical neck
Spine of scapula
Infraglenoid tubercle
Head of humerus
Anatomical neck
Infraspinous fossa
Neck of scapula
Radial n. (spiral) groove
Medial (vertebral) border
Deltoid tuberosity
Lateral (axillary) border
Lateral supracondylar ridge
Olecranon fossa
Medial supra-
condylar ridge
Lateral epicondyle
Spinous process of T8
Head of radius
Medial epicondyle
Neck of radius
Inf. angle of scapula
Spinous process of L1
Olecranon
Ulna
Radius

● Supraspinatus
● Triceps brachii
● Brachialis
● Brachioradialis
● Deltoid
● Teres major
● Trapezius
● Infraspinatus
● Teres minor
● Levator scapulae
● Rhomboid major
● Rhomboid minor
● Anconeus
● Common flexor tendon

Trapezius m.
Deltoid m.
Levator scapulae m.
Biceps brachii m.—long head
Infraspinatus m.
Supraspinatus m.
Teres minor m.
Rhomboid minor m.
Triceps brachii m.—lateral head
Triceps brachii m.—long head
Deltoid m.
Infraspinatus m.
Brachialis m.
Rhomboid major m.
Brachioradialis m.
Triceps brachii m.—medial head
Teres major m.
Triceps brachii m.
Anconeus m.

Common flexor mm. tendon:
  Flexor carpi radialis m.
  Flexor carpi ulnaris m.
  Flexor digitorum superficialis m.—humeroulnar head
  Palmaris longus m.
  Pronator teres m. — humeral head

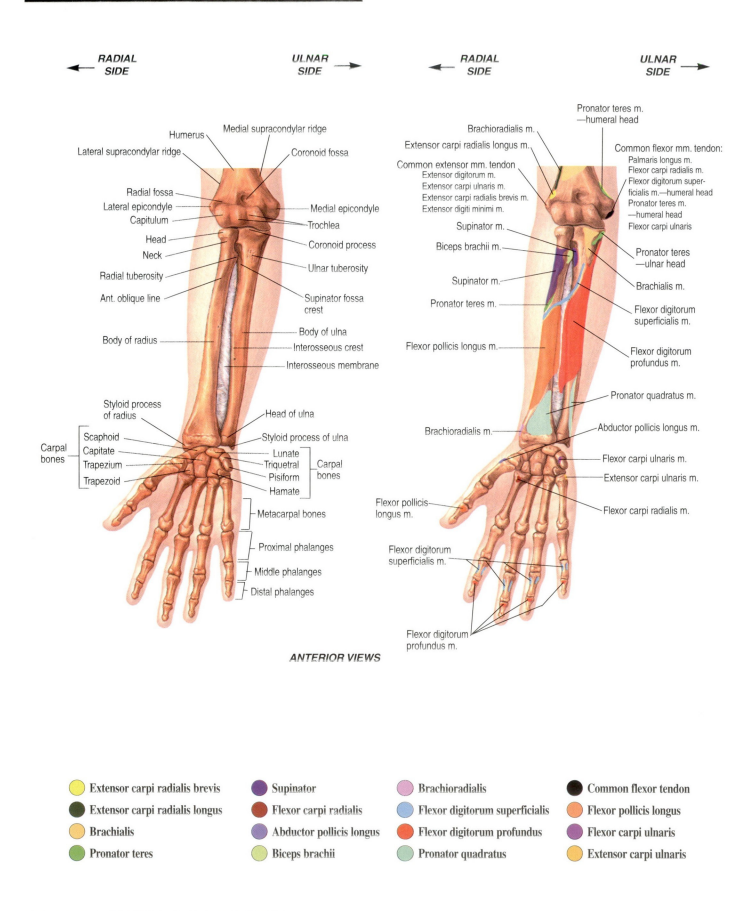

RADIAL SIDE ←   ULNAR SIDE →   ← **RADIAL SIDE**   ULNAR SIDE →

Humerus

Medial supracondylar ridge

Lateral supracondylar ridge

Coronoid fossa

Radial fossa

Lateral epicondyle

Capitulum

Medial epicondyle

Head

Trochlea

Neck

Coronoid process

Radial tuberosity

Ulnar tuberosity

Ant. oblique line

Supinator fossa crest

Body of radius

Body of ulna

Interosseous crest

Interosseous membrane

Styloid process of radius

Head of ulna

Scaphoid

Styloid process of ulna

Capitate

Lunate

Carpal bones

Trapezium

Triquetral

Trapezoid

Pisiform

Carpal bones

Hamate

Metacarpal bones

Proximal phalanges

Middle phalanges

Distal phalanges

Pronator teres m. —humeral head

Brachioradialis m.

Extensor carpi radialis longus m.

Common flexor mm. tendon:
Palmaris longus m.
Flexor carpi radialis m.
Flexor digitorum super-ficialis m.—humeral head
Pronator teres m. —humeral head
Flexor carpi ulnaris

Common extensor mm. tendon
Extensor digitorum m.
Extensor carpi ulnaris m.
Extensor carpi radialis brevis m.
Extensor digiti minimi m.

Supinator m.

Biceps brachii m.

Pronator teres —ulnar head

Supinator m.

Brachialis m.

Pronator teres m.

Flexor digitorum superficialis m.

Flexor pollicis longus m.

Flexor digitorum profundus m.

Pronator quadratus m.

Brachioradialis m.

Abductor pollicis longus m.

Flexor carpi ulnaris m.

Extensor carpi ulnaris m.

Flexor pollicis longus m.

Flexor carpi radialis m.

Flexor digitorum superficialis m.

Flexor digitorum profundus m.

ANTERIOR VIEWS

○ **Extensor carpi radialis brevis**
○ **Extensor carpi radialis longus**
○ **Brachialis**
○ **Pronator teres**

○ **Supinator**
○ **Flexor carpi radialis**
○ **Abductor pollicis longus**
○ **Biceps brachii**

○ **Brachioradialis**
○ **Flexor digitorum superficialis**
○ **Flexor digitorum profundus**
○ **Pronator quadratus**

○ **Common flexor tendon**
○ **Flexor pollicis longus**
○ **Flexor carpi ulnaris**
○ **Extensor carpi ulnaris**

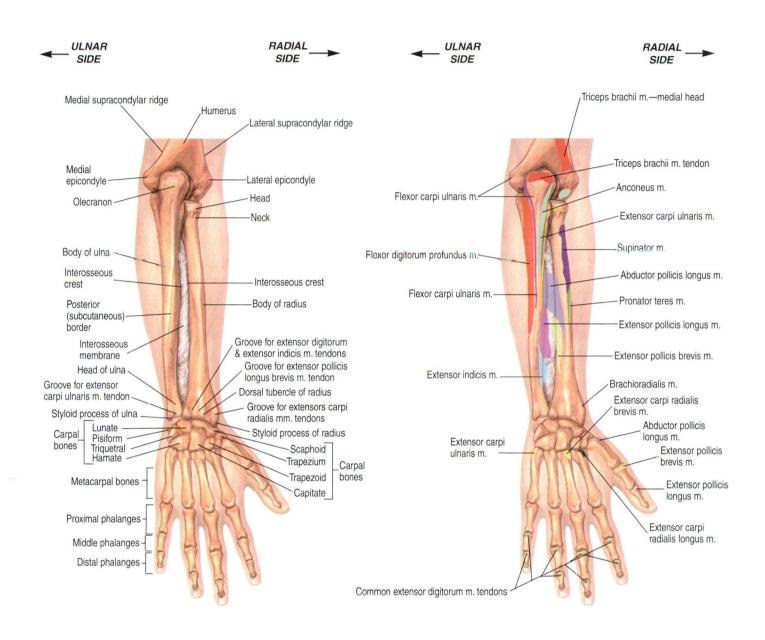

ULNAR SIDE ←   RADIAL SIDE →   ULNAR SIDE ←   RADIAL SIDE →

Medial supracondylar ridge
Humerus
Lateral supracondylar ridge
Medial epicondyle
Lateral epicondyle
Olecranon
Head
Neck
Body of ulna
Interosseous crest
Interosseous crest
Posterior (subcutaneous) border
Body of radius
Interosseous membrane
Head of ulna
Groove for extensor digitorum & extensor indicis m. tendons
Groove for extensor pollicis longus brevis m. tendon
Groove for extensor carpi ulnaris m. tendon
Dorsal tubercle of radius
Styloid process of ulna
Groove for extensors carpi radialis mm. tendons
Lunate
Pisiform
Carpal bones
Triquetral
Hamate
Styloid process of radius
Scaphoid
Trapezium
Carpal bones
Trapezoid
Metacarpal bones
Capitate
Proximal phalanges
Middle phalanges
Distal phalanges

Triceps brachii m.—medial head
Triceps brachii m. tendon
Anconeus m.
Flexor carpi ulnaris m.
Extensor carpi ulnaris m.
Supinator m.
Flexor digitorum profundus m.
Abductor pollicis longus m.
Flexor carpi ulnaris m.
Pronator teres m.
Extensor pollicis longus m.
Extensor pollicis brevis m.
Extensor indicis m.
Brachioradialis m.
Extensor carpi radialis brevis m.
Abductor pollicis longus m.
Extensor carpi ulnaris m.
Extensor pollicis brevis m.
Extensor pollicis longus m.
Extensor carpi radialis longus m.
Common extensor digitorum m. tendons

POSTERIOR VIEWS

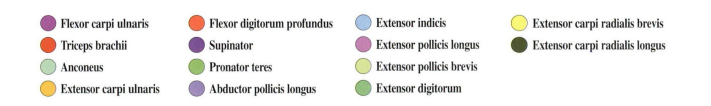

- Flexor carpi ulnaris
- Triceps brachii
- Anconeus
- Extensor carpi ulnaris
- Flexor digitorum profundus
- Supinator
- Pronator teres
- Abductor pollicis longus
- Extensor indicis
- Extensor pollicis longus
- Extensor pollicis brevis
- Extensor digitorum
- Extensor carpi radialis brevis
- Extensor carpi radialis longus

Pectoral & Scapular Muscles
Table 6.1

Muscles in Pectoral Region

Muscle	Proximal Attachment	Distal Attachment	Innervation[a]	Main Actions
Pectoralis major	*Clavicular head:* ant. surface of the medial half of clavicle *Sternocostal head:* ant. surface of sternum, sup. six costal cartilages & aponeurosis of ext. abdominal oblique muscle	Lateral lip of intertubercular groove of humerus	Lateral & medial pectoral n.: clavicular head (C5 & **C6**) Sternocostal head (**C7, C8**, & T1)	Adducts & medially rotates humerus Draws shoulder joint anteriorly & inferiorly *Acting alone:* Clavicular head flexes humerus & sternoclavicular head extends it
Pectoralis minor	Ribs 3–5 near their costal cartilages	Medial border & sup. surface of coracoid process of scapula	Medial pectoral n. (C8 & T1)	Stabilizes scapula by drawing it inferiorly & anteriorly against thoracic wall
Subclavius	Junction of rib 1 & its costal cartilage	Inf. surface of middle third of clavicle	N. to subclavius (**C5** & C6)	(Draws clavicle medially?)
Serratus anterior	Ext. surfaces of lateral parts of ribs 1–8/9	Ant. surface of medial border of scapula	Long thoracic n. (C5, **C6**, & **C7**)	Protracts scapula & holds it against thoracic wall; rotates scapula superiorly

Muscles Connecting Upper Limb to Vertebral Column

Muscle	Medial Attachment	Lateral Attachment	Innervation[a]	Main Actions
Trapezius	Medial third of sup. nuchal line; ext. occipital protuberance, ligamentum nuchae & spinous processes of C7–T12 vertebrae	Lateral thrid of clavicle, acromion & spine of scapula	Spinal root of accessory n. (CN XI) & cervical nn. (C3 & C4)	Elevates, retracts & rotates scapula; *sup. fibers* elevate, *middle fibers* retract, *inf. fibers* depress scapula; sup. & inf. fibers act together in sup. rotation of scapula
Latissimus dorsi	Spinous processes of the inf. six thoracic vertebrae, thoracolumbar fascia, iliac crest & inf. 3 or 4 ribs	Floor of intertubercular groove & crest of lesser tubercle of humerus	Thoracodorsal n. (**C6, C7**, & C8)	Extends, adducts & medially rotates humerus; raises body toward arms during climbing
Levator scapulae	Post. tubercles of transverse processes of C1–C4 vertebrae	Sup. part of medial border of scapula	Dorsal scapular (C5) & cervical (C3 & C4) nn.	Elevates scapula & tilts its glenoid cavity inferiorly by rotating scapula
Rhomboid minor & major	*Minor:* Ligamentum nuchae & spinous processes of C7 & T1 vertebrae *Major:* Spinous processes of T2–T5 vertebrae	Medial border of scapula from level of spine to inf. angle	Dorsal scapular n. (C4 & **C5**) rotate	Retracts scapula & rotates it to depress glenoid cavity; fixes scapula to thoracic wall

[a]In this and subsequent tables, the numbers indicate the spinal cord segmental innervation of the nerves (*e.g.,* C5 and C6 indicate that the nerves supplying the clavicular head of the pectoralis major muscle are derived from the 5th and 6th cervical segments of the spinal cord). **Boldface** indicates the main segmental innervation. Damage to these segments of the spinal cord, or to the motor nerve roots arising from them, results in paralysis of the muscles concerned.

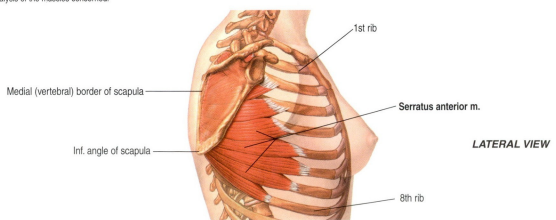

1st rib

Medial (vertebral) border of scapula

Serratus anterior m.

Inf. angle of scapula

LATERAL VIEW

8th rib

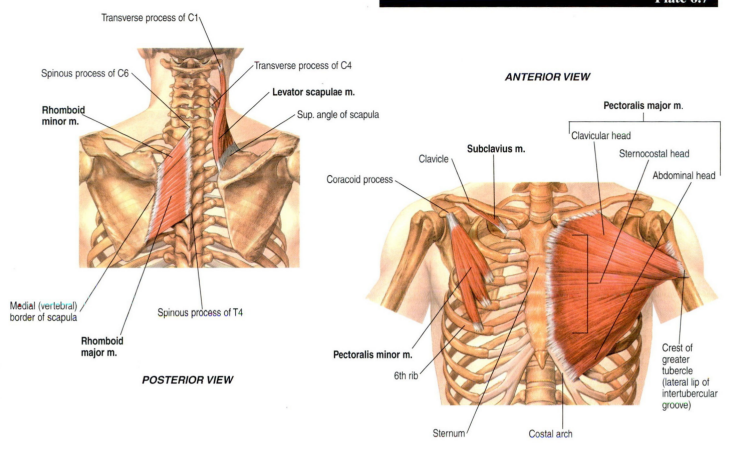

ANTERIOR VIEW

Transverse process of C1

Spinous process of C6

Transverse process of C4

Levator scapulae m.

Rhomboid minor m.

Sup. angle of scapula

Pectoralis major m.

Clavicular head

Subclavius m.

Sternocostal head

Clavicle

Abdominal head

Coracoid process

Medial (vertebral) border of scapula

Spinous process of T4

Rhomboid major m.

POSTERIOR VIEW

Pectoralis minor m.

6th rib

Crest of greater tubercle (lateral lip of intertubercular groove)

Sternum

Costal arch

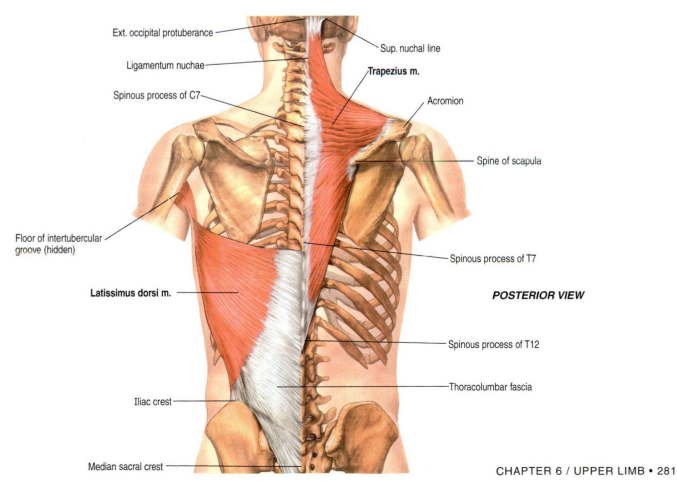

Ext. occipital protuberance

Sup. nuchal line

Ligamentum nuchae

Trapezius m.

Spinous process of C7

Acromion

Spine of scapula

Floor of intertubercular groove (hidden)

Spinous process of T7

POSTERIOR VIEW

Latissimus dorsi m.

Spinous process of T12

Iliac crest

Thoracolumbar fascia

Median sacral crest

CHAPTER 6 / UPPER LIMB • 281

Scapular & Posterior Arm Muscles
Table 6.2

Scapular Muscles

Muscle	Proximal/Medial Attachment	Distal/Lateral Attachment	Innervation[a]	Main Actions
Deltoid	Lateral third of clavicle, acromion & spine of scapula	Deltoid tuberosity of humerus	Axillary n. (**C5** & C6)	*Anterior part:* flexes & medially rotates arm *Middle part:* abducts arm *Posterior part:* extends & laterally rotates arm
Supraspinatus[a]	Supraspinous fossa of scapula	Sup. facet on greater tubercle of humerus	Suprascapular n. (C4, **C5** & C6)	Helps deltoid to abduct arm & acts with rotator cuff muscles[a]
Infraspinatus[a]	Infraspinous fossa of scapula	Middle facet on greater tubercle of humerus	Suprascapular n. (C4, **C5** & C6)	Laterally rotate arm; help to hold humeral head in glenoid cavity of scapula
Teres minor[a]	Sup. part of lateral border of scapula	Inf. facet on greater tubercle of humerus	Axillary n. (**C5** & C6)	
Teres major	Dorsal surface of inf. angle of scapula	Medial lip of intertubular groove of humerus	Lower subscapular n. (**C6** & C7)	Adducts & medially rotates arm
Subscapularis[a]	Subscapular fossa	Lesser tubercle of humerus	Upper & lower subscapular nn. (C5, **C6** & C7)	Medially rotates arm & adducts it; helps to hold humeral head in glenoid cavity

[a]Collectively, the supraspinatus, infraspinatus, teres minor, and subscapularis muscles are referred to as the **rotator cuff muscles**. Their prime function during all movements of the shoulder joint is to hold the head of the humerus in the glenoid cavity of the scapula.

Posterior Arm Muscles

Muscle	Proximal Attachment	Distal Attachment	Innervation	Main Actions
Triceps brachii	*Long head:* infraglenoid tubercle of scapula *Lateral head:* post. surface of humerus, sup. to radial n. groove *Medial head:* post. surface of humerus, inf. to radial n. groove	Proximal end of olecranon ulna & fascia of forearm	Radial n. (**C6, C7,** & C8)	Extends the forearm; it is *chief extensor of forearm;* long head steadies head of abducted humerus
Anconeus	Lateral epicondyle of humerus	Lateral surface of olecranon & sup. part of post. surface of ulna	Radial n. (C7, C8 & T1)	Assists triceps in extending forearm; stabilizes elbow joint; abducts ulna during pronation

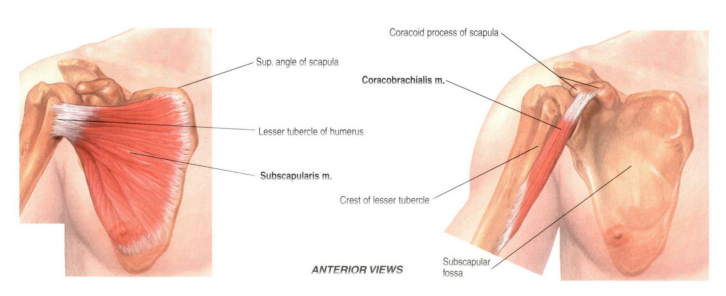

Sup. angle of scapula

Coracoid process of scapula

Coracobrachialis m.

Lesser tubercle of humerus

Subscapularis m.

Crest of lesser tubercle

Subscapular fossa

ANTERIOR VIEWS

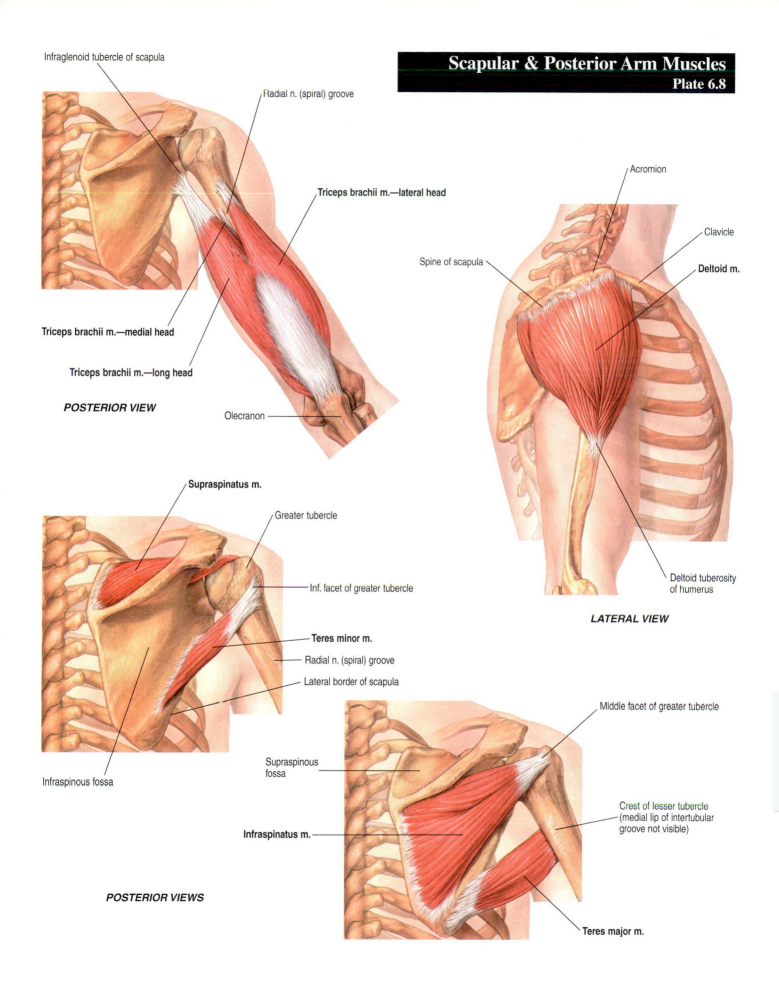

Infraglenoid tubercle of scapula

Radial n. (spiral) groove

Triceps brachii m.—lateral head

Triceps brachii m.—medial head

Triceps brachii m.—long head

POSTERIOR VIEW

Olecranon

Acromion

Clavicle

Spine of scapula

Deltoid m.

Deltoid tuberosity
of humerus

LATERAL VIEW

Supraspinatus m.

Greater tubercle

Inf. facet of greater tubercle

Teres minor m.

Radial n. (spiral) groove

Lateral border of scapula

Infraspinous fossa

POSTERIOR VIEWS

Middle facet of greater tubercle

Supraspinous
fossa

Infraspinatus m.

Crest of lesser tubercle
(medial lip of intertubular
groove not visible)

Teres major m.

Muscles of Anterior Arm

Muscle	Proximal Attachment	Distal Attachment	Innervation[a]	Main Actions
Biceps brachii	*Short head:* Tip of coracoid process of scapula *Long head:* Supraglenoid tubercle of scapula	Tuberosity of radius & fascia of forearm via bicipital aponeurosis	Musculocutaneous n. (C5 & **C6**)	Supinates forearm and, when it is supine, flexes forearm
Brachialis	Distal half of ant. surface of humerus	Coronoid process & tuberosity of ulna		Flexes forearm in all positions
Coracobrachialis	Tip of coracoid process of scapula	Middle third of medial surface of humerus	Musculocutaneous n. (C5, **C6** & C7)	Helps to flex & adduct arm

Superficial and Intermediate Layers of Muscles on Anterior Surface of Forearm[a]

Muscle	Proximal Attachment	Distal Attachment	Innervation[b]	Main Actions
Pronator teres	Medial epicondyle of humerus & coronoid process of ulna	Middle of lateral surface of radius	Median n. (C6 & **C7**)	Pronates forearm & flexes it
Flexor carpi radialis	Medial epicondyle of humerus	Base of 2nd metacarpal bone		Flexes hand & abducts it radially
Palmaris longus	Medial epicondyle of humerus	Distal half of flexor retinanculum & palmar aponeurosis	Median n. (C7 & C8)	Flexes hand & tightens palmar aponeurosis
Flexor carpi ulnaris[b]	*Humeral head:* medial epicondyle of humerus *Ulnar head:* olecranon & post. border of ulna	Pisiform bone (hook of hamate bone & 5th metacarpal bone)	Ulnar n. (C7 & **C8**)	Flexes hand & adducts it ulnarly
Flexor digitorum superficialis[c]	*Humeroulnar head:* medial epicondyle of humerus, ulnar collateral lig. & coronoid process of ulna *Radial head:* sup. half of ant. border of radius	Bodies of the middle phalanges of medial four digits	Median n. (C7, **C8** & T1)	Flexes middle phalanges of medial four digits: acting more strongly, it flexes proximal phalanges & hand

[a]The superficial muscles of the *flexor-pronator group* are attached, in whole or in part, to the anterior surface of the medial epicondyle by a *common flexor tendon.*
[b]In contrast to the other superficial flexor muscles, the flexor carpi ulnaris is supplied by the ulnar nerve.
[c]This muscle comprises the *intermediate muscle layer* in the anterior part of the forearm. In some clinical texts, this muscle is referred to by its old name, "flexor digitorum sublimis."

Deep Layer of Muscles on Anterior Surface of Forearm

Muscle	Proximal Attachment	Distal Attachment	Innervation	Main Actions
Pronator quadratus	Distal fourth of ant. surface of ulna	Distal fourth of ant. surface of radius	Ant. interosseous n. from median (**C8** & T1)	Pronates forearm; deep fibers bind radius & ulna together

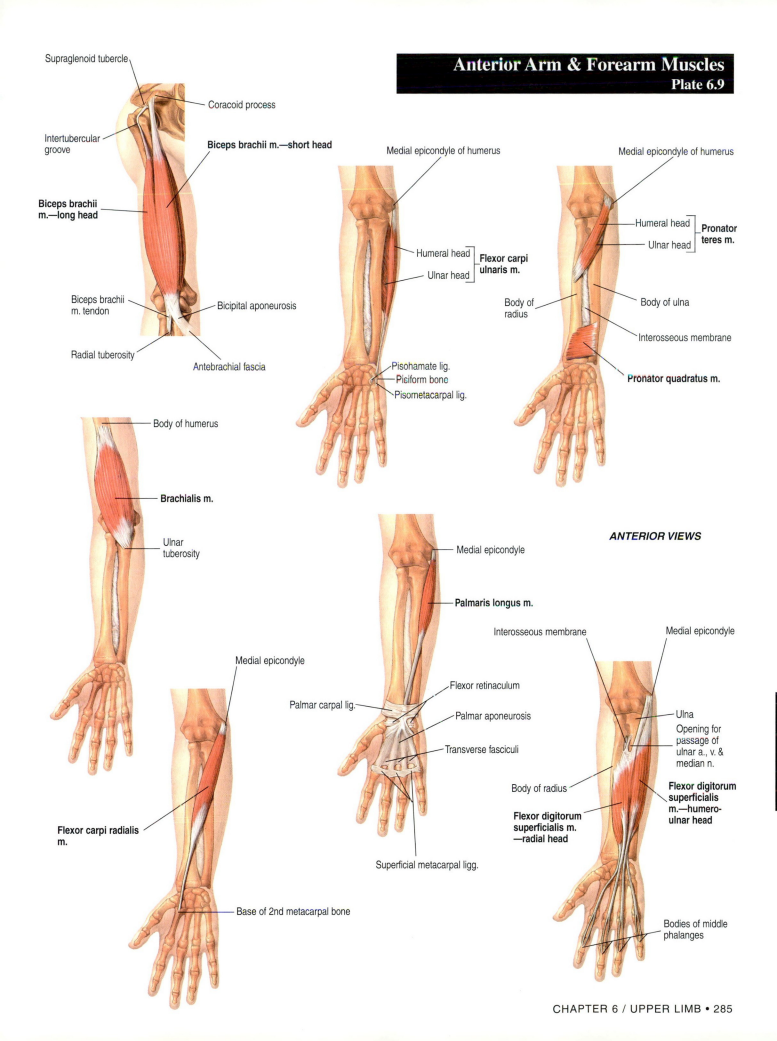

Supraglenoid tubercle

Coracoid process

Intertubercular groove

Biceps brachii m.—short head

Biceps brachii m.—long head

Biceps brachii m. tendon

Bicipital aponeurosis

Radial tuberosity

Antebrachial fascia

Medial epicondyle of humerus

Humeral head

Ulnar head

Flexor carpi ulnaris m.

Pisohamate lig.

Pisiform bone

Pisometacarpal lig.

Medial epicondyle of humerus

Humeral head

Ulnar head

Pronator teres m.

Body of radius

Body of ulna

Interosseous membrane

Pronator quadratus m.

Body of humerus

Brachialis m.

Ulnar tuberosity

ANTERIOR VIEWS

Medial epicondyle

Medial epicondyle

Palmaris longus m.

Palmar carpal lig.

Flexor retinaculum

Palmar aponeurosis

Transverse fasciculi

Superficial metacarpal ligg.

Interosseous membrane

Medial epicondyle

Ulna

Opening for passage of ulnar a., v. & median n.

Body of radius

Flexor digitorum superficialis m. —radial head

Flexor digitorum superficialis m.—humero-ulnar head

Bodies of middle phalanges

Flexor carpi radialis m.

Base of 2nd metacarpal bone

Forearm Muscles
Table 6.4

Deep Layer of Muscles on Anterior Surface of Forearm

Muscle	Proximal Attachment	Distal Attachment	Innervation	Main Actions
Flexor digitorum profundus	Proximal three-fourths of medial & ant. surfaces of ulna & interosseous membrane	Bases of distal phalanges of medial four digits	*Medial part:* Ulnar n. (**C8** & T1) *Lateral part:* Median n. (**C8** & T1)	Flexes distal phalanges of medial four digits (fingers)
Flexor pollicis longus	Ant. surface of the distal radius & adjacent interosseous membrane	Base of distal phalanx of thumb	Ant. interosseous n. from median (**C8** & T1)	Flexes phalanges of first digit (thumb)

Superficial Muscles on Posterior or Extensor Surface of Forearm

Muscle	Proximal Attachment	Distal Attachment	Innervation	Main Actions
Brachioradialis	Proximal two-thirds of lateral supracondylar ridge of humerus, lat. intermuscular septum	Lateral surface of distal end of radius	Radial n. (C5, **C6** & C7)	Flexes forearm
Extensor carpi radialis longus	Lateral supracondylar ridge of humerus, lat. intermuscular septum	Base of 2nd metacarpal bone	Radial n. (C6 & C7)	Extend & abduct hand at wrist joint
Extensor carpi radialis brevis	Lateral epicondyle of humerus	Base of 3rd metacarpal bone	Deep br. of radial n. (**C7** & C8)	Extend & abduct hand at wrist joint
Extensor digitorum	Lateral epicondyle of humerus	Extensor expansions of medial four digits	Post. interosseous n. (**C7** & C8), a br. of the radial n.	Extends medial four digits at metacarpophalangeal joints; extends hand at wrist joint
Extensor carpi ulnaris	Lateral epicondyle of humerus & post. border of ulna	Base of 5th metacarpal bone	Post. interosseous n. (**C7** & C8), a br. of the radial n.	Extends & adducts hand at wrist joint

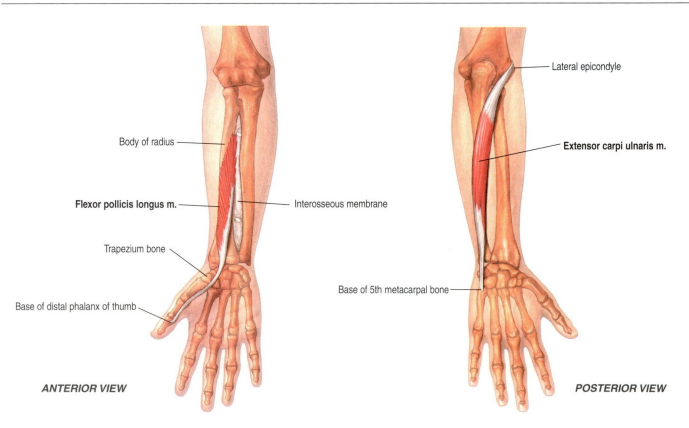

ANTERIOR VIEW

Body of radius

Flexor pollicis longus m. — Interosseous membrane

Trapezium bone

Base of distal phalanx of thumb

POSTERIOR VIEW

Lateral epicondyle

Extensor carpi ulnaris m.

Base of 5th metacarpal bone

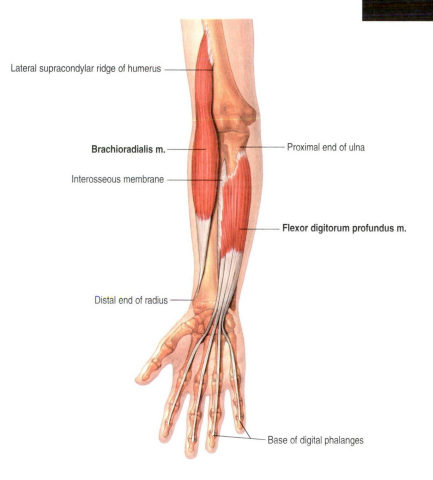

Lateral supracondylar ridge of humerus

Brachioradialis m.

Interosseous membrane

Proximal end of ulna

Flexor digitorum profundus m.

Distal end of radius

Base of digital phalanges

ANTERIOR VIEW

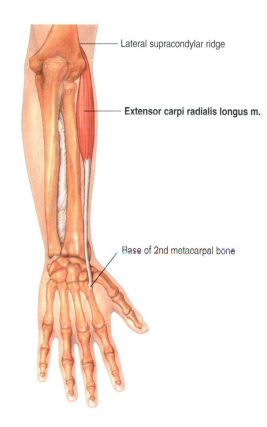

Lateral supracondylar ridge

Extensor carpi radialis longus m.

Base of 2nd metacarpal bone

POSTERIOR VIEW

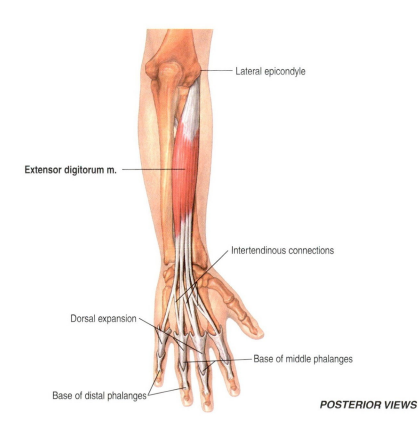

Lateral epicondyle

Extensor digitorum m.

Intertendinous connections

Dorsal expansion

Base of middle phalanges

Base of distal phalanges

POSTERIOR VIEWS

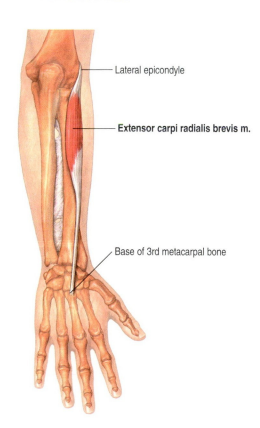

Lateral epicondyle

Extensor carpi radialis brevis m.

Base of 3rd metacarpal bone

Deep Muscles on Posterior or Extensor Surface of Forearm

Muscle	Proximal Attachment	Distal Attachment	Innervation	Main Actions
Supinator	Lateral epicondyle of humerus, radial collateral & anular ligaments, supinator fossa & crest of ulna	Lateral, post. & ant. surfaces of proximal third of radius	Deep br. of radial n. (C5 & **C6**)	Supinates forearm, *i.e.,* rotates radius to turn palm anteriorly
Abductor pollicis longus	Post. surfaces of ulna & radius & interosseous membrane	Base of 1st metacarpal bone		Abducts thumb & extends it at carpometacarpal joint
Extensor pollicis brevis	Post. surface of radius & interosseous membrane	Base of proximal phalanx of thumb	Post. interosseous n. (C7 & **C8**)	Extends proximal phalanx of thumb at carpometacarpal joint
Extensor pollicis longus	Post. surface of middle third of ulnar & interosseous membrane	Base of distal phalanx of thumb		Extends distal phalanx of thumb at metacarpophalangeal & interphalangeal joints
Extensor indicis	Post. surface of ulna & interosseous membrane	Extensor expansion of second digit (index finger)		Extends digit 2 & helps to extend wrist
Extensor digiti minimi	Lateral epicondyle of humerus	Extensor expansion of 5th digit	Post. interosseous n. (**C7** & C8), a br. of the radial n.	Extends digit 5 at metacarpophalangeal & interphalangeal joints

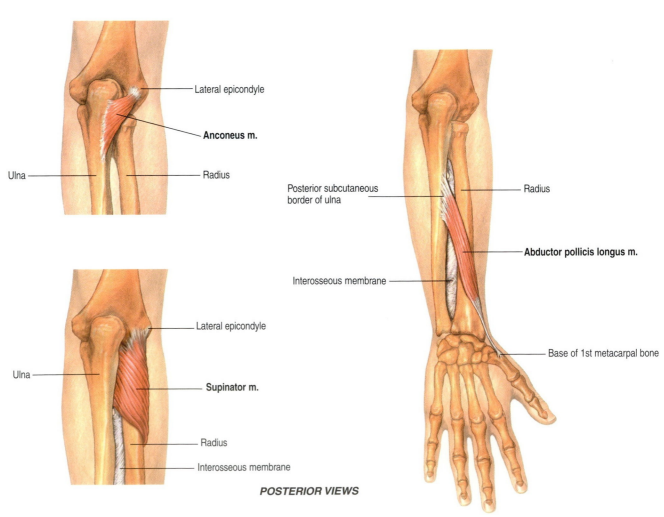

POSTERIOR VIEWS

Posterior Forearm Muscles
Plate 6.11

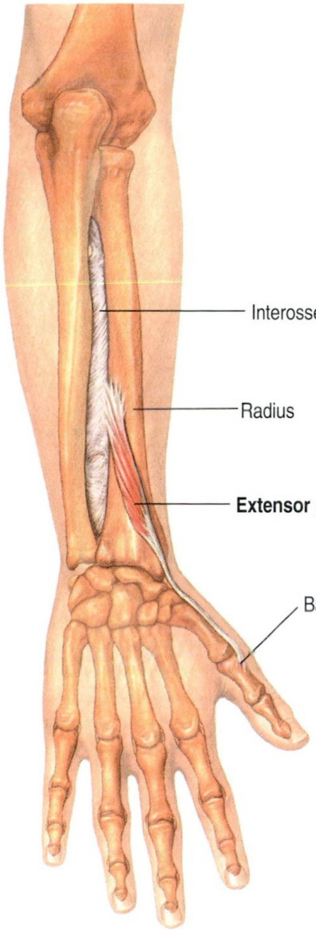

Interosseous membrane
Radius
Extensor pollicis brevis m.
Base of 1st proximal phalanx

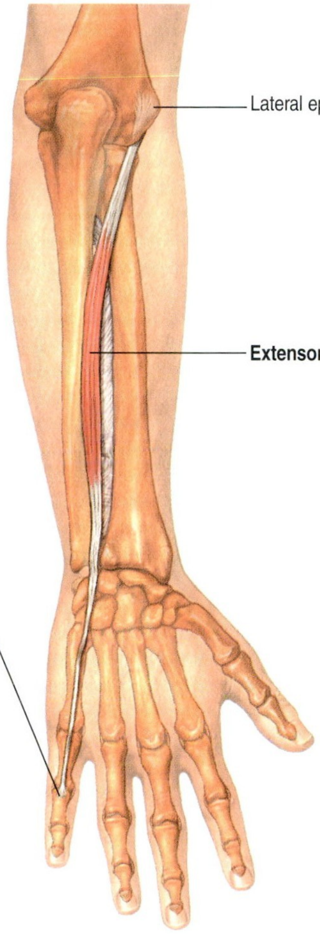

Lateral epicondyle
Extensor digiti minimi m.
Extensor expansion over base of 5th middle phalanx

POSTERIOR VIEWS

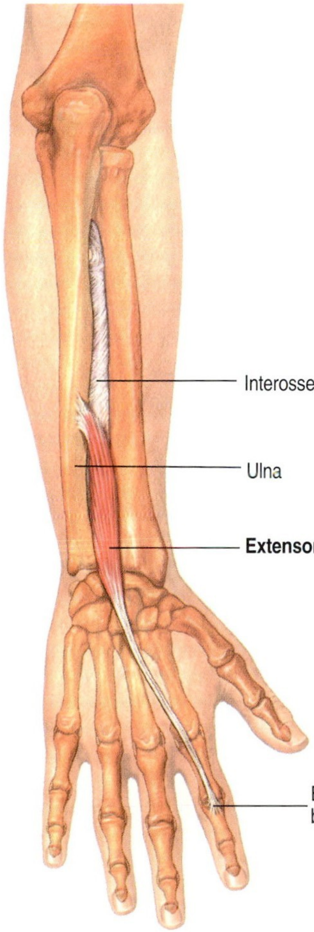

Interosseous membrane
Ulna
Extensor indicis m.
Extensor expansion over base of 2nd middle phalanx

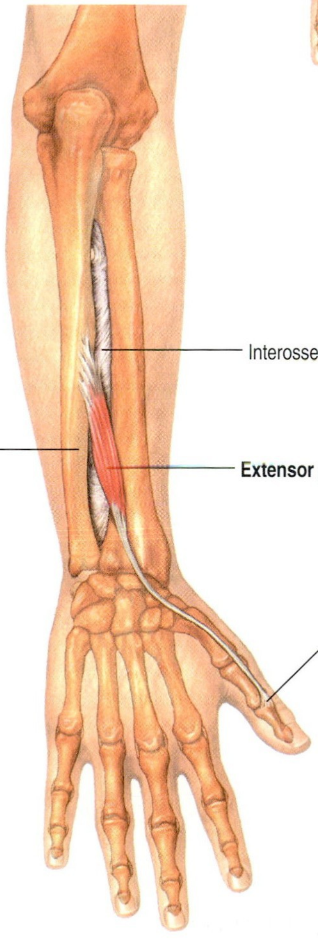

Interosseous membrane
Ulna
Extensor pollicis longus m.
Extensor (dorsal) expansion over base of 1st distal phalanx

Intrinsic Hand Muscles
Table 6.6

Short Muscles of Hand

Muscle	Proximal Attachment	Distal Attachment	Innervation	Main Actions
Lumbricalis 1 & 2	Lateral two tendons of flexor digitorum profundus	Lateral sides of extensor expansions of digits 2 to 5	*Lumbricals 1 & 2*, median n. (C8 & **T1**)	Flex digits at metacarpophalangeal joints & extend interphalangeal joints
Lumbricalis 3 & 4	Medial three tendons of flexor digitorum profundus		*Lumbricals 3 & 4*, deep br. of ulnar n. (C8 & **T1**)	
Dorsal interossei 1–4	Adjacent sides of two metacarpal bones	Extensor expansions & bases of proximal phalanges of digits 2–4	Deep br. of ulnar n. (C8 & **T1**)	Abduct digits 2–4
Palmar interossei 1–3	Palmar surfaces of 1st, 2nd, 4th & 5th metacarpal bones	Extensor expansions of digits and bases of proximal phalanges of digits 1, 2, 4 & 5		Adduct digits 2–4
Abductor digiti minimi	Pisiform bone	Medial side of base of proximal phalanx of digit 5 (little finger)	Deep br. of ulnar n. (C8 & **T1**)	Abducts digit 5 (little finger)
Flexor digiti minimi brevis	Hook of hamate bone & flexor retinaculum			Flexes proximal phalanx of digit 5
Opponens digiti minimi		Medial border of 5th metacarpal bone		Draws 5th metacarpal bone anteriorly & rotates it, bringing digit 5 into opposition with thumb
Abductor pollicis brevis	Flexor retinaculum & tubercles of scaphoid & trapezium bones	Lateral side of base of proximal phalanx of thumb	Recurrent br. of median n. (**C8** & T1)	Abducts thumb & helps oppose it
Flexor pollicis brevis	Flexor retinaculum & tubercle of trapezium bone			Flexes thumb
Opponens pollicis		Lateral side of 1st metacarpal bone		Opposes thumb toward center of palm & rotates it medially
Adductor pollicis	*Oblique head:* Bases of 2nd & 3rd metacarpals, captate & adjacent carpal bones *Transverse head:* Ant. surface of body of 3rd metacarpal bone	Medial side of base of proximal phalanx of thumb	Deep br. of ulnar n. (C8 & **T1**)	Adducts thumb toward middle digit

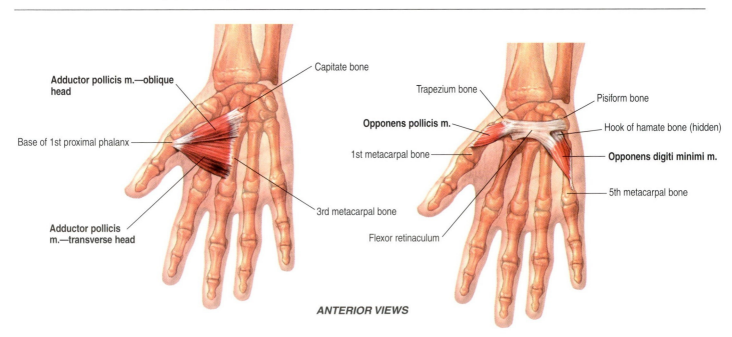

ANTERIOR VIEWS

Dorsal interosseous mm.

Metacarpal bones

4 3 2 1

POSTERIOR VIEW

Bases of proximal phalanges &
extensor (dorsal) expansions
—hidden

Palmar interosseous mm.

ANTERIOR VIEW

Metacarpal bones

1 2 3

Bases of proximal phalanges
extensor (dorsal) expansions
—hidden

Flexor retinaculum

Tubercle of trapezium bone

Flexor pollicis brevis m.

Base of 1st proximal phalanx

Pisiform bone

Hook of hamate bone

Flexor digiti minimi m.

Base of 5th proximal phalanx

ANTERIOR VIEW

Flexor digitorum profundus m. tendons

Lumbrical mm.

1 2 3 4

Bases of proximal phalanges
extensor (dorsal) expansions
—hidden

Scaphoid bone

Trapezium bone

Abductor pollicis brevis m.

Base of 1st proximal phalanx

Flexor retinaculum

Pisiform bone

Abductor digiti minimi m.

Base of 5th proximal phalanx

ANTERIOR VIEWS

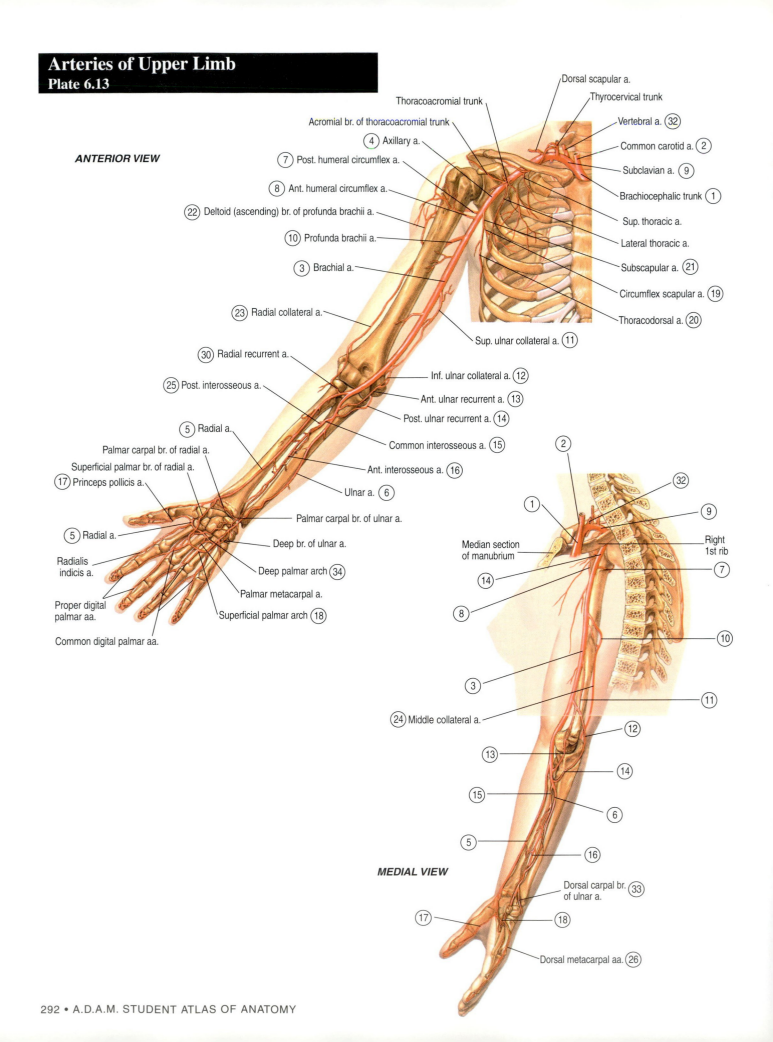

ANTERIOR VIEW

Dorsal scapular a.

Thoracoacromial trunk

Thyrocervical trunk

Acromial br. of thoracoacromial trunk

Vertebral a. (32)

(4) Axillary a.

Common carotid a. (2)

(7) Post. humeral circumflex a.

Subclavian a. (9)

(8) Ant. humeral circumflex a.

Brachiocephalic trunk (1)

(22) Deltoid (ascending) br. of profunda brachii a.

Sup. thoracic a.

(10) Profunda brachii a.

Lateral thoracic a.

(3) Brachial a.

Subscapular a. (21)

Circumflex scapular a. (19)

(23) Radial collateral a.

Thoracodorsal a. (20)

Sup. ulnar collateral a. (11)

(30) Radial recurrent a.

Inf. ulnar collateral a. (12)

(25) Post. interosseous a.

Ant. ulnar recurrent a. (13)

Post. ulnar recurrent a. (14)

(5) Radial a.

Common interosseous a. (15)

Palmar carpal br. of radial a.

Ant. interosseous a. (16)

Superficial palmar br. of radial a.

Ulnar a. (6)

(17) Princeps pollicis a.

Palmar carpal br. of ulnar a.

(5) Radial a.

Deep br. of ulnar a.

Radialis indicis a.

Deep palmar arch (34)

Palmar metacarpal a.

Proper digital palmar aa.

Superficial palmar arch (18)

Common digital palmar aa.

(2)

(32)

(1)

(9)

Median section of manubrium

Right 1st rib

(14)

(7)

(8)

(10)

(3)

(11)

(24) Middle collateral a.

(12)

(13)

(14)

(15)

(6)

(5)

(16)

MEDIAL VIEW

Dorsal carpal br. (33) of ulnar a.

(17)

(18)

Dorsal metacarpal aa. (26)

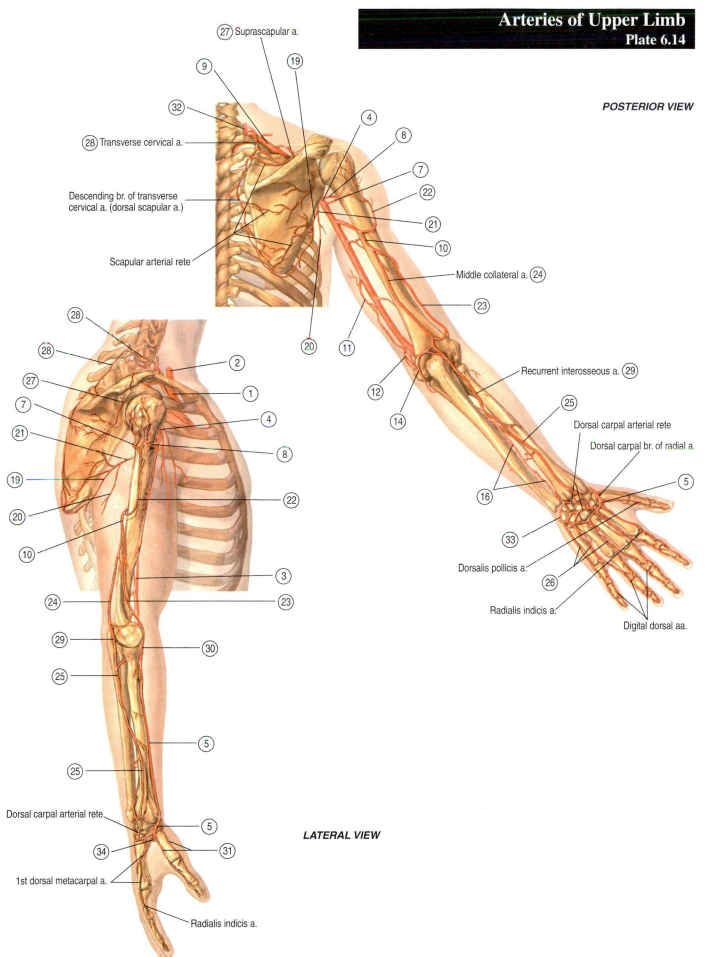

㉗ Suprascapular a.

⑨

⑲

㉜

POSTERIOR VIEW

④

⑧

⑦

㉘ Transverse cervical a.

㉒

㉑

Descending br. of transverse
cervical a. (dorsal scapular a.)

⑩

Middle collateral a. ㉔

Scapular arterial rete

㉓

⑳

⑪

Recurrent interosseous a. ㉙

㉘

⑫

㉕

②

⑭

Dorsal carpal arterial rete

㉘

Dorsal carpal br. of radial a.

①

㉗

⑯

⑤

⑦

④

㉑

⑧

㉝

⑲

㉒

Dorsalis pollicis a.

⑳

㉖

⑩

Radialis indicis a.

Digital dorsal aa.

③

㉓

㉔

㉙

㉚

㉕

⑤

㉕

⑤

Dorsal carpal arterial rete

LATERAL VIEW

㉞

㉛

1st dorsal metacarpal a.

Radialis indicis a.

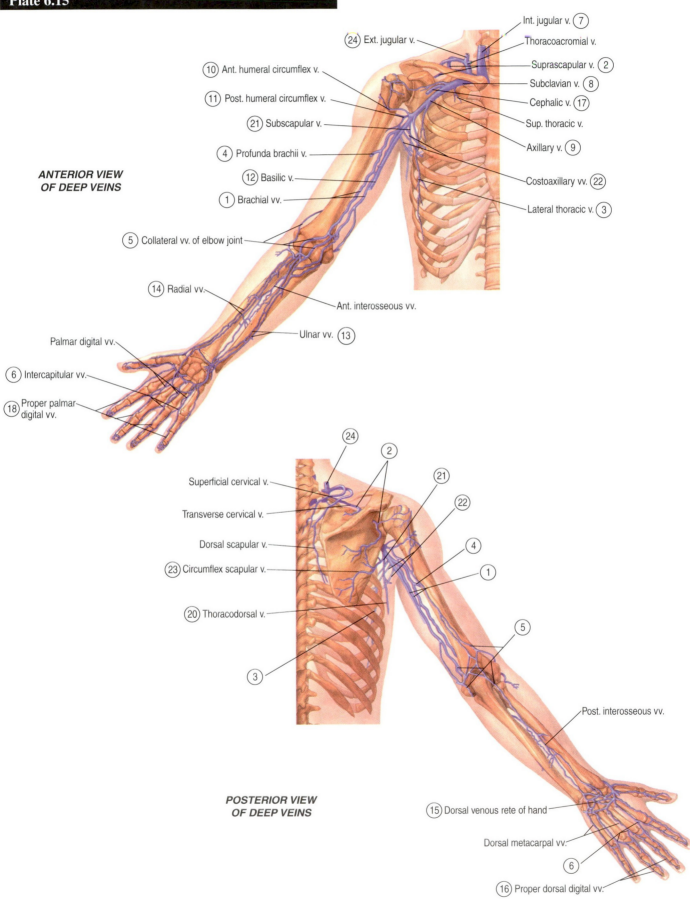

ANTERIOR VIEW
OF DEEP VEINS

(24) Ext. jugular v.
Int. jugular v. (7)
Thoracoacromial v.
(10) Ant. humeral circumflex v.
Suprascapular v. (2)
(11) Post. humeral circumflex v.
Subclavian v. (8)
Cephalic v. (17)
(21) Subscapular v.
Sup. thoracic v.
(4) Profunda brachii v.
Axillary v. (9)
(12) Basilic v.
Costoaxillary vv. (22)
(1) Brachial vv.
Lateral thoracic v. (3)
(5) Collateral vv. of elbow joint
(14) Radial vv.
Ant. interosseous vv.
Palmar digital vv.
Ulnar vv. (13)
(6) Intercapitular vv.
(18) Proper palmar digital vv.

POSTERIOR VIEW
OF DEEP VEINS

(24)
(2)
(21)
(22)
(4)
(1)
Superficial cervical v.
Transverse cervical v.
Dorsal scapular v.
(23) Circumflex scapular v.
(20) Thoracodorsal v.
(5)
(3)
Post. interosseous vv.
(15) Dorsal venous rete of hand
Dorsal metacarpal vv.
(6)
(16) Proper dorsal digital vv.

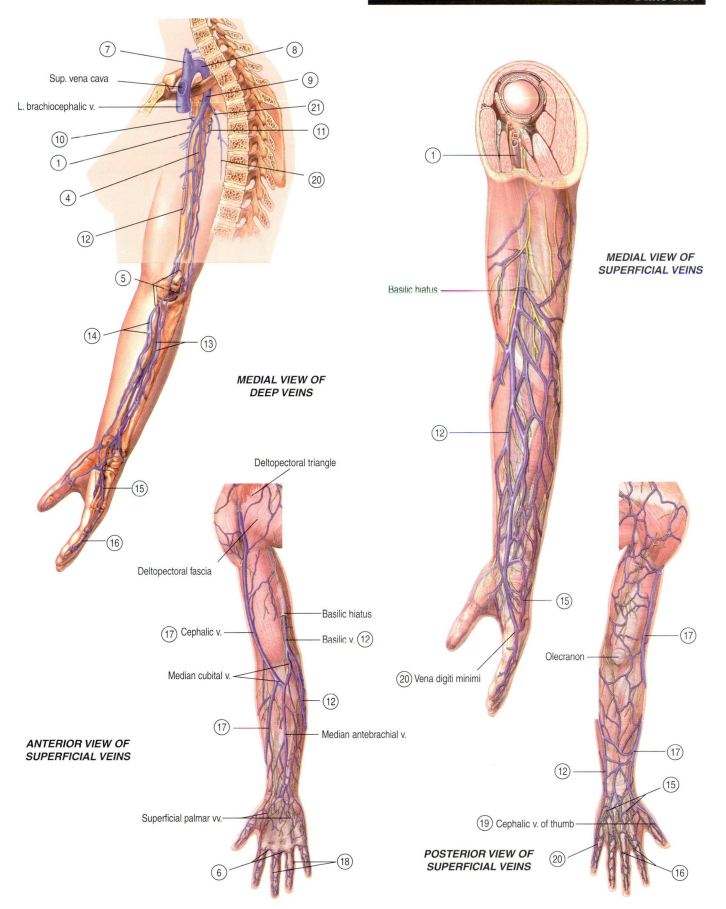

Sup. vena cava

L. brachiocephalic v.

**MEDIAL VIEW OF
DEEP VEINS**

**MEDIAL VIEW OF
SUPERFICIAL VEINS**

Basilic hiatus

Deltopectoral triangle

Deltopectoral fascia

Basilic hiatus

Cephalic v.

Basilic v.

Median cubital v.

Median antebrachial v.

**ANTERIOR VIEW OF
SUPERFICIAL VEINS**

Superficial palmar vv.

Vena digiti minimi

Olecranon

Cephalic v. of thumb

**POSTERIOR VIEW OF
SUPERFICIAL VEINS**

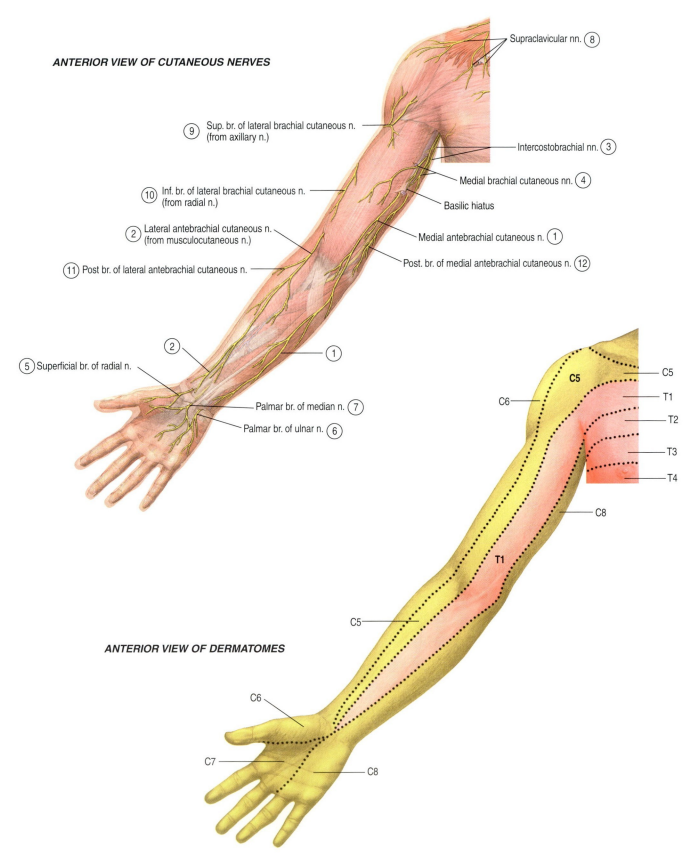

ANTERIOR VIEW OF CUTANEOUS NERVES

Supraclavicular nn. ⑧

⑨ Sup. br. of lateral brachial cutaneous n. (from axillary n.)

Intercostobrachial nn. ③

⑩ Inf. br. of lateral brachial cutaneous n. (from radial n.)

Medial brachial cutaneous nn. ④

Basilic hiatus

② Lateral antebrachial cutaneous n. (from musculocutaneous n.)

Medial antebrachial cutaneous n. ①

⑪ Post br. of lateral antebrachial cutaneous n.

Post. br. of medial antebrachial cutaneous n. ⑫

② ①

⑤ Superficial br. of radial n.

Palmar br. of median n. ⑦

Palmar br. of ulnar n. ⑥

C5

C6

C5

T1

T2

T3

T4

C8

T1

C5

ANTERIOR VIEW OF DERMATOMES

C6

C7

C8

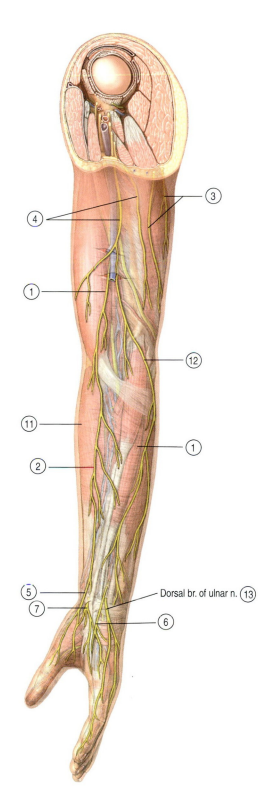

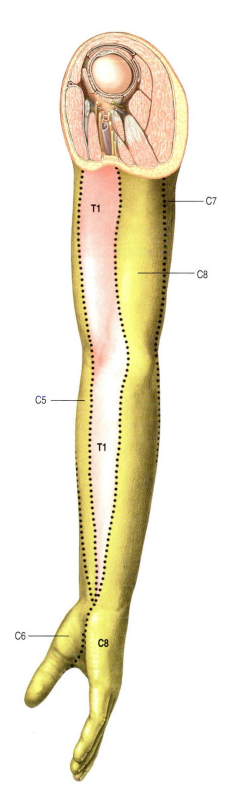

MEDIAL VIEW OF CUTANEOUS NERVES

MEDIAL VIEW OF DERMATOMES

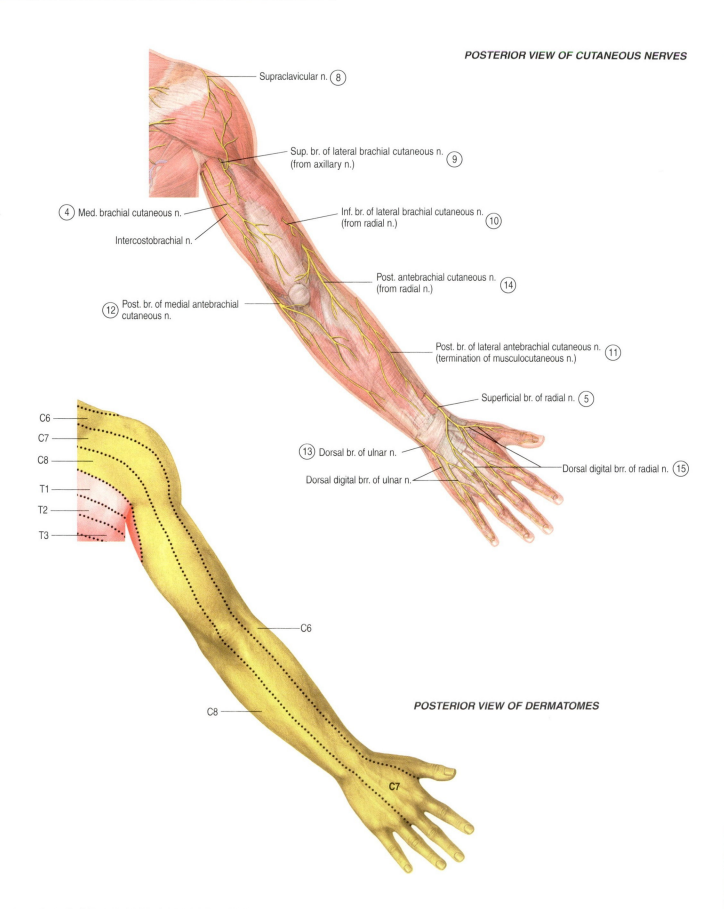

POSTERIOR VIEW OF CUTANEOUS NERVES

Supraclavicular n. (8)

Sup. br. of lateral brachial cutaneous n. (from axillary n.) (9)

(4) Med. brachial cutaneous n.

Intercostobrachial n.

Inf. br. of lateral brachial cutaneous n. (from radial n.) (10)

Post. antebrachial cutaneous n. (from radial n.) (14)

(12) Post. br. of medial antebrachial cutaneous n.

Post. br. of lateral antebrachial cutaneous n. (termination of musculocutaneous n.) (11)

Superficial br. of radial n. (5)

(13) Dorsal br. of ulnar n.

Dorsal digital brr. of ulnar n.

Dorsal digital brr. of radial n. (15)

C6
C7
C8
T1
T2
T3

C6

C8

C7

POSTERIOR VIEW OF DERMATOMES

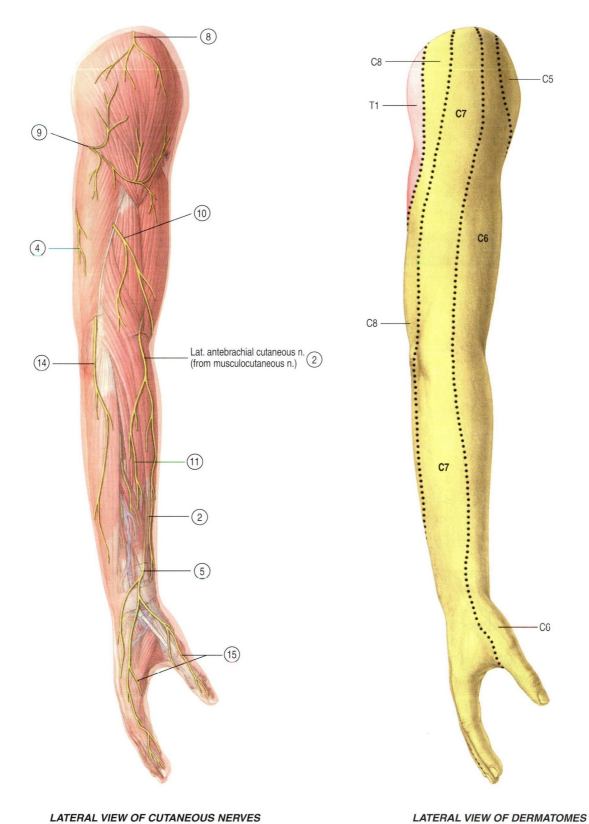

Lat. antebrachial cutaneous n.
(from musculocutaneous n.) ②

LATERAL VIEW OF CUTANEOUS NERVES

LATERAL VIEW OF DERMATOMES

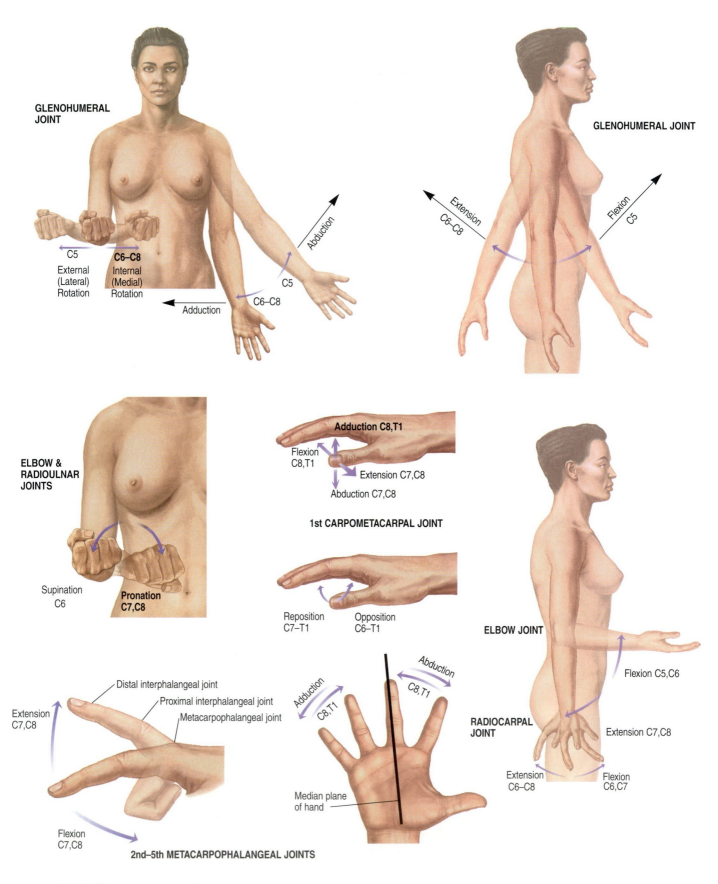

GLENOHUMERAL JOINT

C5
External (Lateral) Rotation

C6–C8
Internal (Medial) Rotation

Abduction
C5

Adduction
C6–C8

GLENOHUMERAL JOINT

Extension
C6–C8

Flexion
C5

ELBOW & RADIOULNAR JOINTS

Supination
C6

Pronation
C7,C8

Adduction C8,T1

Flexion C8,T1

Extension C7,C8

Abduction C7,C8

1st CARPOMETACARPAL JOINT

Reposition C7–T1

Opposition C6–T1

Distal interphalangeal joint

Proximal interphalangeal joint

Metacarpophalangeal joint

Extension C7,C8

Flexion C7,C8

Adduction C8,T1

Abduction C8,T1

Median plane of hand

2nd–5th METACARPOPHALANGEAL JOINTS

ELBOW JOINT

Flexion C5,C6

RADIOCARPAL JOINT

Extension C7,C8

Extension C6–C8

Flexion C6,C7

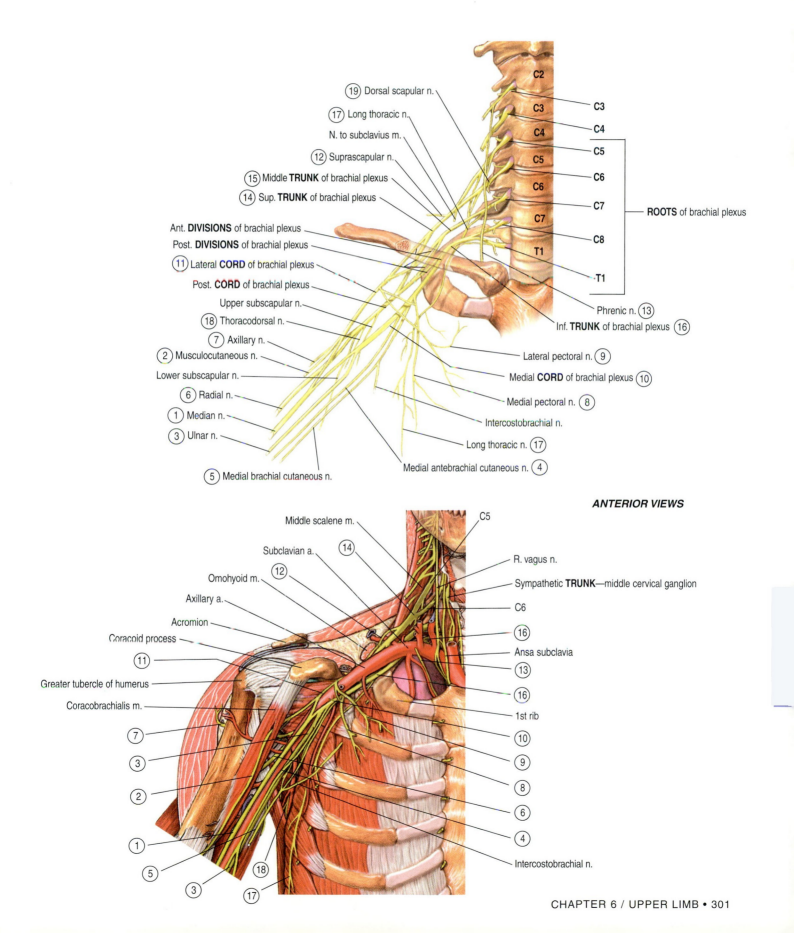

(19) Dorsal scapular n.
(17) Long thoracic n.
N. to subclavius m.
(12) Suprascapular n.
(15) Middle **TRUNK** of brachial plexus
(14) Sup. **TRUNK** of brachial plexus
Ant. **DIVISIONS** of brachial plexus
Post. **DIVISIONS** of brachial plexus
(11) Lateral **CORD** of brachial plexus
Post. **CORD** of brachial plexus
Upper subscapular n.
(18) Thoracodorsal n.
(7) Axillary n.
(2) Musculocutaneous n.
Lower subscapular n.
(6) Radial n.
(1) Median n.
(3) Ulnar n.
(5) Medial brachial cutaneous n.

C2
C3
C4
C5
C6
C7
T1

C3
C4
C5
C6
C7
C8
T1

ROOTS of brachial plexus

Phrenic n. (13)
Inf. **TRUNK** of brachial plexus (16)
Lateral pectoral n. (9)
Medial **CORD** of brachial plexus (10)
Medial pectoral n. (8)
Intercostobrachial n.
Long thoracic n. (17)
Medial antebrachial cutaneous n. (4)

ANTERIOR VIEWS

Middle scalene m.
C5
Subclavian a. (14)
(12)
Omohyoid m.
Axillary a.
Acromion
Coracoid process
(11)
Greater tubercle of humerus
Coracobrachialis m.
(7)
(3)
(2)
(1)
(5)
(18)
(3)
(17)

R. vagus n.
Sympathetic **TRUNK**—middle cervical ganglion
C6
(16)
Ansa subclavia
(13)
(16)
1st rib
(10)
(9)
(8)
(6)
(4)
Intercostobrachial n.

CHAPTER 6 / UPPER LIMB • 301

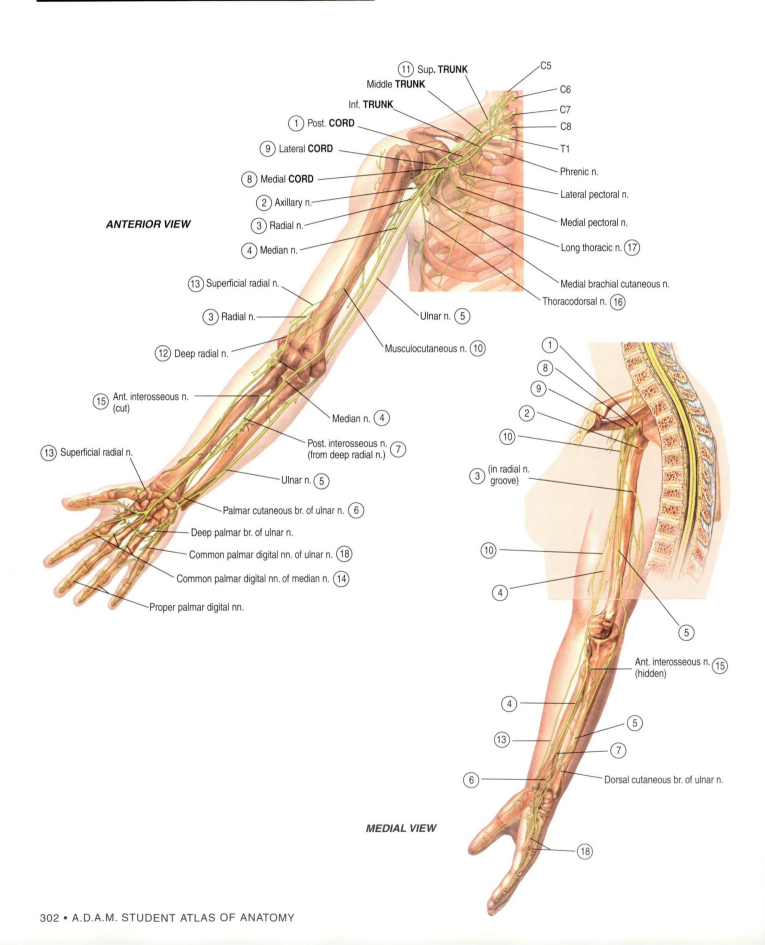

ANTERIOR VIEW

MEDIAL VIEW

(11) Sup. **TRUNK**
Middle **TRUNK**
Inf. **TRUNK**
(1) Post. **CORD**
(9) Lateral **CORD**
(8) Medial **CORD**
(2) Axillary n.
(3) Radial n.
(4) Median n.

C5
C6
C7
C8
T1
Phrenic n.
Lateral pectoral n.
Medial pectoral n.
Long thoracic n. (17)
Medial brachial cutaneous n.
Thoracodorsal n. (16)

(13) Superficial radial n.
(3) Radial n.
(12) Deep radial n.
(15) Ant. interosseous n. (cut)
(13) Superficial radial n.

Ulnar n. (5)
Musculocutaneous n. (10)
Median n. (4)
Post. interosseous n. (7) (from deep radial n.)
Ulnar n. (5)
Palmar cutaneous br. of ulnar n. (6)
Deep palmar br. of ulnar n.
Common palmar digital nn. of ulnar n. (18)
Common palmar digital nn. of median n. (14)
Proper palmar digital nn.

(1)
(8)
(9)
(2)
(10)
(3) (in radial n. groove)
(10)
(4)
(5)
Ant. interosseous n. (15) (hidden)
(4)
(5)
(13)
(7)
(6)
Dorsal cutaneous br. of ulnar n.
(18)

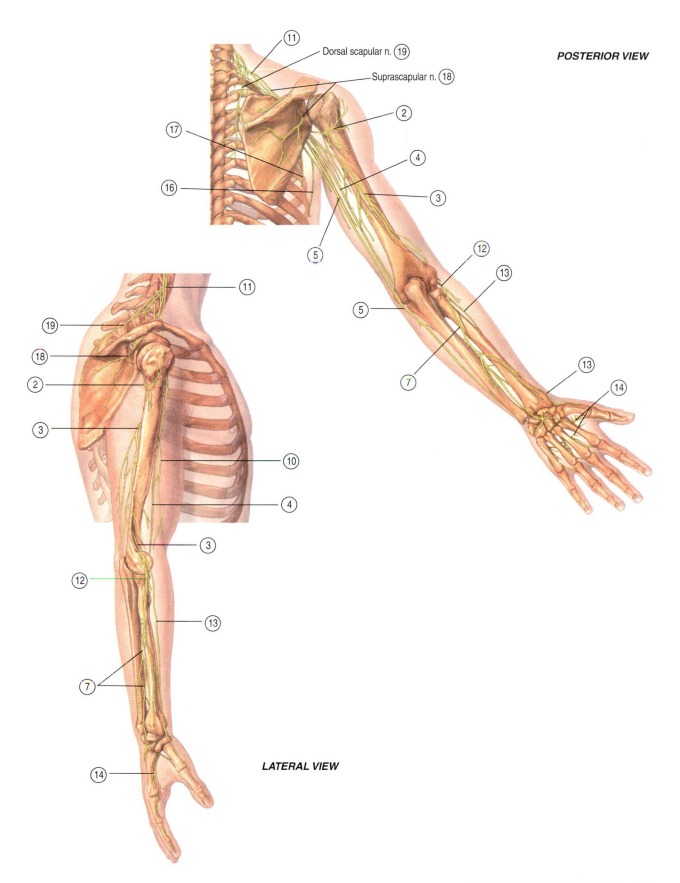

POSTERIOR VIEW

Dorsal scapular n. ⑲

Suprascapular n. ⑱

LATERAL VIEW

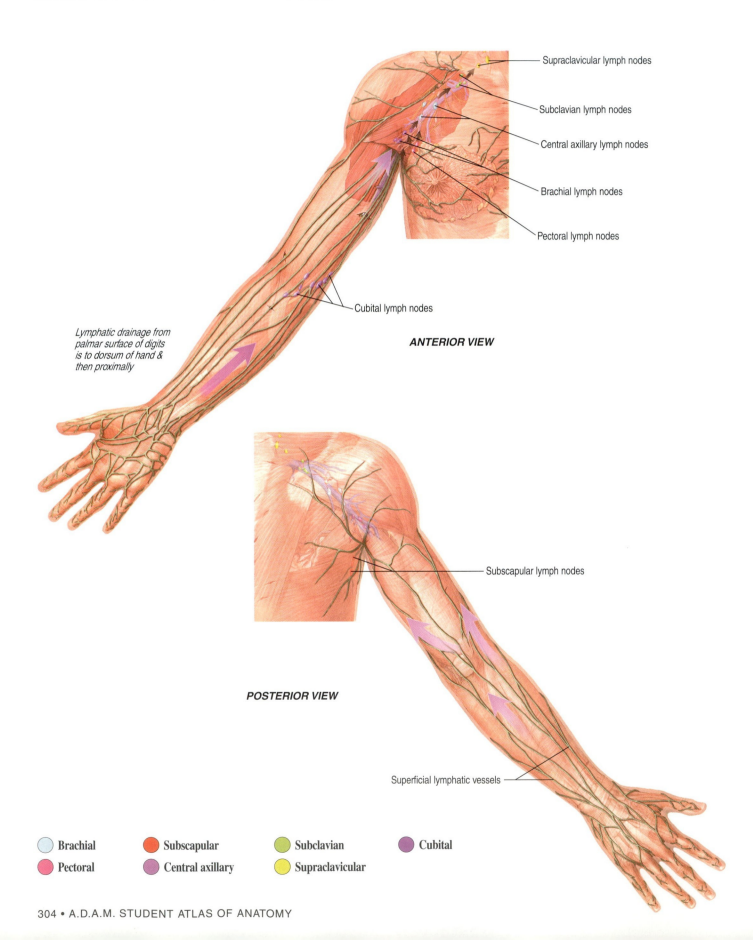

Supraclavicular lymph nodes

Subclavian lymph nodes

Central axillary lymph nodes

Brachial lymph nodes

Pectoral lymph nodes

Cubital lymph nodes

Lymphatic drainage from palmar surface of digits is to dorsum of hand & then proximally

ANTERIOR VIEW

Subscapular lymph nodes

POSTERIOR VIEW

Superficial lymphatic vessels

◯ Brachial   ● Subscapular   ● Subclavian   ● Cubital

● Pectoral   ● Central axillary   ● Supraclavicular

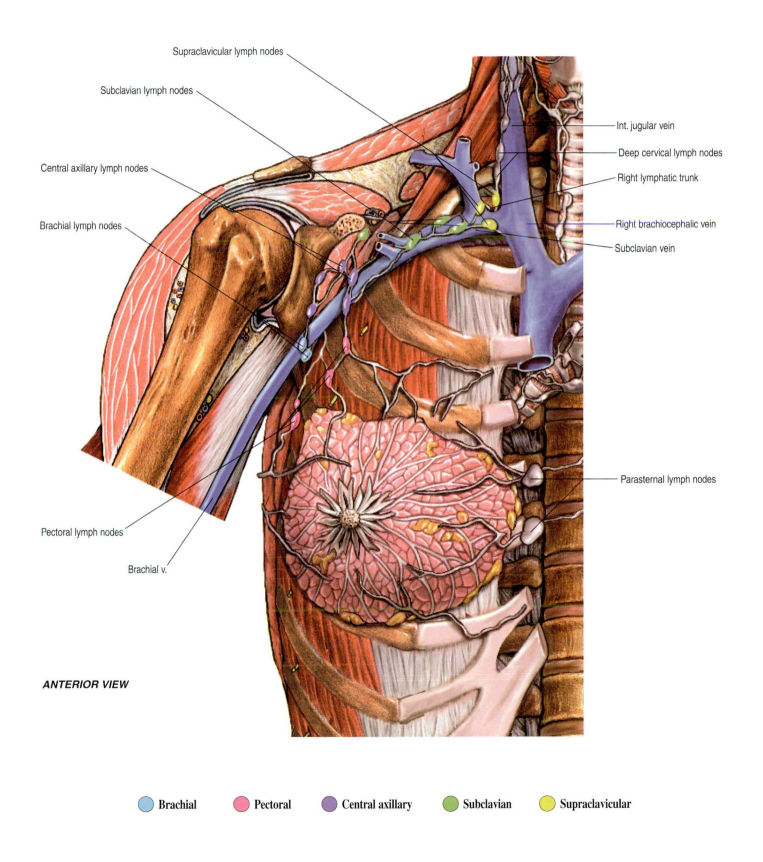

Supraclavicular lymph nodes

Subclavian lymph nodes

Central axillary lymph nodes

Brachial lymph nodes

Int. jugular vein

Deep cervical lymph nodes

Right lymphatic trunk

Right brachiocephalic vein

Subclavian vein

Parasternal lymph nodes

Pectoral lymph nodes

Brachial v.

ANTERIOR VIEW

🔵 **Brachial**   🔴 **Pectoral**   🟣 **Central axillary**   🟢 **Subclavian**   🟡 **Supraclavicular**

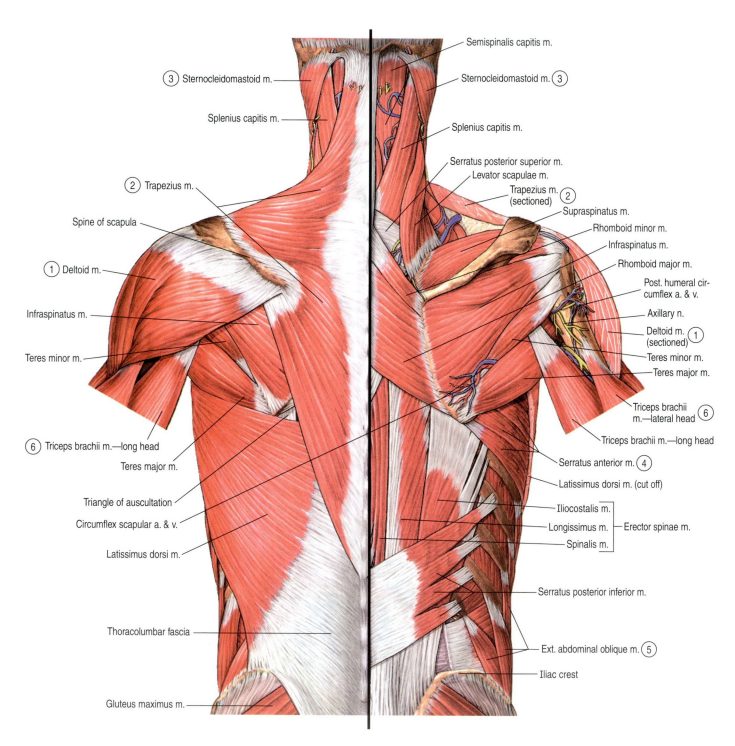

Semispinalis capitis m.

③ Sternocleidomastoid m.

Splenius capitis m.

② Trapezius m.

Spine of scapula

① Deltoid m.

Infraspinatus m.

Teres minor m.

⑥ Triceps brachii m.—long head

Teres major m.

Triangle of auscultation

Circumflex scapular a. & v.

Latissimus dorsi m.

Thoracolumbar fascia

Gluteus maximus m.

Sternocleidomastoid m. ③

Splenius capitis m.

Serratus posterior superior m.

Levator scapulae m.

Trapezius m. (sectioned) ②

Supraspinatus m.

Rhomboid minor m.

Infraspinatus m.

Rhomboid major m.

Post. humeral cir-cumflex a. & v.

Axillary n.

Deltoid m. (sectioned) ①

Teres minor m.

Teres major m.

Triceps brachii m.—lateral head ⑥

Triceps brachii m.—long head

Serratus anterior m. ④

Latissimus dorsi m. (cut off)

Iliocostalis m.

Longissimus m. — Erector spinae m.

Spinalis m.

Serratus posterior inferior m.

Ext. abdominal oblique m. ⑤

Iliac crest

POSTERIOR VIEW

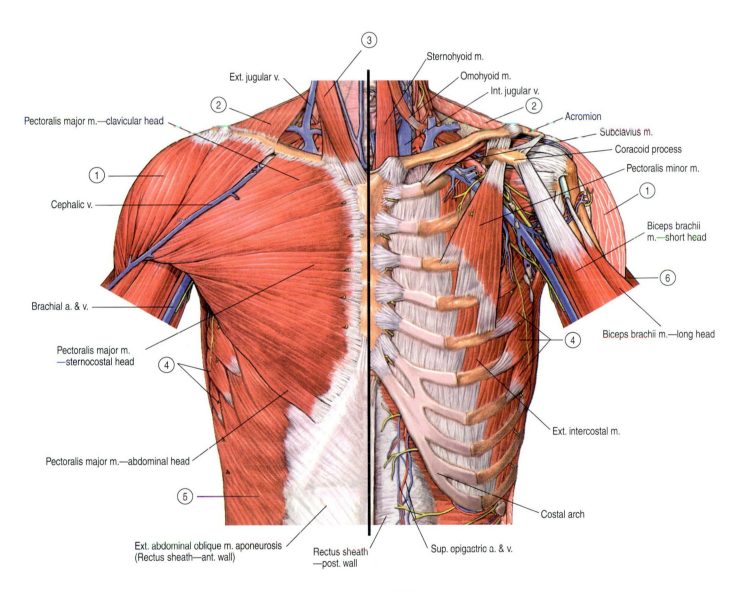

③

Sternohyoid m.

Ext. jugular v.

Omohyoid m.

②

Int. jugular v.

②

Pectoralis major m.—clavicular head

Acromion

Subclavius m.

Coracoid process

Pectoralis minor m.

①

Cephalic v.

①

Biceps brachii
m.—short head

⑥

Brachial a. & v.

Biceps brachii m.—long head

④

Pectoralis major m.
—sternocostal head

④

Ext. intercostal m.

Pectoralis major m.—abdominal head

⑤

Costal arch

Ext. abdominal oblique m. aponeurosis
(Rectus sheath—ant. wall)

Rectus sheath
—post. wall

Sup. epigastric a. & v.

ANTERIOR VIEW

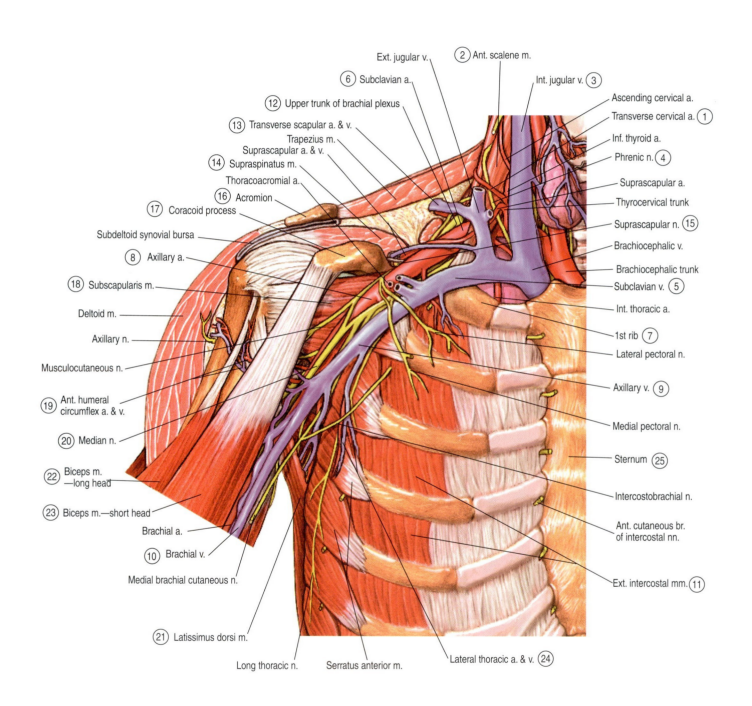

Ext. jugular v.
(2) Ant. scalene m.
(6) Subclavian a.
Int. jugular v. (3)
(12) Upper trunk of brachial plexus
Ascending cervical a.
Transverse cervical a. (1)
(13) Transverse scapular a. & v.
Inf. thyroid a.
Trapezius m.
Phrenic n. (4)
Suprascapular a. & v.
(14) Supraspinatus m.
Suprascapular a.
Thoracoacromial a.
Thyrocervical trunk
(16) Acromion
Suprascapular n. (15)
(17) Coracoid process
Brachiocephalic v.
Subdeltoid synovial bursa
Brachiocephalic trunk
(8) Axillary a.
Subclavian v. (5)
(18) Subscapularis m.
Int. thoracic a.
Deltoid m.
1st rib (7)
Axillary n.
Lateral pectoral n.
Musculocutaneous n.
Axillary v. (9)
(19) Ant. humeral circumflex a. & v.
Medial pectoral n.
(20) Median n.
Sternum (25)
(22) Biceps m. —long head
Intercostobrachial n.
(23) Biceps m.—short head
Ant. cutaneous br. of intercostal nn.
Brachial a.
(10) Brachial v.
Ext. intercostal mm. (11)
Medial brachial cutaneous n.
(21) Latissimus dorsi m.
Long thoracic n.   Serratus anterior m.
Lateral thoracic a. & v. (24)

ANTERIOR VIEW

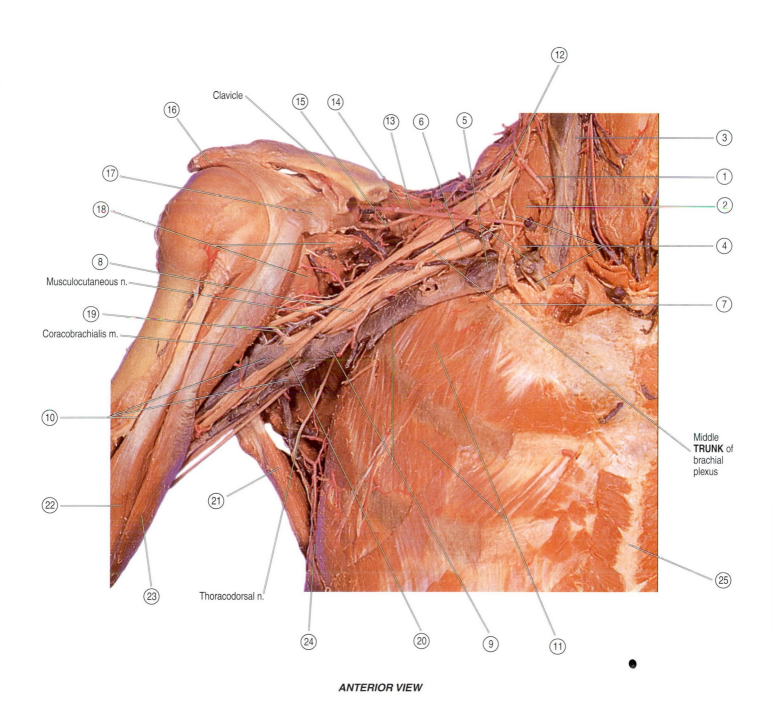

Clavicle

Musculocutaneous n.

Coracobrachialis m.

Middle
TRUNK of
brachial
plexus

Thoracodorsal n.

ANTERIOR VIEW

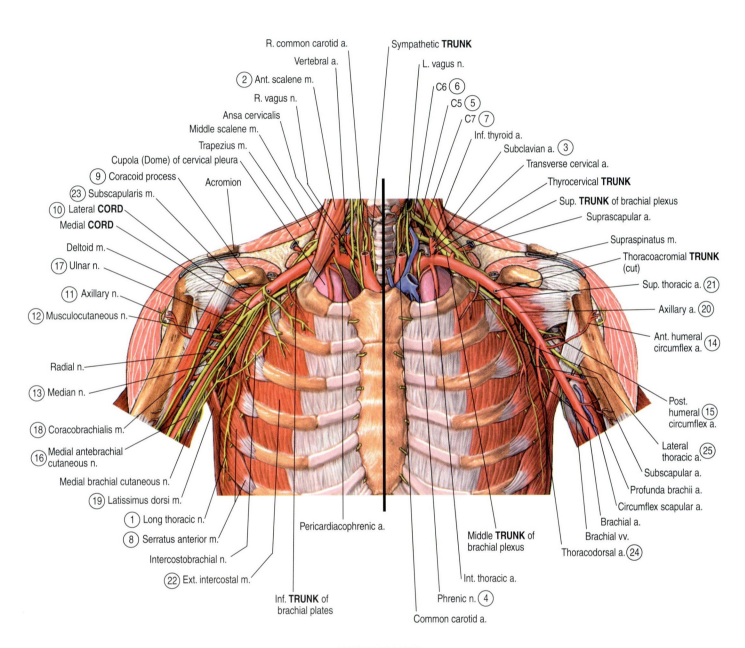

R. common carotid a.
Vertebral a.
② Ant. scalene m.
R. vagus n.
Ansa cervicalis
Middle scalene m.
Trapezius m.
Cupola (Dome) of cervical pleura
⑨ Coracoid process
㉓ Subscapularis m.
⑩ Lateral **CORD**
Medial **CORD**
Deltoid m.
⑰ Ulnar n.
⑪ Axillary n.
⑫ Musculocutaneous n.
Radial n.
⑬ Median n.
⑱ Coracobrachialis m.
⑯ Medial antebrachial cutaneous n.
Medial brachial cutaneous n.
⑲ Latissimus dorsi m.
① Long thoracic n.
⑧ Serratus anterior m.
Intercostobrachial n.
㉒ Ext. intercostal m.

Acromion

Sympathetic **TRUNK**
L. vagus n.
C6 ⑥
C5 ⑤
C7 ⑦
Inf. thyroid a.
Subclavian a. ③
Transverse cervical a.
Thyrocervical **TRUNK**
Sup. **TRUNK** of brachial plexus
Suprascapular a.
Supraspinatus m.
Thoracoacromial **TRUNK** (cut)
Sup. thoracic a. ㉑
Axillary a. ⑳
Ant. humeral circumflex a. ⑭
Post. humeral circumflex a. ⑮
Lateral thoracic a. ㉕
Subscapular a.
Profunda brachii a.
Circumflex scapular a.
Brachial a.
Brachial vv.
Thoracodorsal a. ㉔

Pericardiacophrenic a.

Inf. **TRUNK** of brachial plates

Middle **TRUNK** of brachial plexus

Int. thoracic a.

Phrenic n. ④

Common carotid a.

ANTERIOR VIEW

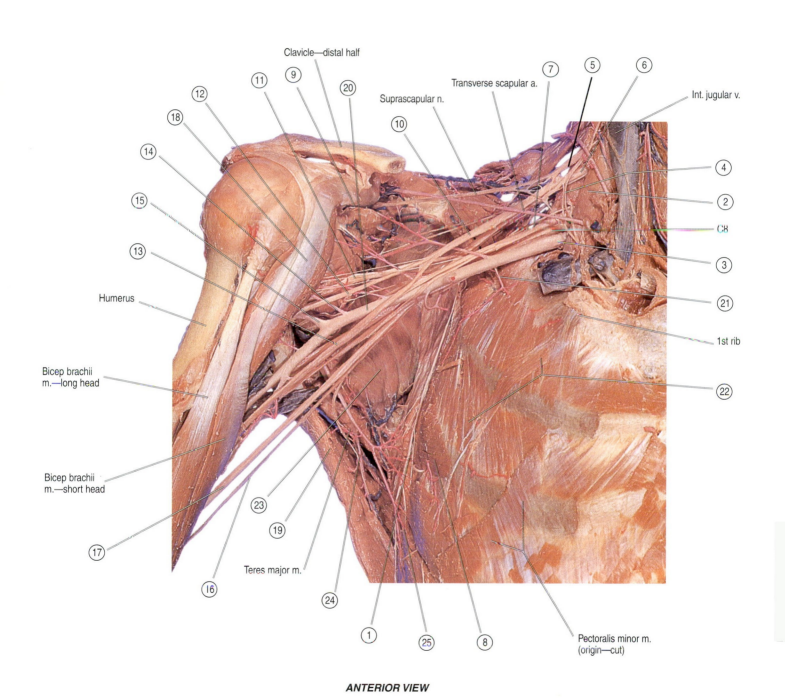

Clavicle—distal half

Transverse scapular a.

Suprascapular n.

Int. jugular v.

Humerus

Bicep brachii
m.—long head

Bicep brachii
m.—short head

Teres major m.

Pectoralis minor m.
(origin—cut)

1st rib

C8

ANTERIOR VIEW

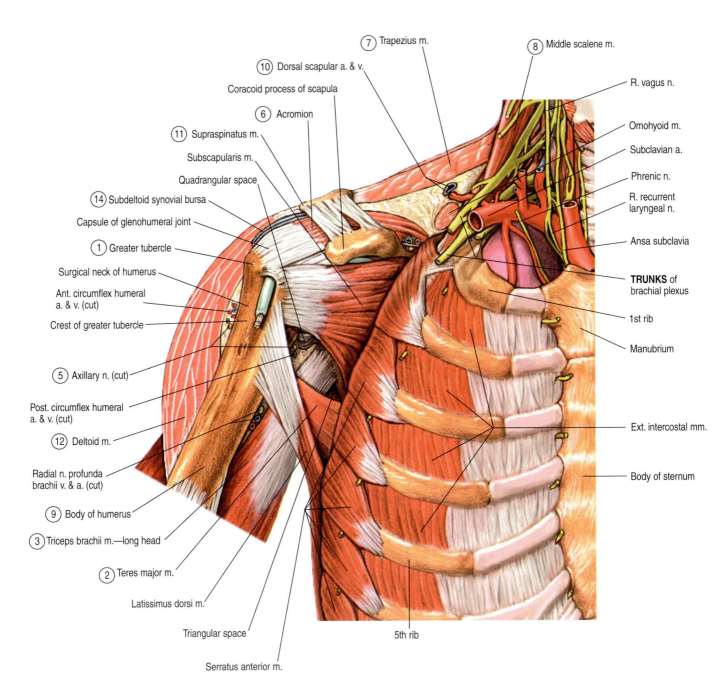

- ⑦ Trapezius m.
- ⑧ Middle scalene m.
- ⑩ Dorsal scapular a. & v.
- R. vagus n.
- Coracoid process of scapula
- Omohyoid m.
- ⑥ Acromion
- Subclavian a.
- ⑪ Supraspinatus m.
- Phrenic n.
- Subscapularis m.
- R. recurrent laryngeal n.
- Quadrangular space
- ⑭ Subdeltoid synovial bursa
- Ansa subclavia
- Capsule of glenohumeral joint
- ① Greater tubercle
- **TRUNKS** of brachial plexus
- Surgical neck of humerus
- 1st rib
- Ant. circumflex humeral a. & v. (cut)
- Manubrium
- Crest of greater tubercle
- ⑤ Axillary n. (cut)
- Post. circumflex humeral a. & v. (cut)
- Ext. intercostal mm.
- ⑫ Deltoid m.
- Radial n. profunda brachii v. & a. (cut)
- Body of sternum
- ⑨ Body of humerus
- ③ Triceps brachii m.—long head
- ② Teres major m.
- Latissimus dorsi m.
- Triangular space
- 5th rib
- Serratus anterior m.

ANTERIOR VIEW

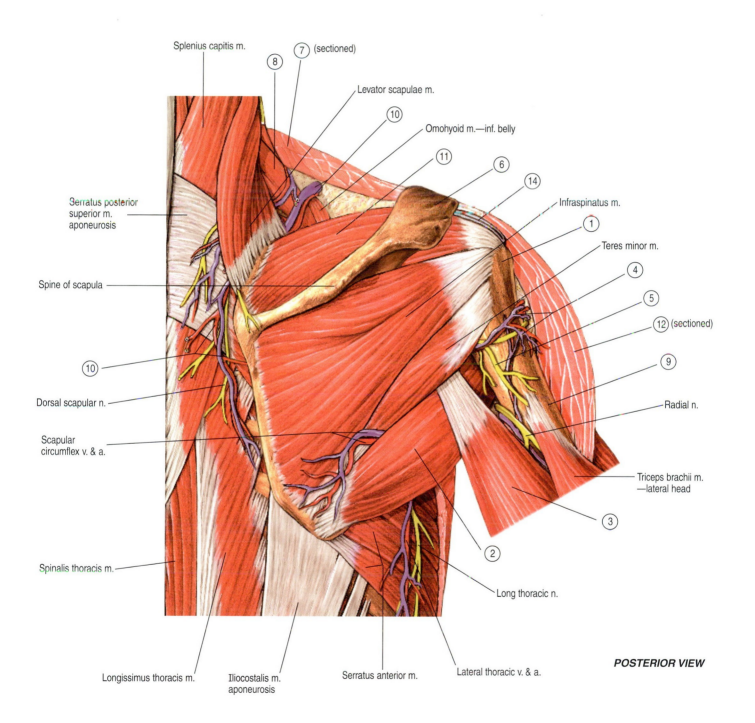

Splenius capitis m.

⑦ (sectioned)

⑧

Levator scapulae m.

⑩

Omohyoid m.—inf. belly

⑪

⑥

⑭

Infraspinatus m.

Serratus posterior
superior m.
aponeurosis

①

Teres minor m.

Spine of scapula

④

⑤

⑫ (sectioned)

⑩

⑨

Dorsal scapular n.

Radial n.

Scapular
circumflex v. & a.

Triceps brachii m.
—lateral head

③

Spinalis thoracis m.

②

Long thoracic n.

Longissimus thoracis m.

Iliocostalis m.
aponeurosis

Serratus anterior m.

Lateral thoracic v. & a.

POSTERIOR VIEW

Shoulder—Coronal Section
Plate 6.35

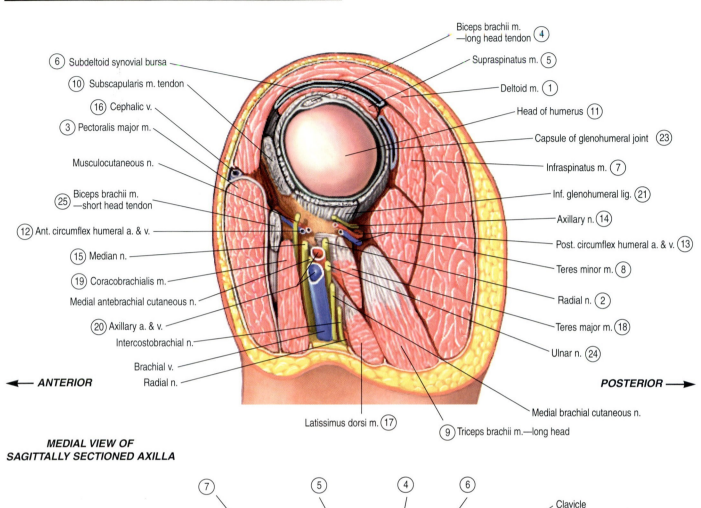

- (6) Subdeltoid synovial bursa
- (10) Subscapularis m. tendon
- (16) Cephalic v.
- (3) Pectoralis major m.
- Musculocutaneous n.
- (25) Biceps brachii m. —short head tendon
- (12) Ant. circumflex humeral a. & v.
- (15) Median n.
- (19) Coracobrachialis m.
- Medial antebrachial cutaneous n.
- (20) Axillary a. & v.
- Intercostobrachial n.
- Brachial v.
- Radial n.

- Biceps brachii m. —long head tendon (4)
- Supraspinatus m. (5)
- Deltoid m. (1)
- Head of humerus (11)
- Capsule of glenohumeral joint (23)
- Infraspinatus m. (7)
- Inf. glenohumeral lig. (21)
- Axillary n. (14)
- Post. circumflex humeral a. & v. (13)
- Teres minor m. (8)
- Radial n. (2)
- Teres major m. (18)
- Ulnar n. (24)
- Medial brachial cutaneous n.

Latissimus dorsi m. (17)

(9) Triceps brachii m.—long head

← **ANTERIOR**

POSTERIOR →

**MEDIAL VIEW OF
SAGITTALLY SECTIONED AXILLA**

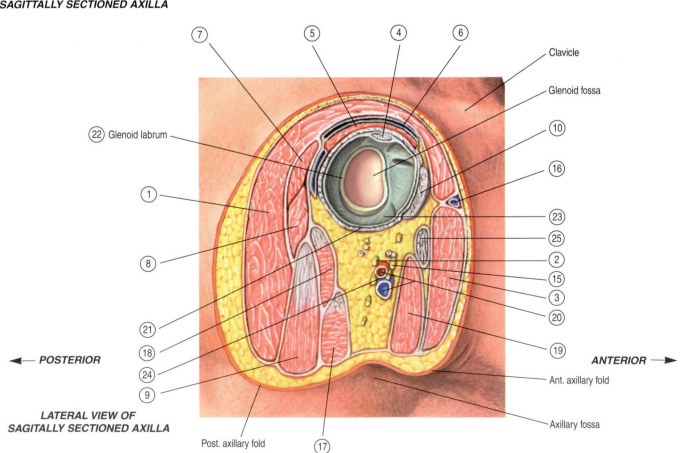

- (22) Glenoid labrum
- (1)
- (8)
- (21)
- (18)
- (24)
- (9)

- (7) (5) (4) (6)

- Clavicle
- Glenoid fossa
- (10)
- (16)
- (23)
- (25)
- (2)
- (15)
- (3)
- (20)
- (19)
- Ant. axillary fold
- Axillary fossa

← **POSTERIOR**

ANTERIOR →

Post. axillary fold

(17)

**LATERAL VIEW OF
SAGITALLY SECTIONED AXILLA**

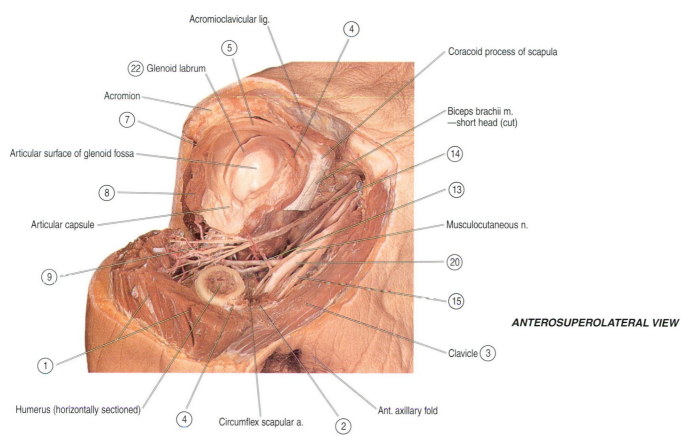

Acromioclavicular lig.

④

⑤

㉒ Glenoid labrum

Acromion

⑦

Articular surface of glenoid fossa

⑧

Articular capsule

⑨

①

Humerus (horizontally sectioned)

④

Circumflex scapular a.

②

Coracoid process of scapula

Biceps brachii m.
—short head (cut)

⑭

⑬

Musculocutaneous n.

⑳

⑮

Clavicle ③

Ant. axillary fold

ANTEROSUPEROLATERAL VIEW

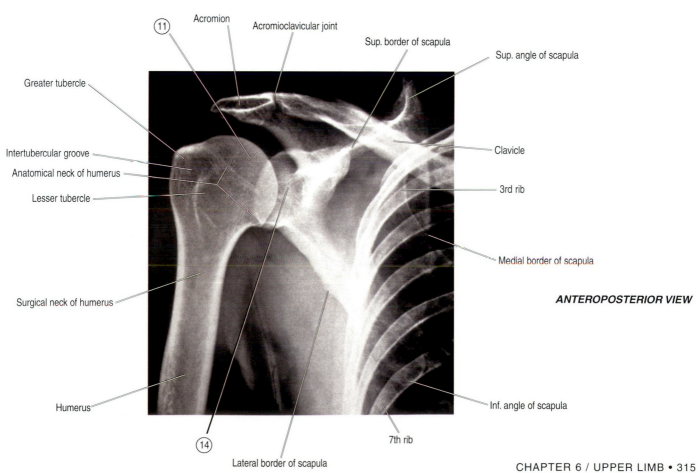

⑪

Acromion

Acromioclavicular joint

Sup. border of scapula

Sup. angle of scapula

Greater tubercle

Clavicle

Intertubercular groove

3rd rib

Anatomical neck of humerus

Lesser tubercle

Medial border of scapula

Surgical neck of humerus

ANTEROPOSTERIOR VIEW

Humerus

Inf. angle of scapula

⑭

Lateral border of scapula

7th rib

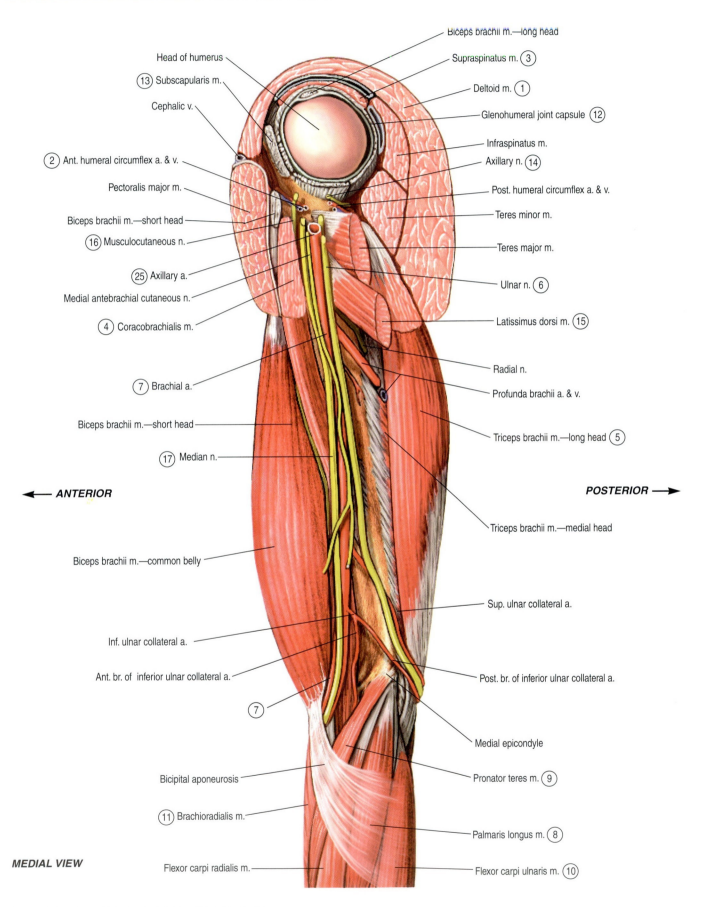

Biceps brachii m.—long head

Head of humerus

(13) Subscapularis m.

Supraspinatus m. (3)

Cephalic v.

Deltoid m. (1)

Glenohumeral joint capsule (12)

Infraspinatus m.

(2) Ant. humeral circumflex a. & v.

Axillary n. (14)

Pectoralis major m.

Post. humeral circumflex a. & v.

Biceps brachii m.—short head

Teres minor m.

(16) Musculocutaneous n.

Teres major m.

(25) Axillary a.

Ulnar n. (6)

Medial antebrachial cutaneous n.

Latissimus dorsi m. (15)

(4) Coracobrachialis m.

Radial n.

(7) Brachial a.

Profunda brachii a. & v.

Biceps brachii m.—short head

Triceps brachii m.—long head (5)

(17) Median n.

← ANTERIOR

POSTERIOR →

Triceps brachii m.—medial head

Biceps brachii m.—common belly

Sup. ulnar collateral a.

Inf. ulnar collateral a.

Ant. br. of inferior ulnar collateral a.

Post. br. of inferior ulnar collateral a.

(7)

Medial epicondyle

Bicipital aponeurosis

Pronator teres m. (9)

(11) Brachioradialis m.

Palmaris longus m. (8)

MEDIAL VIEW

Flexor carpi radialis m.

Flexor carpi ulnaris m. (10)

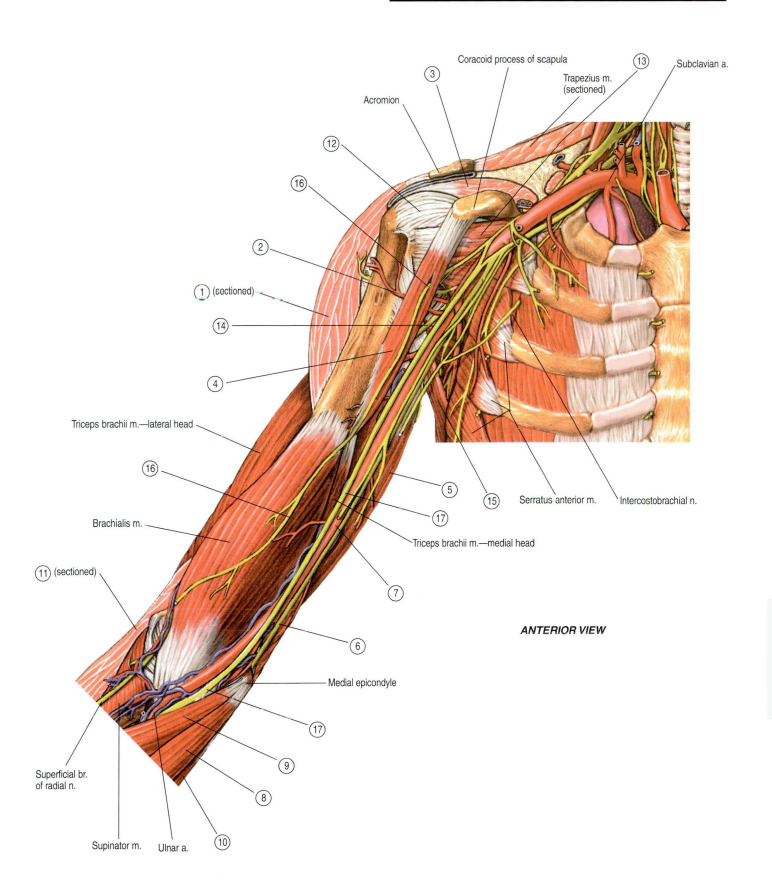

Coracoid process of scapula

③

Trapezius m.
(sectioned)

⑬

Subclavian a.

Acromion

⑫

⑯

②

① (sectioned)

⑭

④

Triceps brachii m.—lateral head

⑯

Brachialis m.

⑪ (sectioned)

⑤

⑰

Triceps brachii m.—medial head

⑦

Serratus anterior m.

⑮

Intercostobrachial n.

ANTERIOR VIEW

⑥

Medial epicondyle

⑰

⑨

Superficial br.
of radial n.

⑧

Supinator m.

Ulnar a.

⑩

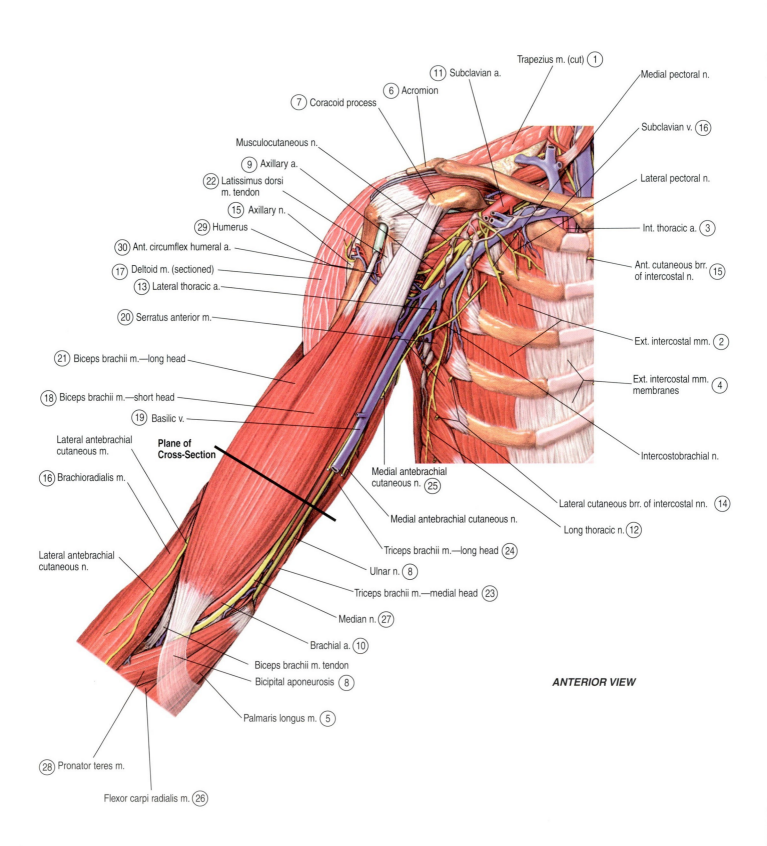

Trapezius m. (cut) (1)

(11) Subclavian a.

(6) Acromion

(7) Coracoid process

Medial pectoral n.

Subclavian v. (16)

Lateral pectoral n.

Musculocutaneous n.

(9) Axillary a.

(22) Latissimus dorsi m. tendon

(15) Axillary n.

(29) Humerus

(30) Ant. circumflex humeral a.

(17) Deltoid m. (sectioned)

(13) Lateral thoracic a.

(20) Serratus anterior m.

(21) Biceps brachii m.—long head

(18) Biceps brachii m.—short head

(19) Basilic v.

Lateral antebrachial cutaneous m.

(16) Brachioradialis m.

Lateral antebrachial cutaneous n.

Plane of Cross-Section

Int. thoracic a. (3)

Ant. cutaneous brr. of intercostal n. (15)

Ext. intercostal mm. (2)

Ext. intercostal mm. membranes (4)

Intercostobrachial n.

Medial antebrachial cutaneous n. (25)

Medial antebrachial cutaneous n.

Lateral cutaneous brr. of intercostal nn. (14)

Long thoracic n. (12)

Triceps brachii m.—long head (24)

Ulnar n. (8)

Triceps brachii m.—medial head (23)

Median n. (27)

Brachial a. (10)

Biceps brachii m. tendon

Bicipital aponeurosis (8)

Palmaris longus m. (5)

(28) Pronator teres m.

Flexor carpi radialis m. (26)

ANTERIOR VIEW

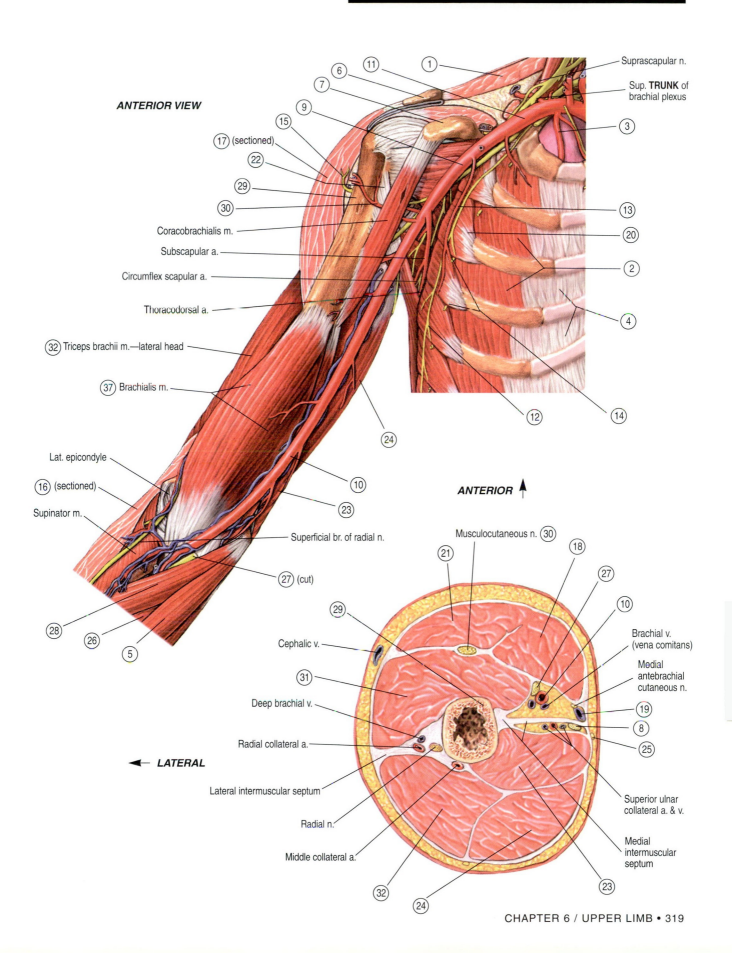

ANTERIOR VIEW

Suprascapular n.

Sup. **TRUNK** of brachial plexus

(17) (sectioned)

Coracobrachialis m.

Subscapular a.

Circumflex scapular a.

Thoracodorsal a.

(32) Triceps brachii m.—lateral head

(37) Brachialis m.

Lat. epicondyle

(16) (sectioned)

Supinator m.

Superficial br. of radial n.

(27) (cut)

ANTERIOR

Musculocutaneous n. (30)

Cephalic v.

Brachial v. (vena comitans)

Medial antebrachial cutaneous n.

Deep brachial v.

Radial collateral a.

LATERAL

Lateral intermuscular septum

Superior ulnar collateral a. & v.

Radial n.

Medial intermuscular septum

Middle collateral a.

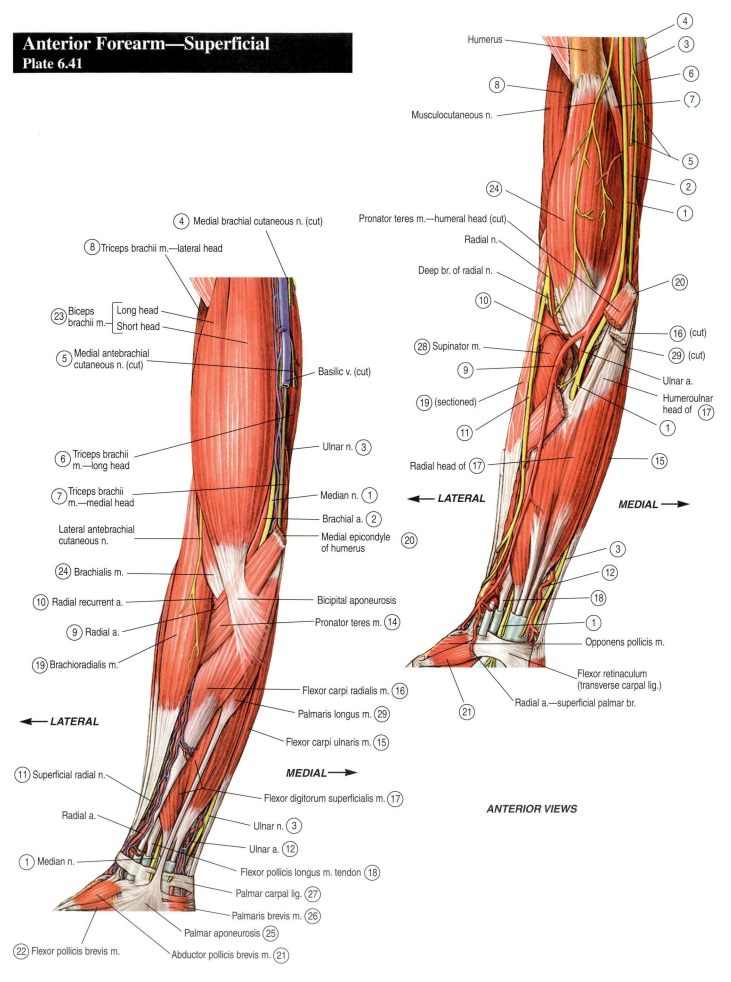

④ Medial brachial cutaneous n. (cut)

⑧ Triceps brachii m.—lateral head

㉓ Biceps brachii m.— { Long head / Short head }

⑤ Medial antebrachial cutaneous n. (cut)

Basilic v. (cut)

⑥ Triceps brachii m.—long head

⑦ Triceps brachii m.—medial head

Ulnar n. ③

Median n. ①

Lateral antebrachial cutaneous n.

Brachial a. ②

Medial epicondyle of humerus ㉘

㉔ Brachialis m.

⑩ Radial recurrent a.

Bicipital aponeurosis

⑨ Radial a.

Pronator teres m. ⑭

⑲ Brachioradialis m.

Flexor carpi radialis m. ⑯

Palmaris longus m. ㉙

Flexor carpi ulnaris m. ⑮

← LATERAL

MEDIAL →

⑪ Superficial radial n.

Flexor digitorum superficialis m. ⑰

Radial a.

Ulnar n. ③

① Median n.

Ulnar a. ⑫

Flexor pollicis longus m. tendon ⑱

Palmar carpal lig. ㉗

Palmaris brevis m. ㉖

Palmar aponeurosis ㉕

㉒ Flexor pollicis brevis m.

Abductor pollicis brevis m. ㉑

Humerus

④
③
⑥
⑦

⑧

Musculocutaneous n.

⑤

②
①

㉔

Pronator teres m.—humeral head (cut)

Radial n.

Deep br. of radial n.

⑩

㉘ Supinator m.

⑨

⑲ (sectioned)

⑪

Radial head of ⑰

← LATERAL

⑳

⑯ (cut)
㉙ (cut)

Ulnar a.

Humeroulnar head of ⑰

①

⑮

MEDIAL →

③
⑫
⑱
①

Opponens pollicis m.

Flexor retinaculum (transverse carpal lig.)

㉑

Radial a.—superficial palmar br.

ANTERIOR VIEWS

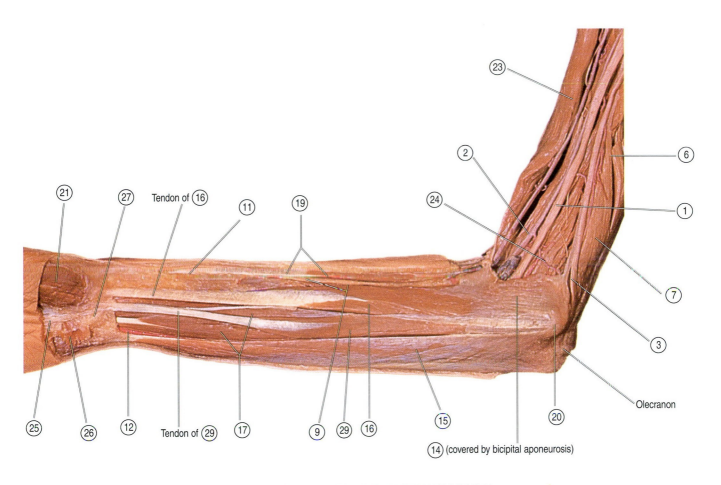

Tendon of (16)

(14) (covered by bicipital aponeurosis)

Tendon of (29)

Olecranon

MEDIAL ARM & ANTERIOR FOREARM & WRIST

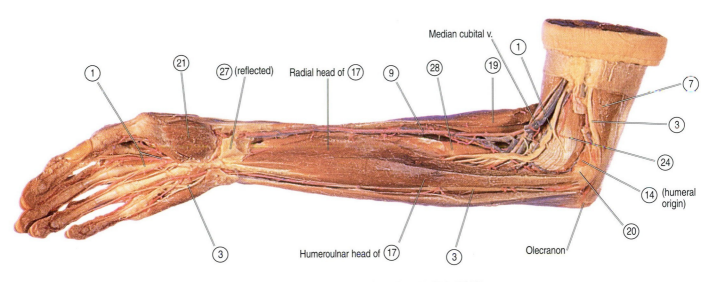

Median cubital v.

(27) (reflected)

Radial head of (17)

Humeroulnar head of (17)

(14) (humeral origin)

Olecranon

MEDIAL ELBOW & ANTERIOR FOREARM & HAND

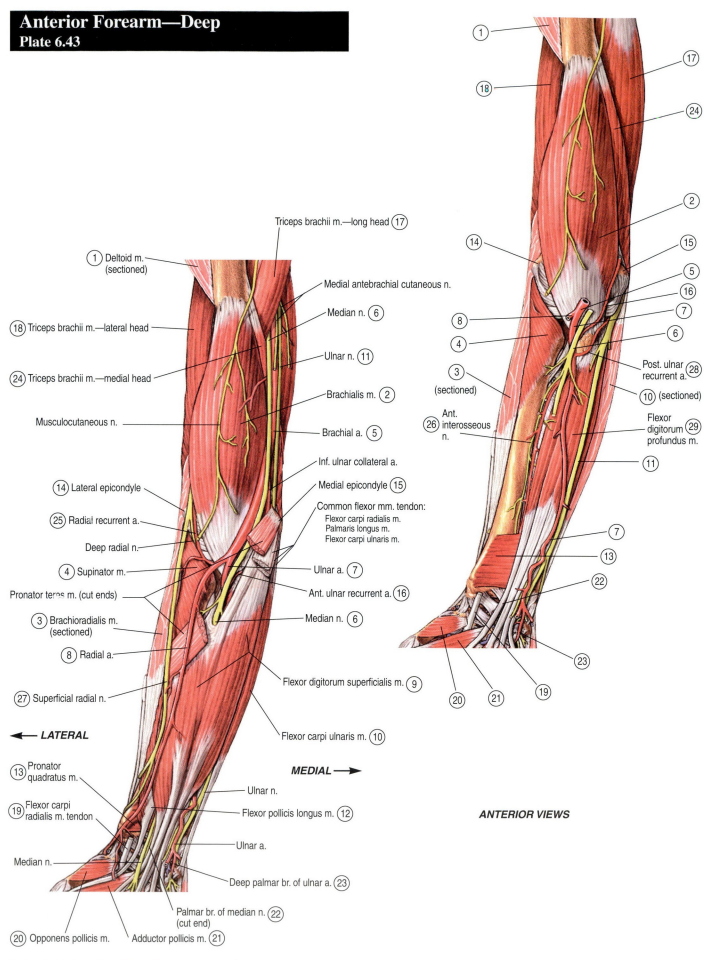

Triceps brachii m.—long head (17)

(1) Deltoid m. (sectioned)

Medial antebrachial cutaneous n.

(18) Triceps brachii m.—lateral head

Median n. (6)

(24) Triceps brachii m.—medial head

Ulnar n. (11)

Musculocutaneous n.

Brachialis m. (2)

Brachial a. (5)

Inf. ulnar collateral a.

(14) Lateral epicondyle

Medial epicondyle (15)

(25) Radial recurrent a.

Common flexor mm. tendon:
Flexor carpi radialis m.
Palmaris longus m.
Flexor carpi ulnaris m.

Deep radial n.

(4) Supinator m.

Ulnar a. (7)

Pronator teres m. (cut ends)

Ant. ulnar recurrent a. (16)

(3) Brachioradialis m. (sectioned)

Median n. (6)

(8) Radial a.

(27) Superficial radial n.

Flexor digitorum superficialis m. (9)

← LATERAL

Flexor carpi ulnaris m. (10)

MEDIAL →

(13) Pronator quadratus m.

Ulnar n.

(19) Flexor carpi radialis m. tendon

Flexor pollicis longus m. (12)

Median n.

Ulnar a.

Deep palmar br. of ulnar a. (23)

Palmar br. of median n. (22) (cut end)

(20) Opponens pollicis m.

Adductor pollicis m. (21)

---

(1)
(18)
(17)
(24)

(14)
(2)
(15)
(5)
(16)
(8)
(7)
(4)
(6)

(3) (sectioned)

Post. ulnar recurrent a. (28)

(26) Ant. interosseous n.

(10) (sectioned)

Flexor digitorum profundus m. (29)

(11)

(7)
(13)
(22)

(20)
(21)
(19)
(23)

ANTERIOR VIEWS

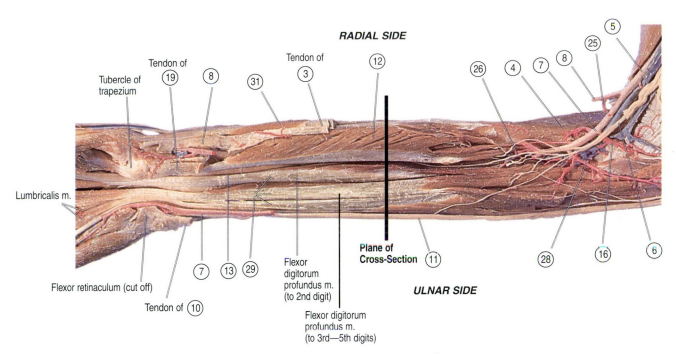

RADIAL SIDE

Tubercle of trapezium

Tendon of ⑲   ⑧   ㉛   Tendon of ③   ⑫   ㉖   ④   ⑦   ⑧   ㉕   ⑤

Lumbricalis m.

Flexor retinaculum (cut off)

⑦   ⑬   ㉙

Tendon of ⑩

Flexor digitorum profundus m. (to 2nd digit)

Flexor digitorum profundus m. (to 3rd—5th digits)

Plane of Cross-Section

⑪   ㉘   ⑯   ⑥

ULNAR SIDE

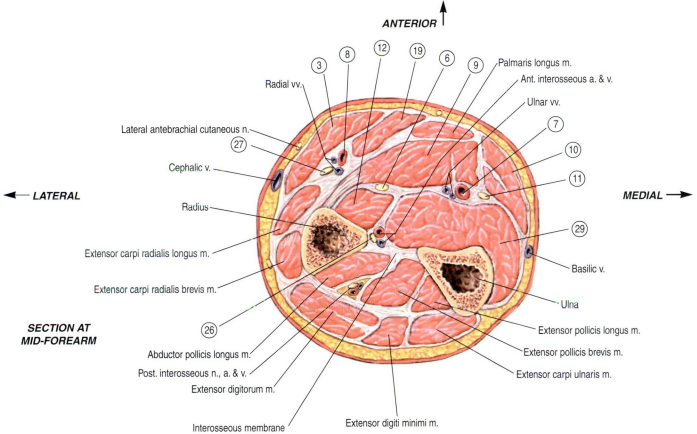

ANTERIOR ↑

Radial vv.

Lateral antebrachial cutaneous n.

㉗

Cephalic v.

Radius

Extensor carpi radialis longus m.

Extensor carpi radialis brevis m.

③   ⑧   ⑫   ⑲   ⑥   ⑨   Palmaris longus m.

Ant. interosseous a. & v.

Ulnar vv.

⑦

⑩

⑪

㉙

Basilic v.

Ulna

Extensor pollicis longus m.

Extensor pollicis brevis m.

Extensor carpi ulnaris m.

SECTION AT MID-FOREARM

◄— LATERAL   MEDIAL —►

㉖

Abductor pollicis longus m.

Post. interosseous n., a. & v.

Extensor digitorum m.

Interosseous membrane

Extensor digiti minimi m.

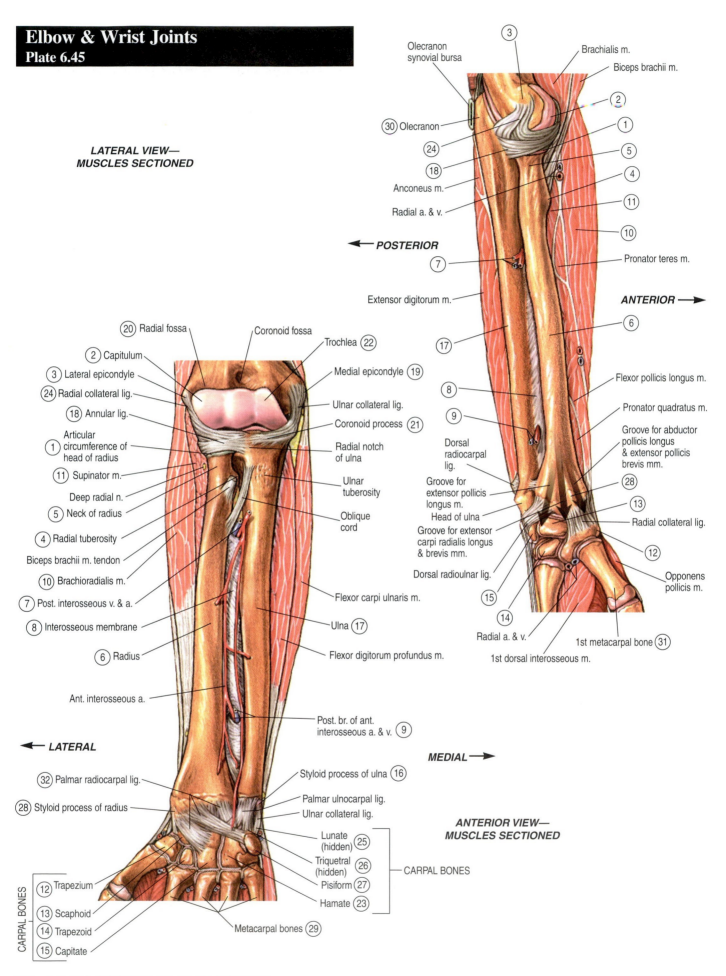

LATERAL VIEW—MUSCLES SECTIONED

Olecranon synovial bursa
③
Brachialis m.
Biceps brachii m.
③⓪ Olecranon
②
②④
①
①⑧
⑤
Anconeus m.
④
Radial a. & v.
①①
①⓪

POSTERIOR ←

⑦

Extensor digitorum m.

ANTERIOR →

①⑦

⑥

⑧

Flexor pollicis longus m.

⑨

Pronator quadratus m.

Dorsal radiocarpal lig.

Groove for abductor pollicis longus & extensor pollicis brevis mm.

Groove for extensor pollicis longus m.

②⑧

Head of ulna

①③

Groove for extensor carpi radialis longus & brevis mm.

Radial collateral lig.

Dorsal radioulnar lig.

①②

①⑤

Opponens pollicis m.

①④

Radial a. & v.

1st metacarpal bone ③①

1st dorsal interosseous m.

Pronator teres m.

MEDIAL →

ANTERIOR VIEW—MUSCLES SECTIONED

②⓪ Radial fossa
Coronoid fossa
Trochlea ②②

② Capitulum
③ Lateral epicondyle
Medial epicondyle ①⑨
②④ Radial collateral lig.
Ulnar collateral lig.
①⑧ Annular lig.
Coronoid process ②①
① Articular circumference of head of radius
Radial notch of ulna
①① Supinator m.
Deep radial n.
Ulnar tuberosity
⑤ Neck of radius
Oblique cord
④ Radial tuberosity
Biceps brachii m. tendon
①⓪ Brachioradialis m.
⑦ Post. interosseous v. & a.
Flexor carpi ulnaris m.
⑧ Interosseous membrane
Ulna ①⑦
⑥ Radius
Flexor digitorum profundus m.

Ant. interosseous a.

Post. br. of ant. interosseous a. & v. ⑨

LATERAL ←

Styloid process of ulna ①⑥

③② Palmar radiocarpal lig.

Palmar ulnocarpal lig.
②⑧ Styloid process of radius
Ulnar collateral lig.

Lunate (hidden) ②⑤

Triquetral (hidden) ②⑥

CARPAL BONES

①② Trapezium
Pisiform ②⑦
①③ Scaphoid
Hamate ②③
①④ Trapezoid
①⑤ Capitate

CARPAL BONES

Metacarpal bones ②⑨

LATERAL VIEW

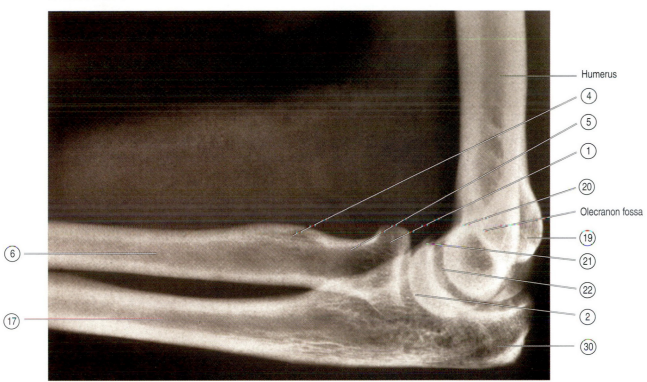

Humerus

(4)

(5)

(1)

(20)

Olecranon fossa

(19)

(21)

(22)

(2)

(30)

(6)

(17)

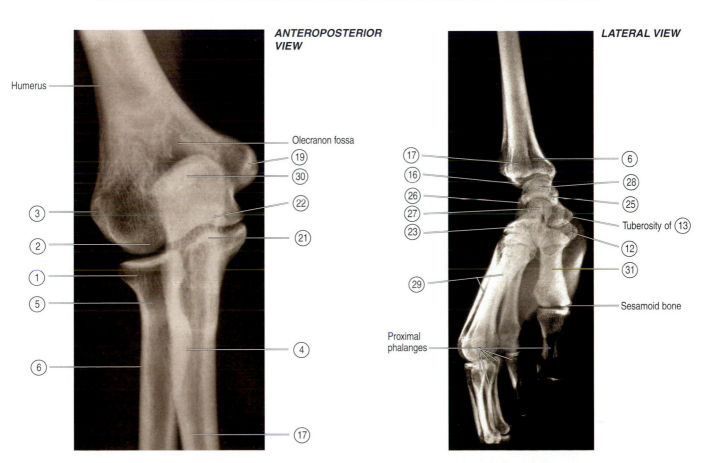

ANTEROPOSTERIOR
VIEW

Humerus

Olecranon fossa

(19)

(30)

(22)

(21)

(4)

(17)

(3)

(2)

(1)

(5)

(6)

LATERAL VIEW

(17)

(16)

(26)

(27)

(23)

(29)

(6)

(28)

(25)

Tuberosity of (13)

(12)

(31)

Sesamoid bone

Proximal
phalanges

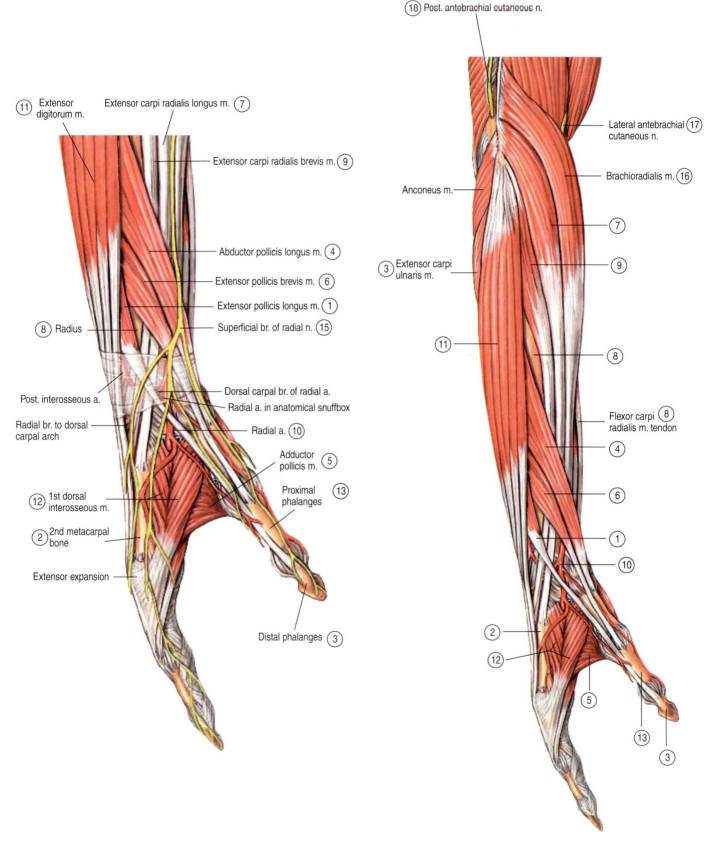

⑱ Post. antebrachial cutaneous n.

⑪ Extensor digitorum m.

Extensor carpi radialis longus m. ⑦

Extensor carpi radialis brevis m. ⑨

Lateral antebrachial ⑰ cutaneous n.

Brachioradialis m. ⑯

Anconeus m.

⑦

③ Extensor carpi ulnaris m.

⑨

Abductor pollicis longus m. ④

Extensor pollicis brevis m. ⑥

Extensor pollicis longus m. ①

⑧ Radius

Superficial br. of radial n. ⑮

⑪

⑧

Post. interosseous a.

Dorsal carpal br. of radial a.

Radial a. in anatomical snuffbox

Flexor carpi ⑧ radialis m. tendon

Radial br. to dorsal carpal arch

Radial a. ⑩

④

Adductor pollicis m. ⑤

⑥

Proximal phalanges ⑬

①

⑫ 1st dorsal interosseous m.

⑩

② 2nd metacarpal bone

Extensor expansion

②

⑫

Distal phalanges ③

⑤

⑬

③

LATERAL VIEWS

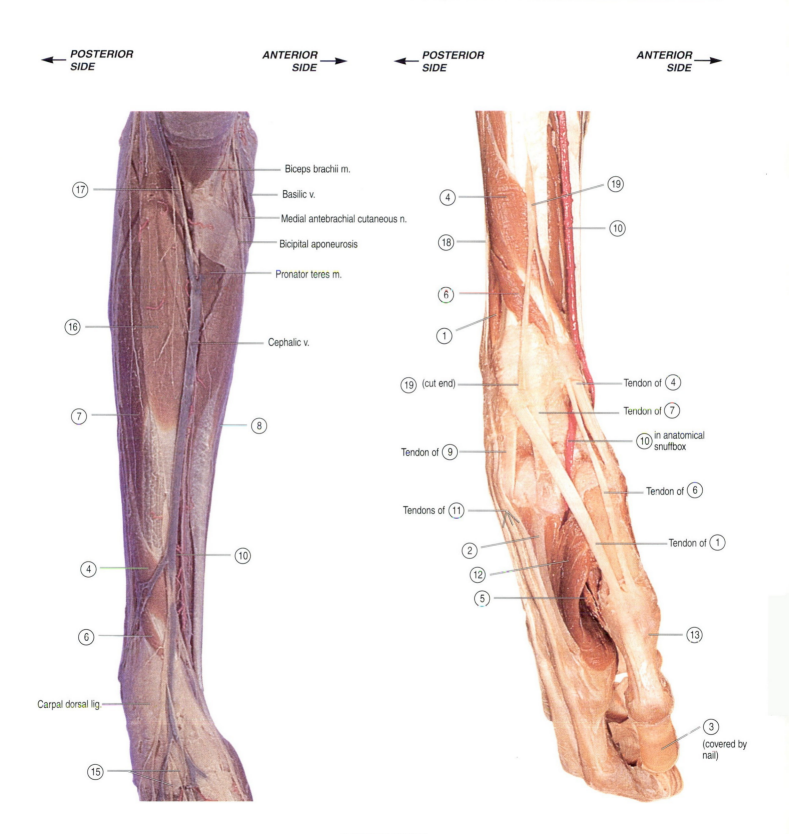

POSTERIOR SIDE ← — ANTERIOR SIDE →   ← POSTERIOR SIDE — ANTERIOR SIDE →

Biceps brachii m.

Basilic v.

Medial antebrachial cutaneous n.

Bicipital aponeurosis

Pronator teres m.

Cephalic v.

Carpal dorsal lig.

Tendon of (4)

Tendon of (7)

(10) in anatomical snuffbox

Tendon of (6)

Tendon of (9)

Tendons of (11)

Tendon of (1)

(19) (cut end)

(3) (covered by nail)

LATERAL VIEWS

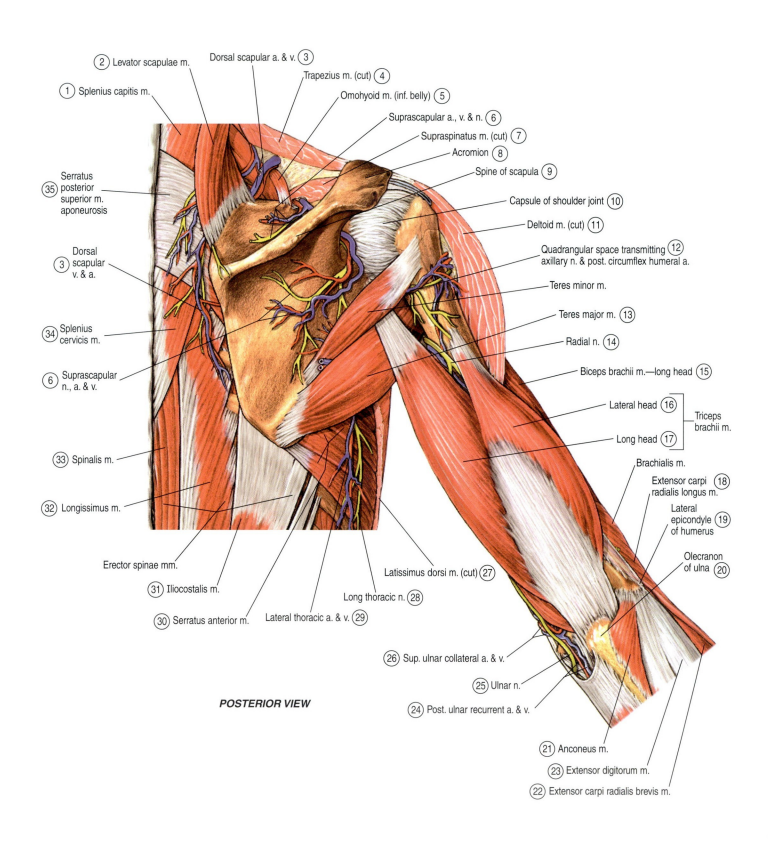

② Levator scapulae m.

Dorsal scapular a. & v. ③

Trapezius m. (cut) ④

① Splenius capitis m.

Omohyoid m. (inf. belly) ⑤

Suprascapular a., v. & n. ⑥

Supraspinatus m. (cut) ⑦

Acromion ⑧

Spine of scapula ⑨

③⑤ Serratus posterior superior m. aponeurosis

Capsule of shoulder joint ⑩

Deltoid m. (cut) ⑪

Quadrangular space transmitting ⑫ axillary n. & post. circumflex humeral a.

③ Dorsal scapular v. & a.

Teres minor m.

Teres major m. ⑬

③④ Splenius cervicis m.

Radial n. ⑭

Biceps brachii m.—long head ⑮

⑥ Suprascapular n., a. & v.

Lateral head ⑯ ⎫ Triceps brachii m.

Long head ⑰ ⎭

Brachialis m.

Extensor carpi ⑱ radialis longus m.

③③ Spinalis m.

Lateral epicondyle ⑲ of humerus

③② Longissimus m.

Olecranon of ulna ⑳

Erector spinae mm.

Latissimus dorsi m. (cut) ㉗

③① Iliocostalis m.

Long thoracic n. ㉘

③⓪ Serratus anterior m.

Lateral thoracic a. & v. ㉙

㉖ Sup. ulnar collateral a. & v.

POSTERIOR VIEW

㉕ Ulnar n.

㉔ Post. ulnar recurrent a. & v.

㉑ Anconeus m.

㉓ Extensor digitorum m.

㉒ Extensor carpi radialis brevis m.

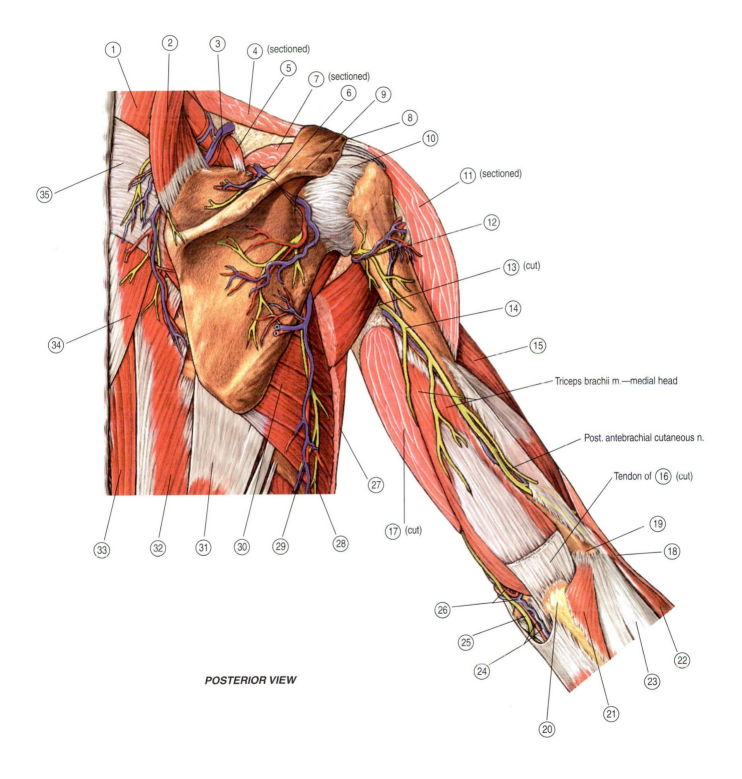

Triceps brachii m.—medial head

Post. antebrachial cutaneous n.

Tendon of (16) (cut)

POSTERIOR VIEW

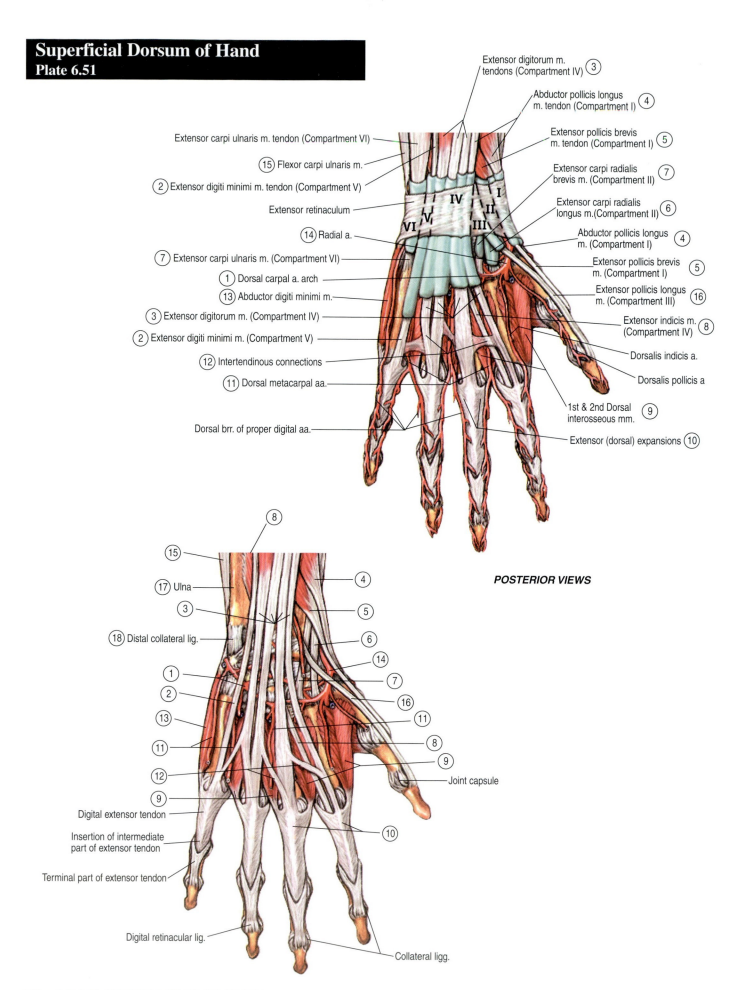

Extensor digitorum m. tendons (Compartment IV) ③

Abductor pollicis longus m. tendon (Compartment I) ④

Extensor pollicis brevis m. tendon (Compartment I) ⑤

Extensor carpi radialis brevis m. (Compartment II) ⑦

Extensor carpi radialis longus m.(Compartment II) ⑥

Abductor pollicis longus m. (Compartment I) ④

Extensor pollicis brevis m. (Compartment I) ⑤

Extensor pollicis longus m. (Compartment III) ⑯

Extensor indicis m. (Compartment IV) ⑧

Dorsalis indicis a.

Dorsalis pollicis a

1st & 2nd Dorsal interosseous mm. ⑨

Extensor (dorsal) expansions ⑩

Extensor carpi ulnaris m. tendon (Compartment VI)

⑮ Flexor carpi ulnaris m.

② Extensor digiti minimi m. tendon (Compartment V)

Extensor retinaculum

⑭ Radial a.

⑦ Extensor carpi ulnaris m. (Compartment VI)

① Dorsal carpal a. arch

⑬ Abductor digiti minimi m.

③ Extensor digitorum m. (Compartment IV)

② Extensor digiti minimi m. (Compartment V)

⑫ Intertendinous connections

⑪ Dorsal metacarpal aa.

Dorsal brr. of proper digital aa.

IV   I
VI V   II
III

POSTERIOR VIEWS

⑧

⑮

⑰ Ulna

③

⑱ Distal collateral lig.

①

②

⑬

⑪

⑫

⑨

Digital extensor tendon

Insertion of intermediate part of extensor tendon

Terminal part of extensor tendon

Digital retinacular lig.

④

⑤

⑥

⑭

⑦

⑯

⑪

⑧

⑨

Joint capsule

⑩

Collateral ligg.

(3)

(17)

(8)

(20) Post. interosseous a. & v.

(19) Distal ulnar collateral lig.

(23) Dorsal carpal br. of ulnar a.

(1)

(26) Dorsal carpometacarpal lig.

(2)

(13)

(24) 4th dorsal interosseous m.

(4)

(5)

(7)

(6)

(14)

Dorsal carpal venous arch

Radial a.—dorsal carpal br. (27)

Dorsal pollicis a. (25)

(11)

(9)

(8)

Metacarpophalangeal joint capsule (22)

Proximal phalanx (28)

Triangular aponeuroses

Middle phalanx (19)

Distal phalanx (21)

(10)

Proximal interphalangeal joint capsule

Distal interphalangeal joint capsule

Lateral bands

Insertion of extensor tendon at base of distal phalanges

POSTERIOR VIEWS

Post. interosseous n.

Interosseous membrane

Dorsal tubercle of radius

Dorsal radiocarpal lig.

Distal radial collateral lig.

(14)

Scaphoid bone

(27)

(25)

(9)

Dorsal radioulnar lig.

(20)

(19)

(23)

(26)

(1)

(13)

(11)

(24)

(22)

(28)

(19)

(21)

Hamate bone

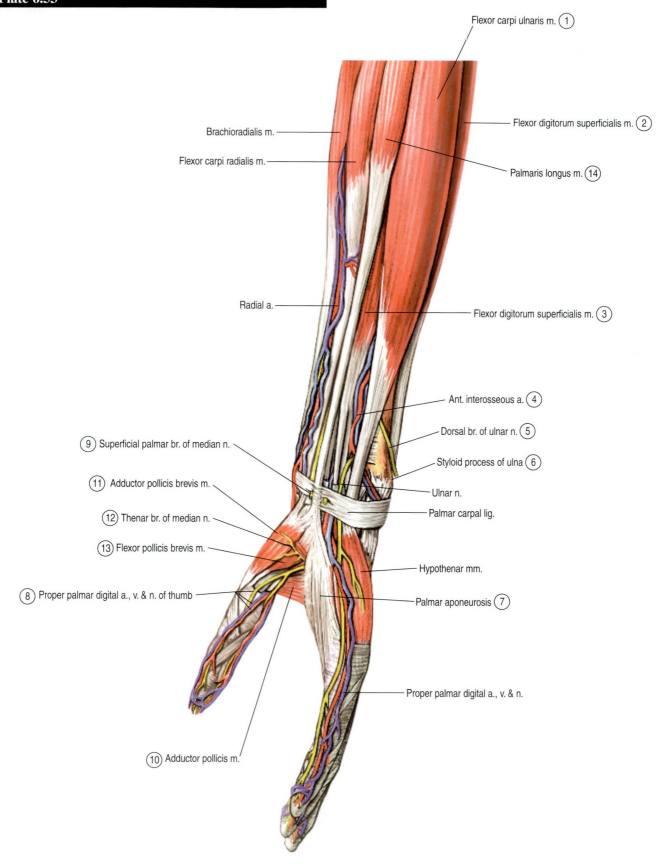

Flexor carpi ulnaris m. (1)

Flexor digitorum superficialis m. (2)

Brachioradialis m.

Flexor carpi radialis m.

Palmaris longus m. (14)

Radial a.

Flexor digitorum superficialis m. (3)

Ant. interosseous a. (4)

Dorsal br. of ulnar n. (5)

(9) Superficial palmar br. of median n.

Styloid process of ulna (6)

(11) Adductor pollicis brevis m.

Ulnar n.

(12) Thenar br. of median n.

Palmar carpal lig.

(13) Flexor pollicis brevis m.

Hypothenar mm.

(8) Proper palmar digital a., v. & n. of thumb

Palmar aponeurosis (7)

Proper palmar digital a., v. & n.

(10) Adductor pollicis m.

MEDIAL VIEW

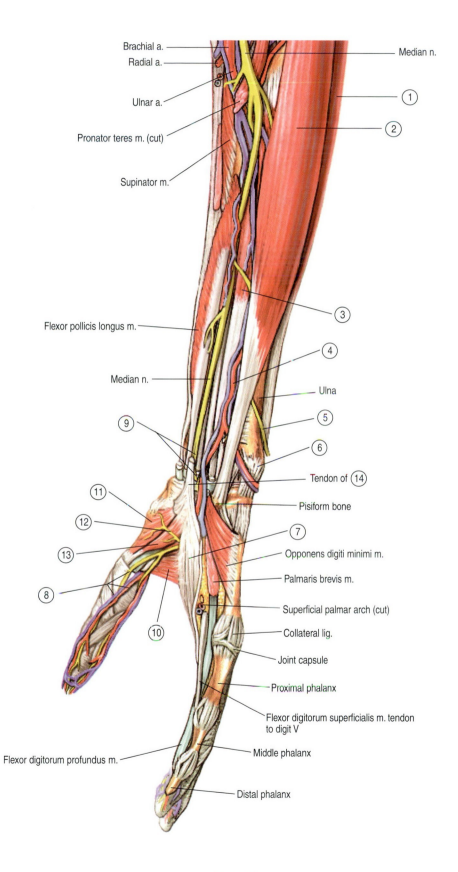

Brachial a.

Radial a.

Median n.

①

②

Ulnar a.

Pronator teres m. (cut)

Supinator m.

③

Flexor pollicis longus m.

④

Ulna

Median n.

⑤

⑨

⑥

Tendon of ⑭

Pisiform bone

⑪

⑫

⑬

⑦

Opponens digiti minimi m.

⑧

Palmaris brevis m.

Superficial palmar arch (cut)

⑩

Collateral lig.

Joint capsule

Proximal phalanx

Flexor digitorum superficialis m. tendon to digit V

Flexor digitorum profundus m.

Middle phalanx

Distal phalanx

MEDIAL VIEW

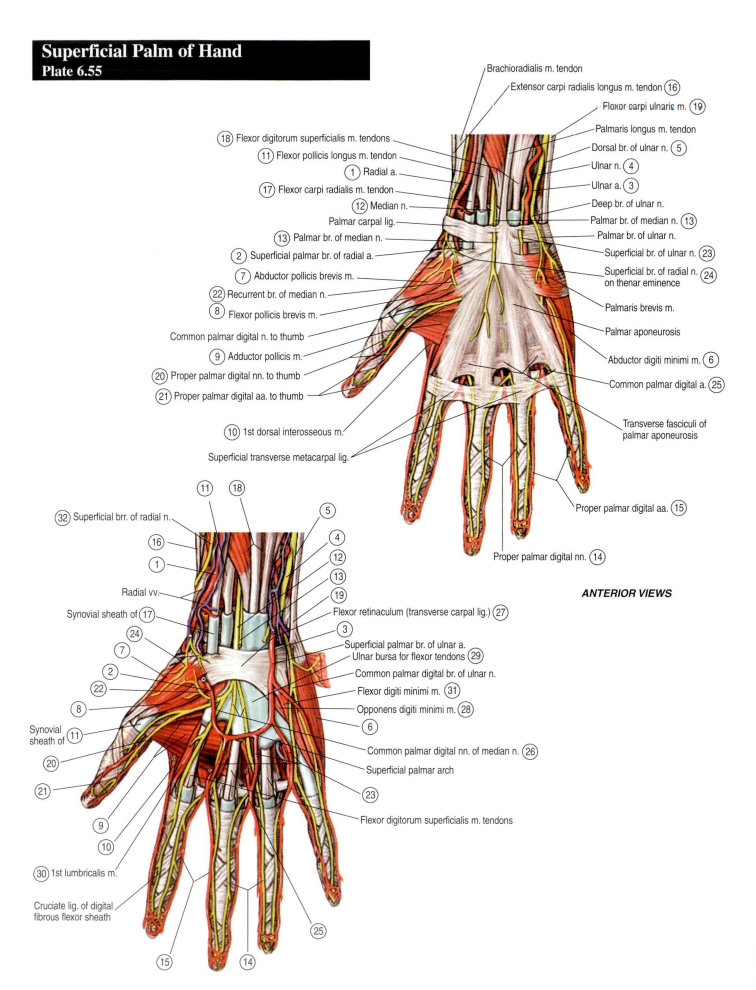

Brachioradialis m. tendon

Extensor carpi radialis longus m. tendon (16)

Flexor carpi ulnaris m. (19)

(18) Flexor digitorum superficialis m. tendons

(11) Flexor pollicis longus m. tendon

(1) Radial a.

(17) Flexor carpi radialis m. tendon

(12) Median n.

Palmar carpal lig.

(13) Palmar br. of median n.

(2) Superficial palmar br. of radial a.

(7) Abductor pollicis brevis m.

(22) Recurrent br. of median n.

(8) Flexor pollicis brevis m.

Common palmar digital n. to thumb

(9) Adductor pollicis m.

(20) Proper palmar digital nn. to thumb

(21) Proper palmar digital aa. to thumb

(10) 1st dorsal interosseous m.

Superficial transverse metacarpal lig.

Palmaris longus m. tendon

Dorsal br. of ulnar n. (5)

Ulnar n. (4)

Ulnar a. (3)

Deep br. of ulnar n.

Palmar br. of median n. (13)

Palmar br. of ulnar n.

Superficial br. of ulnar n. (23)

Superficial br. of radial n. (24) on thenar eminence

Palmaris brevis m.

Palmar aponeurosis

Abductor digiti minimi m. (6)

Common palmar digital a. (25)

Transverse fasciculi of palmar aponeurosis

Proper palmar digital aa. (15)

Proper palmar digital nn. (14)

ANTERIOR VIEWS

(32) Superficial brr. of radial n.

(16)

(1)

Radial vv.

Synovial sheath of (17)

(24)

(7)

(2)

(22)

(8)

Synovial sheath of (11)

(20)

(21)

(9)

(10)

(30) 1st lumbricalis m.

Cruciate lig. of digital fibrous flexor sheath

(11) (18)

(5)

(4)

(12)

(13)

(19)

Flexor retinaculum (transverse carpal lig.) (27)

(3)

Superficial palmar br. of ulnar a.

Ulnar bursa for flexor tendons (29)

Common palmar digital br. of ulnar n.

Flexor digiti minimi m. (31)

Opponens digiti minimi m. (28)

(6)

Common palmar digital nn. of median n. (26)

Superficial palmar arch

(23)

Flexor digitorum superficialis m. tendons

(15) (14)

(25)

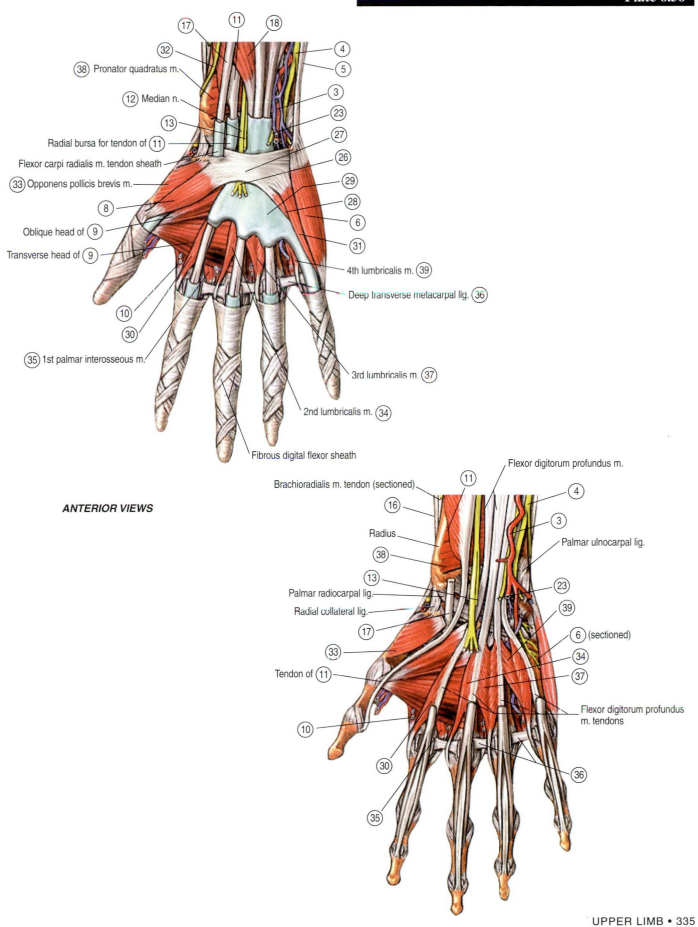

(17) (11) (18)

(32)

(38) Pronator quadratus m.

(12) Median n.

(13)

Radial bursa for tendon of (11)

Flexor carpi radialis m. tendon sheath

(33) Opponens pollicis brevis m.

(8)

Oblique head of (9)

Transverse head of (9)

(10)

(30)

(35) 1st palmar interosseous m.

(4)
(5)
(3)
(23)
(27)
(26)
(29)
(28)
(6)
(31)

4th lumbricalis m. (39)

Deep transverse metacarpal lig. (36)

3rd lumbricalis m. (37)

2nd lumbricalis m. (34)

Fibrous digital flexor sheath

ANTERIOR VIEWS

Brachioradialis m. tendon (sectioned)

(16)

Radius

(38)

(13)

Palmar radiocarpal lig.

Radial collateral lig.

(17)

(33)

Tendon of (11)

(10)

(30)

(35)

Flexor digitorum profundus m.

(11)

(4)

(3)

Palmar ulnocarpal lig.

(23)

(39)

(6) (sectioned)

(34)

(37)

Flexor digitorum profundus m. tendons

(36)

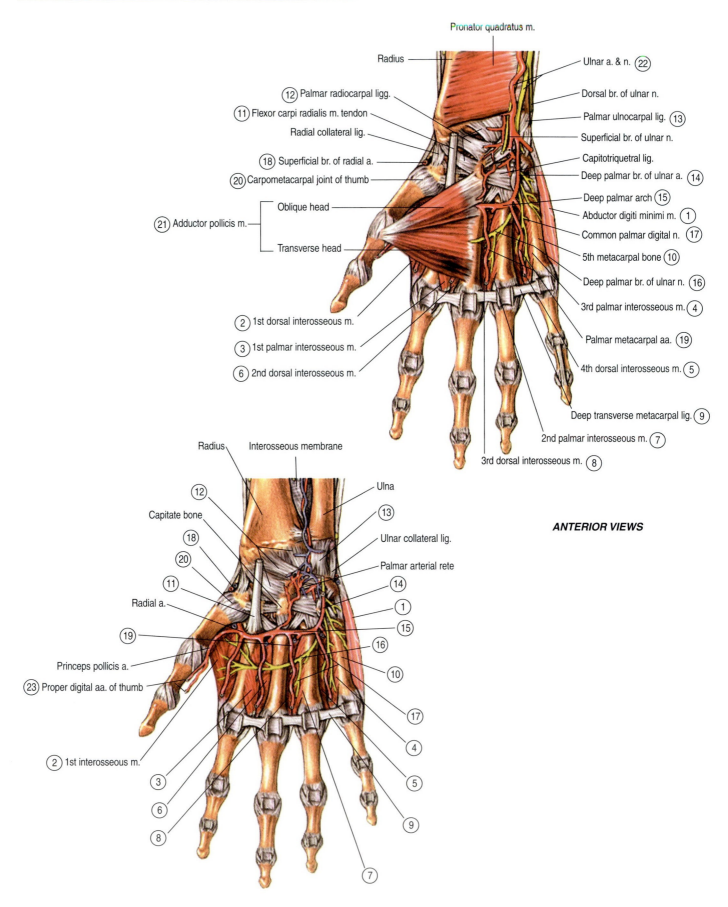

Pronator quadratus m.

Radius

⑫ Palmar radiocarpal ligg.

⑪ Flexor carpi radialis m. tendon

Radial collateral lig.

⑱ Superficial br. of radial a.

⑳ Carpometacarpal joint of thumb

⑪ Adductor pollicis m.

Oblique head

Transverse head

② 1st dorsal interosseous m.

③ 1st palmar interosseous m.

⑥ 2nd dorsal interosseous m.

Ulnar a. & n. ㉒

Dorsal br. of ulnar n.

Palmar ulnocarpal lig. ⑬

Superficial br. of ulnar n.

Capitotriquetral lig.

Deep palmar br. of ulnar a. ⑭

Deep palmar arch ⑮

Abductor digiti minimi m. ①

Common palmar digital n. ⑰

5th metacarpal bone ⑩

Deep palmar br. of ulnar n. ⑯

3rd palmar interosseous m. ④

Palmar metacarpal aa. ⑲

4th dorsal interosseous m. ⑤

Deep transverse metacarpal lig. ⑨

2nd palmar interosseous m. ⑦

3rd dorsal interosseous m. ⑧

ANTERIOR VIEWS

Radius Interosseous membrane

⑫

Capitate bone

⑱

⑳

⑪

Radial a.

⑲

Princeps pollicis a.

㉓ Proper digital aa. of thumb

② 1st interosseous m.

③

⑥

⑧

Ulna

⑬

Ulnar collateral lig.

Palmar arterial rete

⑭

①

⑮

⑯

⑩

⑰

④

⑤

⑨

⑦

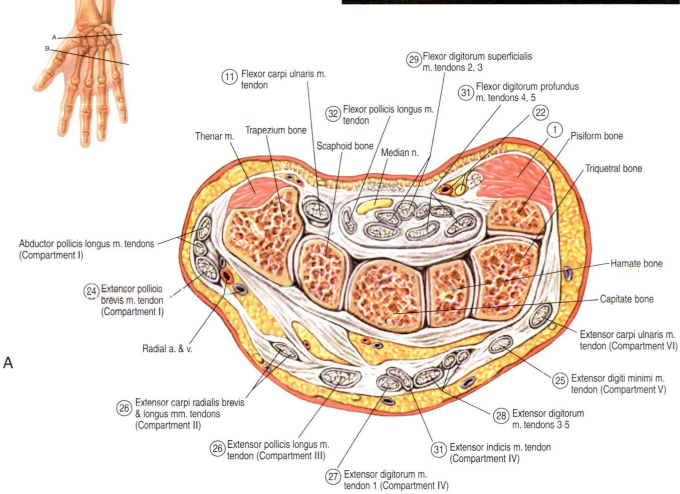

Flexor digitorum superficialis m. tendons 2, 3 — (29)

Flexor digitorum profundus m. tendons 4, 5 — (31)

(11) Flexor carpi ulnaris m. tendon

(32) Flexor pollicis longus m. tendon

(22)

(1)

Thenar m.

Trapezium bone

Scaphoid bone

Median n.

Pisiform bone

Triquetral bone

Abductor pollicis longus m. tendons (Compartment I)

(24) Extensor pollicis brevis m. tendon (Compartment I)

Hamate bone

Capitate bone

Radial a. & v.

Extensor carpi ulnaris m. tendon (Compartment VI)

(26) Extensor carpi radialis brevis & longus mm. tendons (Compartment II)

(25) Extensor digiti minimi m. tendon (Compartment V)

(26) Extensor pollicis longus m. tendon (Compartment III)

(28) Extensor digitorum m. tendons 3-5

(31) Extensor indicis m. tendon (Compartment IV)

(27) Extensor digitorum m. tendon 1 (Compartment IV)

A

◄— RADIAL SIDE

DISTAL VIEW OF SECTIONS THROUGH RIGHT WRIST & HAND

ULNAR SIDE —►

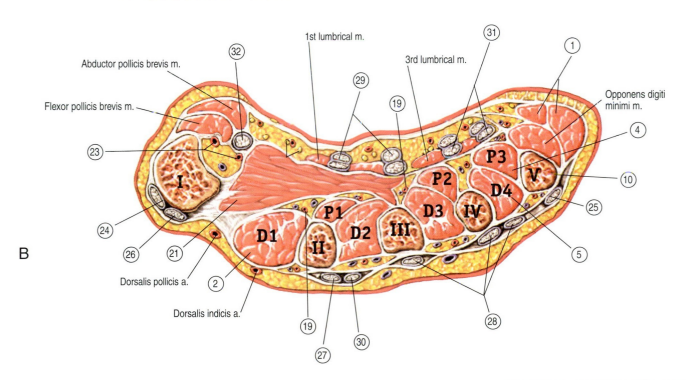

1st lumbrical m.

(31)

(1)

(32)

(29)

3rd lumbrical m.

(19)

Opponens digiti minimi m.

Abductor pollicis brevis m.

Flexor pollicis brevis m.

(4)

(23)

P3

V

(10)

P2

(25)

P1

D4

I

D3

IV

(24)

D1

D2

III

(5)

(26)

II

(21)

(2)

Dorsalis pollicis a.

(28)

Dorsalis indicis a.

(19)

(30)

B

(27)

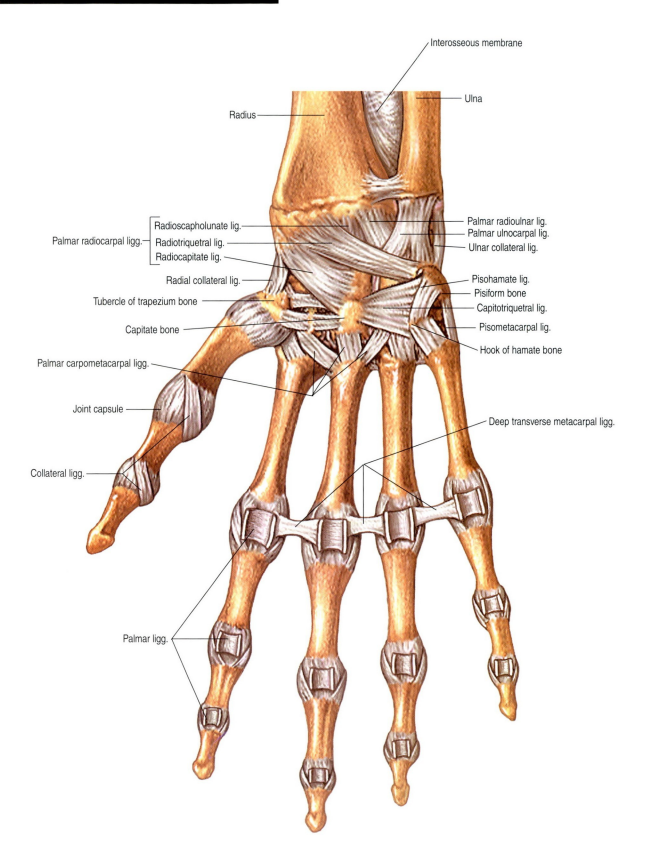

Interosseous membrane

Ulna

Radius

Palmar radioulnar lig.

Palmar radiocarpal ligg.

Radioscapholunate lig.

Radiotriquetral lig.

Radiocapitate lig.

Palmar ulnocarpal lig.

Ulnar collateral lig.

Radial collateral lig.

Pisohamate lig.

Tubercle of trapezium bone

Pisiform bone

Capitate bone

Capitotriquetral lig.

Pisometacarpal lig.

Hook of hamate bone

Palmar carpometacarpal ligg.

Joint capsule

Deep transverse metacarpal ligg.

Collateral ligg.

Palmar ligg.

ANTERIOR VIEW OF PALMAR SURFACE

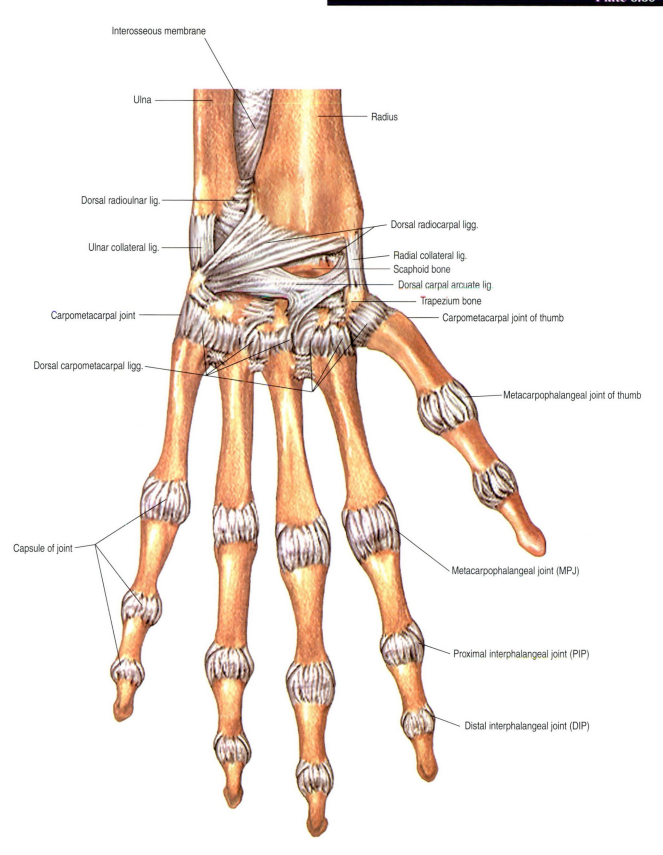

Interosseous membrane

Ulna

Radius

Dorsal radioulnar lig.

Dorsal radiocarpal ligg.

Ulnar collateral lig.

Radial collateral lig.

Scaphoid bone

Dorsal carpal arcuate lig.

Trapezium bone

Carpometacarpal joint

Carpometacarpal joint of thumb

Dorsal carpometacarpal ligg.

Metacarpophalangeal joint of thumb

Capsule of joint

Metacarpophalangeal joint (MPJ)

Proximal interphalangeal joint (PIP)

Distal interphalangeal joint (DIP)

POSTERIOR VIEW OF DORSAL SURFACE

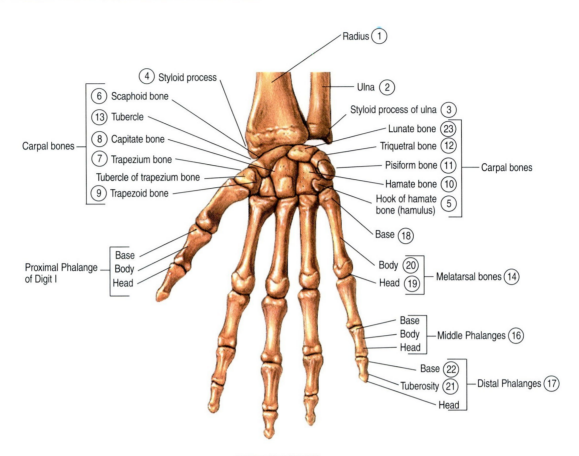

Radius ①
④ Styloid process
⑥ Scaphoid bone
Ulna ②
⑬ Tubercle
Styloid process of ulna ③
⑧ Capitate bone
Lunate bone ㉓
Carpal bones
⑦ Trapezium bone
Triquetral bone ⑫
Tubercle of trapezium bone
Pisiform bone ⑪
Carpal bones
⑨ Trapezoid bone
Hamate bone ⑩
Hook of hamate bone (hamulus) ⑤

Proximal Phalange of Digit I
Base
Body
Head

Base ⑱
Body ⑳
Head ⑲
Melatarsal bones ⑭

Base
Body
Head
Middle Phalanges ⑯

Base ㉒
Tuberosity ㉑
Head
Distal Phalanges ⑰

ANTERIOR VIEW

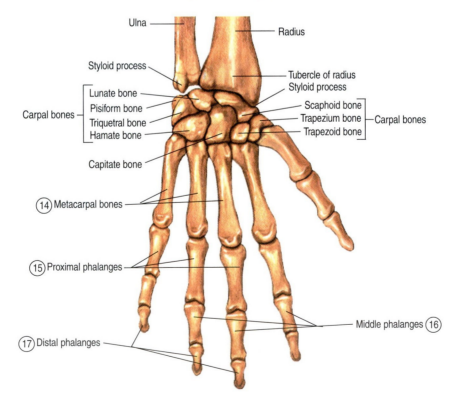

Ulna
Radius
Styloid process
Tubercle of radius
Styloid process
Lunate bone
Pisiform bone
Triquetral bone
Hamate bone
Carpal bones
Scaphoid bone
Trapezium bone
Trapezoid bone
Carpal bones
Capitate bone

⑭ Metacarpal bones

⑮ Proximal phalanges

Middle phalanges ⑯

⑰ Distal phalanges

POSTERIOR VIEW

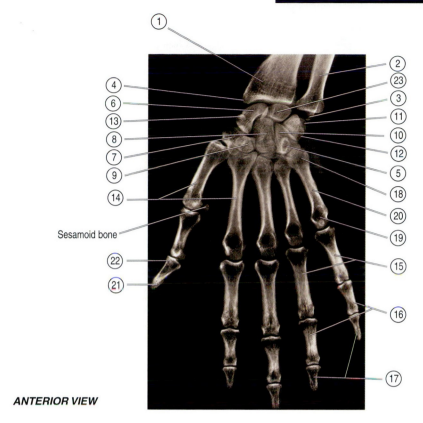

ANTERIOR VIEW

Sesamoid bone

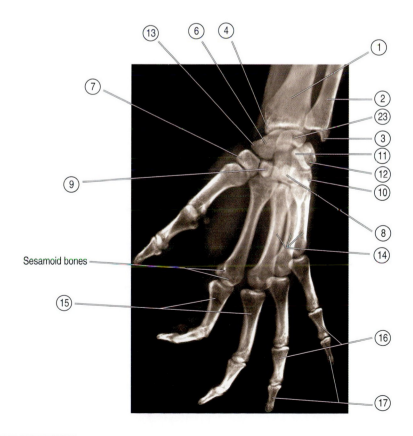

Sesamoid bones

OBLIQUE VIEW

Head and Neck

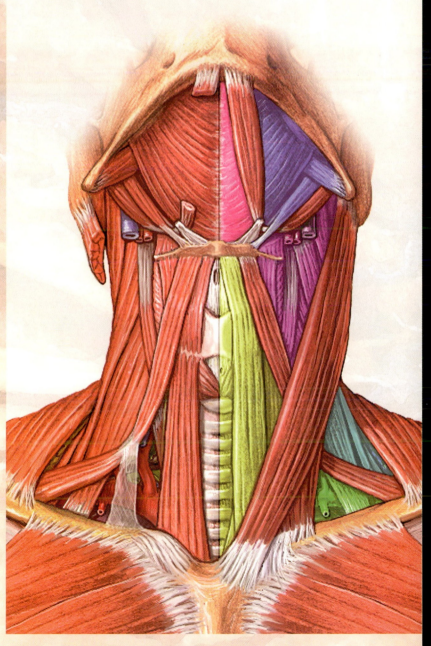

Chapter 7

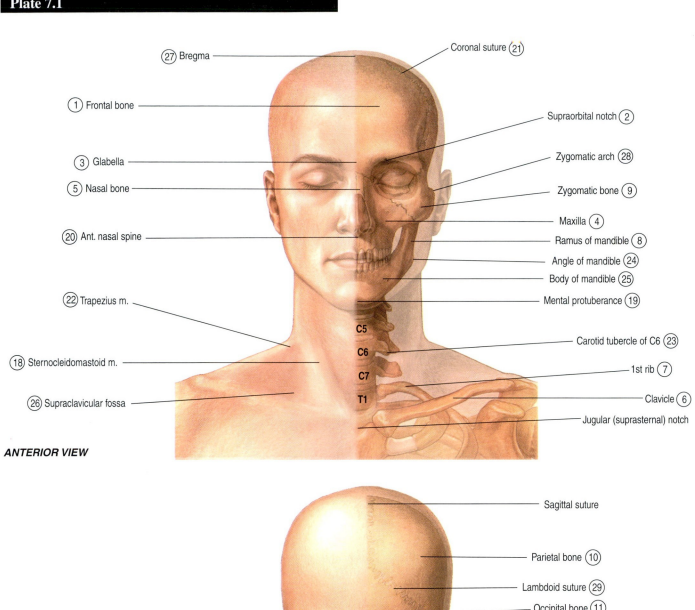

27 Bregma — Coronal suture 21

1 Frontal bone

Supraorbital notch 2

3 Glabella

Zygomatic arch 28

5 Nasal bone

Zygomatic bone 9

Maxilla 4

20 Ant. nasal spine

Ramus of mandible 8

Angle of mandible 24

Body of mandible 25

22 Trapezius m.

Mental protuberance 19

C5

18 Sternocleidomastoid m.

C6

Carotid tubercle of C6 23

C7

1st rib 7

26 Supraclavicular fossa

T1

Clavicle 6

Jugular (suprasternal) notch

ANTERIOR VIEW

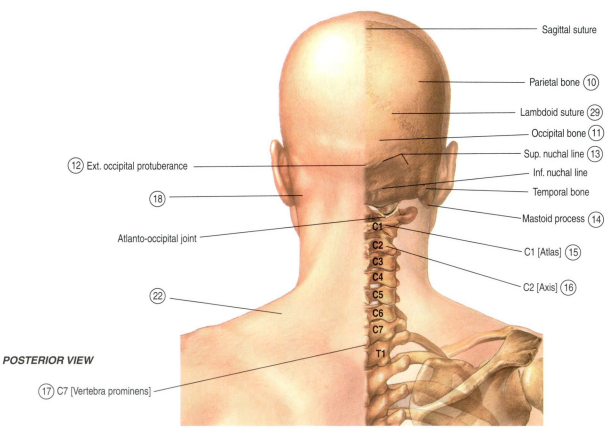

Sagittal suture

Parietal bone 10

Lambdoid suture 29

Occipital bone 11

Sup. nuchal line 13

12 Ext. occipital protuberance

Inf. nuchal line

Temporal bone

18

Mastoid process 14

Atlanto-occipital joint

C1

C1 [Atlas] 15

C2

C3

C4

C2 [Axis] 16

C5

22

C6

C7

T1

POSTERIOR VIEW

17 C7 [Vertebra prominens]

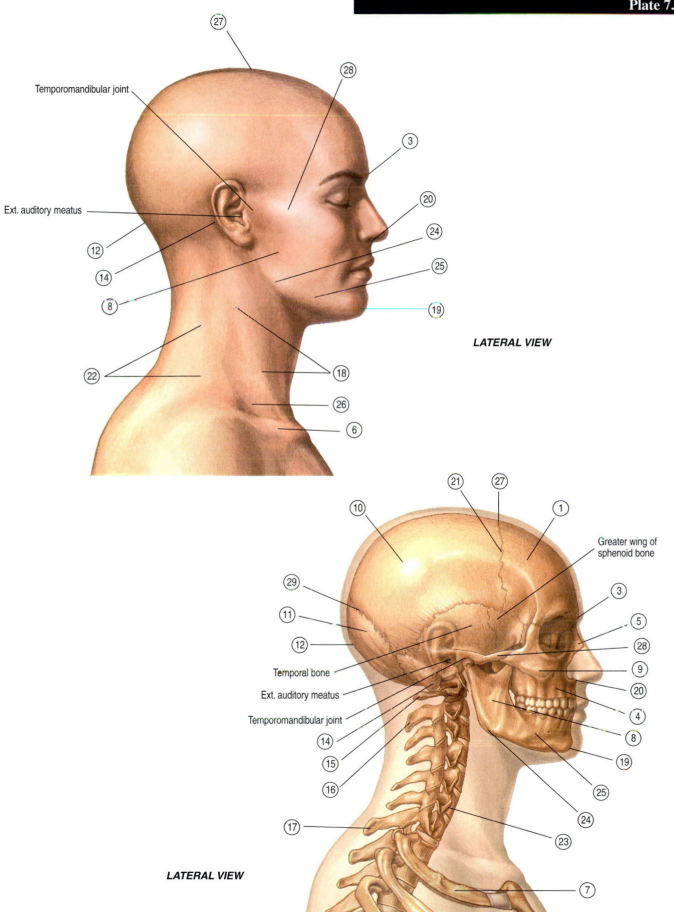

Temporomandibular joint

Ext. auditory meatus

LATERAL VIEW

Greater wing of
sphenoid bone

Temporal bone

Ext. auditory meatus

Temporomandibular joint

LATERAL VIEW

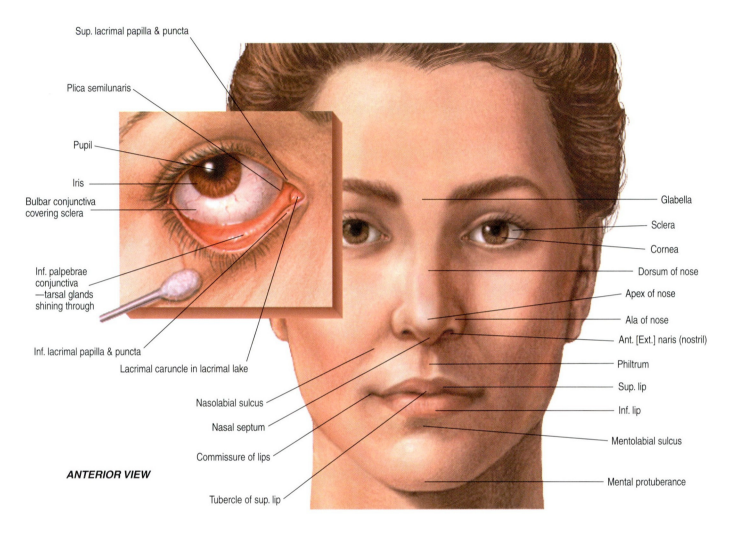

Sup. lacrimal papilla & puncta

Plica semilunaris

Pupil

Iris

Bulbar conjunctiva covering sclera

Inf. palpebrae conjunctiva —tarsal glands shining through

Inf. lacrimal papilla & puncta

Lacrimal caruncle in lacrimal lake

Glabella

Sclera

Cornea

Dorsum of nose

Apex of nose

Ala of nose

Ant. [Ext.] naris (nostril)

Philtrum

Sup. lip

Inf. lip

Mentolabial sulcus

Mental protuberance

Nasolabial sulcus

Nasal septum

Commissure of lips

Tubercle of sup. lip

ANTERIOR VIEW

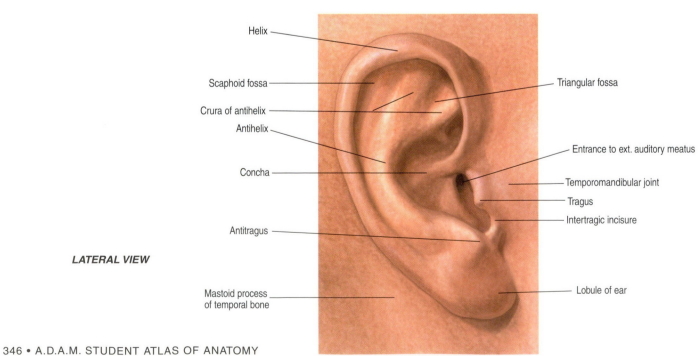

Helix

Scaphoid fossa

Crura of antihelix

Antihelix

Concha

Antitragus

Triangular fossa

Entrance to ext. auditory meatus

Temporomandibular joint

Tragus

Intertragic incisure

Lobule of ear

Mastoid process of temporal bone

LATERAL VIEW

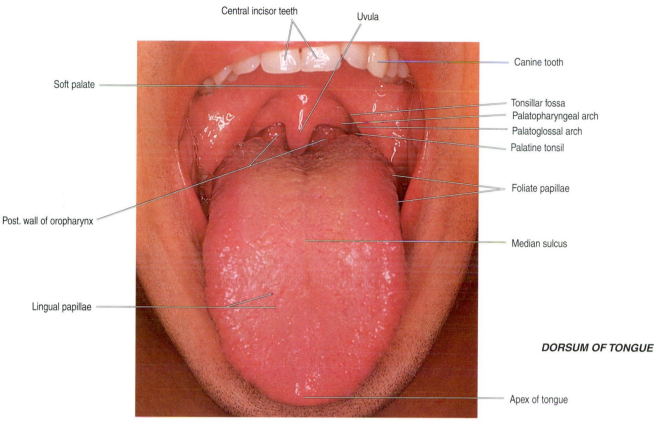

Central incisor teeth

Uvula

Canine tooth

Soft palate

Tonsillar fossa
Palatopharyngeal arch
Palatoglossal arch
Palatine tonsil

Foliate papillae

Post. wall of oropharynx

Median sulcus

Lingual papillae

DORSUM OF TONGUE

Apex of tongue

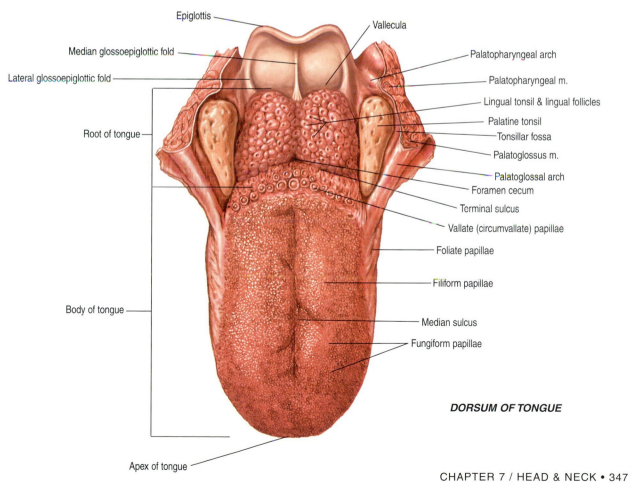

Epiglottis

Vallecula

Median glossoepiglottic fold

Palatopharyngeal arch

Lateral glossoepiglottic fold

Palatopharyngeal m.

Lingual tonsil & lingual follicles

Root of tongue

Palatine tonsil

Tonsillar fossa

Palatoglossus m.

Palatoglossal arch

Foramen cecum

Terminal sulcus

Vallate (circumvallate) papillae

Foliate papillae

Filiform papillae

Body of tongue

Median sulcus

Fungiform papillae

DORSUM OF TONGUE

Apex of tongue

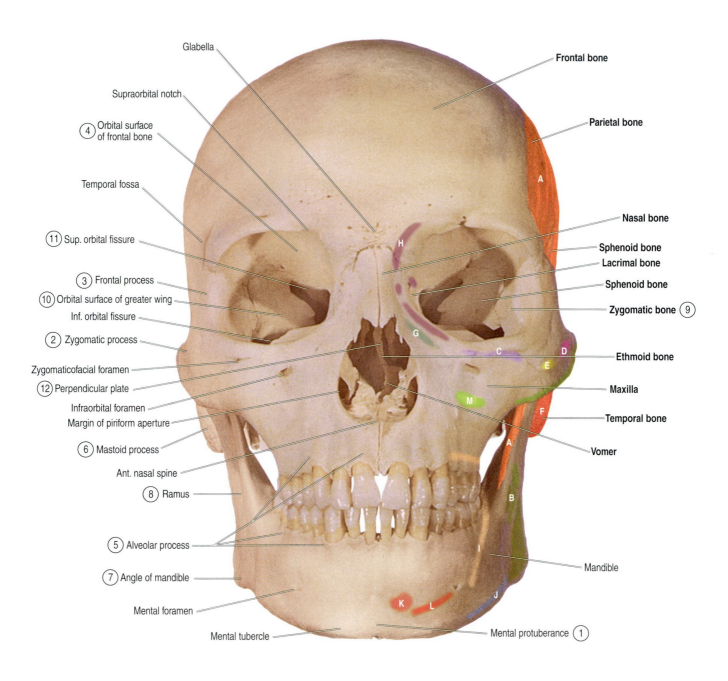

Glabella

Supraorbital notch

④ Orbital surface of frontal bone

Temporal fossa

⑪ Sup. orbital fissure

③ Frontal process

⑩ Orbital surface of greater wing

Inf. orbital fissure

② Zygomatic process

Zygomaticofacial foramen

⑫ Perpendicular plate

Infraorbital foramen

Margin of piriform aperture

⑥ Mastoid process

Ant. nasal spine

⑧ Ramus

⑤ Alveolar process

⑦ Angle of mandible

Mental foramen

Mental tubercle

Frontal bone

Parietal bone

Nasal bone

Sphenoid bone

Lacrimal bone

Sphenoid bone

Zygomatic bone ⑨

Ethmoid bone

Maxilla

Temporal bone

Vomer

Mandible

Mental protuberance ①

ANTERIOR VIEW

Ⓐ Temporalis

Ⓑ Masseter

Ⓒ Levator labii superioris

Ⓓ Zygomaticus major

Ⓔ Zygomaticus minor

Ⓕ Sternocleidomastoid

Ⓖ Levator labii superioris alaeque nasi

Ⓗ Orbicularis oculi

Ⓘ Buccinator

Ⓙ Platysma

Ⓚ Mentalis

Ⓛ Depressor labii inferioris & Depressor anguli oris

Ⓜ Levator anguli oris

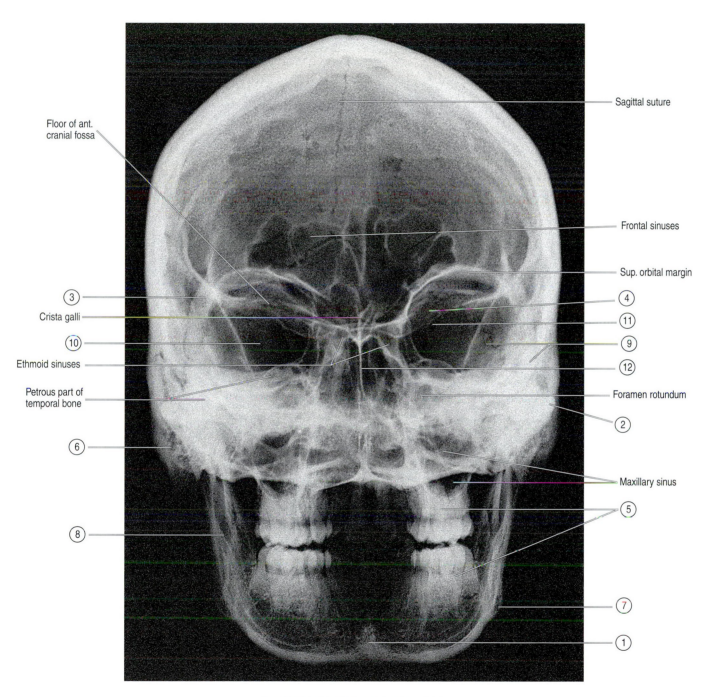

Floor of ant. cranial fossa

Crista galli

Ethmoid sinuses

Petrous part of temporal bone

Sagittal suture

Frontal sinuses

Sup. orbital margin

Foramen rotundum

Maxillary sinus

③ ④ ⑪ ⑩ ⑨ ⑫ ② ⑥ ⑤ ⑧ ⑦ ①

ANTEROPOSTERIOR VIEW OF SKULL

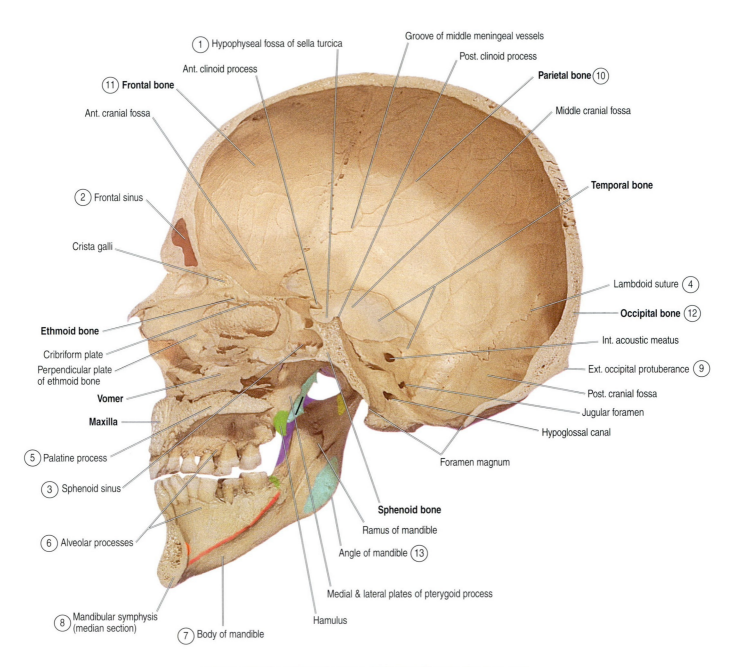

① Hypophyseal fossa of sella turcica

Ant. clinoid process

⑪ **Frontal bone**

Ant. cranial fossa

② Frontal sinus

Crista galli

Ethmoid bone

Cribriform plate

Perpendicular plate of ethmoid bone

Vomer

Maxilla

⑤ Palatine process

③ Sphenoid sinus

⑥ Alveolar processes

⑧ Mandibular symphysis (median section)

⑦ Body of mandible

Hamulus

Medial & lateral plates of pterygoid process

Angle of mandible ⑬

Ramus of mandible

Sphenoid bone

Foramen magnum

Hypoglossal canal

Jugular foramen

Post. cranial fossa

Ext. occipital protuberance ⑨

Int. acoustic meatus

Occipital bone ⑫

Lambdoid suture ④

Temporal bone

Middle cranial fossa

Parietal bone ⑩

Post. clinoid process

Groove of middle meningeal vessels

LEFT LATERAL VIEW OF SKULL SECTIONED IN MEDIAN PLANE

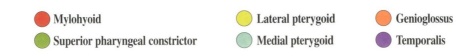

● Mylohyoid

● Superior pharyngeal constrictor

● Lateral pterygoid

● Medial pterygoid

● Genioglossus

● Temporalis

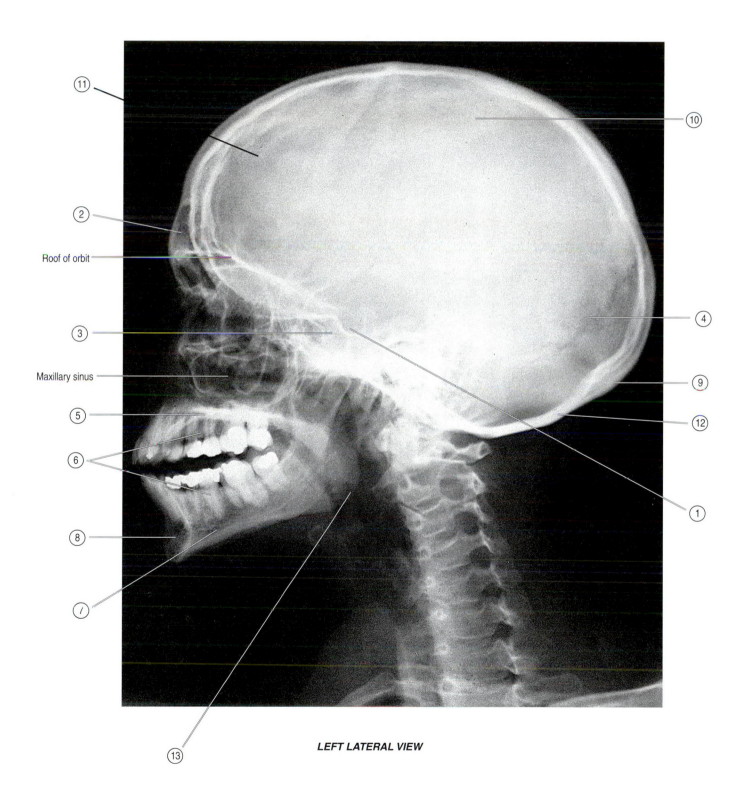

Roof of orbit

Maxillary sinus

LEFT LATERAL VIEW

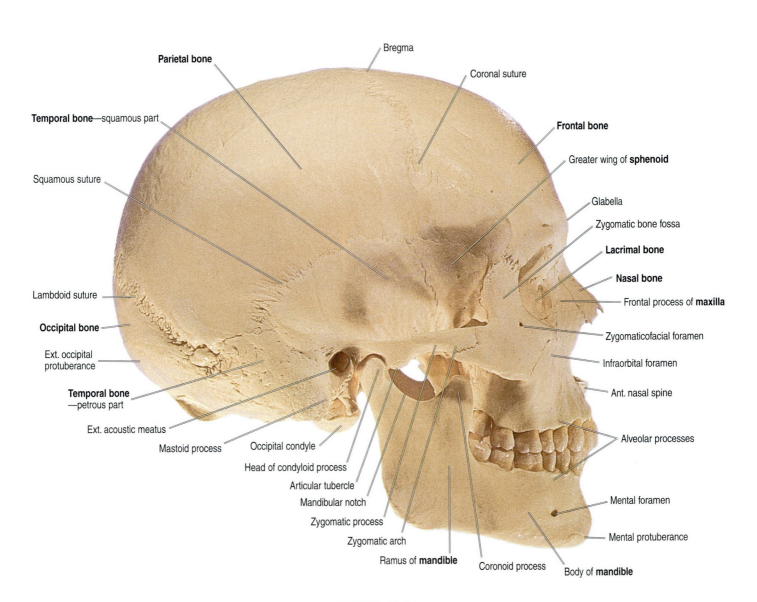

Bregma

Parietal bone

Coronal suture

Temporal bone—squamous part

Frontal bone

Greater wing of sphenoid

Squamous suture

Glabella

Zygomatic bone fossa

Lacrimal bone

Nasal bone

Lambdoid suture

Frontal process of maxilla

Occipital bone

Zygomaticofacial foramen

Ext. occipital protuberance

Infraorbital foramen

Temporal bone —petrous part

Ant. nasal spine

Ext. acoustic meatus

Alveolar processes

Mastoid process

Occipital condyle

Head of condyloid process

Articular tubercle

Mental foramen

Mandibular notch

Zygomatic process

Mental protuberance

Zygomatic arch

Ramus of mandible

Coronoid process

Body of mandible

LATERAL VIEW

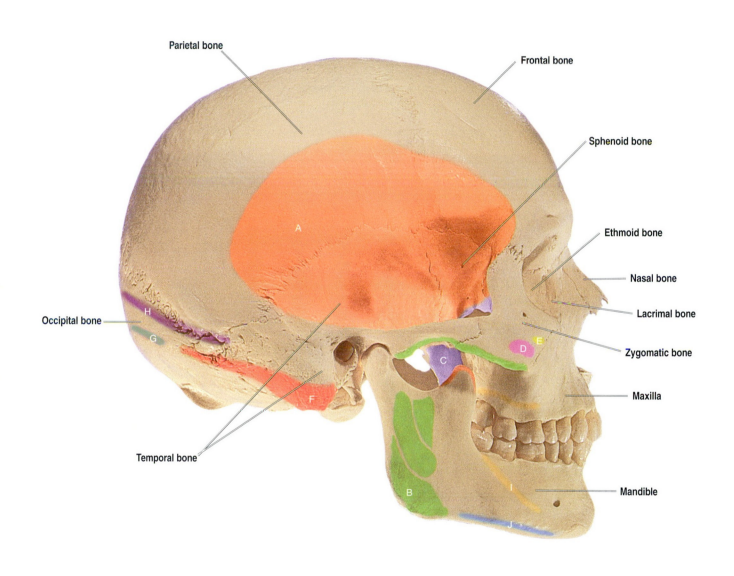

Parietal bone

Frontal bone

Sphenoid bone

Ethmoid bone

Nasal bone

Lacrimal bone

Zygomatic bone

Maxilla

Mandible

Occipital bone

Temporal bone

A **Temporalis**

B **Masseter**

C **Lateral pterygoid**

D **Zygomaticus major**

E **Zygomaticus minor**

F **Sternocleidomastoid**

G **Trapezius**

H **Epicranius-occipital belly**

Buccinator

I **Platysma**

J

Cranial Foramina, Fissures & Canals
Table 7.1

Foramina/Openings	Contents
FACE	
Supraorbital notch/foramen	CN V^1 - supraorbital n. & vessels
Infraorbital notch/foramen	CN V^2 - infraorbital n. & vessels
Mental foramen	CN V^3 - mental n. & vessels
Zygomaticofacial foramen	CN V^2 - zygomaticofacial n. & vessels
ORBIT	
Superior orbital fissure	Passage between middle cranial fossa & orbit for CN III, V, VI, V^1 — lacrimal n., V^1 — frontal n., V^1—nasociliary n., postganglionic sympathetic n. fibers, & ophthalmic v.
Optic canal	CN II, & ophthalmic a.
Inferior orbital fissure	Passage between pterygopalatine fossa & orbit for CN V^2 — infraorbital n. & vessels, & nerves from pterygopalatine ganglion
Anterior ethmoidal foramen	CN V^1— ant. ethmoidal br. of nasociliary n. & vessels
Posterior ethmoidal foramen	CN V^1— post. ethmoidal br. of nasociliary n. & vessels
Nasolacrimal canal	Nasolacrimal duct
NASAL CAVITY	
Piriform aperture (anterior nasal aperture)	Anterior opening into nasal cavity
Incisive canals	CN V^1— nasopalatine n. & greater palatine vessels
Foramina in cribriform plates	CN I — Sensory axons from olfactory epithelium that collectively constitute olfactory nn.
Sphenoethmoidal recess	Duct from sphenoid sinuses
Superior meatus	Duct from post. ethmoid sinuses
Middle meatus	Ducts from frontal sinus, ant. & middle ethmoidl sinuses, & duct from maxillary sinus through semilunar hiatus
Anterior meatus	Nasolacrimal duct
Sphenopalatine foramen	CN V^2 — nasopalatine n. & sphenopalatine vessels
Choana (posterior nasal aperture)	Opening between nasal cavity & nasopharynx
LATERAL CRANIAL SURFACE	
Zygomaticofacial foramen	CN V^2 — zygomaticofacial n. & vessels
Pterygomaxillary fissure	Passage between infratemporal & pterygopalatine fossae for CN V^2 — post. sup. alveolar nn. & vessels, & 3rd part of maxillary a.
External acoustic meatus—bony part	Opening in temporal bone leading to tympanic membrane
Mastoid foramen	Mastoid br. of occipital a. & mastoid emissary v. to sigmoid sinus & diploic vv.
CRANIAL BASE	
Incisive fossa & canals	CN V^1 — nasopalatine n., & greater palatine vessels
Greater palatine foramen/canal	Passage between oral cavity & pterygopalatine fossa for CN V^2 — greater palatine n. & vessels
Lesser palatine foramina	Passages between greater palatine canal & oral cavity for CN V^2 — lesser palatine n. & vessels
Mandibular canal	CN V^3 — inf. alveolar n. & vessels
Foramen lacerum	Closed inferoexternally by fibrocartilage plug
Auditory tube - bony portion	Passage between nasopharynx & middle ear, tensor tympani m., & sup. tympanic a.
Pterygoid (vidian) canal	Passage through base of median pterygoid process between foramen lacerum & pterygopalatine fossa for CN VII — n. & vessels of pterygoid (vidian) canal
Foramen ovale	CN V^3 — mandibular n., CH IX — lesser petrosal n. & accessory meningeal a.
Foramen spinosum	CN V^3 — meningeal br. & middle meningeal vessels
Carotid canal	Internal carotid a. & sympathetic n. plexus
Stylomastoid foramen	CN VII — facial n., & stylomastoid vessels
Petrotympanic fissure	CN VII — chorda tympani n., & ant. tympanic a.
Mastoid canaliculus	CN IX — auricular br.
Tympanic canaliculus	CN IX — tympanic br., & inf. tympanic a.
Jugular fossa & foramen	CN IX, X & XI, sup. bulb of internal jugular v., inferior petrosal & sigmoid sinuses, & meningeal brr. of ascending pharyngeal & occipital aa.
Condylar fossa & canal	*Inconsistent* passage for condylar emissary v. between sigmoid sinus & vertebral venous plexi
Hypoglossal canal	CN XII — hypoglossal n., meningeal br. of ascending pharyngeal a.
Foramen magnum	Medulla & meninges of spinal cord, CN XI — spinal roots, vertebral aa., ant. & post. spinal aa., & brr. ofinternal vertebral venous plexus

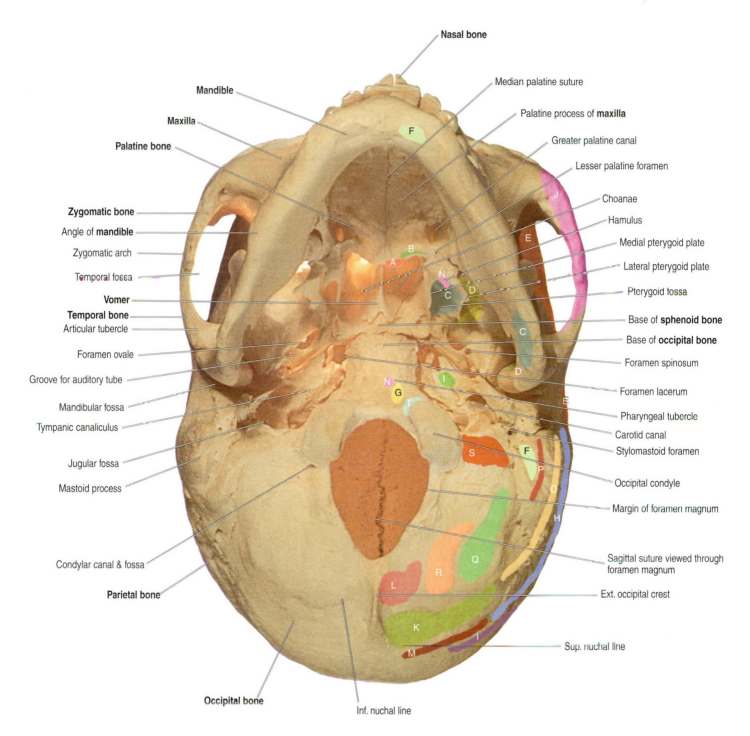

Nasal bone

Median palatine suture

Palatine process of **maxilla**

Greater palatine canal

Lesser palatine foramen

Choanae

Hamulus

Medial pterygoid plate

Lateral pterygoid plate

Pterygoid fossa

Base of **sphenoid bone**

Base of **occipital bone**

Foramen spinosum

Foramen lacerum

Pharyngeal tubercle

Carotid canal

Stylomastoid foramen

Occipital condyle

Margin of foramen magnum

Sagittal suture viewed through foramen magnum

Ext. occipital crest

Sup. nuchal line

Mandible

Maxilla

Palatine bone

Zygomatic bone

Angle of **mandible**

Zygomatic arch

Temporal fossa

Vomer

Temporal bone

Articular tubercle

Foramen ovale

Groove for auditory tube

Mandibular fossa

Tympanic canaliculus

Jugular fossa

Mastoid process

Condylar canal & fossa

Parietal bone

Occipital bone

Inf. nuchal line

INFERIOR VIEW OF CRANIAL BASE

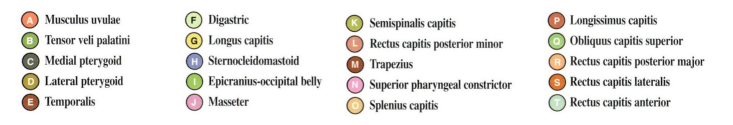

- **A** Musculus uvulae
- **B** Tensor veli palatini
- **C** Medial pterygoid
- **D** Lateral pterygoid
- **E** Temporalis
- **F** Digastric
- **G** Longus capitis
- **H** Sternocleidomastoid
- **I** Epicranius-occipital belly
- **J** Masseter
- **K** Semispinalis capitis
- **L** Rectus capitis posterior minor
- **M** Trapezius
- **N** Superior pharyngeal constrictor
- **O** Splenius capitis
- **P** Longissimus capitis
- **Q** Obliquus capitis superior
- **R** Rectus capitis posterior major
- **S** Rectus capitis lateralis
- **T** Rectus capitis anterior

Internal Neurocranial Foramina, Fissures & Canals
Table 7.2

Foramina/Openings	Contents
ANTERIOR CRANIAL FOSSA	
Foramen cecum	Inconsistent passage for nasal emissary vv. tributaries of superior sagittal sinus
Foramina in cribriform plates	CN I — Sensory axons from olfactory epithelium that collectively constitute the olfactory nn.
Anterior ethmoidal foramen	CN V^1 — anterior ethmoidal br. of nasociliary n. & vessels
Posterior ethmoidal foramen	CN V^1 — posterior ethmoidal br. of nasociliary n. & vessels
MIDDLE CRANIAL FOSSA	
Optic canal	CN II, & ophthalmic a.
Superior orbital fissure	Passage between middle cranial fossa & orbit for CN III, IV, VI, V1 — lacrimal n., V1 — frontal n., V^1 — nasociliary n., postganglionic sympathetic n. fibers, & ophthalmic v.
Foramen rotundum	CN V^2 — maxillary n.
Foramen ovale	CN V^3 — mandibular n., CH IX - lesser petrosal n. & accessory meningeal a.
Foramen spinosum	CN V^3 — meningeal br. & middle meningeal vessels
Foramen lacerum	Internal carotid a., sympathetic nn. & venous plexi from carotid canal, & CN VII — greater petrosal n.. Closed inferoexternally by fibrocartilage plug
Hiatus for greater petrosal n. (Facial hiatus)	CN VII — greater petrosal n., & petrosal br. of middle meningeal a.
Hiatus for lesser petrosal n.	CN IX — lesser petrosal n.
POSTERIOR CRANIAL FOSSA	
Internal acoustic meatus	CN VII & VIII, labyrinthine a.
Jugular fossa & foramen	CN IX, X & XI, superior bulb of internal jugular v., inferior petrosal & sigmoid sinuses, & meningeal brr. of ascendingpharyngeal & occipital aa.
Condylar fossa & canal	*Inconsistent* passage for condylar emissary v. between sigmoid sinus & vertebral venous plexi
Mastoid foramen	Mastoid br. of occipital a. & mastoid emissary v. to sigmoid sinus & diploic vv.
Hypoglossal canal	CN XII — hypoglossal n.
Foramen magnum	Medulla & meninges of spinal cord, CN XI— spinal roots, vertebral aa., ant. & post. spinal aa., & brr. of internal vertebral venous plexus

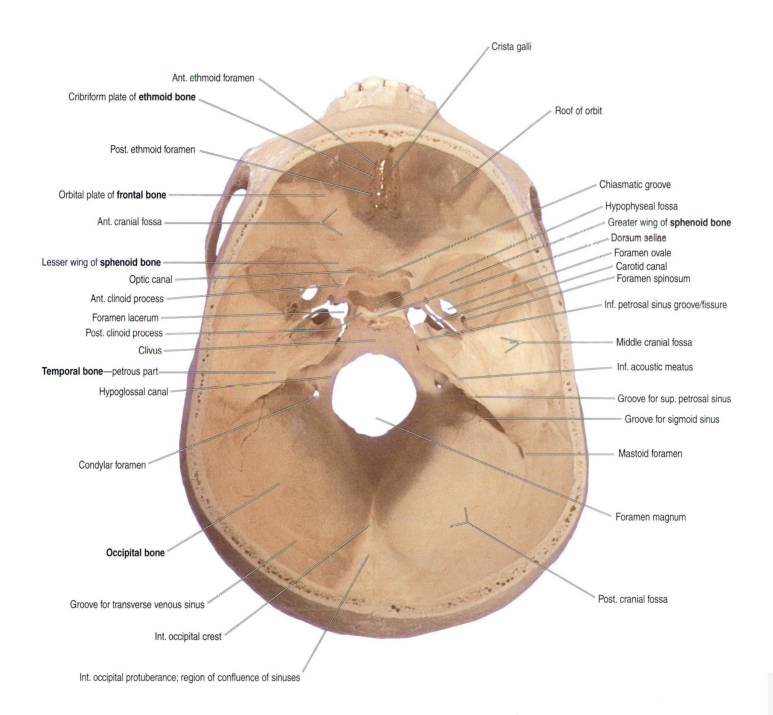

Crista galli

Ant. ethmoid foramen

Cribriform plate of **ethmoid bone**

Roof of orbit

Post. ethmoid foramen

Orbital plate of **frontal bone**

Chiasmatic groove

Ant. cranial fossa

Hypophyseal fossa

Greater wing of **sphenoid bone**

Lesser wing of **sphenoid bone**

Dorsum sellae

Optic canal

Foramen ovale

Ant. clinoid process

Carotid canal

Foramen spinosum

Foramen lacerum

Inf. petrosal sinus groove/fissure

Post. clinoid process

Clivus

Middle cranial fossa

Temporal bone—petrous part

Inf. acoustic meatus

Hypoglossal canal

Groove for sup. petrosal sinus

Groove for sigmoid sinus

Condylar foramen

Mastoid foramen

Foramen magnum

Occipital bone

Post. cranial fossa

Groove for transverse venous sinus

Int. occipital crest

Int. occipital protuberance; region of confluence of sinuses

SUPERIOR VIEW WITH CALVARIA REMOVED

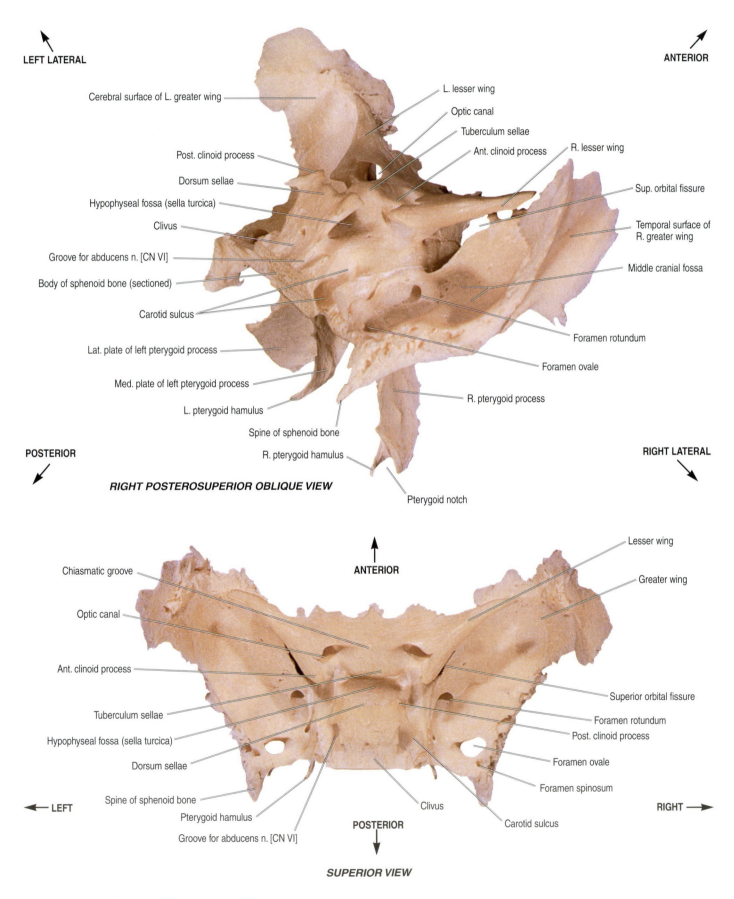

LEFT LATERAL

ANTERIOR

Cerebral surface of L. greater wing

L. lesser wing

Optic canal

Tuberculum sellae

Ant. clinoid process

R. lesser wing

Post. clinoid process

Dorsum sellae

Sup. orbital fissure

Hypophyseal fossa (sella turcica)

Temporal surface of R. greater wing

Clivus

Groove for abducens n. [CN VI]

Middle cranial fossa

Body of sphenoid bone (sectioned)

Carotid sulcus

Lat. plate of left pterygoid process

Foramen rotundum

Med. plate of left pterygoid process

Foramen ovale

L. pterygoid hamulus

R. pterygoid process

Spine of sphenoid bone

POSTERIOR

R. pterygoid hamulus

RIGHT LATERAL

Pterygoid notch

RIGHT POSTEROSUPERIOR OBLIQUE VIEW

ANTERIOR

Lesser wing

Chiasmatic groove

Greater wing

Optic canal

Ant. clinoid process

Superior orbital fissure

Tuberculum sellae

Foramen rotundum

Hypophyseal fossa (sella turcica)

Post. clinoid process

Dorsum sellae

Foramen ovale

Spine of sphenoid bone

Foramen spinosum

LEFT

Pterygoid hamulus

Clivus

RIGHT

Groove for abducens n. [CN VI]

Carotid sulcus

POSTERIOR

SUPERIOR VIEW

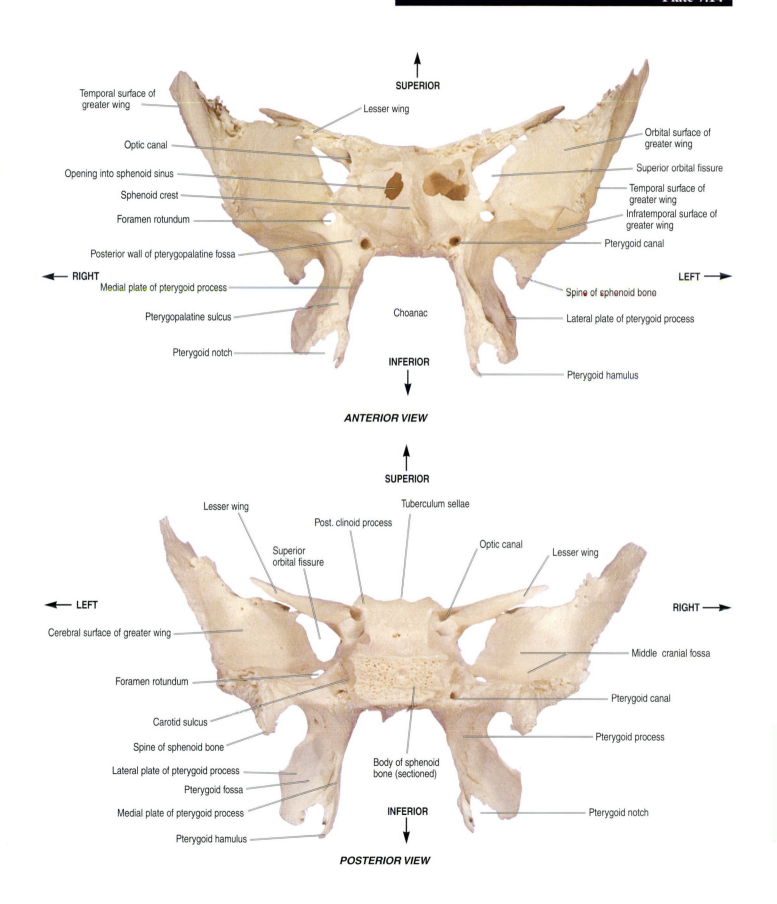

ANTERIOR VIEW

- Temporal surface of greater wing
- Optic canal
- Opening into sphenoid sinus
- Sphenoid crest
- Foramen rotundum
- Posterior wall of pterygopalatine fossa
- Medial plate of pterygoid process
- Pterygopalatine sulcus
- Pterygoid notch

SUPERIOR

Lesser wing

- Orbital surface of greater wing
- Superior orbital fissure
- Temporal surface of greater wing
- Infratemporal surface of greater wing
- Pterygoid canal
- Spine of sphenoid bone
- Lateral plate of pterygoid process
- Pterygoid hamulus

RIGHT

LEFT

Choanac

INFERIOR

POSTERIOR VIEW

SUPERIOR

- Lesser wing
- Superior orbital fissure
- Post. clinoid process
- Tuberculum sellae
- Optic canal
- Lesser wing

LEFT

RIGHT

- Cerebral surface of greater wing
- Foramen rotundum
- Carotid sulcus
- Spine of sphenoid bone
- Lateral plate of pterygoid process
- Pterygoid fossa
- Medial plate of pterygoid process
- Pterygoid hamulus

- Middle cranial fossa
- Pterygoid canal
- Pterygoid process
- Body of sphenoid bone (sectioned)
- Pterygoid notch

INFERIOR

Orbital plate of frontal bone

Zygomatic process of frontal bone

Lesser wing of sphenoid bone

Sup. orbital fissure

Optic canal

Orbital surface of zygomatic bone

Orbital process of palatine bone

Orbital surface of greater wing of sphenoid bone

Inf. orbital fissure

Supraorbital foramen

Post. & ant. ethmoidal foramen

Nasal bone

Orbital plate of ethmoid bone

Lacrimal bone

Fossa for lacrimal sac

Frontal process of maxilla

Infraorbital groove

Maxilla

Infraorbital foramen

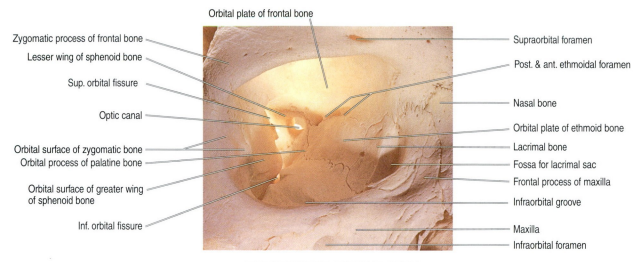

ANTERIOR VIEW OF RIGHT ORBIT

Frontal bone

Sup. orbital fissure

Maxilla

Inf. orbital fissure

Zygomatic bone

Infraorbital foramen

Inf. nasal concha

Mastoid process

Medial incisor teeth

Orbital plate of frontal bone

Nasal bones

Orbital surface of greater wing of sphenoid bone

Middle nasal concha

Perpendicular plate of ethmoid bone — Nasal septum

Vomer

Canine tooth

Lateral incisor tooth

ANTERIOR VIEW

Crista galli

Nasal bone

Sup. concha

Sphenopalatine foramen

Middle concha

Middle meatus

Maxilla

Inf. concha

Inf. meatus

Ant. nasal spine

Palatine process of maxilla

Incisive canal

Cribriform plate of ethmoid bone

Sphenoethmoidal recess

Hypophyseal fossa

Sphenoid sinus

Body of sphenoid bone (sectioned)

Sup. meatus

Perpendicular plate of palatine bone

Lateral pterygoid plate

Medial pterygoid plate

Horizontal plate of palatine bone

Pterygoid hamulus

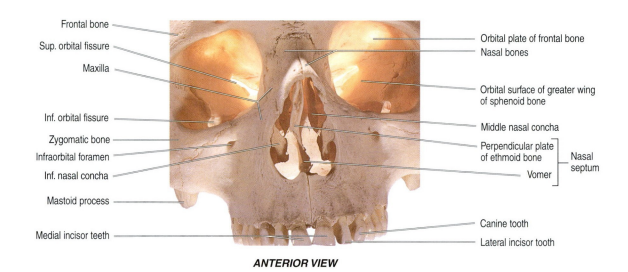

MEDIAL VIEW OF RIGHT NASAL CAVITY

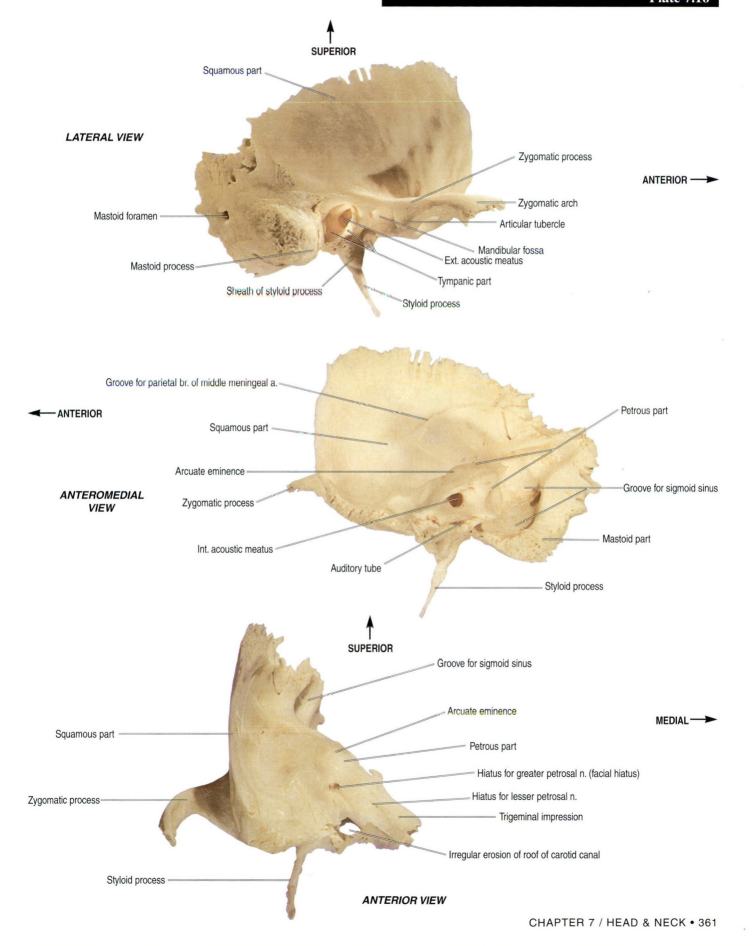

SUPERIOR

Squamous part

LATERAL VIEW

ANTERIOR →

Zygomatic process

Zygomatic arch

Articular tubercle

Mastoid foramen

Mandibular fossa

Ext. acoustic meatus

Mastoid process

Tympanic part

Sheath of styloid process

Styloid process

Groove for parietal br. of middle meningeal a.

← ANTERIOR

Petrous part

Squamous part

**ANTEROMEDIAL
VIEW**

Arcuate eminence

Groove for sigmoid sinus

Zygomatic process

Int. acoustic meatus

Mastoid part

Auditory tube

Styloid process

SUPERIOR

Groove for sigmoid sinus

Arcuate eminence

MEDIAL →

Squamous part

Petrous part

Hiatus for greater petrosal n. (facial hiatus)

Zygomatic process

Hiatus for lesser petrosal n.

Trigeminal impression

Irregular erosion of roof of carotid canal

Styloid process

ANTERIOR VIEW

ANTERIOR

RIGHT SIDE   **LEFT SIDE**

OBLIQUE BASAL VIEW OF CHOANAE

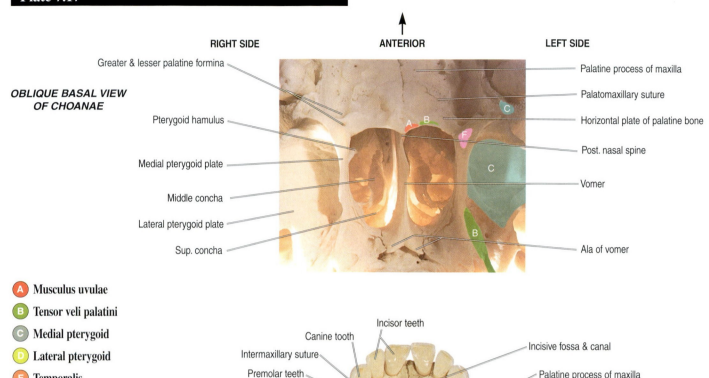

Greater & lesser palatine formina

Pterygoid hamulus

Medial pterygoid plate

Middle concha

Lateral pterygoid plate

Sup. concha

Palatine process of maxilla

Palatomaxillary suture

Horizontal plate of palatine bone

Post. nasal spine

Vomer

Ala of vomer

- **A** Musculus uvulae
- **B** Tensor veli palatini
- **C** Medial pterygoid
- **D** Lateral pterygoid
- **E** Temporalis
- **F** Superior pharyngeal constrictor
- **G** Tensor tympani
- **H** Levator veli palatini

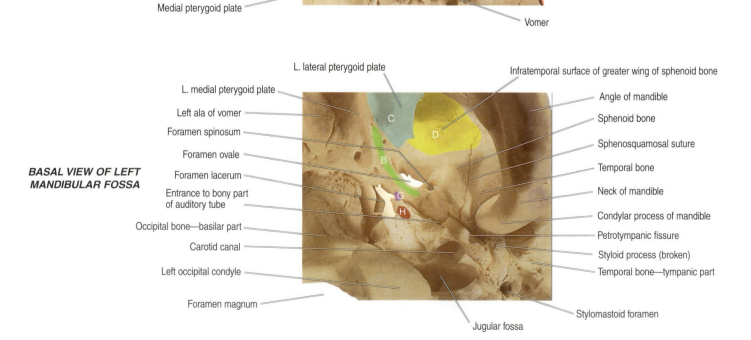

Incisor teeth

Canine tooth

Intermaxillary suture

Premolar teeth

Palatomaxillary suture

Molar teeth

Greater & lesser palatine foramina

Pterygoid hamulus

Lateral pterygoid plate

Medial pterygoid plate

Incisive fossa & canal

Palatine process of maxilla

BASAL VIEW

Zygomatic process of maxilla

Horizontal plate of palatine bone

Post. nasal spine

Choanae

Sphenoid bone

Vomer

BASAL VIEW OF LEFT MANDIBULAR FOSSA

L. lateral pterygoid plate

L. medial pterygoid plate

Left ala of vomer

Foramen spinosum

Foramen ovale

Foramen lacerum

Entrance to bony part of auditory tube

Occipital bone—basilar part

Carotid canal

Left occipital condyle

Foramen magnum

Infratemporal surface of greater wing of sphenoid bone

Angle of mandible

Sphenoid bone

Sphenosquamosal suture

Temporal bone

Neck of mandible

Condylar process of mandible

Petrotympanic fissure

Styloid process (broken)

Temporal bone—tympanic part

Stylomastoid foramen

Jugular fossa

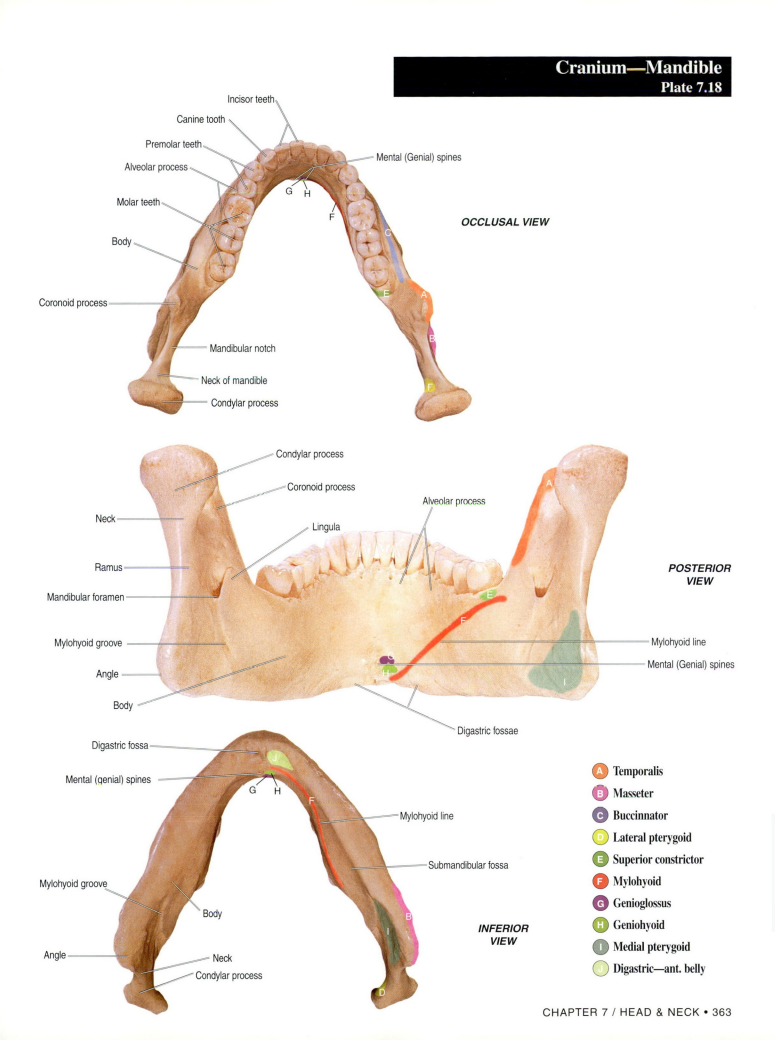

Incisor teeth

Canine tooth

Premolar teeth

Alveolar process

Mental (Genial) spines

Molar teeth

G H

F

OCCLUSAL VIEW

C

Body

E

A

Coronoid process

B

Mandibular notch

Neck of mandible

Condylar process

F

Condylar process

Coronoid process

Alveolar process

Neck

A

Lingula

Ramus

POSTERIOR
VIEW

Mandibular foramen

E

Mylohyoid line

F

Mylohyoid groove

Mylohyoid line

Angle

H

Mental (Genial) spines

I

Body

Digastric fossae

Digastric fossa

J

Mental (genial) spines

G H

F

Mylohyoid groove

Mylohyoid line

Submandibular fossa

Body

B

Mylohyoid groove

I

Angle

INFERIOR
VIEW

Neck

Condylar process

D

A Temporalis

B Masseter

C Buccinnator

D Lateral pterygoid

E Superior constrictor

F Mylohyoid

G Genioglossus

H Geniohyoid

I Medial pterygoid

J Digastric—ant. belly

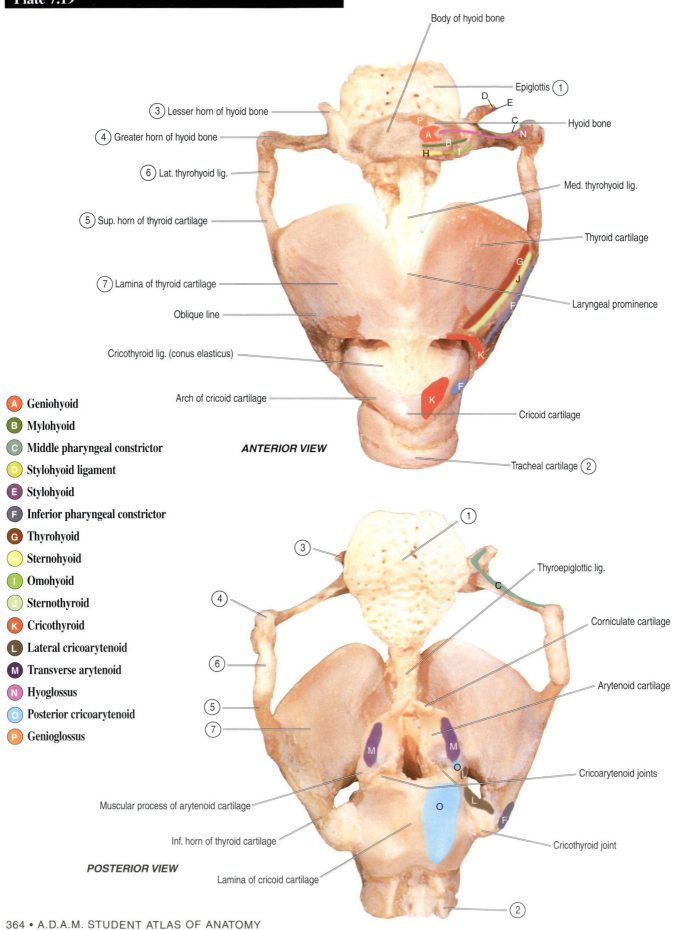

Body of hyoid bone

Epiglottis ①

D
E

③ Lesser horn of hyoid bone

Hyoid bone

④ Greater horn of hyoid bone

⑥ Lat. thyrohyoid lig.

Med. thyrohyoid lig.

⑤ Sup. horn of thyroid cartilage

Thyroid cartilage

⑦ Lamina of thyroid cartilage

Laryngeal prominence

Oblique line

Cricothyroid lig. (conus elasticus)

Arch of cricoid cartilage

Cricoid cartilage

ANTERIOR VIEW

Tracheal cartilage ②

Ⓐ **Geniohyoid**

Ⓑ **Mylohyoid**

Ⓒ **Middle pharyngeal constrictor**

Ⓓ **Stylohyoid ligament**

Ⓔ **Stylohyoid**

Ⓕ **Inferior pharyngeal constrictor**

Ⓖ **Thyrohyoid**

Ⓗ **Sternohyoid**

Ⓘ **Omohyoid**

Ⓙ **Sternothyroid**

Ⓚ **Cricothyroid**

Ⓛ **Lateral cricoarytenoid**

Ⓜ **Transverse arytenoid**

Ⓝ **Hyoglossus**

Ⓞ **Posterior cricoarytenoid**

Ⓟ **Genioglossus**

Thyroepiglottic lig.

Corniculate cartilage

Arytenoid cartilage

Cricoarytenoid joints

Muscular process of arytenoid cartilage

Cricothyroid joint

Inf. horn of thyroid cartilage

POSTERIOR VIEW

Lamina of cricoid cartilage

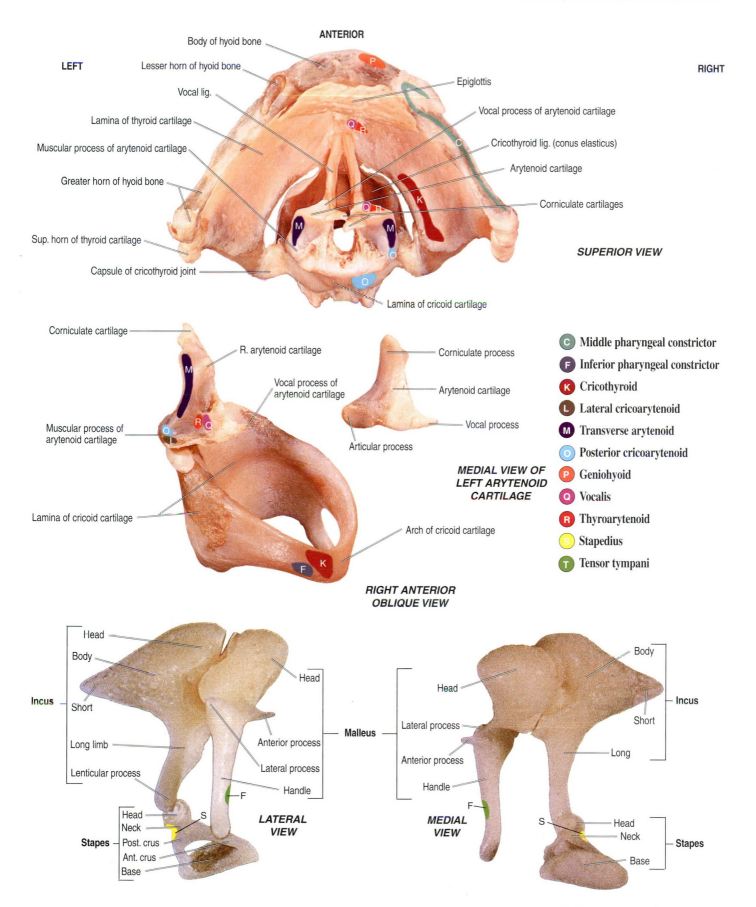

ANTERIOR

LEFT

RIGHT

Body of hyoid bone

Lesser horn of hyoid bone

Vocal lig.

Lamina of thyroid cartilage

Muscular process of arytenoid cartilage

Greater horn of hyoid bone

Sup. horn of thyroid cartilage

Capsule of cricothyroid joint

Epiglottis

Vocal process of arytenoid cartilage

Cricothyroid lig. (conus elasticus)

Arytenoid cartilage

Corniculate cartilages

SUPERIOR VIEW

Lamina of cricoid cartilage

Corniculate cartilage

R. arytenoid cartilage

Corniculate process

Arytenoid cartilage

Vocal process of arytenoid cartilage

Vocal process

Muscular process of arytenoid cartilage

Articular process

Lamina of cricoid cartilage

Arch of cricoid cartilage

MEDIAL VIEW OF LEFT ARYTENOID CARTILAGE

RIGHT ANTERIOR OBLIQUE VIEW

C Middle pharyngeal constrictor
F Inferior pharyngeal constrictor
K Cricothyroid
L Lateral cricoarytenoid
M Transverse arytenoid
O Posterior cricoarytenoid
P Geniohyoid
Q Vocalis
R Thyroarytenoid
S Stapedius
T Tensor tympani

Head

Body

Incus

Short

Long limb

Lenticular process

Head

Body

Head

Anterior process

Lateral process

Handle

F

Malleus

Stapes — Head
Neck
Post. crus
Ant. crus
Base

S

LATERAL VIEW

Body

Head

Lateral process

Anterior process

Handle

F

Incus

Short

Long

Malleus

MEDIAL VIEW

S

Head

Neck

Base

Stapes

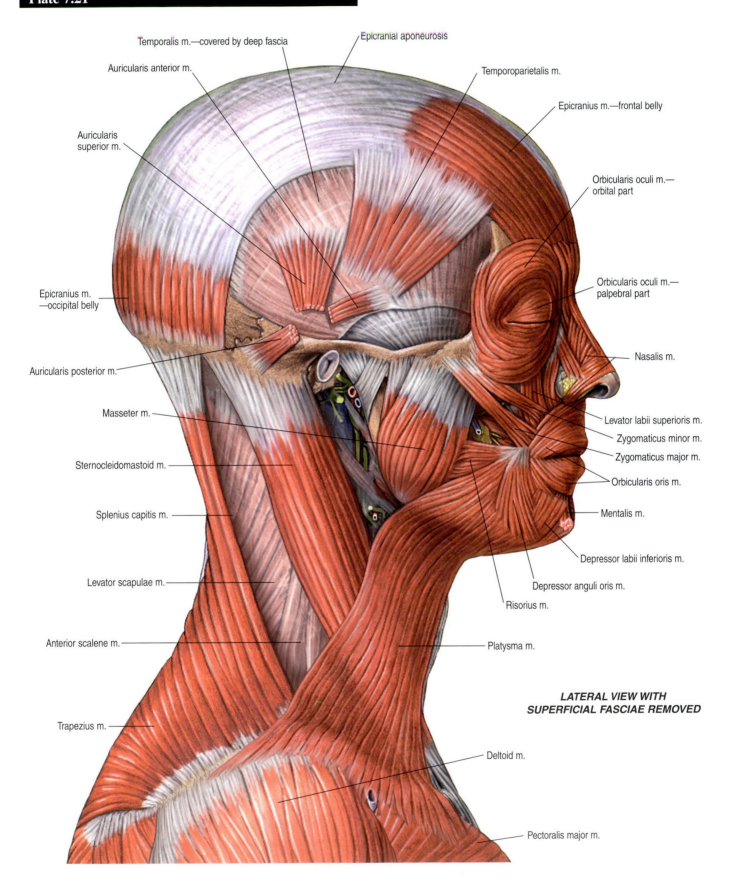

Temporalis m.—covered by deep fascia

Epicranial aponeurosis

Auricularis anterior m.

Temporoparietalis m.

Auricularis superior m.

Epicranius m.—frontal belly

Orbicularis oculi m.—orbital part

Epicranius m.—occipital belly

Orbicularis oculi m.—palpebral part

Auricularis posterior m.

Nasalis m.

Masseter m.

Levator labii superioris m.

Zygomaticus minor m.

Sternocleidomastoid m.

Zygomaticus major m.

Orbicularis oris m.

Splenius capitis m.

Mentalis m.

Levator scapulae m.

Depressor labii inferioris m.

Anterior scalene m.

Depressor anguli oris m.

Risorius m.

Platysma m.

Trapezius m.

LATERAL VIEW WITH SUPERFICIAL FASCIAE REMOVED

Deltoid m.

Pectoralis major m.

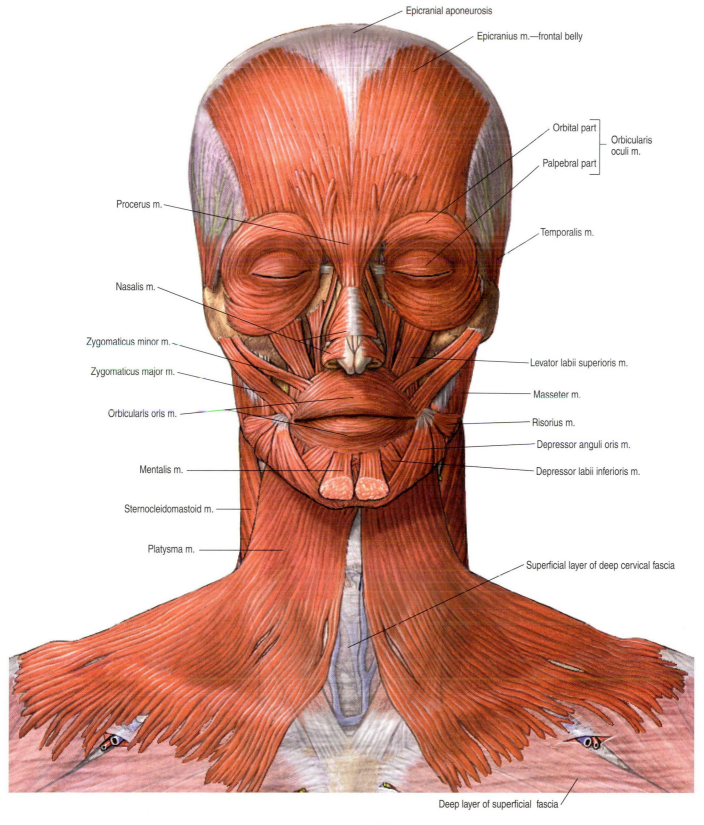

Epicranial aponeurosis

Epicranius m.—frontal belly

Orbital part ⎤
⎥ Orbicularis
Palpebral part ⎦ oculi m.

Procerus m.

Temporalis m.

Nasalis m.

Zygomaticus minor m.

Levator labii superioris m.

Zygomaticus major m.

Masseter m.

Orbicularis oris m.

Risorius m.

Depressor anguli oris m.

Mentalis m.

Depressor labii inferioris m.

Sternocleidomastoid m.

Platysma m.

Superficial layer of deep cervical fascia

Deep layer of superficial fascia

ANTERIOR VIEW

Muscles Acting on the Temporomandibular Joint

Muscle	Stable Attachment	Mobile Attachment	Innervation	Main Actions
Temporalis	Floor of temporal fossa & deep surface of temporal fascia	Tip & medial surface of coronoid process & ant. border of ramus of mandible	Deep temporal br. of mandibular n. (CN V^3)	Elevates mandible, closing jaws; its posterior fibers retrude mandible after protrusion
Masseter	Inf. border & medial surface of zygomatic arch	Lateral surface of ramus of mandible & its coronoid process	Mandibular n. (CN V^3) via masseteric nerve that enters its deep surface	Elevates & protrudes mandible, thus closing jaws;
Lateral pterygoid	*Superior head:* Infratemporal surface & infratemporal crest of greater wing of sphenoid bone	Articular disc & capsule of temporomandibular joint	Mandibular n. (CN V^3) via lateral pterygoid n. from ant. trunk, which enters it unilaterally deep surface	*Acting bilaterally,* they protrude mandible & depress chin *Acting unilaterally* & alternately, they produce side-to-side movements of mandible
	Inferior head: Lateral surface of lateral pterygoid plate	Neck of mandible		
Medial pterygoid	*Deep head:* Medial surface of lateral pterygoid plate & pyramidal process of palatine bone	Medial surface of ramus of mandible, inf. to mandibular foramen	Mandibular n. (CN V^3) via medial pterygoid n.	Helps to elevate mandible, closing jaws *Acting bilaterally,* they help to protrude mandible *Acting unilaterally,* it protrudes side of jaw *Acting alternately,* they produce a grinding motion
	Superficial head: Tuberosity of maxilla			

Actions and Nerve Supply of the Ocular Muscles

Muscle	Action(s) on the Eyeball	Nerve Supply
Medial rectus[a]	Adducts	CN III
Lateral rectus[a]	Abducts	CN VI[b]
Superior rectus	Elevates, adducts & rotate medially	CN III
Inferior rectus	Depresses, adducts & rotates laterally	CN III
Superior oblique[c]	Abducts, depresses & rotates eye medially (intorsion), depresses adducted eye	CN IV[b]
Inferior oblique[c]	Abducts, elevates & rotates eye laterally (extorsion), elevates adducted eye	CN III

[a]The medial and lateral rectus muscles move the eyeball in one axis only, whereas each of the other four muscles moves it in all three axes.
[b]CN IV and VI each supply one muscle, whereas CN III supplies the other four muscles.
[c]The superior and inferior oblique muscles are used with the medial rectus muscle in adducting both eyes medially for near vision. This movement, accompanied by pupillary construction, is known as accommodation.

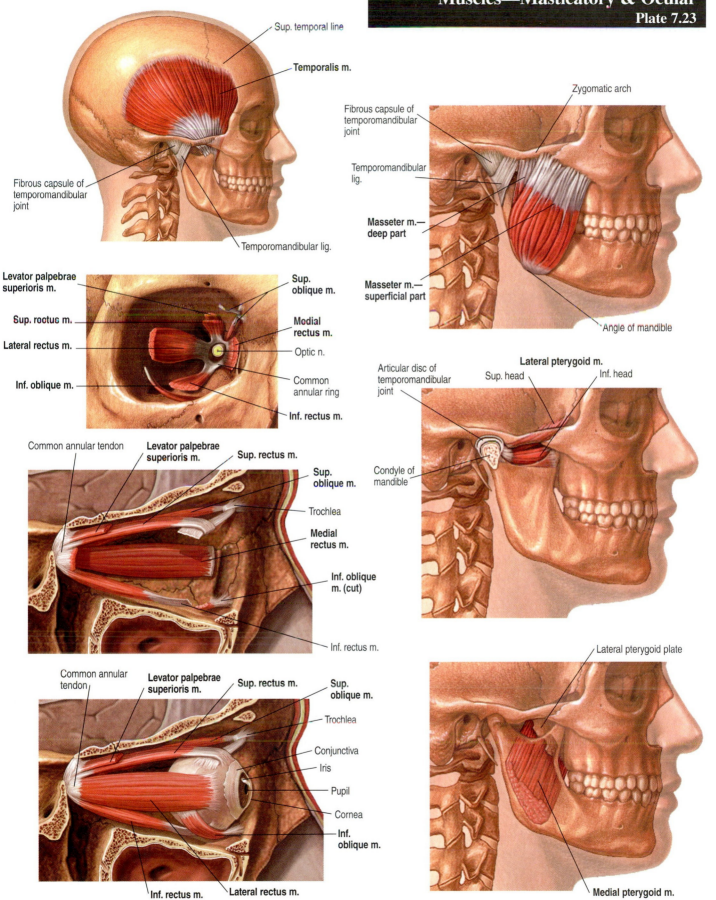

Sup. temporal line

Temporalis m.

Fibrous capsule of temporomandibular joint

Temporomandibular lig.

Zygomatic arch

Fibrous capsule of temporomandibular joint

Temporomandibular lig.

Masseter m.— deep part

Masseter m.— superficial part

Angle of mandible

Levator palpebrae superioris m.

Sup. rectus m.

Lateral rectus m.

Inf. oblique m.

Sup. oblique m.

Medial rectus m.

Optic n.

Common annular ring

Inf. rectus m.

Articular disc of temporomandibular joint

Condyle of mandible

Lateral pterygoid m.

Sup. head

Inf. head

Common annular tendon

Levator palpebrae superioris m.

Sup. rectus m.

Sup. oblique m.

Trochlea

Medial rectus m.

Inf. oblique m. (cut)

Inf. rectus m.

Lateral pterygoid plate

Common annular tendon

Levator palpebrae superioris m.

Sup. rectus m.

Sup. oblique m.

Trochlea

Conjunctiva

Iris

Pupil

Cornea

Inf. oblique m.

Inf. rectus m.

Lateral rectus m.

Medial pterygoid m.

Muscles—Soft Palate & Tongue
Table 7.4

Muscles of the Soft Palate

Muscle	Superior Attachment	Inferior Attachment	Innervation	Main Actions
Levator veli palatini	Cartilage of auditory tube & petrous part of temporal bone		Pharyngeal br. of vagus n. via pharyngeal plexus (CN X)	Elevates soft palate during swallowing & yawning
		Palatine aponeurosis		
Tensor veli palatini	Scaphoid fossa of medial pterygoid plate, spine of sphenoid bone & cartilage of auditory tube		Medial pterygoid n. (a br. of the mandibular n.) via otic ganglion (CN V^3)	Tenses soft palate & opens cartilagenous part of auditory tube during swallowing & yawning
Palatoglossus	Palatine aponeurosis	Side of tongue		Elevates posterior part of tongue & draws soft palate onto tongue
Palatopharyngeus	Hard palate & palatine aponeurosis	Lateral wall of pharynx	Cranial part of CN XI through pharyngeal br. of vagus n. (CN X) via pharyngeal plexus	Tenses soft palate & pulls walls of pharynx superiorly, anteriorly, and medially during swallowing
Musculus uvulae	Posterior nasal spine & palatine aponeurosis	Mucosa of uvula		Shortens uvula & pulls it superiorly

Extrinsic Muscles of the Tongue

Muscle	Stable Attachment	Mobile Attachment	Innervation	Actions
Genioglossus	Sup. part of mental spine of mandible	Dorsum of tongue & body of hyoid bone		Protrudes, retracts & depresses tongue; its post. part protrudes tongue
Hyoglossus	Body & greater horn of hyoid bone	Side of tongue	Hypoglossal n. CN XII	Depresses & retracts tongue
Styloglossus	Styloid process & stylohyoid lig.	Side & inf. aspect of tongue		Retracts tongue & draws it up to create a trough for swallowing
Palatoglossus	Palatine aponeurosis of soft palate	Side of tongue	Cranial root of CN XI via pharyngeal br. CN X & pharyngeal plexus	Elevates post. part of tongue

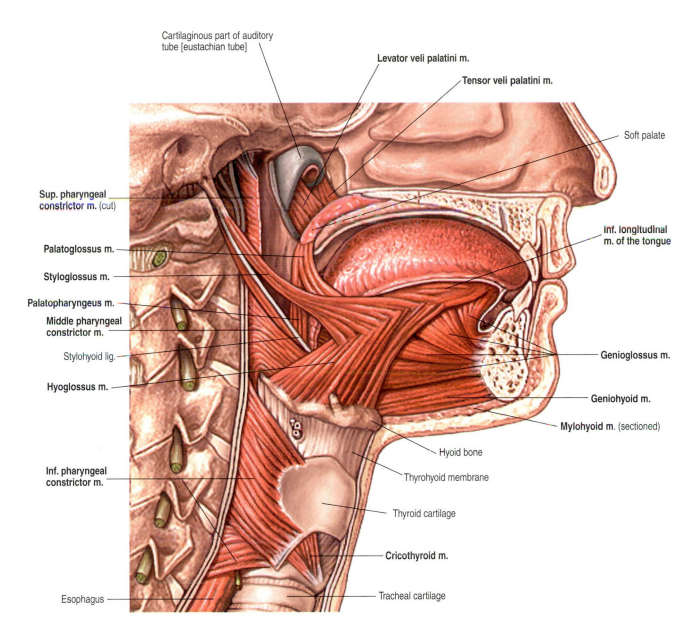

Cartilaginous part of auditory tube [eustachian tube]

Levator veli palatini m.

Tensor veli palatini m.

Soft palate

Sup. pharyngeal constrictor m. (cut)

Inf. longitudinal m. of the tongue

Palatoglossus m.

Styloglossus m.

Palatopharyngeus m.

Middle pharyngeal constrictor m.

Stylohyoid lig.

Hyoglossus m.

Genioglossus m.

Geniohyoid m.

Mylohyoid m. (sectioned)

Inf. pharyngeal constrictor m.

Hyoid bone

Thyrohyoid membrane

Thyroid cartilage

Cricothyroid m.

Esophagus

Tracheal cartilage

LATERAL VIEW OF TONGUE & PHARYNGEAL MUSCLES

Muscles—Hyoid
Table 7.5

Suprahyoid Muscles[a]

Muscle	Superior Attachment	Inferior Attachment	Innervation	Main Actions
Mylohyoid	Mylohyoid line of mandible	Oral raphe & body of hyoid bone	Mylohyoid n., a br. of inf. alveolar n. (CN V³)	Elevates hyoid bone, floor of mouth & tongue during swallowing & speaking
Geniohyoid	Inf. mental spine of mandible	Body of hyoid bone	C1 via the hypoglossal n. (CN XII)	Pulls hyoid bone anterosuperiorly, shortens floor of mouth & widens pharynx
Stylohyoid	Styloid process of temporal bone	Body of hyoid bone	Cervical br. of facial n. (CN VII)	Elevates & retracts hyoid bone, thereby elongating floor of mouth
Digastric	*Anterior belly:* Digastric fossa of mandible *Posterior belly:* Mastoid notch of temporal bone	Intermediate tendon to body & greater horn of hyoid bone	*Anterior belly:* Mylohyoid n., a br. of inf. alveolar n. (CN V³) *Posterior belly:* Facial n. (CN VII)	Depresses mandible, raises hyoid bone & steadies it during swallowing & speaking

[a]These muscles connect the hyoid bone to the skull.

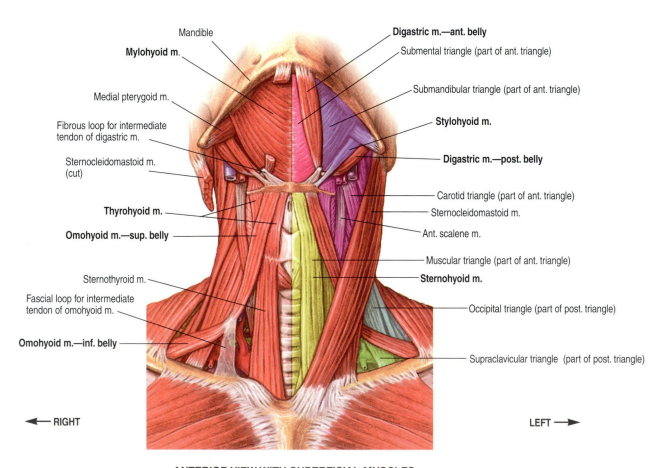

ANTERIOR VIEW WITH SUPERFICIAL MUSCLES ON LEFT & DEEPER MUSCLES ON RIGHT

Infrahyoid Muscles[a]

Muscle	Origin	Insertion	Innervation	Actions
Sternohyoid	Manubrium of sternum & medial end of clavicle	Body of hyoid bone	C1, C2 & C3 from ansa cervicalis	Depresses hyoid bone after it has been elevated during swallowing
Sternothyroid	Post. surface of manubrium of sternum	Oblique line of thyroid cartilage	C2 & C3 by a br. of ansa cervicalis	Depresses hyoid bone & larynx
Thyrohyoid	Oblique line of thyroid cartilage	Inf. border of body & greater horn of hyoid bone	C1 via hypoglossal n. (CN XII)	Depresses hyoid bone & elevates larynx
Omohyoid	Sup. border of scapula near suprascapular notch	Inf. border of hyoid bone	C1, C2 & C3 by a br. of ansa cervicalis	Depresses, retracts & steadies hyoid bone

[a]These four step-like muscles anchor the hyoid bone (*i.e.,* they fix and steady it). They are concerned with the suprahyoid muscles in movements of the tongue, hyoid bone, and larynx in both swallowing and speaking.

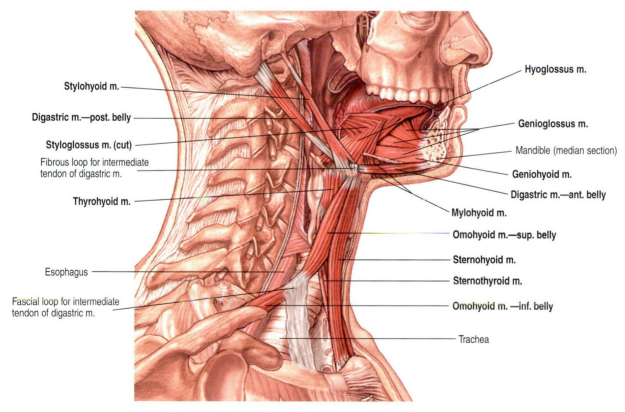

LATERAL VIEW WITH RIGHT HALF OF MANDIBLE REMOVED

Muscle	Lateral Attachments	Medial Attachments	Innervation	Main Actions
CIRCULAR PHARYNGEAL MUSCLES				
Superior constrictor	Pterygoid hamulus, ptergomandibular raphe, post. end of mylohyoid line of mandible & side of tongue	Median raphe of pharynx & pharyngeal tubercle	Pharyngeal & sup. laryngeal brr. of vagus n. [CN X] through pharyngeal plexus	Constrict wall of pharynx during swallowing
Middle constrictor	Stylohyoid lig. and greater & lesser horns of hyoid bone	Median raphe of pharynx		
Inferior constrictor	Oblique line of thyroid cartilage & side of cricoid cartilage			
LONGITUDINAL PHARYNGEAL MUSCLES				
Palatopharyngeus	Hard palate & palatine aponeurosis	Post. border of lamina of thyroid cartilage & side of pharynx & esophagus		Elevate pharynx & larynx during swallowing & speaking[a]
Salpingopharynegeus	Cartilaginous part of auditory tube	Blends with palatopharynegeus		
Stylopharyngeus	Styloid process of temporal bone	Post. & sup. borders of thyroid cartilage with palatopharynegus m.	Glossopharyngeal n.[CN IX]	

[a]The salpingopharyngeus muscle also opens the auditory tube.

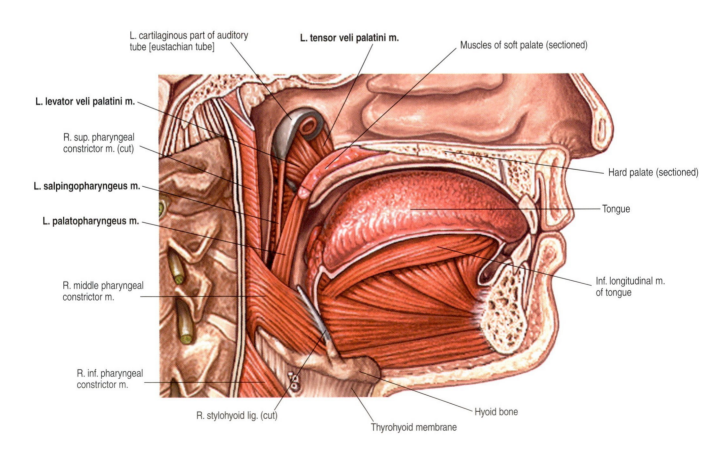

L. cartilaginous part of auditory tube [eustachian tube]

L. tensor veli palatini m.

Muscles of soft palate (sectioned)

L. levator veli palatini m.

R. sup. pharyngeal constrictor m. (cut)

L. salpingopharyngeus m.

L. palatopharyngeus m.

R. middle pharyngeal constrictor m.

R. inf. pharyngeal constrictor m.

Hard palate (sectioned)

Tongue

Inf. longitudinal m. of tongue

R. stylohyoid lig. (cut)

Thyrohyoid membrane

Hyoid bone

LATERAL VIEW OF NECK & MEDIAN SECTIONED SKULL

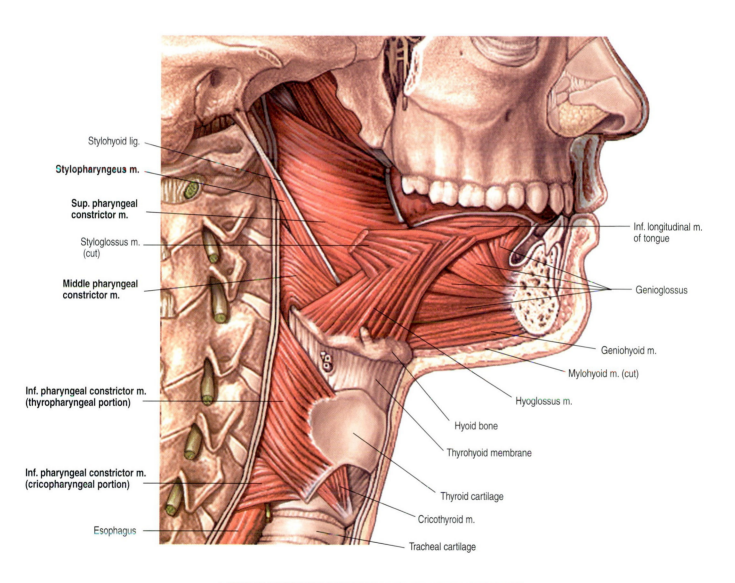

Stylohyoid lig.

Stylopharyngeus m.

**Sup. pharyngeal
constrictor m.**

Styloglossus m.
(cut)

**Middle pharyngeal
constrictor m.**

**Inf. pharyngeal constrictor m.
(thyropharyngeal portion)**

**Inf. pharyngeal constrictor m.
(cricopharyngeal portion)**

Esophagus

Inf. longitudinal m.
of tongue

Genioglossus

Geniohyoid m.

Mylohyoid m. (cut)

Hyoglossus m.

Hyoid bone

Thyrohyoid membrane

Thyroid cartilage

Cricothyroid m.

Tracheal cartilage

LATERAL VIEW WITH RIGHT HALF OF MANDIBLE REMOVED

Muscles of the Larynx

Muscle	Origin	Insertion	Innervation	Main Actions
Cricothyroid	Anterolateral part of cricoid cartilage	Inf. margin & inf. horn of thyroid cartilage	Ext. laryngeal n. (CN X)	Stretches & tenses the vocal fold
Posterior cricoarytenoid	Post. surface of laminae of cricoid cartilage	Muscular process of arytenoid cartilage		Abducts vocal fold
Lateral cricoarytenoid	Arch of cricoid cartilage			Adducts vocal fold
Thyroarytenoid[a]	Post. surface of thyroid cartilage	Muscular process of arytenoid process	Recurrent laryngeal n. (CN X)	Relaxes vocal fold
Transverse & oblique arytenoids	One arytenoid cartilage	Opposition arytenoid cartilage		Close laryngeal aditus by approximating arytenoid cartilages
Vocalis[b]	Angle between laminae of thyroid cartilage	Vocal process of arytenoid cartilage		Alters vocal fold during phonation

[a]The superior fibers of the thyroarytenoid muscle pass into the aryepiglottic fold, and some of them reach the epiglottic cartilage. These fibers constitute the *thyroepiglottic muscle*, which widens the inlet of the larynx.
[b]These short fine muscular slips are derived from the most medial fibers of the thyroarytenoid muscle.

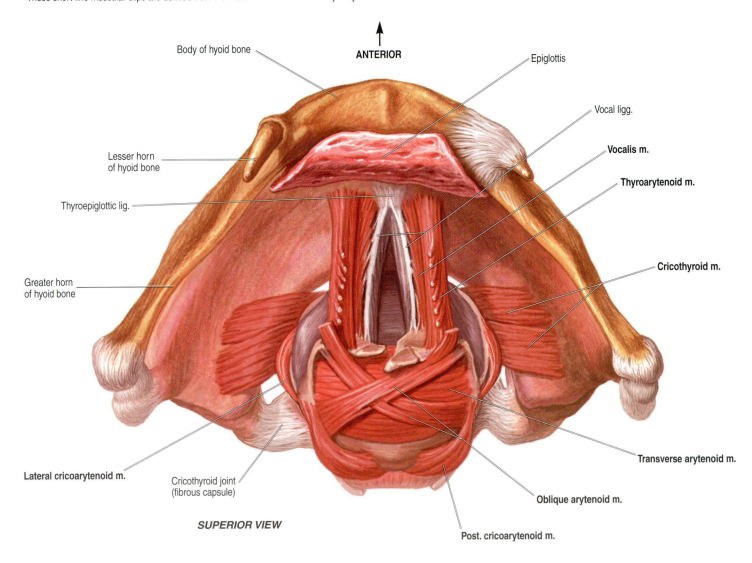

ANTERIOR

Body of hyoid bone

Epiglottis

Vocal ligg.

Lesser horn of hyoid bone

Vocalis m.

Thyroarytenoid m.

Thyroepiglottic lig.

Greater horn of hyoid bone

Cricothyroid m.

Lateral cricoarytenoid m.

Transverse arytenoid m.

Cricothyroid joint (fibrous capsule)

Oblique arytenoid m.

Post. cricoarytenoid m.

SUPERIOR VIEW

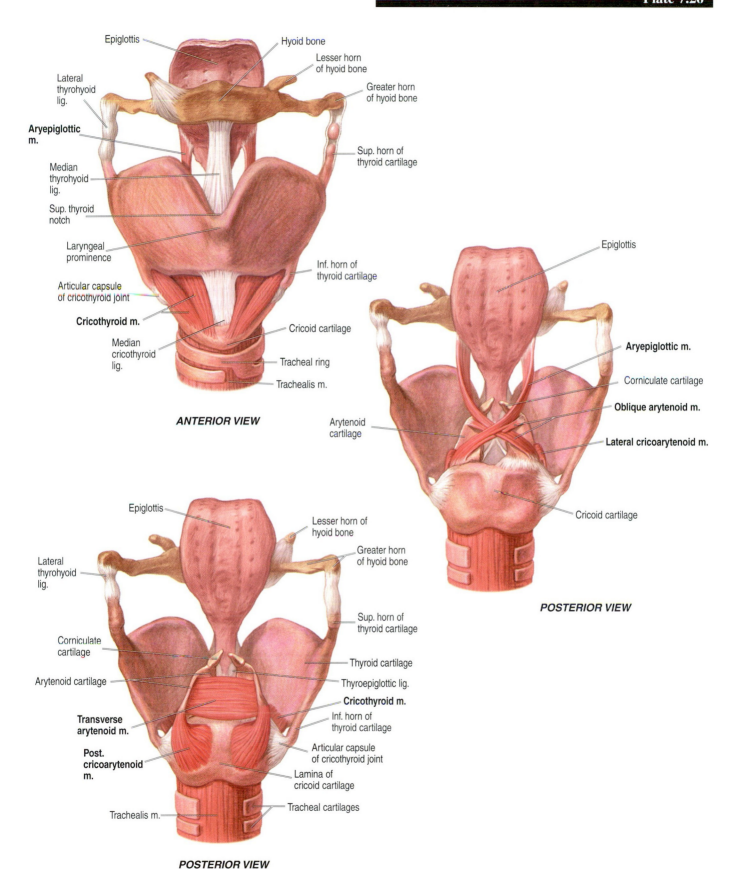

Epiglottis

Hyoid bone

Lesser horn
of hyoid bone

Lateral
thyrohyoid
lig.

Greater horn
of hyoid bone

**Aryepiglottic
m.**

Sup. horn of
thyroid cartilage

Median
thyrohyoid
lig.

Sup. thyroid
notch

Laryngeal
prominence

Inf. horn of
thyroid cartilage

Articular capsule
of cricothyroid joint

Cricothyroid m.

Cricoid cartilage

Median
cricothyroid
lig.

Tracheal ring

Trachealis m.

ANTERIOR VIEW

Epiglottis

Arytenoid
cartilage

Aryepiglottic m.

Corniculate cartilage

Oblique arytenoid m.

Lateral cricoarytenoid m.

Cricoid cartilage

POSTERIOR VIEW

Epiglottis

Lesser horn of
hyoid bone

Lateral
thyrohyoid
lig.

Greater horn
of hyoid bone

Sup. horn of
thyroid cartilage

Corniculate
cartilage

Arytenoid cartilage

Thyroid cartilage

Thyroepiglottic lig.

Cricothyroid m.

**Transverse
arytenoid m.**

Inf. horn of
thyroid cartilage

Articular capsule
of cricothyroid joint

**Post.
cricoarytenoid
m.**

Lamina of
cricoid cartilage

Trachealis m.

Tracheal cartilages

POSTERIOR VIEW

Muscles—Lateral & Prevertebral
Table 7.9

Muscle	Inferior Attachment	Superior Attachment	Innervation	Main Actions
Sternocleidomastoid				
Sternal head	Ventral surface of the manubrium sterni	Lateral surface of mastoid process; sup. nuchal line of occipital bone	Spinal accessory n. (motor); sensory fibers of C2 n.	Various: both sides together support head, move chin upward, and pull back of head down. One side alone turns chin upward and to opposite side.
Clavicular head	Cranial surface of medial third of clavicle			
Splenius capitis	Inf. half of ligamentum nuchae & spinous process of sup. six thoracic vertebrae	Lateral aspect of mastoid process & lateral third of sup. nuchal line	Dorsal rami of middle cervical spinal nn.	Laterally flexes & rotates head & neck to same side; acting bilaterally, they extend head & neck
Splenius cervicis	Spines of 3rd (or 4th) to 6th thoracic vertebrae	Posterior tubercles of the transverse process of the upper three cervical vertebrae	Dorsal rami of nerves C2-C5, lateral brr. (same as splenius capitis m.)	
Posterior scalene	Post. tubercles of transverse processes of C4-C6	Ext. border of second rib	Ventral rami of cervical spinal nn. (C7 & C8)	Flexes neck laterally; elevates second rib during forced inspiration
Middle scalene	Posterior tubercles of transverse processes of C2 & C7	Sup. surface of first rib, posterior to groove for subclavian a.	Ventral rami of cervical spinal nn. (C3-C8)	Flexes neck laterally; elevates first rib during forced inspiration
Anterior scalene	Ant. tubercles of transverse processes of C3-C6	Scalene tubercle of 1st rib	Long thoracic n. (C5-C7)	
Longus colli				
Vertical portion	Body of first three thoracic & last three cervical vertebrae	Bodies of C2-C4	Ventral rami of C2-C6	Bilaterally acting to flex neck and head anteriorly, unilaterally to flex head and neck laterally and to rotate the head toward the same side
Superior oblique	Ant. tubercles of transverse process of C3-C5	Tubercle on ant. arch of the atlas & body axis	Ventral rami of C1 to C4	
Inferior oblique	Ant. surface of bodies of first two or three thoracic vertebrae	Ant. tubercles of the transverse processes of C5 & C6		
Longus capitis	Ant. tubercle of transverse processes of C3-C6	Inf. border of basilar part of occipital		

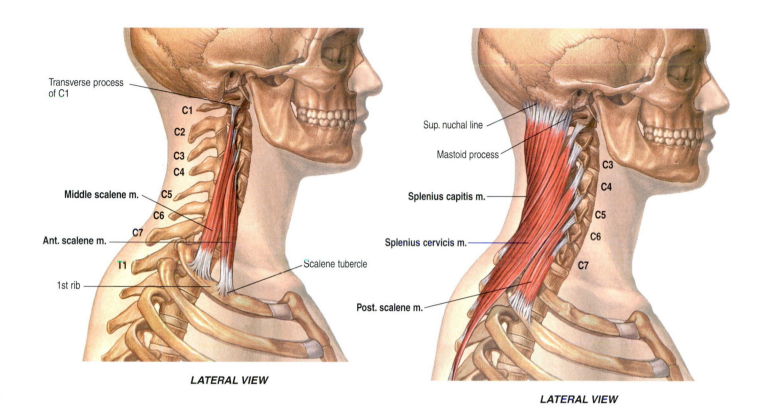

Transverse process of C1

C1
C2
C3
C4
Middle scalene m.
C5
C6
Ant. scalene m.
C7
T1
1st rib

Scalene tubercle

LATERAL VIEW

Sup. nuchal line

Mastoid process

C3
C4
C5
C6
C7

Splenius capitis m.

Splenius cervicis m.

Post. scalene m.

LATERAL VIEW

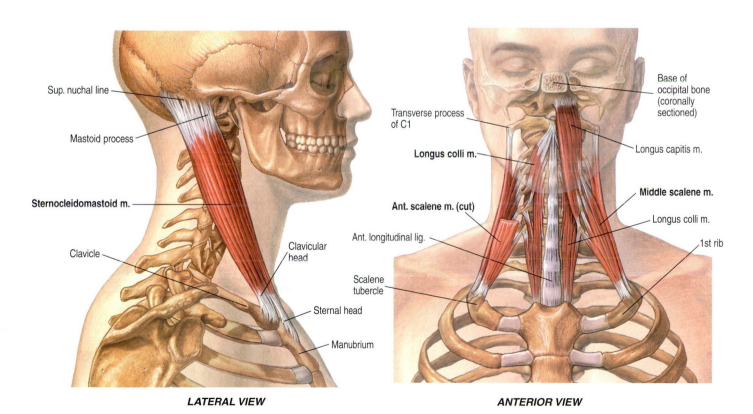

Sup. nuchal line

Mastoid process

Sternocleidomastoid m.

Clavicle

Clavicular head

Sternal head

Manubrium

LATERAL VIEW

Base of occipital bone (coronally sectioned)

Transverse process of C1

Longus colli m.

Longus capitis m.

Middle scalene m.

Ant. scalene m. (cut)

Longus colli m.

Ant. longitudinal lig.

1st rib

Scalene tubercle

ANTERIOR VIEW

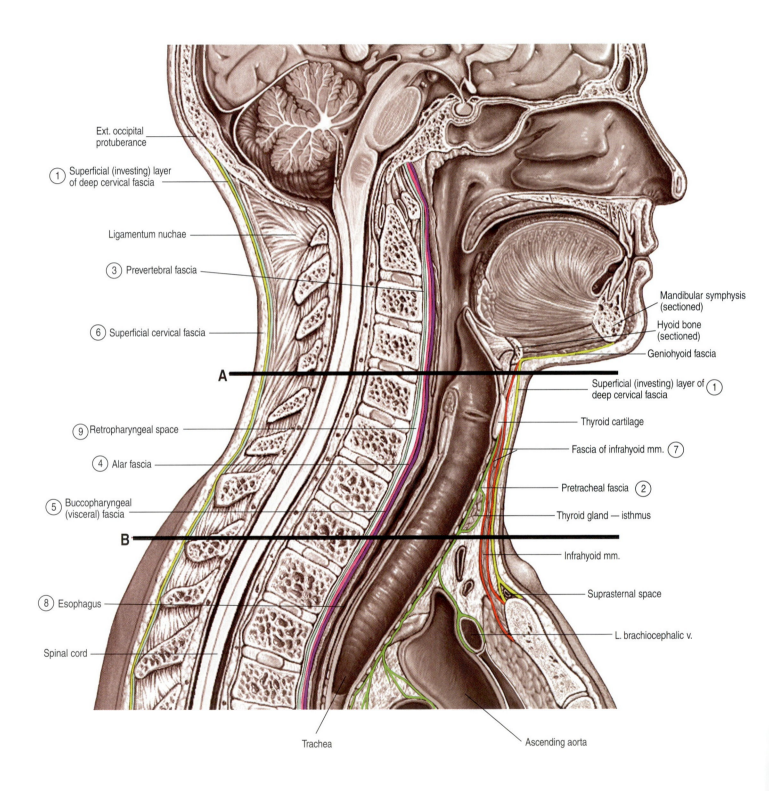

Ext. occipital protuberance

1 Superficial (investing) layer of deep cervical fascia

Ligamentum nuchae

3 Prevertebral fascia

6 Superficial cervical fascia

A

9 Retropharyngeal space

4 Alar fascia

5 Buccopharyngeal (visceral) fascia

B

8 Esophagus

Spinal cord

Trachea

Mandibular symphysis (sectioned)

Hyoid bone (sectioned)

Geniohyoid fascia

Superficial (investing) layer of 1 deep cervical fascia

Thyroid cartilage

Fascia of infrahyoid mm. 7

Pretracheal fascia 2

Thyroid gland — isthmus

Infrahyoid mm.

Suprasternal space

L. brachiocephalic v.

Ascending aorta

LATERAL VIEW OF MEDIAN SECTION

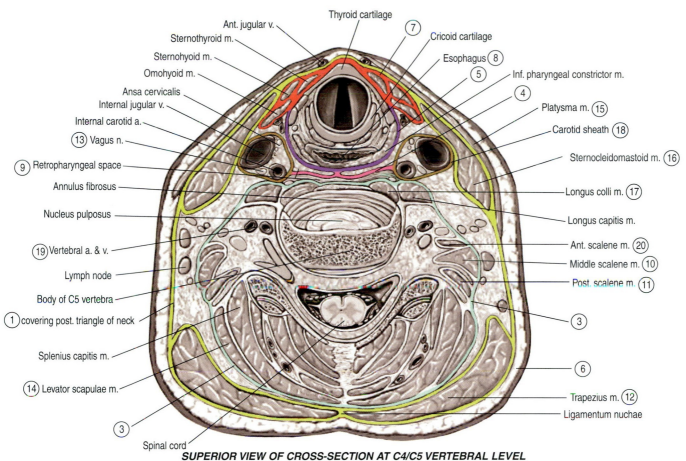

Thyroid cartilage

Ant. jugular v.

Sternothyroid m.

Sternohyoid m.

Omohyoid m.

Ansa cervicalis

Internal jugular v.

Internal carotid a.

(13) Vagus n.

(9) Retropharyngeal space

Annulus fibrosus

Nucleus pulposus

(19) Vertebral a. & v.

Lymph node

Body of C5 vertebra

(1) covering post. triangle of neck

Splenius capitis m.

(14) Levator scapulae m.

(3)

Spinal cord

(7)

Cricoid cartilage

Esophagus (8)

(5)

Inf. pharyngeal constrictor m.

(4)

Platysma m. (15)

Carotid sheath (18)

Sternocleidomastoid m. (16)

Longus colli m. (17)

Longus capitis m.

Ant. scalene m. (20)

Middle scalene m. (10)

Post. scalene m. (11)

(3)

(6)

Trapezius m. (12)

Ligamentum nuchae

SUPERIOR VIEW OF CROSS-SECTION AT C4/C5 VERTEBRAL LEVEL

A

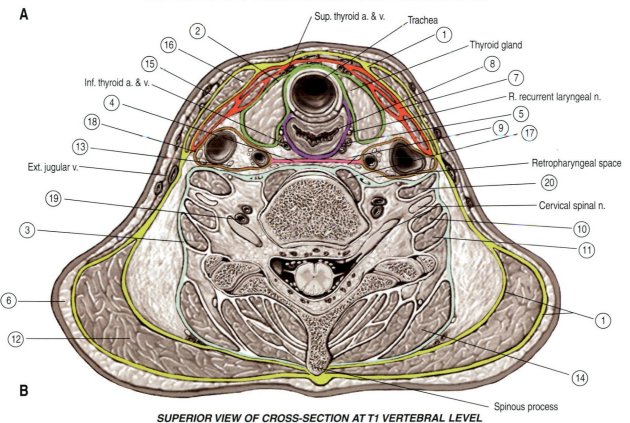

Sup. thyroid a. & v.

Trachea

(2)

(16)

(15)

Inf. thyroid a. & v.

(4)

(18)

(13)

Ext. jugular v.

(19)

(3)

(6)

(12)

(1)

Thyroid gland

(8)

(7)

R. recurrent laryngeal n.

(5)

(9) (17)

Retropharyngeal space

(20)

Cervical spinal n.

(10)

(11)

(1)

(14)

Spinous process

B

SUPERIOR VIEW OF CROSS-SECTION AT T1 VERTEBRAL LEVEL

LATERAL VIEW

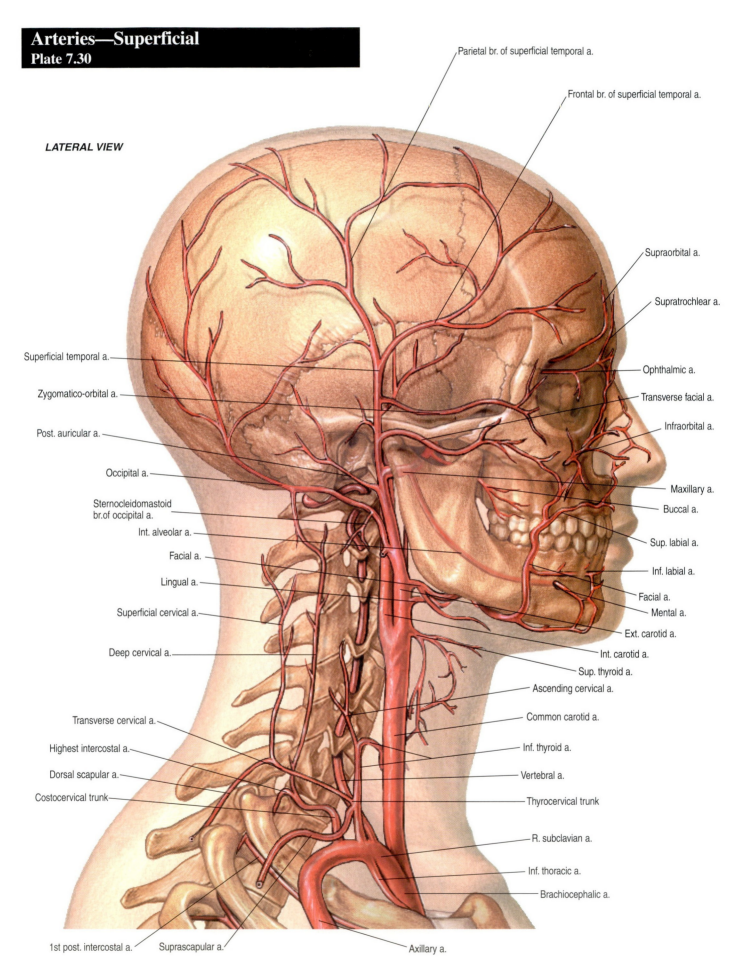

Parietal br. of superficial temporal a.

Frontal br. of superficial temporal a.

Supraorbital a.

Supratrochlear a.

Ophthalmic a.

Transverse facial a.

Infraorbital a.

Superficial temporal a.

Zygomatico-orbital a.

Post. auricular a.

Occipital a.

Sternocleidomastoid br. of occipital a.

Int. alveolar a.

Facial a.

Lingual a.

Superficial cervical a.

Deep cervical a.

Maxillary a.

Buccal a.

Sup. labial a.

Inf. labial a.

Facial a.

Mental a.

Ext. carotid a.

Int. carotid a.

Sup. thyroid a.

Ascending cervical a.

Common carotid a.

Inf. thyroid a.

Vertebral a.

Thyrocervical trunk

R. subclavian a.

Inf. thoracic a.

Brachiocephalic a.

Transverse cervical a.

Highest intercostal a.

Dorsal scapular a.

Costocervical trunk

1st post. intercostal a.

Suprascapular a.

Axillary a.

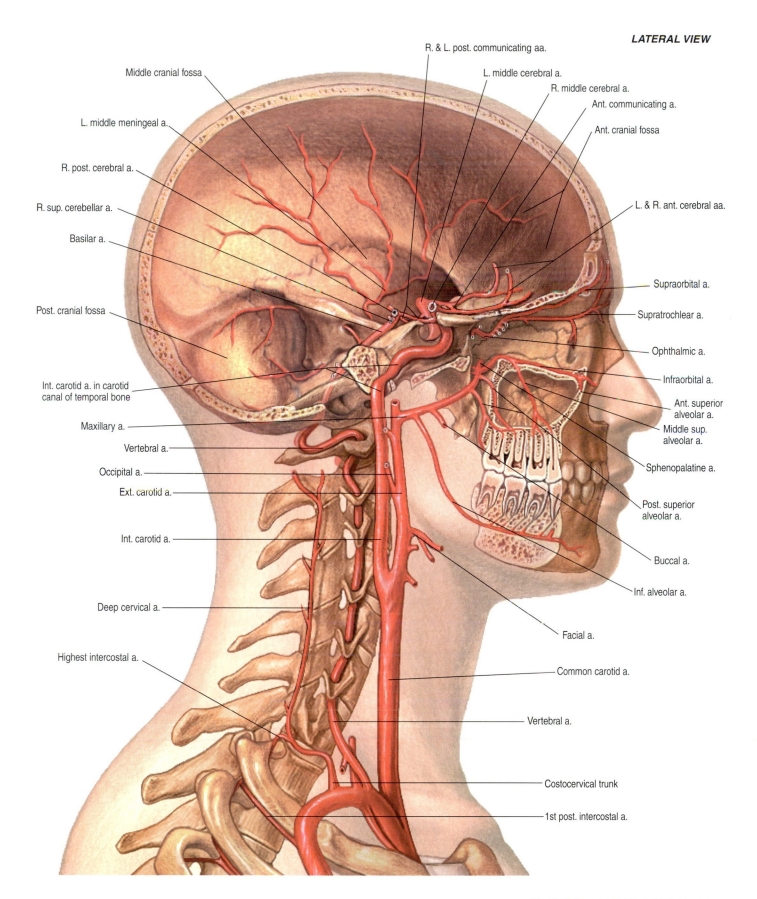

LATERAL VIEW

R. & L. post. communicating aa.

L. middle cerebral a.

R. middle cerebral a.

Ant. communicating a.

Ant. cranial fossa

Middle cranial fossa

L. middle meningeal a.

R. post. cerebral a.

R. sup. cerebellar a.

Basilar a.

Post. cranial fossa

Int. carotid a. in carotid canal of temporal bone

Maxillary a.

Vertebral a.

Occipital a.

Ext. carotid a.

Int. carotid a.

Deep cervical a.

Highest intercostal a.

L. & R. ant. cerebral aa.

Supraorbital a.

Supratrochlear a.

Ophthalmic a.

Infraorbital a.

Ant. superior alveolar a.

Middle sup. alveolar a.

Sphenopalatine a.

Post. superior alveolar a.

Buccal a.

Inf. alveolar a.

Facial a.

Common carotid a.

Vertebral a.

Costocervical trunk

1st post. intercostal a.

LATERAL VIEW

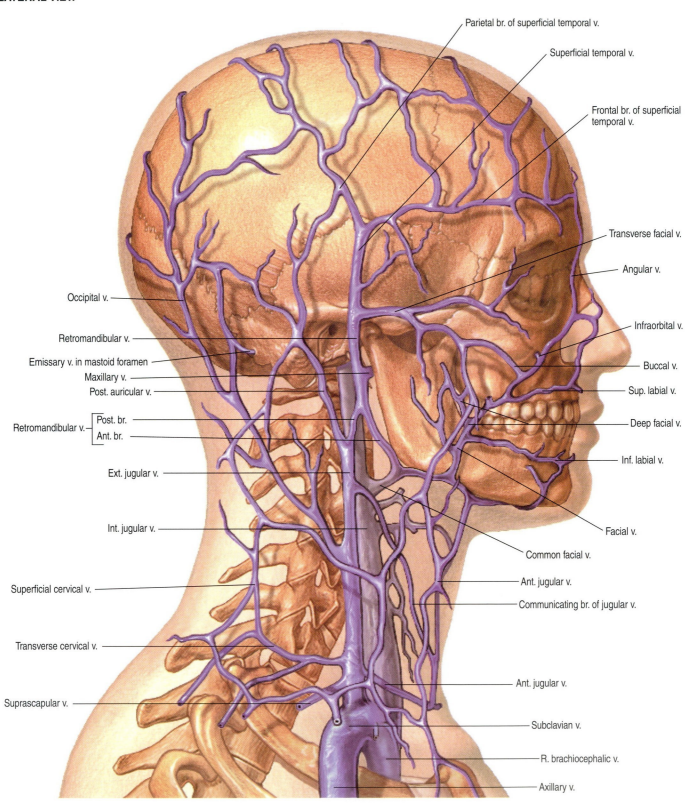

Parietal br. of superficial temporal v.

Superficial temporal v.

Frontal br. of superficial temporal v.

Transverse facial v.

Angular v.

Infraorbital v.

Buccal v.

Sup. labial v.

Deep facial v.

Inf. labial v.

Facial v.

Common facial v.

Ant. jugular v.

Communicating br. of jugular v.

Ant. jugular v.

Subclavian v.

R. brachiocephalic v.

Axillary v.

Occipital v.

Retromandibular v.

Emissary v. in mastoid foramen

Maxillary v.

Post. auricular v.

Retromandibular v. — Post. br.
Ant. br.

Ext. jugular v.

Int. jugular v.

Superficial cervical v.

Transverse cervical v.

Suprascapular v.

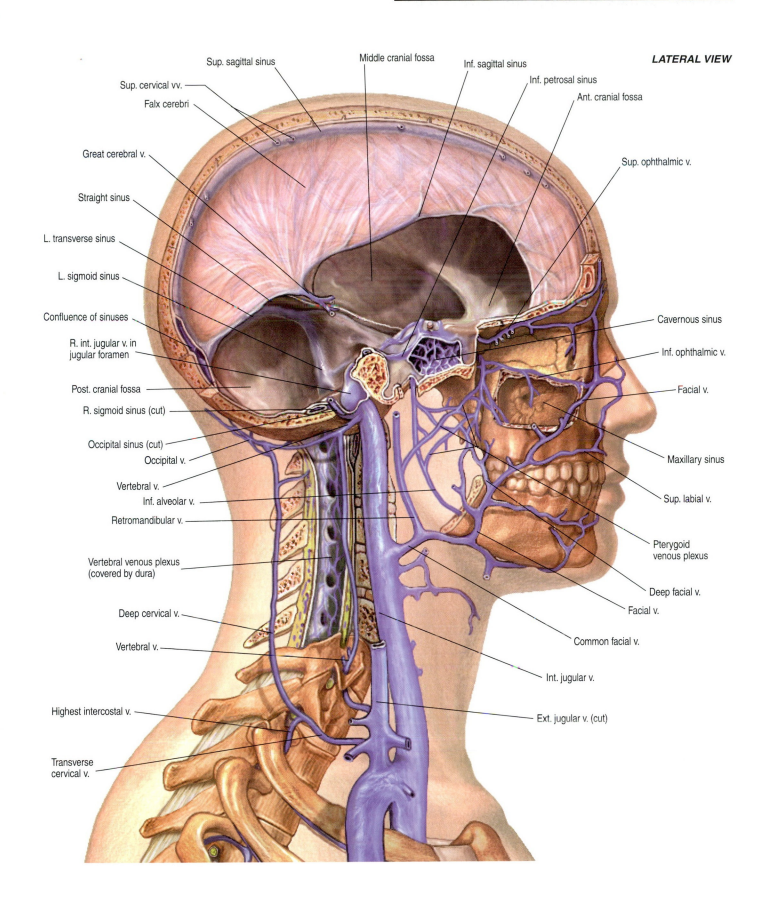

LATERAL VIEW

Sup. sagittal sinus

Sup. cervical vv.

Falx cerebri

Great cerebral v.

Straight sinus

L. transverse sinus

L. sigmoid sinus

Confluence of sinuses

R. int. jugular v. in jugular foramen

Post. cranial fossa

R. sigmoid sinus (cut)

Occipital sinus (cut)

Occipital v.

Vertebral v.

Inf. alveolar v.

Retromandibular v.

Vertebral venous plexus (covered by dura)

Deep cervical v.

Vertebral v.

Highest intercostal v.

Transverse cervical v.

Middle cranial fossa

Inf. sagittal sinus

Inf. petrosal sinus

Ant. cranial fossa

Sup. ophthalmic v.

Cavernous sinus

Inf. ophthalmic v.

Facial v.

Maxillary sinus

Sup. labial v.

Pterygoid venous plexus

Deep facial v.

Facial v.

Common facial v.

Int. jugular v.

Ext. jugular v. (cut)

Dermatomes & Cutaneous Innervation
Plate 7.34

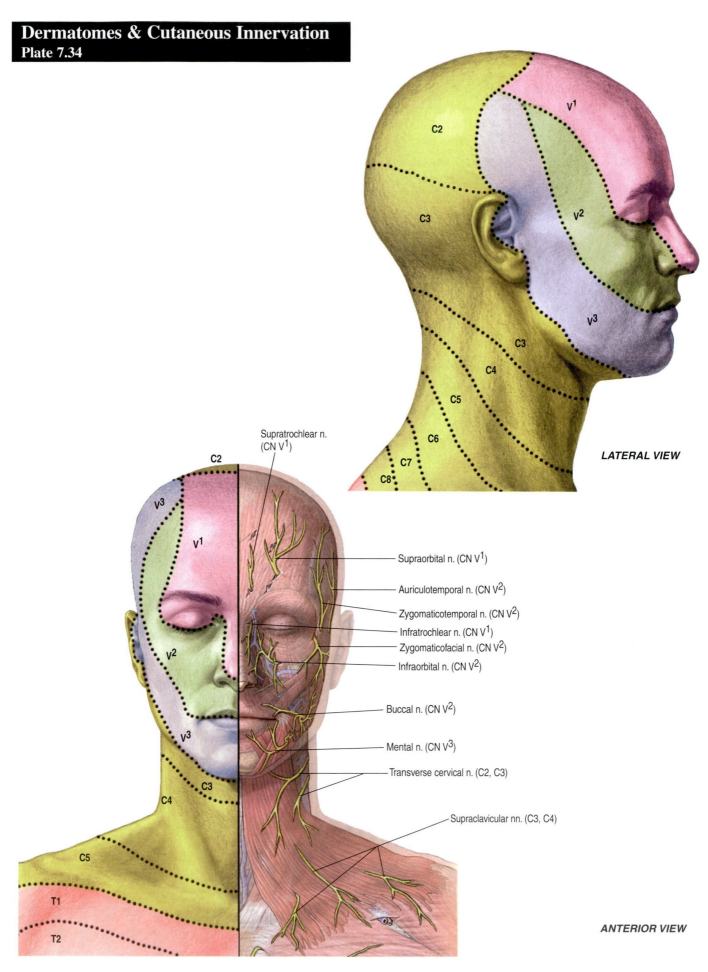

LATERAL VIEW

Supratrochlear n. (CN V^1)

C2

V^3

V^1

V^2

V^3

C3

C4

C5

T1

T2

Supraorbital n. (CN V^1)

Auriculotemporal n. (CN V^2)

Zygomaticotemporal n. (CN V^2)

Infratrochlear n. (CN V^1)

Zygomaticofacial n. (CN V^2)

Infraorbital n. (CN V^2)

Buccal n. (CN V^2)

Mental n. (CN V^3)

Transverse cervical n. (C2, C3)

Supraclavicular nn. (C3, C4)

ANTERIOR VIEW

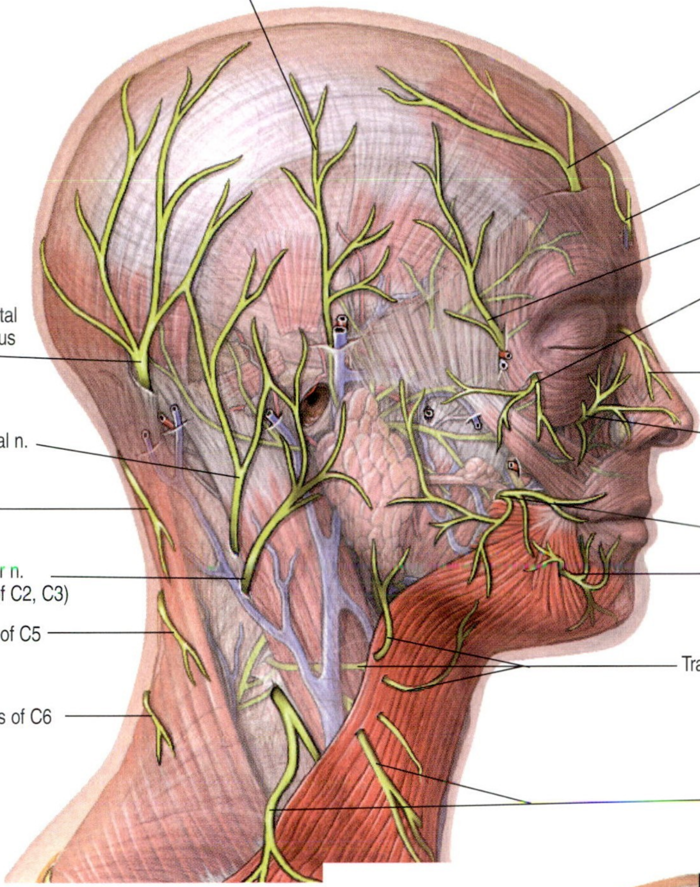

Auriculotemporal n.

Supraorbital n. (CN V^1)

Supratrochlear n. (CN V^1)

Zygomaticotemporal n. (CN V^2)

Zygomaticofacial n. (CN V^2)

Infratrochlear n. (CN V^1)

Infraorbital n. (CN V^2)

Greater occipital n. (dorsal ramus of C2)

Lesser occipital n.

Dorsal ramus of C4

Great auricular n. (ventral rami of C2, C3)

Dorsal ramus of C5

Dorsal ramus of C6

Buccal n. (CN V^2)

Mental n. (CN V^3)

Transverse cervical n. (C2, C3)

LATERAL VIEW

Supraclavicular nn. (C3, C4)

Greater occipital n. (dorsal ramus of C2)

3rd occipital n. (dorsal ramus of C3)

Lesser auricular n. (cervical plexus C2, C3)

Greater occipital n. (cervical plexus C2, C3)

Dorsal ramus of C4

Dorsal ramus of C5

Dorsal ramus of C6

C2

C3

C4

C5

C6

C7

C8

T1

T2

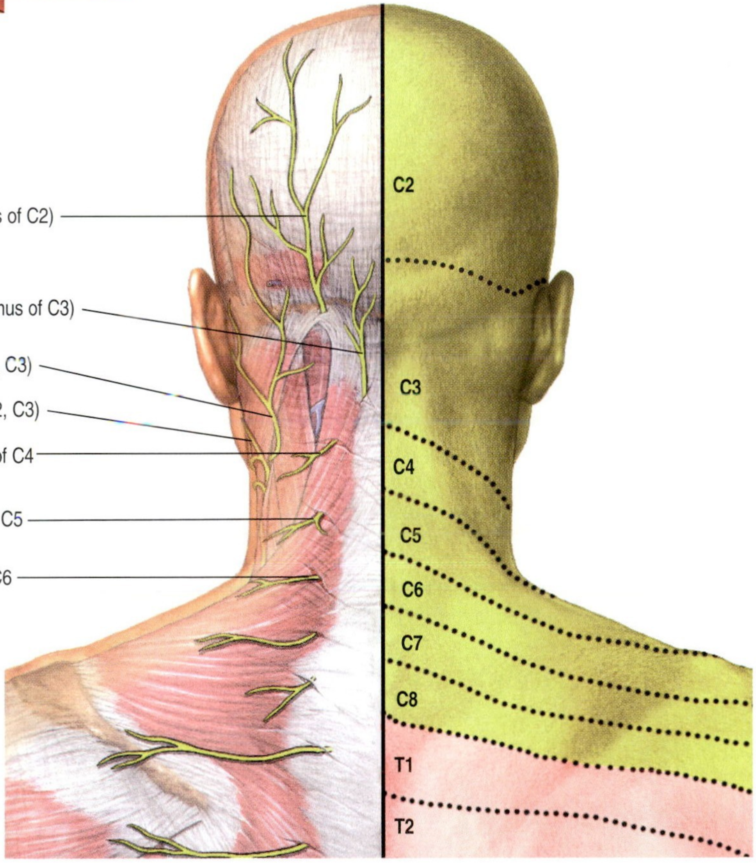

POSTERIOR VIEW

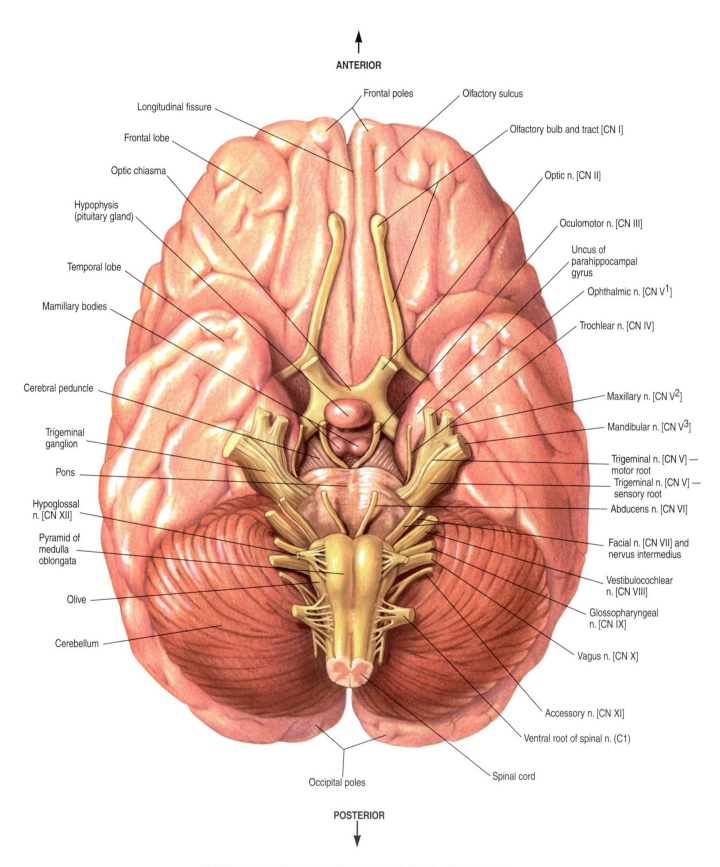

ANTERIOR

Frontal poles

Olfactory sulcus

Longitudinal fissure

Olfactory bulb and tract [CN I]

Frontal lobe

Optic n. [CN II]

Optic chiasma

Oculomotor n. [CN III]

Hypophysis
(pituitary gland)

Uncus of
parahippocampal
gyrus

Temporal lobe

Ophthalmic n. [CN V¹]

Mamillary bodies

Trochlear n. [CN IV]

Cerebral peduncle

Maxillary n. [CN V²]

Mandibular n. [CN V³]

Trigeminal
ganglion

Trigeminal n. [CN V] —
motor root

Pons

Trigeminal n. [CN V] —
sensory root

Abducens n. [CN VI]

Hypoglossal
n. [CN XII]

Facial n. [CN VII] and
nervus intermedius

Pyramid of
medulla
oblongata

Vestibulocochlear
n. [CN VIII]

Olive

Glossopharyngeal
n. [CN IX]

Cerebellum

Vagus n. [CN X]

Accessory n. [CN XI]

Ventral root of spinal n. (C1)

Occipital poles

Spinal cord

POSTERIOR

INFERIOR SURFACE OF BRAIN, BRAINSTEM & SPINAL CORD

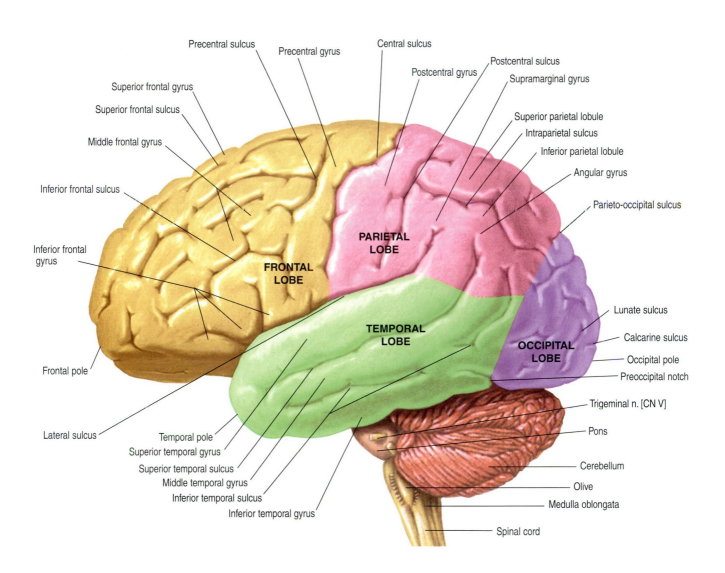

Precentral sulcus
Precentral gyrus
Central sulcus
Postcentral gyrus
Postcentral sulcus
Supramarginal gyrus
Superior frontal gyrus
Superior frontal sulcus
Superior parietal lobule
Intraparietal sulcus
Middle frontal gyrus
Inferior parietal lobule
Angular gyrus
Inferior frontal sulcus
Parieto-occipital sulcus
Inferior frontal gyrus
PARIETAL LOBE
FRONTAL LOBE
Lunate sulcus
TEMPORAL LOBE
Calcarine sulcus
OCCIPITAL LOBE
Occipital pole
Preoccipital notch
Frontal pole
Trigeminal n. [CN V]
Pons
Lateral sulcus
Temporal pole
Superior temporal gyrus
Cerebellum
Superior temporal sulcus
Olive
Middle temporal gyrus
Medulla oblongata
Inferior temporal sulcus
Spinal cord
Inferior temporal gyrus

LEFT LATERAL VIEW OF BRAIN & BRAINSTEM

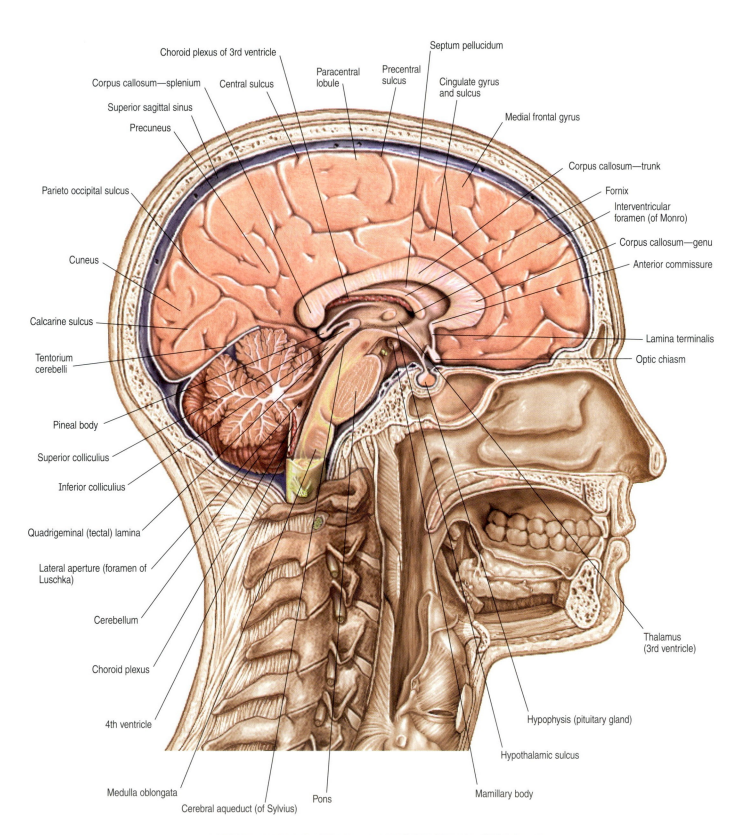

Choroid plexus of 3rd ventricle

Corpus callosum—splenium

Central sulcus

Paracentral lobule

Precentral sulcus

Septum pellucidum

Cingulate gyrus and sulcus

Medial frontal gyrus

Superior sagittal sinus

Precuneus

Corpus callosum—trunk

Fornix

Interventricular foramen (of Monro)

Parieto occipital sulcus

Corpus callosum—genu

Anterior commissure

Cuneus

Calcarine sulcus

Lamina terminalis

Optic chiasm

Tentorium cerebelli

Pineal body

Superior colliculius

Inferior colliculius

Quadrigeminal (tectal) lamina

Lateral aperture (foramen of Luschka)

Cerebellum

Choroid plexus

Thalamus (3rd ventricle)

4th ventricle

Hypophysis (pituitary gland)

Hypothalamic sulcus

Medulla oblongata

Mamillary body

Cerebral aqueduct (of Sylvius)

Pons

LATERAL VIEW WITH BRAIN & BRAINSTEM MEDIAN SECTIONED

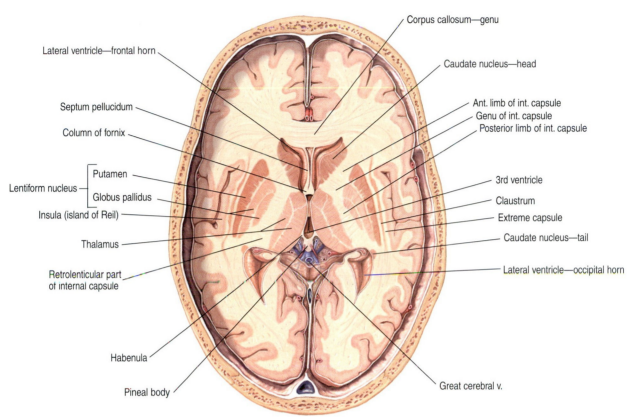

Corpus callosum—genu

Lateral ventricle—frontal horn

Caudate nucleus—head

Septum pellucidum

Ant. limb of int. capsule
Genu of int. capsule
Posterior limb of int. capsule

Column of fornix

Putamen

Lentiform nucleus

Globus pallidus

Insula (island of Reil)

3rd ventricle

Claustrum

Extreme capsule

Caudate nucleus—tail

Thalamus

Retrolenticular part
of internal capsule

Lateral ventricle—occipital horn

Habenula

Pineal body

Great cerebral v.

HORIZONTAL SECTIONS OF BRAIN

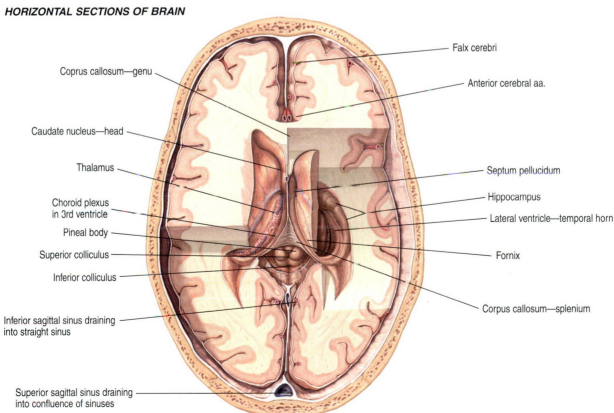

Coprus callosum—genu

Falx cerebri

Anterior cerebral aa.

Caudate nucleus—head

Thalamus

Septum pellucidum

Choroid plexus
in 3rd ventricle

Hippocampus

Lateral ventricle—temporal horn

Pineal body

Superior colliculus

Fornix

Inferior colliculus

Inferior sagittal sinus draining
into straight sinus

Corpus callosum—splenium

Superior sagittal sinus draining
into confluence of sinuses

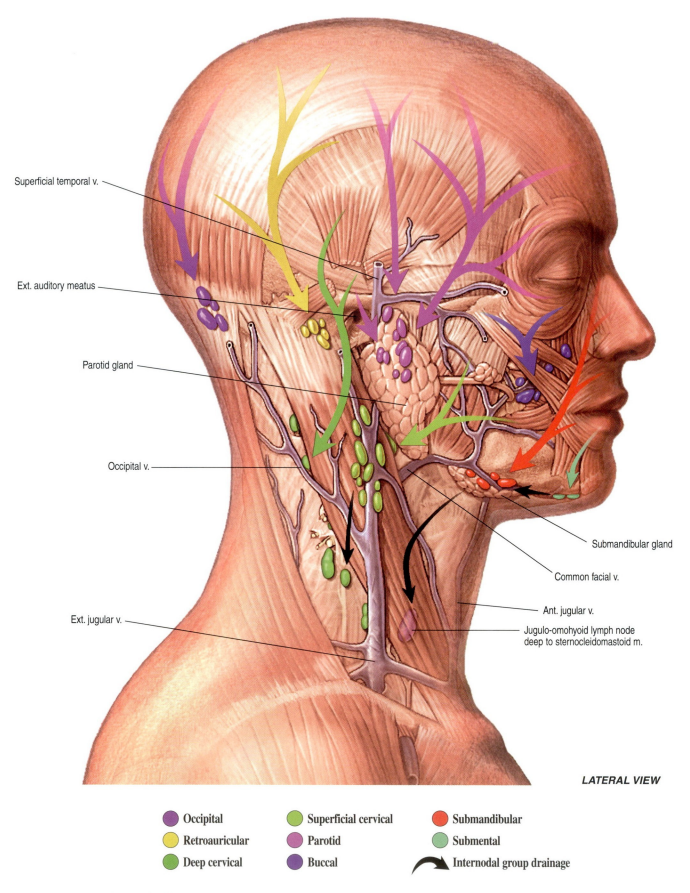

Superficial temporal v.

Ext. auditory meatus

Parotid gland

Occipital v.

Ext. jugular v.

Submandibular gland

Common facial v.

Ant. jugular v.

Jugulo-omohyoid lymph node
deep to sternocleidomastoid m.

LATERAL VIEW

● Occipital	● Superficial cervical	● Submandibular
● Retroauricular	● Parotid	● Submental
● Deep cervical	● Buccal	↱ Internodal group drainage

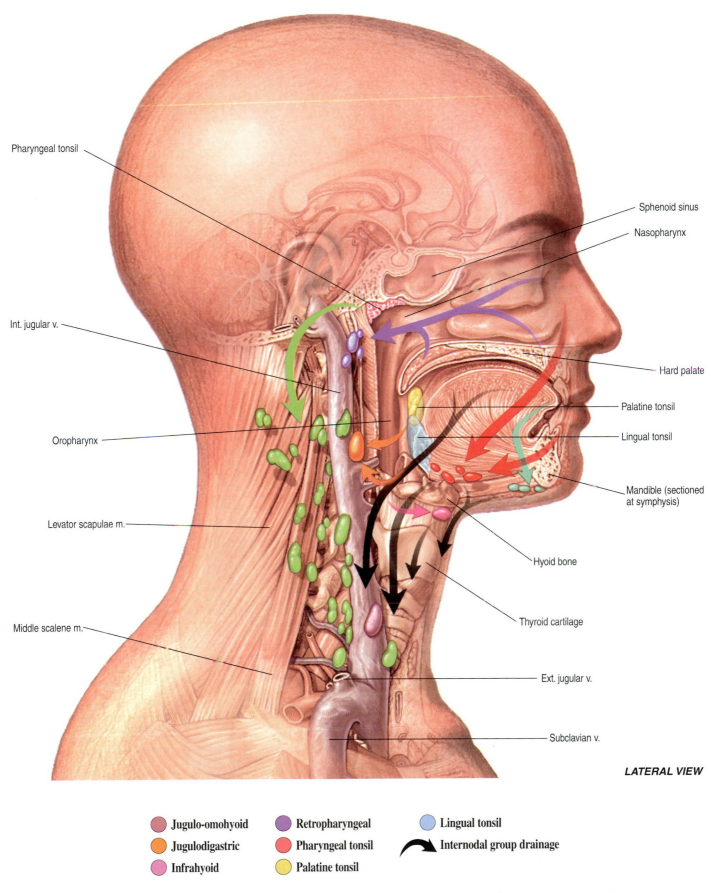

Pharyngeal tonsil

Int. jugular v.

Oropharynx

Levator scapulae m.

Middle scalene m.

Sphenoid sinus

Nasopharynx

Hard palate

Palatine tonsil

Lingual tonsil

Mandible (sectioned at symphysis)

Hyoid bone

Thyroid cartilage

Ext. jugular v.

Subclavian v.

LATERAL VIEW

🔴 **Jugulo-omohyoid**	🟣 **Retropharyngeal**	🔵 **Lingual tonsil**
🟠 **Jugulodigastric**	🔴 **Pharyngeal tonsil**	➤ **Internodal group drainage**
🩷 **Infrahyoid**	🟡 **Palatine tonsil**	

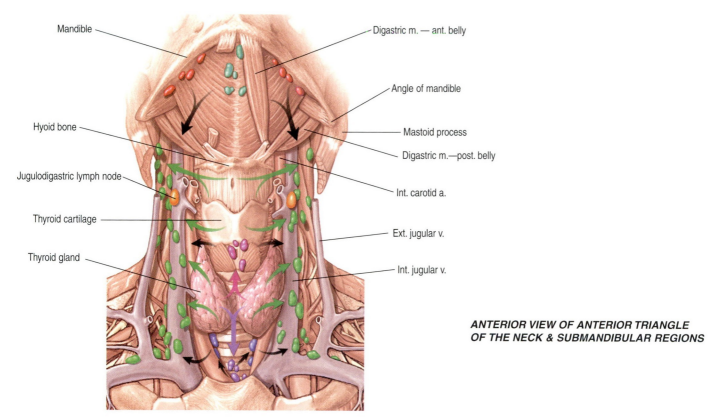

Mandible

Hyoid bone

Jugulodigastric lymph node

Thyroid cartilage

Thyroid gland

Digastric m. — ant. belly

Angle of mandible

Mastoid process

Digastric m.—post. belly

Int. carotid a.

Ext. jugular v.

Int. jugular v.

*ANTERIOR VIEW OF ANTERIOR TRIANGLE
OF THE NECK & SUBMANDIBULAR REGIONS*

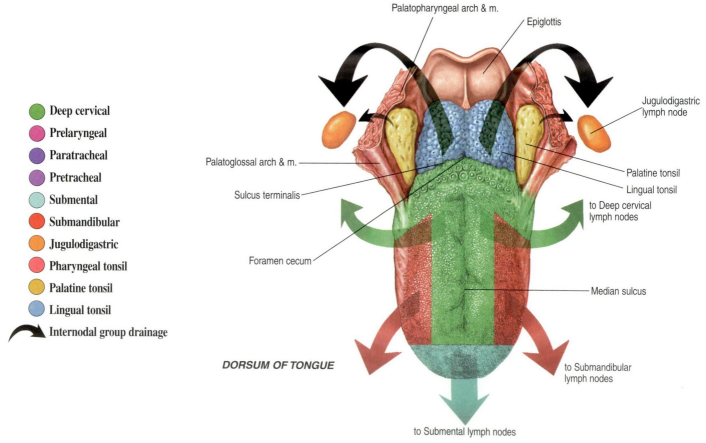

Palatopharyngeal arch & m.

Epiglottis

Jugulodigastric lymph node

Palatoglossal arch & m.

Palatine tonsil

Lingual tonsil

Sulcus terminalis

to Deep cervical lymph nodes

Foramen cecum

Median sulcus

to Submandibular lymph nodes

to Submental lymph nodes

DORSUM OF TONGUE

- ● Deep cervical
- ● Prelaryngeal
- ● Paratracheal
- ● Pretracheal
- ● Submental
- ● Submandibular
- ● Jugulodigastric
- ● Pharyngeal tonsil
- ● Palatine tonsil
- ● Lingual tonsil
- ➤ Internodal group drainage

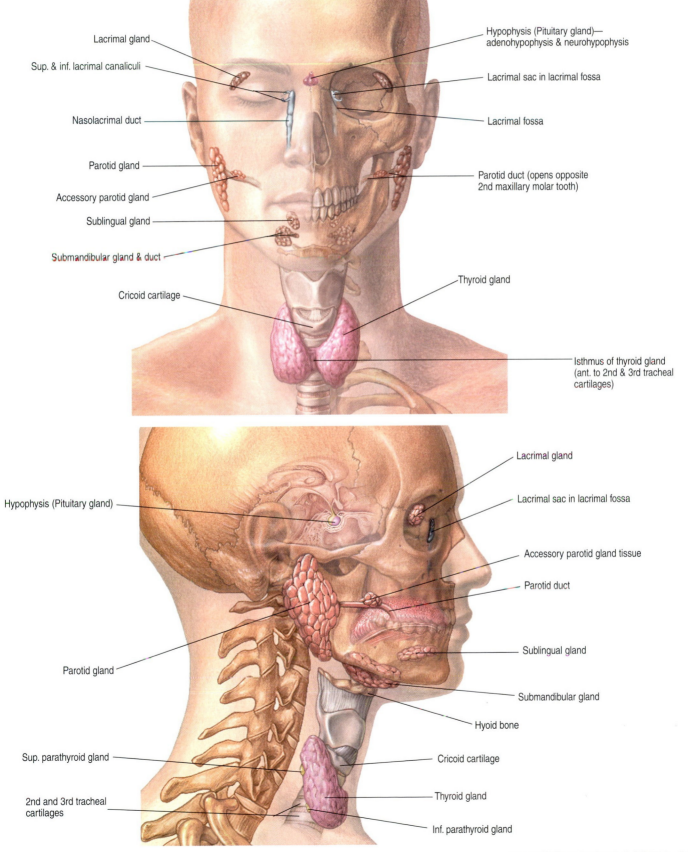

Lacrimal gland

Sup. & inf. lacrimal canaliculi

Nasolacrimal duct

Parotid gland

Accessory parotid gland

Sublingual gland

Submandibular gland & duct

Cricoid cartilage

Hypophysis (Pituitary gland)—adenohypophysis & neurohypophysis

Lacrimal sac in lacrimal fossa

Lacrimal fossa

Parotid duct (opens opposite 2nd maxillary molar tooth)

Thyroid gland

Isthmus of thyroid gland (ant. to 2nd & 3rd tracheal cartilages)

Hypophysis (Pituitary gland)

Parotid gland

Sup. parathyroid gland

2nd and 3rd tracheal cartilages

Lacrimal gland

Lacrimal sac in lacrimal fossa

Accessory parotid gland tissue

Parotid duct

Sublingual gland

Submandibular gland

Hyoid bone

Cricoid cartilage

Thyroid gland

Inf. parathyroid gland

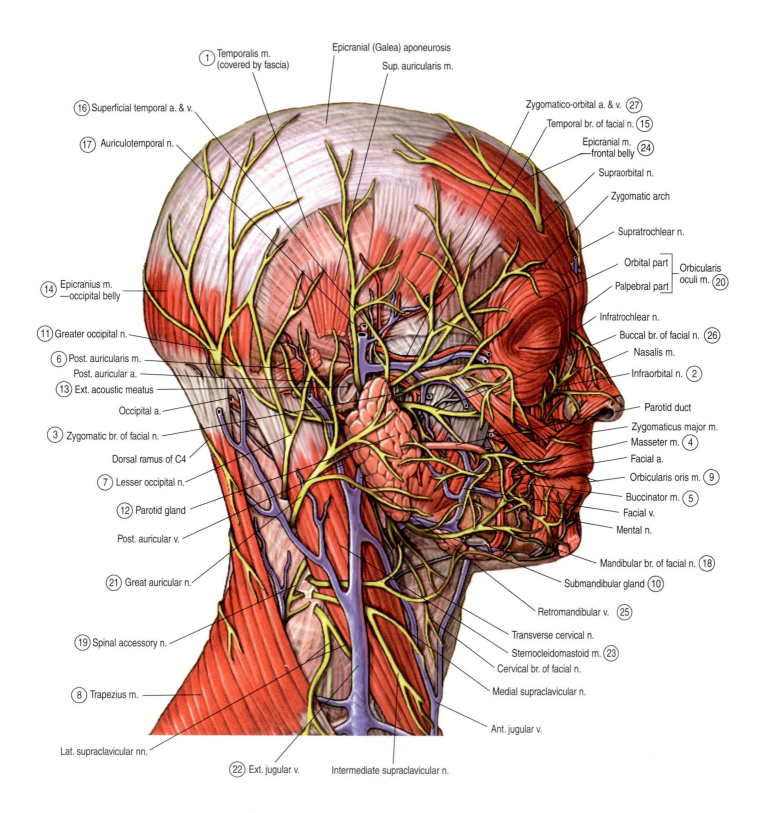

① Temporalis m. (covered by fascia)

Epicranial (Galea) aponeurosis

Sup. auricularis m.

⑯ Superficial temporal a. & v.

⑰ Auriculotemporal n.

Zygomatico-orbital a. & v. ㉗

Temporal br. of facial n. ⑮

Epicranial m. ㉔ —frontal belly

Supraorbital n.

Zygomatic arch

Supratrochlear n.

Orbital part ⎱ Orbicularis
Palpebral part ⎰ oculi m. ⑳

⑭ Epicranius m. —occipital belly

Infratrochlear n.

Buccal br. of facial n. ㉖

⑪ Greater occipital n.

Nasalis m.

⑥ Post. auricularis m.

Infraorbital n. ②

Post. auricular a.

⑬ Ext. acoustic meatus

Occipital a.

Parotid duct

Zygomaticus major m.

③ Zygomatic br. of facial n.

Masseter m. ④

Dorsal ramus of C4

Facial a.

Orbicularis oris m. ⑨

⑦ Lesser occipital n.

Buccinator m. ⑤

⑫ Parotid gland

Facial v.

Post. auricular v.

Mental n.

Mandibular br. of facial n. ⑱

㉑ Great auricular n.

Submandibular gland ⑩

Retromandibular v. ㉕

⑲ Spinal accessory n.

Transverse cervical n.

Sternocleidomastoid m. ㉓

Cervical br. of facial n.

Medial supraclavicular n.

⑧ Trapezius m.

Ant. jugular v.

Lat. supraclavicular nn.

㉒ Ext. jugular v.

Intermediate supraclavicular n.

LATERAL VIEW

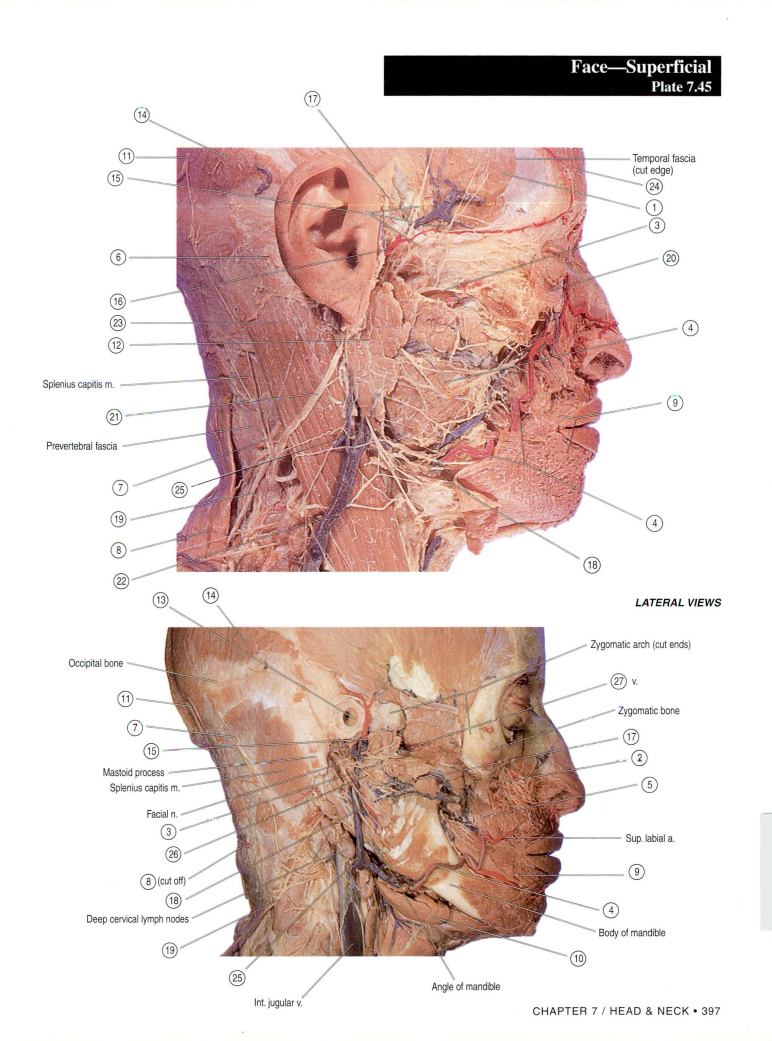

Temporal fascia (cut edge)

Splenius capitis m.

Prevertebral fascia

LATERAL VIEWS

Occipital bone

Zygomatic arch (cut ends)

Zygomatic bone

Mastoid process
Splenius capitis m.

Facial n.

Sup. labial a.

Deep cervical lymph nodes

Body of mandible

Angle of mandible

Int. jugular v.

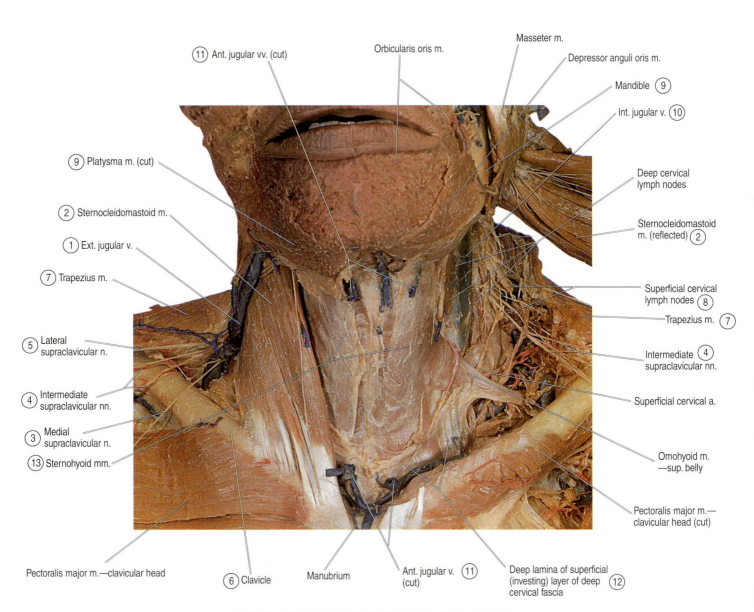

⑪ Ant. jugular vv. (cut)

Orbicularis oris m.

Masseter m.

Depressor anguli oris m.

Mandible ⑨

Int. jugular v. ⑩

Deep cervical lymph nodes

Sternocleidomastoid m. (reflected) ②

⑨ Platysma m. (cut)

② Sternocleidomastoid m.

① Ext. jugular v.

⑦ Trapezius m.

Superficial cervical lymph nodes ⑧

Trapezius m. ⑦

⑤ Lateral supraclavicular n.

Intermediate ④ supraclavicular nn.

④ Intermediate supraclavicular nn.

Superficial cervical a.

③ Medial supraclavicular n.

⑬ Sternohyoid mm.

Omohyoid m. —sup. belly

Pectoralis major m.— clavicular head (cut)

Pectoralis major m.—clavicular head

⑥ Clavicle

Manubrium

Ant. jugular v. ⑪ (cut)

Deep lamina of superficial (investing) layer of deep cervical fascia ⑫

**ANTERIOR VIEW OF NECK WITH DEEPER STRUCTURES
EXPOSED ON LEFT SIDE**

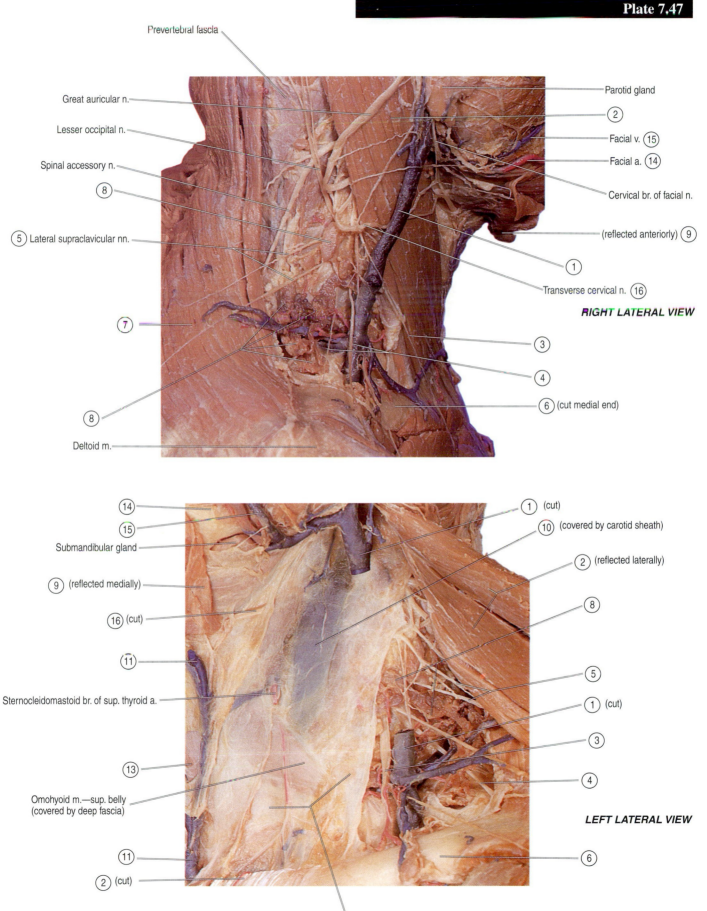

Prevertebral fascia

Great auricular n.

Lesser occipital n.

Spinal accessory n.

⑧

⑤ Lateral supraclavicular nn.

⑦

⑧

Deltoid m.

Parotid gland

②

Facial v. ⑮

Facial a. ⑭

Cervical br. of facial n.

(reflected anteriorly) ⑨

①

Transverse cervical n. ⑯

RIGHT LATERAL VIEW

③

④

⑥ (cut medial end)

⑭
⑮

Submandibular gland

⑨ (reflected medially)

⑯ (cut)

⑪

Sternocleidomastoid br. of sup. thyroid a.

⑬

Omohyoid m.—sup. belly
(covered by deep fascia)

⑪

② (cut)

① (cut)

⑩ (covered by carotid sheath)

② (reflected laterally)

⑧

⑤

① (cut)

③

④

LEFT LATERAL VIEW

⑥

⑫

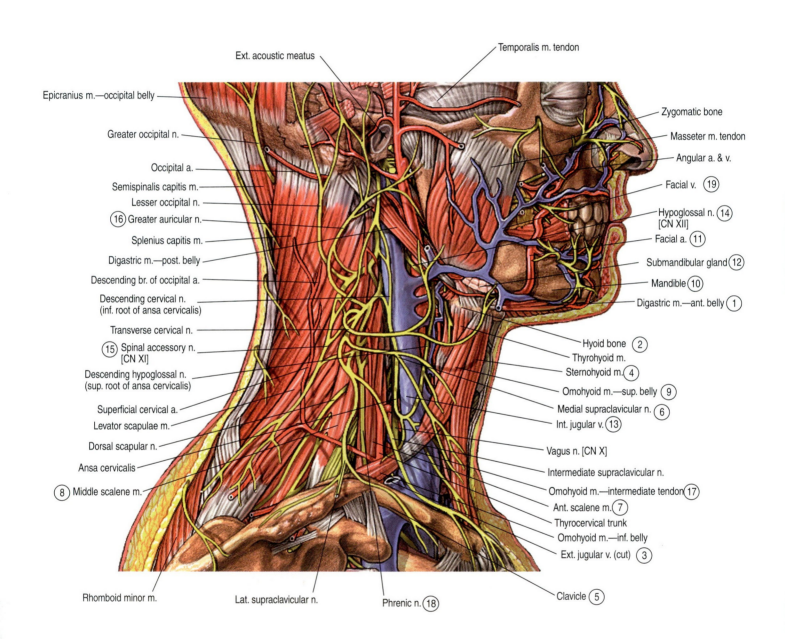

Ext. acoustic meatus

Temporalis m. tendon

Epicranius m.—occipital belly

Zygomatic bone

Greater occipital n.

Masseter m. tendon

Occipital a.

Angular a. & v.

Semispinalis capitis m.

Facial v. (19)

Lesser occipital n.

Hypoglossal n. (14)
[CN XII]

(16) Greater auricular n.

Facial a. (11)

Splenius capitis m.

Submandibular gland (12)

Digastric m.—post. belly

Mandible (10)

Descending br. of occipital a.

Digastric m.—ant. belly (1)

Descending cervical n.
(inf. root of ansa cervicalis)

Transverse cervical n.

Hyoid bone (2)

(15) Spinal accessory n.
[CN XI]

Thyrohyoid m.

Sternohyoid m. (4)

Descending hypoglossal n.
(sup. root of ansa cervicalis)

Omohyoid m.—sup. belly (9)

Medial supraclavicular n. (6)

Superficial cervical a.

Int. jugular v. (13)

Levator scapulae m.

Dorsal scapular n.

Vagus n. [CN X]

Ansa cervicalis

Intermediate supraclavicular n.

(8) Middle scalene m.

Omohyoid m.—intermediate tendon (17)

Ant. scalene m. (7)

Thyrocervical trunk

Omohyoid m.—inf. belly

Ext. jugular v. (cut) (3)

Rhomboid minor m.

Lat. supraclavicular n.

Phrenic n. (18)

Clavicle (5)

LATERAL VIEW

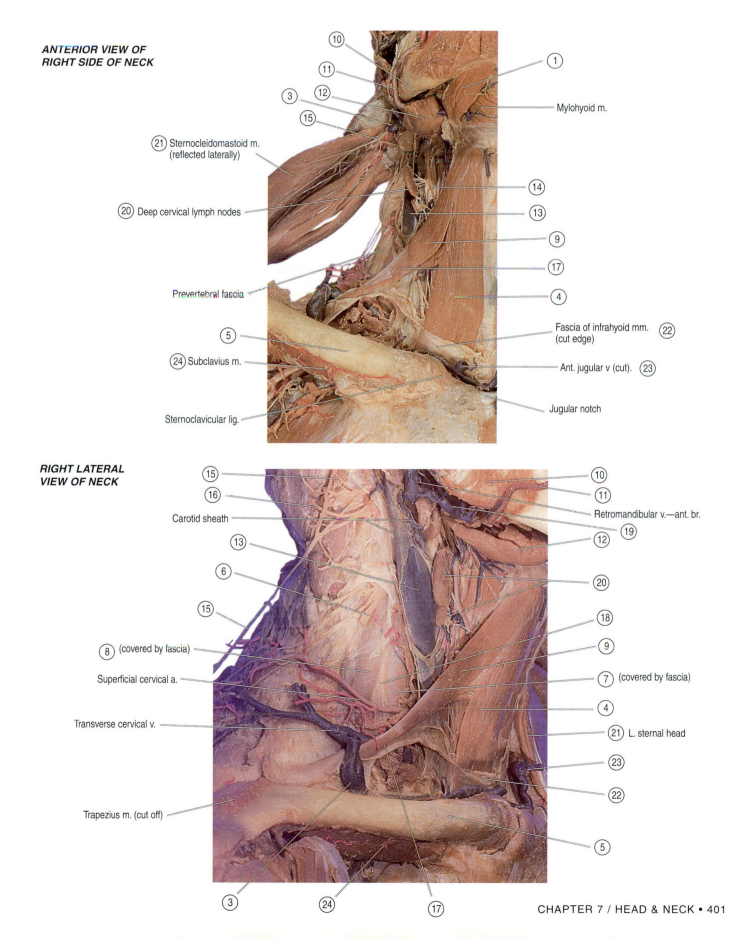

ANTERIOR VIEW OF
RIGHT SIDE OF NECK

⑩
⑪
③ ⑫
⑮
① — Mylohyoid m.
㉑ Sternocleidomastoid m.
(reflected laterally)
⑳ Deep cervical lymph nodes
⑭
⑬
⑨
⑰
④
Prevertebral fascia
⑤
㉔ Subclavius m.
Fascia of infrahyoid mm. ㉒
(cut edge)
Ant. jugular v (cut). ㉓
Sternoclavicular lig.
Jugular notch

RIGHT LATERAL
VIEW OF NECK

⑮
⑯
Carotid sheath
⑬
⑥
⑮
⑧ (covered by fascia)
Superficial cervical a.
Transverse cervical v.
Trapezius m. (cut off)

⑩
⑪
Retromandibular v.—ant. br.
⑫
⑲
⑳
⑱
⑨
⑦ (covered by fascia)
④
㉑ L. sternal head
㉓
㉒
⑤

③ ㉔ ⑰

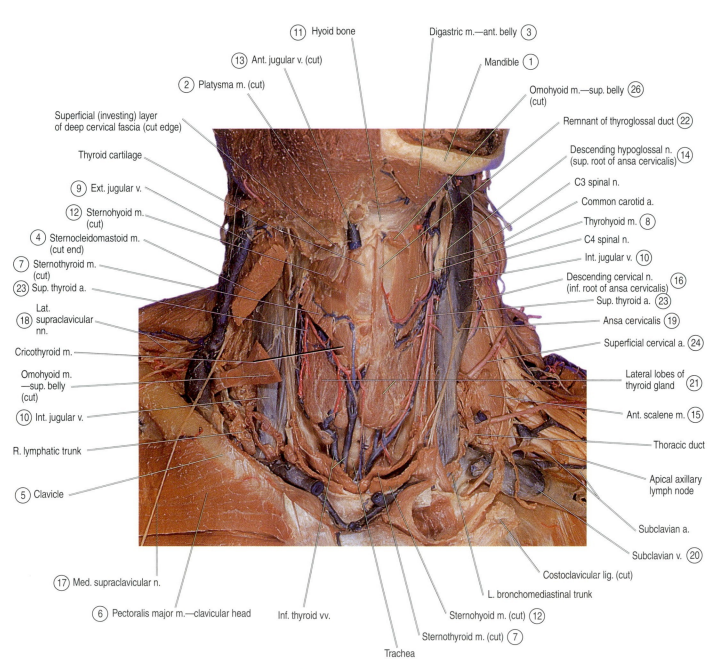

(11) Hyoid bone

(13) Ant. jugular v. (cut)

(2) Platysma m. (cut)

Superficial (investing) layer
of deep cervical fascia (cut edge)

Thyroid cartilage

(9) Ext. jugular v.

(12) Sternohyoid m. (cut)

(4) Sternocleidomastoid m. (cut end)

(7) Sternothyroid m. (cut)

(23) Sup. thyroid a.

Lat. (18) supraclavicular nn.

Cricothyroid m.

Omohyoid m. —sup. belly (cut)

(10) Int. jugular v.

R. lymphatic trunk

(5) Clavicle

(17) Med. supraclavicular n.

(6) Pectoralis major m.—clavicular head

Inf. thyroid vv.

Trachea

Sternothyroid m. (cut) (7)

Sternohyoid m. (cut) (12)

L. bronchomediastinal trunk

Costoclavicular lig. (cut)

Subclavian v. (20)

Subclavian a.

Apical axillary lymph node

Thoracic duct

Ant. scalene m. (15)

Lateral lobes of thyroid gland (21)

Superficial cervical a. (24)

Ansa cervicalis (19)

Sup. thyroid a. (23)

Descending cervical n. (inf. root of ansa cervicalis) (16)

Int. jugular v. (10)

C4 spinal n.

Thyrohyoid m. (8)

Common carotid a.

C3 spinal n.

Descending hypoglossal n. (sup. root of ansa cervicalis) (14)

Remnant of thyroglossal duct (22)

Omohyoid m.—sup. belly (26) (cut)

Mandible (1)

Digastric m.—ant. belly (3)

**ANTERIOR VIEW OF NECK
WITH DEEP STRUCTURES ON RIGHT SIDE**

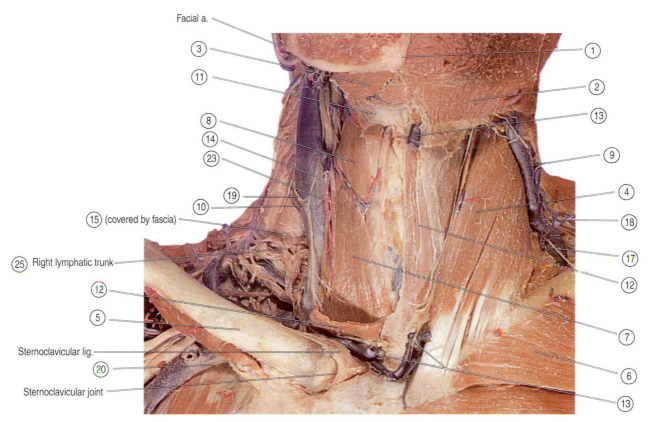

Facial a.

③
⑪
⑧
⑭
㉓
⑲
⑩
⑮ (covered by fascia)
㉕ Right lymphatic trunk
⑫
⑤
Sternoclavicular lig.
⑳
Sternoclavicular joint

①
②
⑬
⑨
④
⑱
⑰
⑫
⑦
⑥
⑬

**ANTERIOR VIEW OF NECK WITH DEEPER STRUCTURES
ON RIGHT SIDE**

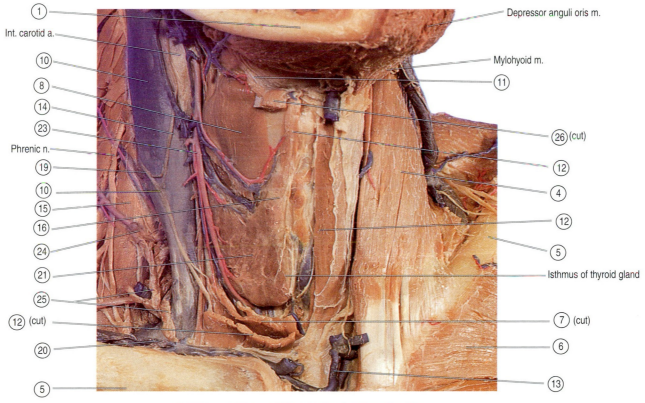

①
Int. carotid a.
⑩
⑧
⑭
㉓
Phrenic n.
⑲
⑩
⑮
⑯
㉔
㉑
㉕
⑫ (cut)
⑳
⑤

Depressor anguli oris m.
Mylohyoid m.
⑪
㉖ (cut)
⑫
④
⑫
⑤
Isthmus of thyroid gland
⑦ (cut)
⑥
⑬

ANTEROLATERAL VIEW OF RIGHT SIDE OF NECK

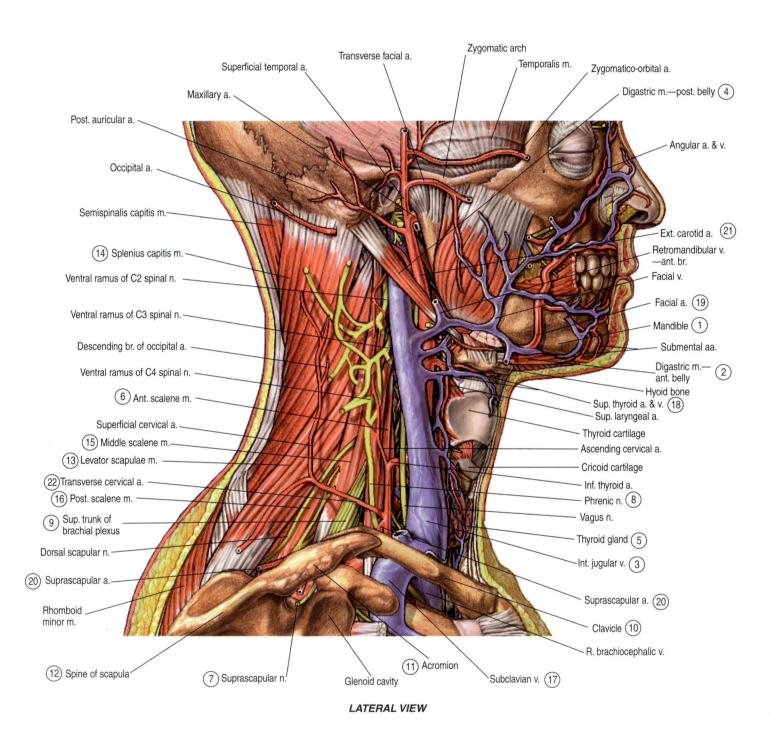

Superficial temporal a.

Transverse facial a.

Zygomatic arch

Temporalis m.

Zygomatico-orbital a.

Maxillary a.

Digastric m.—post. belly (4)

Post. auricular a.

Angular a. & v.

Occipital a.

Semispinalis capitis m.

Ext. carotid a. (21)

(14) Splenius capitis m.

Retromandibular v.—ant. br.

Ventral ramus of C2 spinal n.

Facial v.

Ventral ramus of C3 spinal n.

Facial a. (19)

Descending br. of occipital a.

Mandible (1)

Ventral ramus of C4 spinal n.

Submental aa.

(6) Ant. scalene m.

Digastric m.—ant. belly (2)

Hyoid bone

Superficial cervical a.

Sup. thyroid a. & v. (18)

(15) Middle scalene m.

Sup. laryngeal a.

Thyroid cartilage

(13) Levator scapulae m.

Ascending cervical a.

(22) Transverse cervical a.

Cricoid cartilage

(16) Post. scalene m.

Inf. thyroid a.

Phrenic n. (8)

(9) Sup. trunk of brachial plexus

Vagus n.

Dorsal scapular n.

Thyroid gland (5)

(20) Suprascapular a.

Int. jugular v. (3)

Rhomboid minor m.

Suprascapular a. (20)

Clavicle (10)

R. brachiocephalic v.

(12) Spine of scapula

(7) Suprascapular n.

Glenoid cavity

(11) Acromion

Subclavian v. (17)

LATERAL VIEW

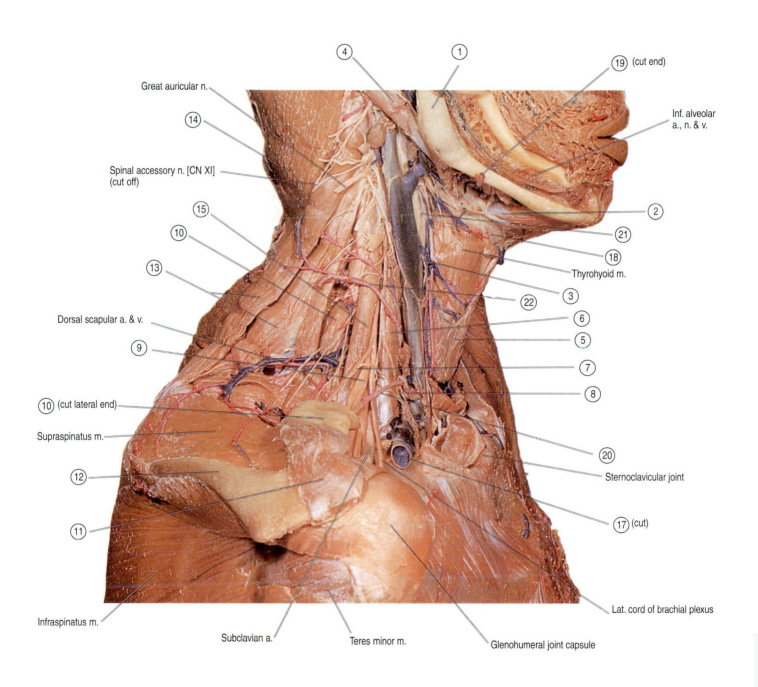

Great auricular n.

Spinal accessory n. [CN XI]
(cut off)

Dorsal scapular a. & v.

Supraspinatus m.

Infraspinatus m.

Inf. alveolar
a., n. & v.

Thyrohyoid m.

Sternoclavicular joint

Lat. cord of brachial plexus

Subclavian a.

Teres minor m.

Glenohumeral joint capsule

(19) (cut end)

(10) (cut lateral end)

(17) (cut)

LATERAL VIEW

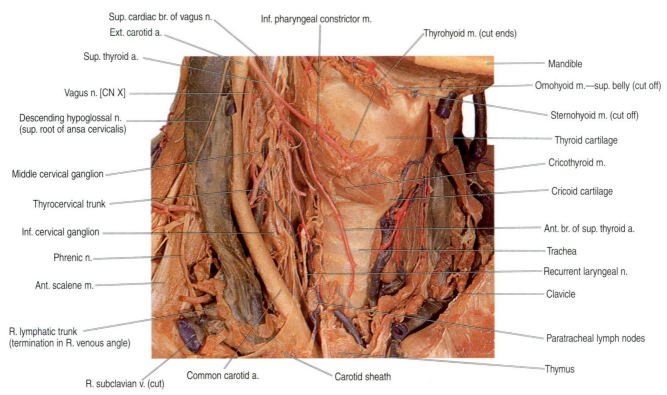

Sup. cardiac br. of vagus n.

Ext. carotid a.

Sup. thyroid a.

Vagus n. [CN X]

Descending hypoglossal n.
(sup. root of ansa cervicalis)

Middle cervical ganglion

Thyrocervical trunk

Inf. cervical ganglion

Phrenic n.

Ant. scalene m.

R. lymphatic trunk
(termination in R. venous angle)

R. subclavian v. (cut)

Common carotid a.

Inf. pharyngeal constrictor m.

Thyrohyoid m. (cut ends)

Mandible

Omohyoid m.—sup. belly (cut off)

Sternohyoid m. (cut off)

Thyroid cartilage

Cricothyroid m.

Cricoid cartilage

Ant. br. of sup. thyroid a.

Trachea

Recurrent laryngeal n.

Clavicle

Paratracheal lymph nodes

Thymus

Carotid sheath

ANTEROLATERAL VIEW OF RELATIONSHIPS OF LARYNX

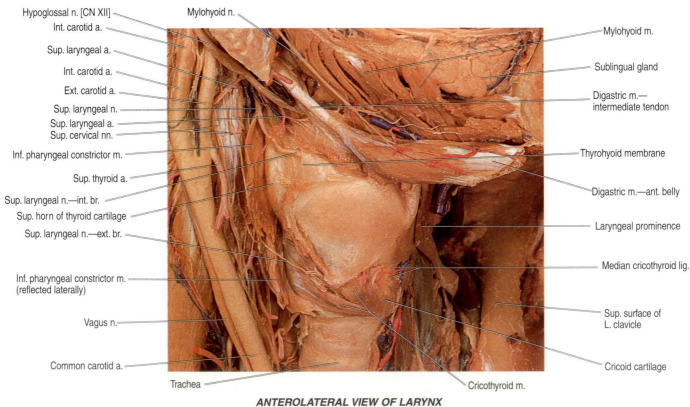

Hypoglossal n. [CN XII]

Int. carotid a.

Sup. laryngeal a.

Int. carotid a.

Ext. carotid a.

Sup. laryngeal n.

Sup. laryngeal a.

Sup. cervical nn.

Inf. pharyngeal constrictor m.

Sup. thyroid a.

Sup. laryngeal n.—int. br.

Sup. horn of thyroid cartilage

Sup. laryngeal n.—ext. br.

Inf. pharyngeal constrictor m.
(reflected laterally)

Vagus n.

Common carotid a.

Trachea

Mylohyoid n.

Mylohyoid m.

Sublingual gland

Digastric m.—
intermediate tendon

Thyrohyoid membrane

Digastric m.—ant. belly

Laryngeal prominence

Median cricothyroid lig.

Sup. surface of
L. clavicle

Cricoid cartilage

Cricothyroid m.

**ANTEROLATERAL VIEW OF LARYNX
WITH BODY OF MANDIBLE REMOVED**

ANTEROLATERAL VIEW OF LARYNX

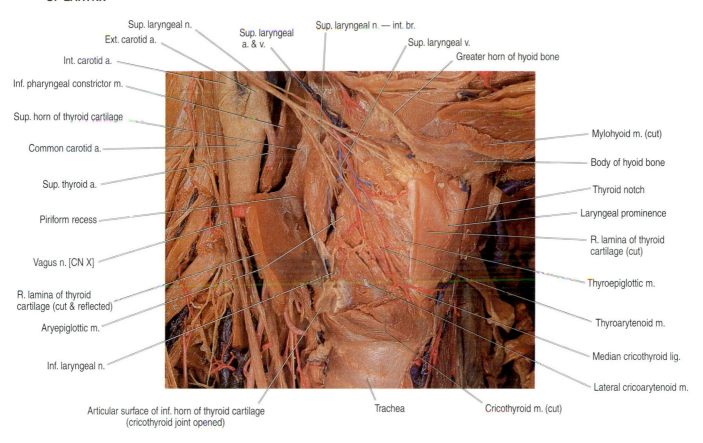

- Sup. laryngeal n.
- Ext. carotid a.
- Int. carotid a.
- Inf. pharyngeal constrictor m.
- Sup. horn of thyroid cartilage
- Common carotid a.
- Sup. thyroid a.
- Piriform recess
- Vagus n. [CN X]
- R. lamina of thyroid cartilage (cut & reflected)
- Aryepiglottic m.
- Inf. laryngeal n.
- Sup. laryngeal a. & v.
- Sup. laryngeal n. — int. br.
- Sup. laryngeal v.
- Greater horn of hyoid bone
- Mylohyoid m. (cut)
- Body of hyoid bone
- Thyroid notch
- Laryngeal prominence
- R. lamina of thyroid cartilage (cut)
- Thyroepiglottic m.
- Thyroarytenoid m.
- Median cricothyroid lig.
- Lateral cricoarytenoid m.
- Articular surface of inf. horn of thyroid cartilage (cricothyroid joint opened)
- Trachea
- Cricothyroid m. (cut)

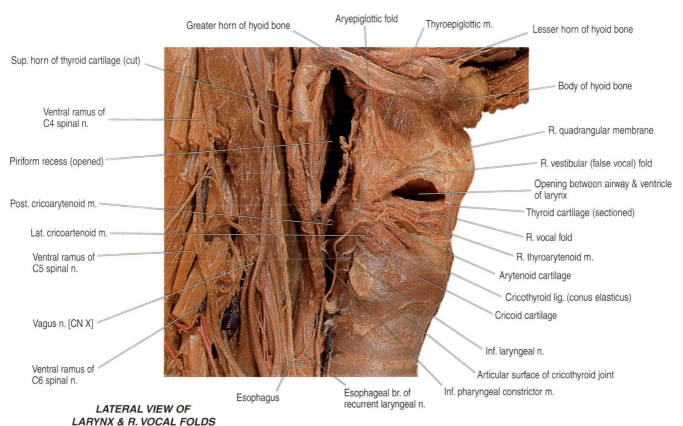

- Sup. horn of thyroid cartilage (cut)
- Ventral ramus of C4 spinal n.
- Piriform recess (opened)
- Post. cricoarytenoid m.
- Lat. cricoartenoid m.
- Ventral ramus of C5 spinal n.
- Vagus n. [CN X]
- Ventral ramus of C6 spinal n.
- Greater horn of hyoid bone
- Aryepiglottic fold
- Thyroepiglottic m.
- Lesser horn of hyoid bone
- Body of hyoid bone
- R. quadrangular membrane
- R. vestibular (false vocal) fold
- Opening between airway & ventricle of larynx
- Thyroid cartilage (sectioned)
- R. vocal fold
- R. thyroarytenoid m.
- Arytenoid cartilage
- Cricothyroid lig. (conus elasticus)
- Cricoid cartilage
- Inf. laryngeal n.
- Articular surface of cricothyroid joint
- Inf. pharyngeal constrictor m.
- Esophagus
- Esophageal br. of recurrent laryngeal n.

LATERAL VIEW OF LARYNX & R. VOCAL FOLDS

POSTERIOR VIEW OF LARYNX

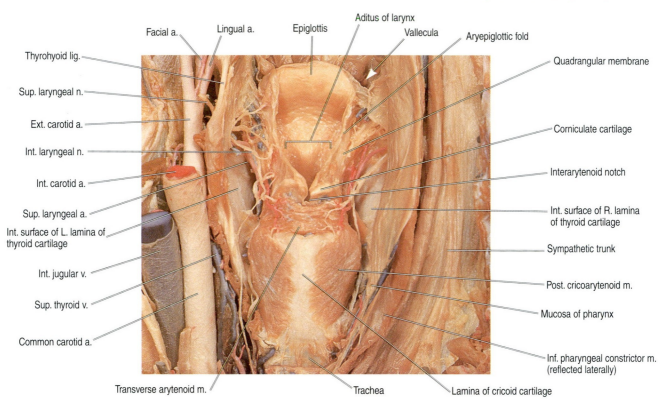

Facial a.

Lingual a.

Epiglottis

Aditus of larynx

Vallecula

Aryepiglottic fold

Thyrohyoid lig.

Sup. laryngeal n.

Ext. carotid a.

Int. laryngeal n.

Int. carotid a.

Sup. laryngeal a.

Int. surface of L. lamina of thyroid cartilage

Int. jugular v.

Sup. thyroid v.

Common carotid a.

Quadrangular membrane

Corniculate cartilage

Interarytenoid notch

Int. surface of R. lamina of thyroid cartilage

Sympathetic trunk

Post. cricoarytenoid m.

Mucosa of pharynx

Inf. pharyngeal constrictor m. (reflected laterally)

Transverse arytenoid m.

Trachea

Lamina of cricoid cartilage

ANTERIOR

Epiglottis

Sup. laryngeal v.

SUPERIOR VIEW OF LARYNX

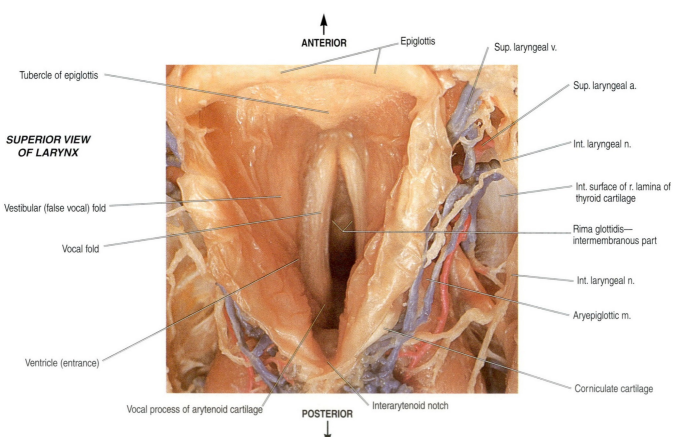

Tubercle of epiglottis

Vestibular (false vocal) fold

Vocal fold

Ventricle (entrance)

Sup. laryngeal a.

Int. laryngeal n.

Int. surface of r. lamina of thyroid cartilage

Rima glottidis— intermembranous part

Int. laryngeal n.

Aryepiglottic m.

Corniculate cartilage

Vocal process of arytenoid cartilage

POSTERIOR

Interarytenoid notch

MEDIAL VIEW OF LEFT HALF OF LARYNX

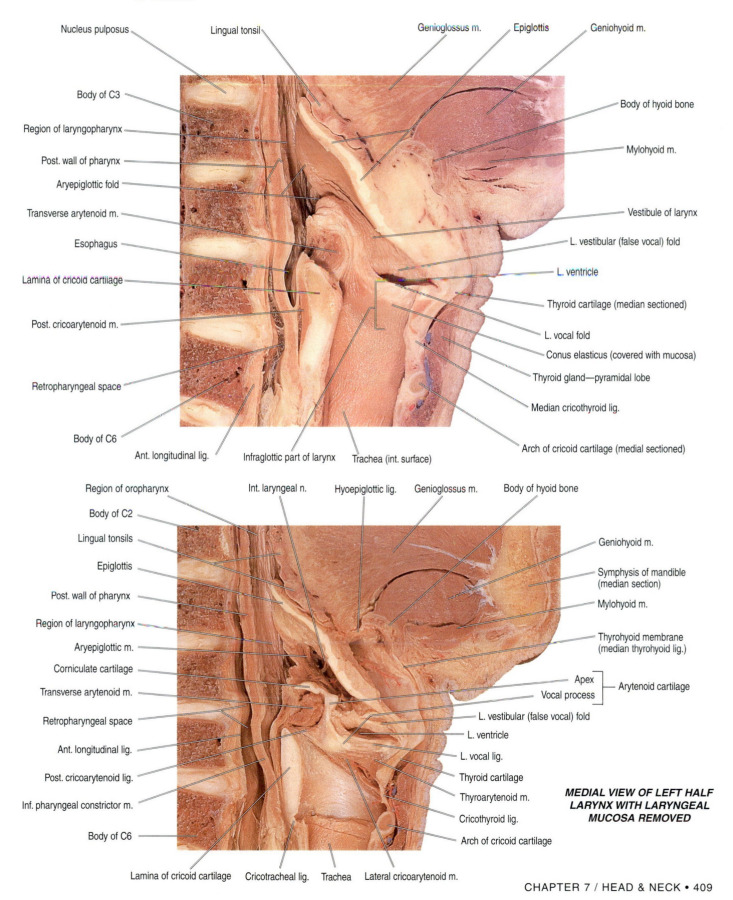

Nucleus pulposus

Lingual tonsil

Genioglossus m.

Epiglottis

Geniohyoid m.

Body of C3

Body of hyoid bone

Region of laryngopharynx

Mylohyoid m.

Post. wall of pharynx

Aryepiglottic fold

Vestibule of larynx

Transverse arytenoid m.

L. vestibular (false vocal) fold

Esophagus

L. ventricle

Lamina of cricoid cartilage

Thyroid cartilage (median sectioned)

Post. cricoarytenoid m.

L. vocal fold

Conus elasticus (covered with mucosa)

Thyroid gland—pyramidal lobe

Retropharyngeal space

Median cricothyroid lig.

Body of C6

Arch of cricoid cartilage (medial sectioned)

Ant. longitudinal lig.

Infraglottic part of larynx

Trachea (int. surface)

Region of oropharynx

Int. laryngeal n.

Hyoepiglottic lig.

Genioglossus m.

Body of hyoid bone

Body of C2

Lingual tonsils

Geniohyoid m.

Epiglottis

Symphysis of mandible (median section)

Post. wall of pharynx

Mylohyoid m.

Region of laryngopharynx

Thyrohyoid membrane (median thyrohyoid lig.)

Aryepiglottic m.

Corniculate cartilage

Apex

Arytenoid cartilage

Transverse arytenoid m.

Vocal process

Retropharyngeal space

L. vestibular (false vocal) fold

Ant. longitudinal lig.

L. ventricle

Post. cricoarytenoid lig.

L. vocal lig.

Inf. pharyngeal constrictor m.

Thyroid cartilage

Thyroarytenoid m.

Body of C6

Cricothyroid lig.

Arch of cricoid cartilage

Lamina of cricoid cartilage

Cricotracheal lig.

Trachea

Lateral cricoarytenoid m.

MEDIAL VIEW OF LEFT HALF LARYNX WITH LARYNGEAL MUCOSA REMOVED

**POSTERIOR VIEW OF POST. WALL
OF PHARYNX & ESOPHAGUS**

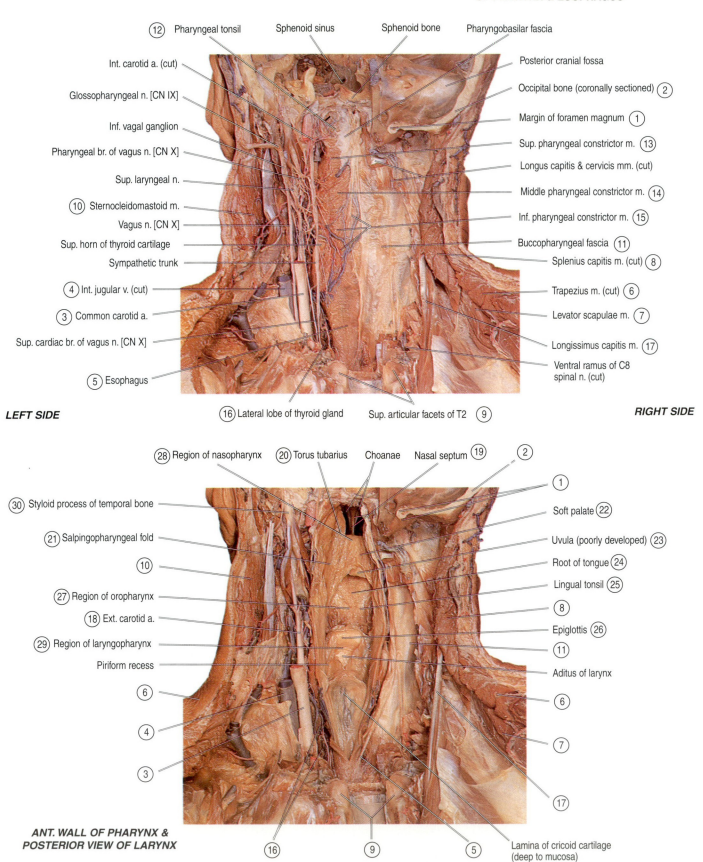

⑫ Pharyngeal tonsil
Sphenoid sinus
Sphenoid bone
Pharyngobasilar fascia

Int. carotid a. (cut)

Glossopharyngeal n. [CN IX]

Inf. vagal ganglion

Pharyngeal br. of vagus n. [CN X]

Sup. laryngeal n.

⑩ Sternocleidomastoid m.

Vagus n. [CN X]

Sup. horn of thyroid cartilage

Sympathetic trunk

④ Int. jugular v. (cut)

③ Common carotid a.

Sup. cardiac br. of vagus n. [CN X]

⑤ Esophagus

Posterior cranial fossa

Occipital bone (coronally sectioned) ②

Margin of foramen magnum ①

Sup. pharyngeal constrictor m. ⑬

Longus capitis & cervicis mm. (cut)

Middle pharyngeal constrictor m. ⑭

Inf. pharyngeal constrictor m. ⑮

Buccopharyngeal fascia ⑪

Splenius capitis m. (cut) ⑧

Trapezius m. (cut) ⑥

Levator scapulae m. ⑦

Longissimus capitis m. ⑰

Ventral ramus of C8
spinal n. (cut)

LEFT SIDE

⑯ Lateral lobe of thyroid gland
Sup. articular facets of T2 ⑨

RIGHT SIDE

⑱ Region of nasopharynx
⑳ Torus tubarius
Choanae
Nasal septum ⑲
②

①

⑳ Styloid process of temporal bone

㉑ Salpingopharyngeal fold

⑩

㉗ Region of oropharynx

⑱ Ext. carotid a.

㉙ Region of laryngopharynx

Piriform recess

⑥

④

③

Soft palate ㉒

Uvula (poorly developed) ㉓

Root of tongue ㉔

Lingual tonsil ㉕

⑧

Epiglottis ㉖

⑪

Aditus of larynx

⑥

⑦

⑰

**ANT. WALL OF PHARYNX &
POSTERIOR VIEW OF LARYNX**

⑯
⑨
⑤
Lamina of cricoid cartilage
(deep to mucosa)

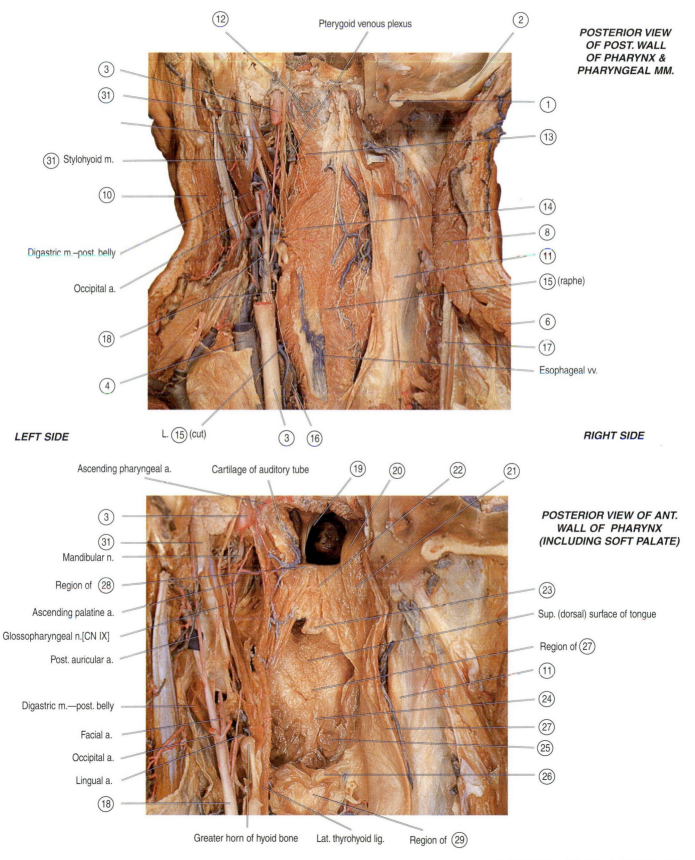

POSTERIOR VIEW OF POST. WALL OF PHARYNX & PHARYNGEAL MM.

12 — Pterygoid venous plexus — 2

3
31
31 Stylohoid m.
10
Digastric m.—post. belly
Occipital a.
18
4

1
13
14
8
11
15 (raphe)
6
17
Esophageal vv.

LEFT SIDE

L. 15 (cut) — 3 — 16

RIGHT SIDE

Ascending pharyngeal a. — Cartilage of auditory tube — 19 — 20 — 22 — 21

POSTERIOR VIEW OF ANT. WALL OF PHARYNX (INCLUDING SOFT PALATE)

3
31
Mandibular n.
Region of 28
Ascending palatine a.
Glossopharyngeal n.[CN IX]
Post. auricular a.
Digastric m.—post. belly
Facial a.
Occipital a.
Lingual a.
18

23
Sup. (dorsal) surface of tongue
Region of 27
11
24
27
25
26

Greater horn of hyoid bone — Lat. thyrohyoid lig. — Region of 29

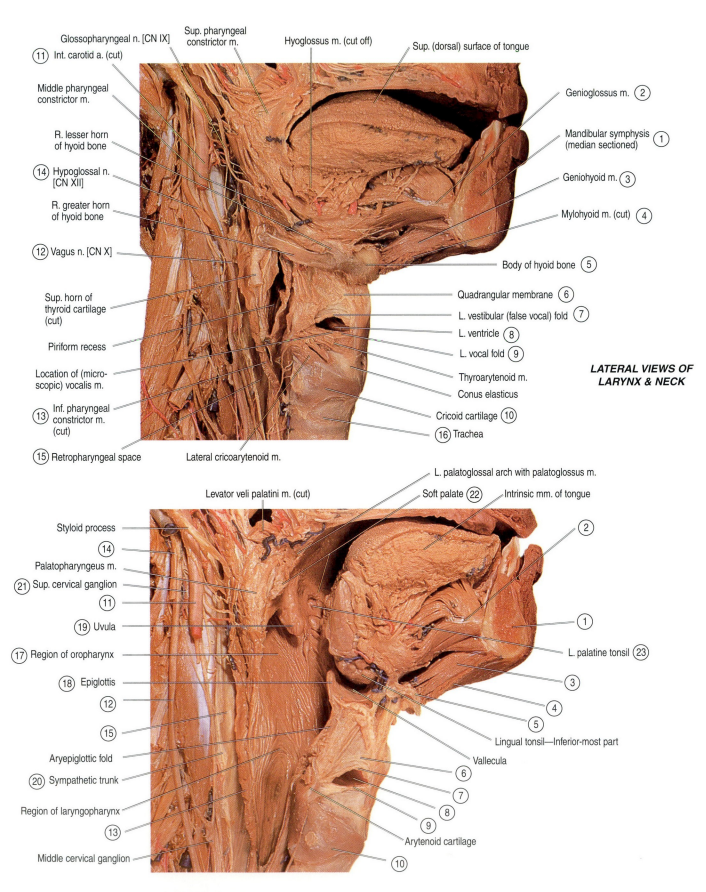

Glossopharyngeal n. [CN IX]

Sup. pharyngeal constrictor m.

Hyoglossus m. (cut off)

Sup. (dorsal) surface of tongue

⑪ Int. carotid a. (cut)

Middle pharyngeal constrictor m.

R. lesser horn of hyoid bone

⑭ Hypoglossal n. [CN XII]

R. greater horn of hyoid bone

⑫ Vagus n. [CN X]

Sup. horn of thyroid cartilage (cut)

Piriform recess

Location of (microscopic) vocalis m.

⑬ Inf. pharyngeal constrictor m. (cut)

⑮ Retropharyngeal space

Lateral cricoarytenoid m.

Genioglossus m. ②

Mandibular symphysis (median sectioned) ①

Geniohyoid m. ③

Mylohyoid m. (cut) ④

Body of hyoid bone ⑤

Quadrangular membrane ⑥

L. vestibular (false vocal) fold ⑦

L. ventricle ⑧

L. vocal fold ⑨

Thyroarytenoid m.

Conus elasticus

Cricoid cartilage ⑩

⑯ Trachea

LATERAL VIEWS OF LARYNX & NECK

Levator veli palatini m. (cut)

L. palatoglossal arch with palatoglossus m.

Soft palate ㉒

Intrinsic mm. of tongue

Styloid process

⑭

Palatopharyngeus m.

㉑ Sup. cervical ganglion

⑪

⑲ Uvula

⑰ Region of oropharynx

⑱ Epiglottis

⑫

⑮

Aryepiglottic fold

⑳ Sympathetic trunk

Region of laryngopharynx

⑬

Middle cervical ganglion

②

①

L. palatine tonsil ㉓

③

④

⑤

Lingual tonsil—Inferior-most part

Vallecula

⑥

⑦

⑧

⑨

Arytenoid cartilage

⑩

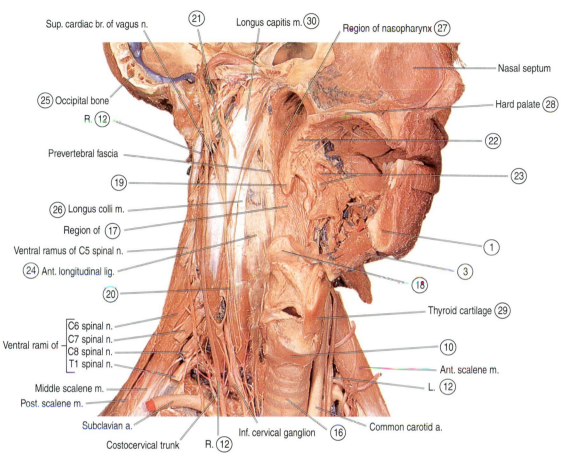

Sup. cardiac br. of vagus n.
(21)
Longus capitis m. (30)
Region of nasopharynx (27)
Nasal septum

(25) Occipital bone
R. (12)
Hard palate (28)

Prevertebral fascia
(22)

(19)
(23)

(26) Longus colli m.
Region of (17)
Ventral ramus of C5 spinal n.
(1)

(24) Ant. longitudinal lig.
(3)

(20)
(18)

Thyroid cartilage (29)

C6 spinal n.
C7 spinal n.
Ventral rami of — C8 spinal n.
T1 spinal n.
(10)

Middle scalene m.
Ant. scalene m.
L. (12)

Post. scalene m.

Subclavian a.
Inf. cervical ganglion
(16)
Common carotid a.

Costocervical trunk
R. (12)

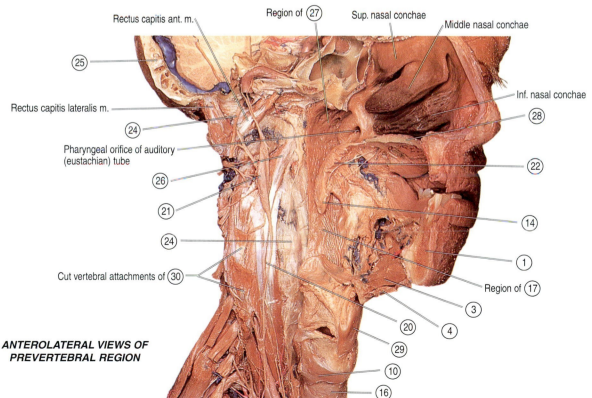

Rectus capitis ant. m.
Region of (27)
Sup. nasal conchae
Middle nasal conchae

(25)

Rectus capitis lateralis m.
Inf. nasal conchae

(24)
(28)

Pharyngeal orifice of auditory
(eustachian) tube
(22)

(26)

(21)
(14)

(24)
(1)

Cut vertebral attachments of (30)
Region of (17)

(3)

(20)
(4)

**ANTEROLATERAL VIEWS OF
PREVERTEBRAL REGION**
(29)

(10)

(16)

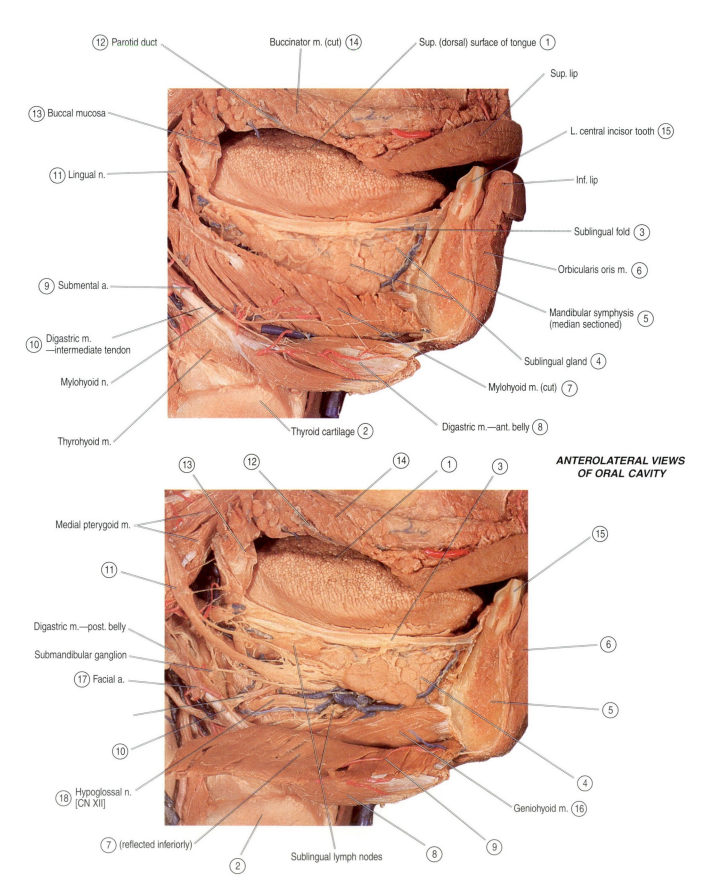

12 Parotid duct

Buccinator m. (cut) 14

Sup. (dorsal) surface of tongue 1

Sup. lip

13 Buccal mucosa

L. central incisor tooth 15

11 Lingual n.

Inf. lip

Sublingual fold 3

Orbicularis oris m. 6

9 Submental a.

Mandibular symphysis 5
(median sectioned)

10 Digastric m.
—intermediate tendon

Sublingual gland 4

Mylohyoid n.

Mylohyoid m. (cut) 7

Thyrohyoid m.

Thyroid cartilage 2

Digastric m.—ant. belly 8

**ANTEROLATERAL VIEWS
OF ORAL CAVITY**

13   12   14   1   3

Medial pterygoid m.

15

11

Digastric m.—post. belly

6

Submandibular ganglion

17 Facial a.

5

10

4

18 Hypoglossal n.
[CN XII]

Geniohyoid m. 16

7 (reflected inferiorly)

Sublingual lymph nodes

8   9

2

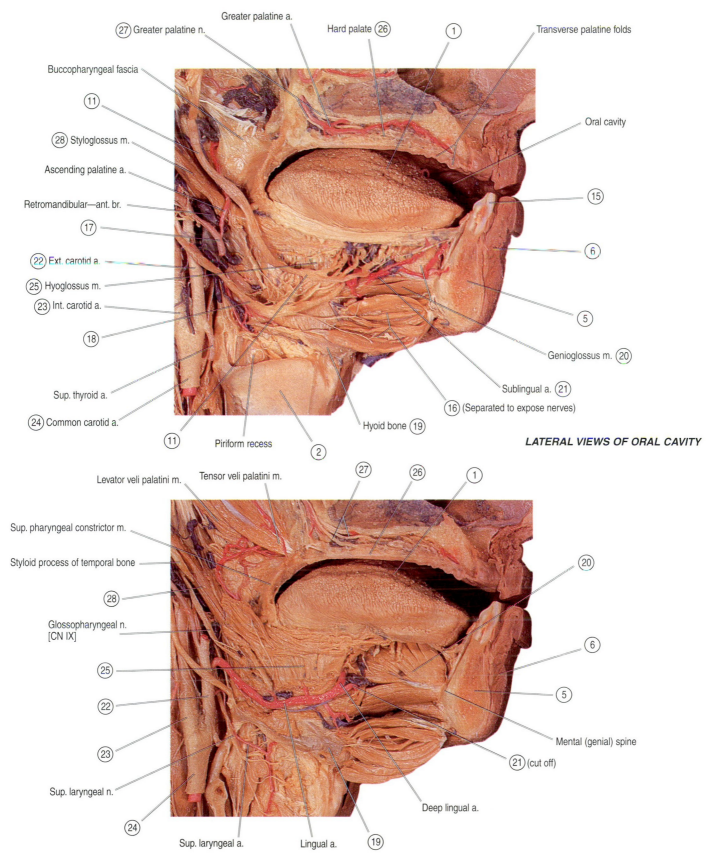

Greater palatine a.

㉗ Greater palatine n.

Hard palate ㉖

①

Transverse palatine folds

Buccopharyngeal fascia

⑪

㉘ Styloglossus m.

Ascending palatine a.

Retromandibular—ant. br.

⑰

㉒ Ext. carotid a.

㉕ Hyoglossus m.

㉓ Int. carotid a.

⑱

Sup. thyroid a.

㉔ Common carotid a.

⑪

Piriform recess

②

Hyoid bone ⑲

⑯ (Separated to expose nerves)

Sublingual a. ㉑

Genioglossus m. ⑳

⑤

⑥

⑮

Oral cavity

LATERAL VIEWS OF ORAL CAVITY

Levator veli palatini m.

Tensor veli palatini m.

㉗

㉖

①

Sup. pharyngeal constrictor m.

Styloid process of temporal bone

㉘

Glossopharyngeal n.
[CN IX]

㉕

㉒

㉓

Sup. laryngeal n.

㉔

Sup. laryngeal a.

Lingual a.

⑲

Deep lingual a.

㉑ (cut off)

Mental (genial) spine

⑤

⑥

⑳

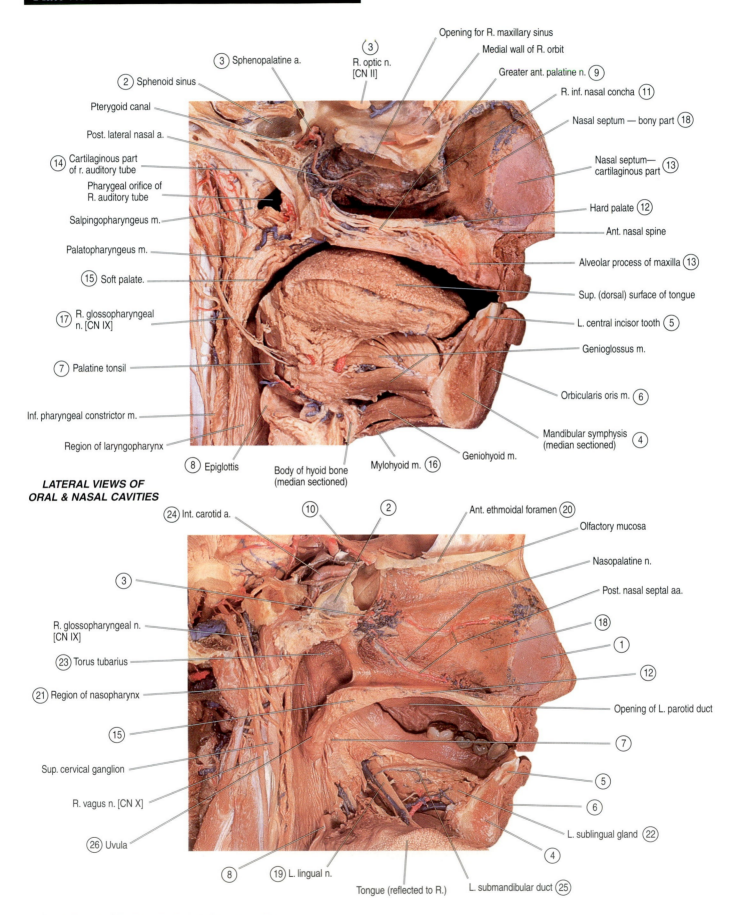

③ Sphenopalatine a.

② Sphenoid sinus

Pterygoid canal

Post. lateral nasal a.

⑭ Cartilaginous part of r. auditory tube

Pharygeal orifice of R. auditory tube

Salpingopharyngeus m.

Palatopharyngeus m.

⑮ Soft palate.

⑰ R. glossopharyngeal n. [CN IX]

⑦ Palatine tonsil

Inf. pharyngeal constrictor m.

Region of laryngopharynx

⑧ Epiglottis

③ R. optic n. [CN II]

Opening for R. maxillary sinus

Medial wall of R. orbit

Greater ant. palatine n. ⑨

R. inf. nasal concha ⑪

Nasal septum — bony part ⑱

Nasal septum — cartilaginous part ⑬

Hard palate ⑫

Ant. nasal spine

Alveolar process of maxilla ⑬

Sup. (dorsal) surface of tongue

L. central incisor tooth ⑤

Genioglossus m.

Orbicularis oris m. ⑥

Mandibular symphysis (median sectioned) ④

Geniohyoid m.

Body of hyoid bone (median sectioned)

Mylohyoid m. ⑯

LATERAL VIEWS OF ORAL & NASAL CAVITIES

⑭ Int. carotid a.

③

R. glossopharyngeal n. [CN IX]

㉓ Torus tubarius

㉑ Region of nasopharynx

⑮

Sup. cervical ganglion

R. vagus n. [CN X]

㉖ Uvula

⑧   ⑲ L. lingual n.

⑩   ②

Ant. ethmoidal foramen ⑳

Olfactory mucosa

Nasopalatine n.

Post. nasal septal aa.

⑱

①

⑫

Opening of L. parotid duct

⑦

⑤

⑥

L. sublingual gland ㉒

④

Tongue (reflected to R.)   L. submandibular duct ㉕

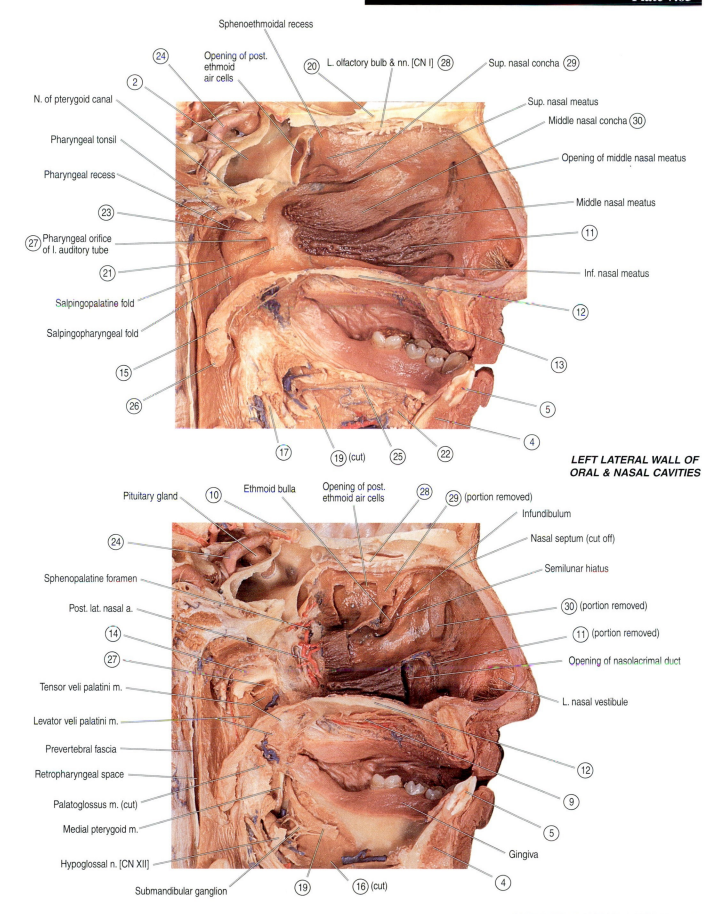

Sphenoethmoidal recess

(24)

Opening of post. ethmoid air cells

(2)

(20) L. olfactory bulb & nn. [CN I] (28)

Sup. nasal concha (29)

N. of pterygoid canal

Sup. nasal meatus

Middle nasal concha (30)

Pharyngeal tonsil

Opening of middle nasal meatus

Pharyngeal recess

Middle nasal meatus

(23)

(27) Pharyngeal orifice of l. auditory tube

(21)

(11)

Inf. nasal meatus

Salpingopalatine fold

(12)

Salpingopharyngeal fold

(13)

(15)

(5)

(26)

(4)

(17) (19) (cut) (25) (22)

LEFT LATERAL WALL OF ORAL & NASAL CAVITIES

Pituitary gland

(10)

Ethmoid bulla

Opening of post. ethmoid air cells

(28)

(29) (portion removed)

Infundibulum

(24)

Nasal septum (cut off)

Sphenopalatine foramen

Semilunar hiatus

Post. lat. nasal a.

(30) (portion removed)

(14)

(11) (portion removed)

(27)

Opening of nasolacrimal duct

Tensor veli palatini m.

L. nasal vestibule

Levator veli palatini m.

Prevertebral fascia

(12)

Retropharyngeal space

Palatoglossus m. (cut)

(9)

Medial pterygoid m.

(5)

Hypoglossal n. [CN XII]

Gingiva

(4)

Submandibular ganglion

(19) (16) (cut)

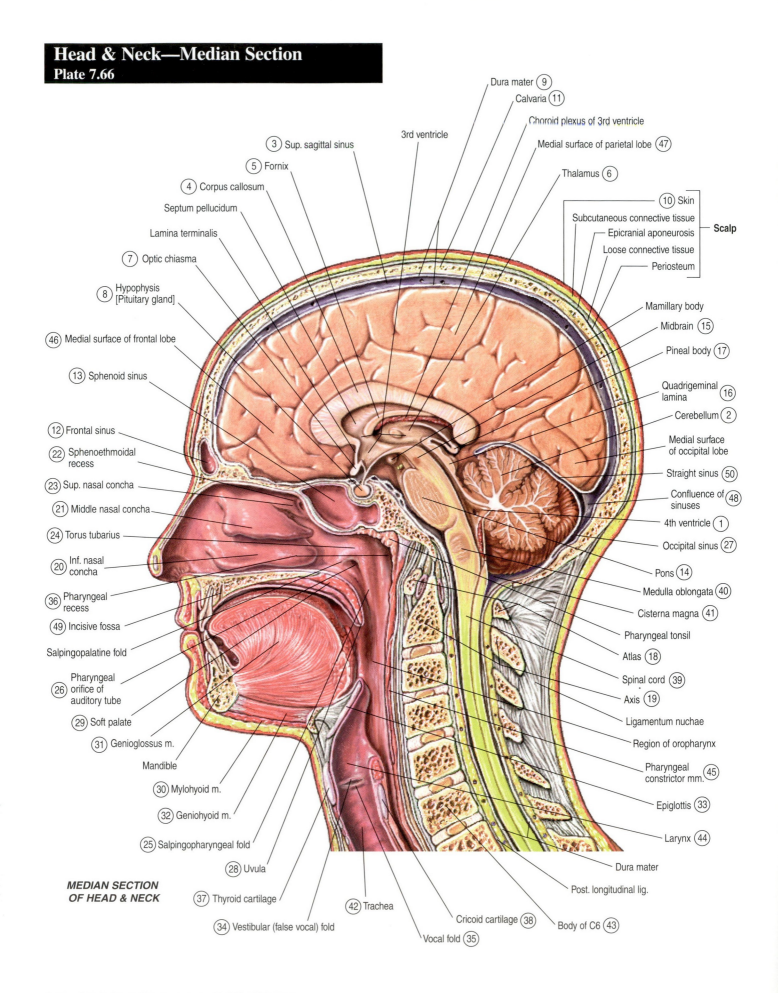

Dura mater (9)
Calvaria (11)
Choroid plexus of 3rd ventricle
3rd ventricle
Medial surface of parietal lobe (47)
(3) Sup. sagittal sinus
Thalamus (6)
(5) Fornix
(10) Skin
Subcutaneous connective tissue
(4) Corpus callosum
Epicranial aponeurosis **Scalp**
Septum pellucidum
Loose connective tissue
Lamina terminalis
Periosteum
(7) Optic chiasma
Mamillary body
Midbrain (15)
(8) Hypophysis [Pituitary gland]
Pineal body (17)
(46) Medial surface of frontal lobe
Quadrigeminal lamina (16)
(13) Sphenoid sinus
Cerebellum (2)
Medial surface of occipital lobe
(12) Frontal sinus
(22) Sphenoethmoidal recess
Straight sinus (50)
(23) Sup. nasal concha
Confluence of sinuses (48)
(21) Middle nasal concha
4th ventricle (1)
(24) Torus tubarius
Occipital sinus (27)
(20) Inf. nasal concha
Pons (14)
Medulla oblongata (40)
(36) Pharyngeal recess
Cisterna magna (41)
(49) Incisive fossa
Pharyngeal tonsil
Salpingopalatine fold
Atlas (18)
Pharyngeal orifice of auditory tube (26)
Spinal cord (39)
(29) Soft palate
Axis (19)
(31) Genioglossus m.
Ligamentum nuchae
Mandible
Region of oropharynx
(30) Mylohyoid m.
Pharyngeal constrictor mm. (45)
(32) Geniohyoid m.
Epiglottis (33)
(25) Salpingopharyngeal fold
Larynx (44)
(28) Uvula
Dura mater

MEDIAN SECTION OF HEAD & NECK

Post. longitudinal lig.
(37) Thyroid cartilage
(42) Trachea
Cricoid cartilage (38)
Body of C6 (43)
(34) Vestibular (false vocal) fold
Vocal fold (35)

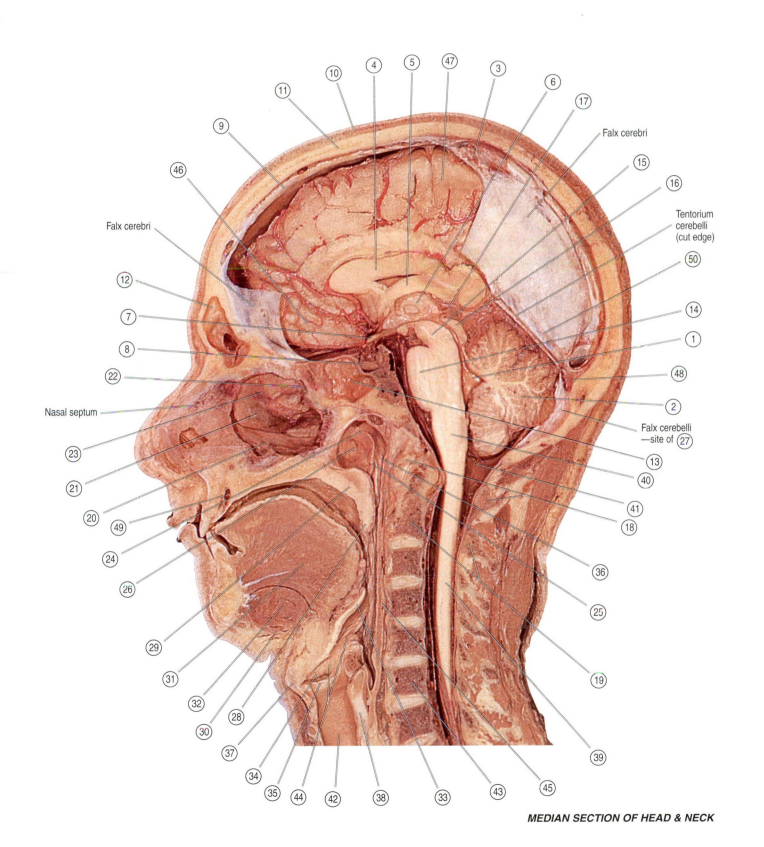

Falx cerebri

Tentorium
cerebelli
(cut edge)

Falx cerebri

Nasal septum

Falx cerebelli
—site of ㉗

MEDIAN SECTION OF HEAD & NECK

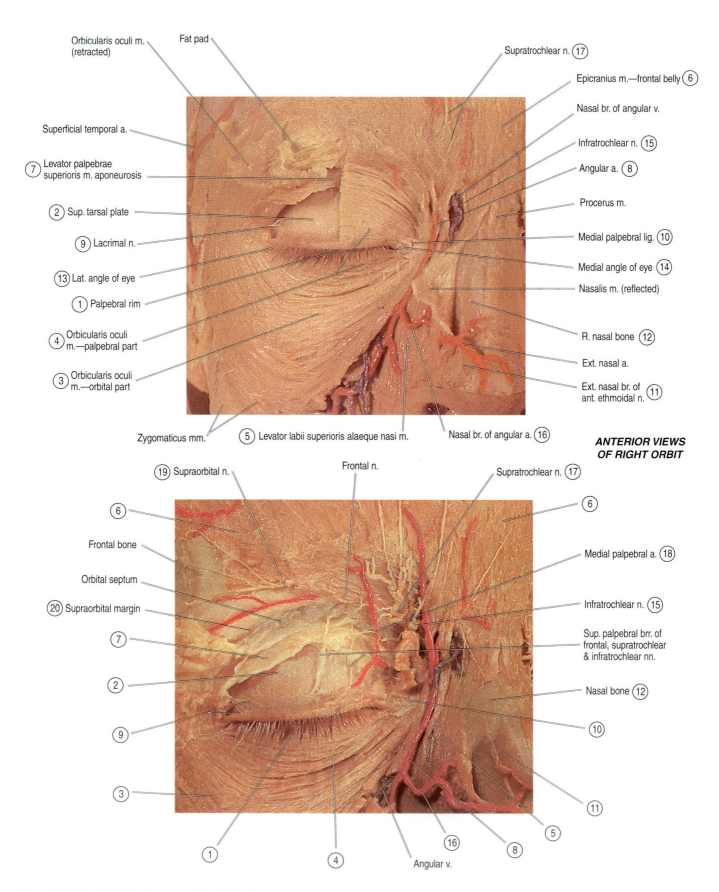

Orbicularis oculi m. (retracted)

Fat pad

Supratrochlear n. (17)

Epicranius m.—frontal belly (6)

Nasal br. of angular v.

Superficial temporal a.

Infratrochlear n. (15)

Angular a. (8)

(7) Levator palpebrae superioris m. aponeurosis

Procerus m.

(2) Sup. tarsal plate

Medial palpebral lig. (10)

(9) Lacrimal n.

Medial angle of eye (14)

(13) Lat. angle of eye

Nasalis m. (reflected)

(1) Palpebral rim

(4) Orbicularis oculi m.—palpebral part

R. nasal bone (12)

Ext. nasal a.

(3) Orbicularis oculi m.—orbital part

Ext. nasal br. of ant. ethmoidal n. (11)

Zygomaticus mm.

(5) Levator labii superioris alaeque nasi m.

Nasal br. of angular a. (16)

ANTERIOR VIEWS OF RIGHT ORBIT

(19) Supraorbital n.

Frontal n.

Supratrochlear n. (17)

(6)

(6)

Frontal bone

Medial palpebral a. (18)

Orbital septum

Infratrochlear n. (15)

(20) Supraorbital margin

(7)

Sup. palpebral brr. of frontal, supratrochlear & infratrochlear nn.

(2)

Nasal bone (12)

(9)

(10)

(3)

(11)

(1)

(4)

(16)

(8)

(5)

Angular v.

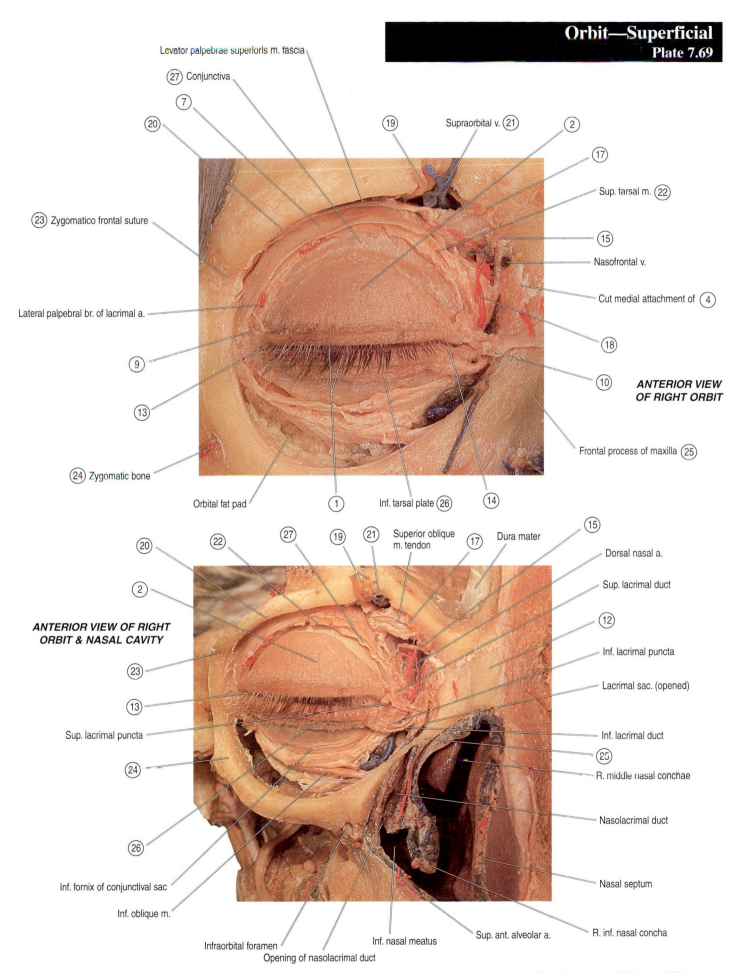

Levator palpebrae superioris m. fascia

(27) Conjunctiva

(7)

(20)

(23) Zygomatico frontal suture

Lateral palpebral br. of lacrimal a.

(9)

(13)

(24) Zygomatic bone

Orbital fat pad

(1)

(19)

Supraorbital v. (21)

(2)

(17)

Sup. tarsal m. (22)

(15)

Nasofrontal v.

Cut medial attachment of (4)

(18)

(10)

**ANTERIOR VIEW
OF RIGHT ORBIT**

Frontal process of maxilla (25)

Inf. tarsal plate (26)

(14)

**ANTERIOR VIEW OF RIGHT
ORBIT & NASAL CAVITY**

(20)

(22)

(27)

(19)

(21)

Superior oblique
m. tendon

(17)

Dura mater

(15)

Dorsal nasal a.

Sup. lacrimal duct

(12)

(2)

(23)

(13)

Sup. lacrimal puncta

(24)

(26)

Inf. fornix of conjunctival sac

Inf. oblique m.

Infraorbital foramen

Opening of nasolacrimal duct

Inf. nasal meatus

Sup. ant. alveolar a.

Inf. lacrimal puncta

Lacrimal sac. (opened)

Inf. lacrimal duct

(25)

R. middle nasal conchae

Nasolacrimal duct

Nasal septum

R. inf. nasal concha

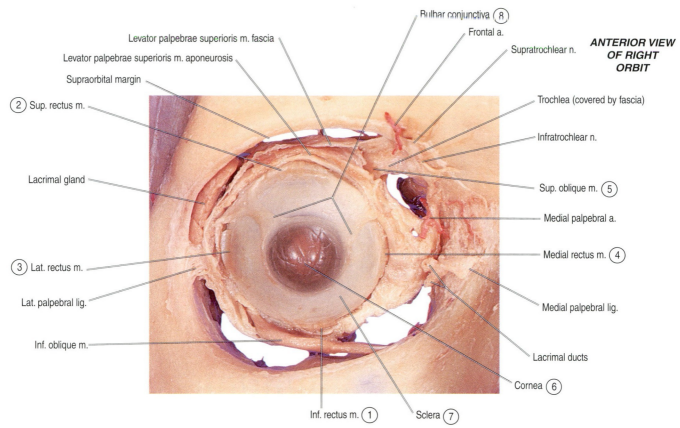

ANTERIOR VIEW OF RIGHT ORBIT

Bulbar conjunctiva (8)
Frontal a.
Supratrochlear n.
Levator palpebrae superioris m. fascia
Levator palpebrae superioris m. aponeurosis
Supraorbital margin
(2) Sup. rectus m.
Lacrimal gland
(3) Lat. rectus m.
Lat. palpebral lig.
Inf. oblique m.
Trochlea (covered by fascia)
Infratrochlear n.
Sup. oblique m. (5)
Medial palpebral a.
Medial rectus m. (4)
Medial palpebral lig.
Lacrimal ducts
Cornea (6)
Inf. rectus m. (1)
Sclera (7)

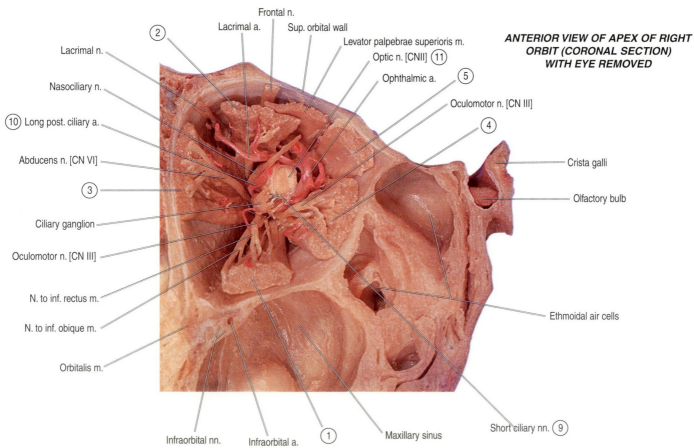

ANTERIOR VIEW OF APEX OF RIGHT ORBIT (CORONAL SECTION) WITH EYE REMOVED

Frontal n.
Lacrimal a.
Sup. orbital wall
(2)
Lacrimal n.
Nasociliary n.
Levator palpebrae superioris m.
Optic n. [CN II] (11)
Ophthalmic a.
(5)
(10) Long post. ciliary a.
Abducens n. [CN VI]
(3)
Oculomotor n. [CN III]
(4)
Ciliary ganglion
Oculomotor n. [CN III]
N. to inf. rectus m.
N. to inf. obique m.
Orbitalis m.
Crista galli
Olfactory bulb
Ethmoidal air cells
Infraorbital nn.
Infraorbital a.
(1)
Maxillary sinus
Short ciliary nn. (9)

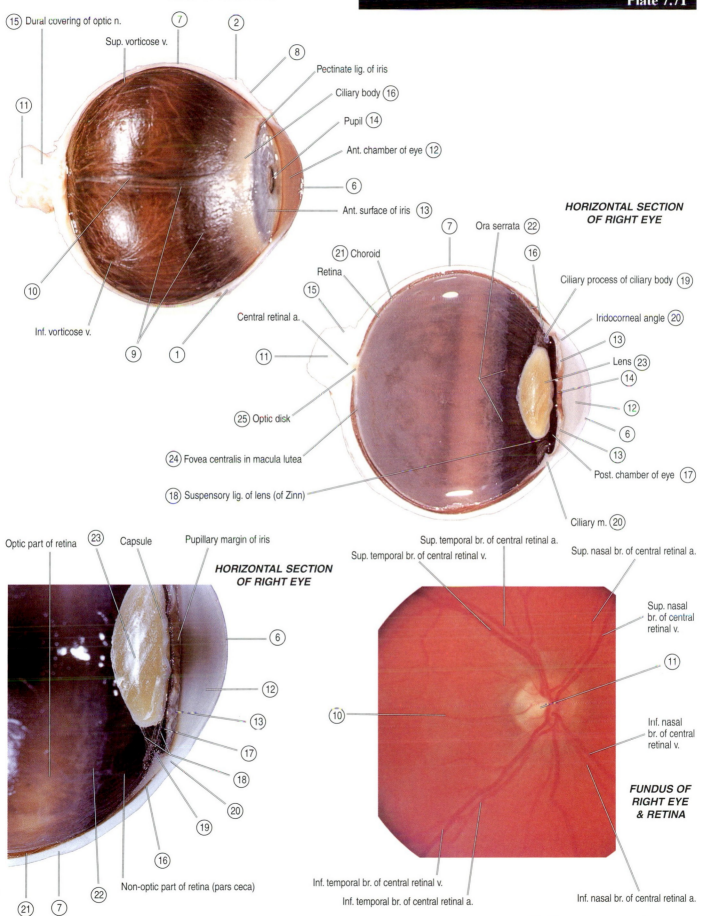

LATERAL VIEW OF VASCULAR TUNIC OF RIGHT EYE

(15) Dural covering of optic n.
(7)
(2)
Sup. vorticose v.
(8)
(11)
Pectinate lig. of iris
Ciliary body (16)
Pupil (14)
Ant. chamber of eye (12)
(6)
Ant. surface of iris (13)
(10)
Inf. vorticose v.
(9)
(1)

Eye
Plate 7.71

HORIZONTAL SECTION OF RIGHT EYE

(7)
Ora serrata (22)
(16)
Ciliary process of ciliary body (19)
(21) Choroid
Iridocorneal angle (20)
Retina
(13)
(15)
Lens (23)
(14)
Central retinal a.
(12)
(11)
(6)
(25) Optic disk
(13)
Post. chamber of eye (17)
(24) Fovea centralis in macula lutea
Ciliary m. (20)
(18) Suspensory lig. of lens (of Zinn)

Optic part of retina
(23)
Capsule
Pupillary margin of iris

HORIZONTAL SECTION OF RIGHT EYE

(6)
(12)
(13)
(17)
(18)
(20)
(19)
(16)
Non-optic part of retina (pars ceca)
(21)
(7)
(22)

Sup. temporal br. of central retinal a.
Sup. temporal br. of central retinal v.
Sup. nasal br. of central retinal a.

Sup. nasal br. of central retinal v.

(11)

(10)

Inf. nasal br. of central retinal v.

FUNDUS OF RIGHT EYE & RETINA

Inf. temporal br. of central retinal v.
Inf. temporal br. of central retinal a.
Inf. nasal br. of central retinal a.

LATERAL VIEW OF RIGHT ORBIT

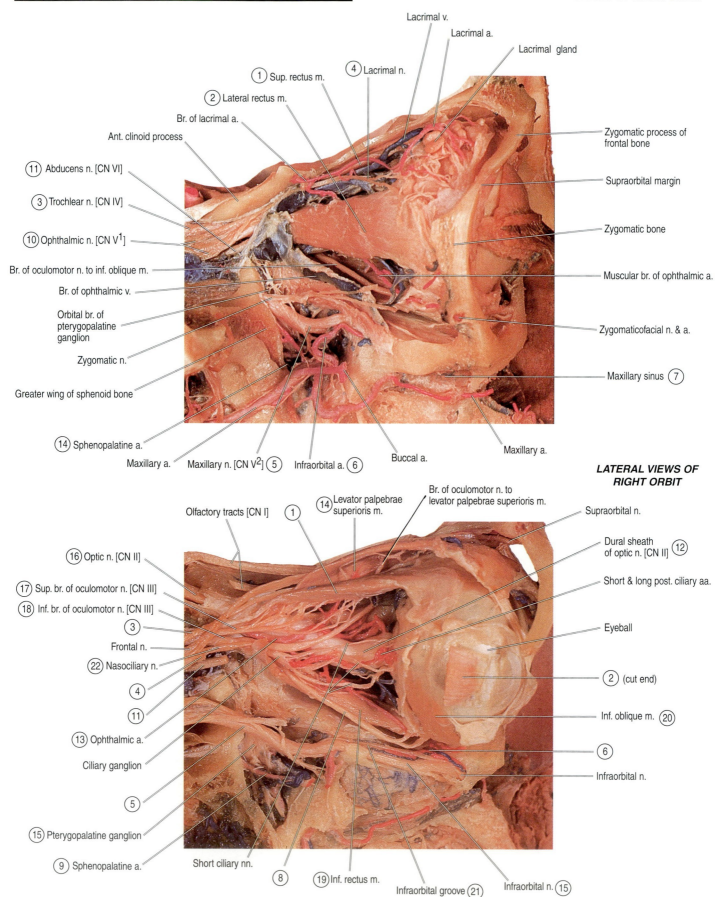

Lacrimal v.

Lacrimal a.

Lacrimal gland

④ Lacrimal n.

① Sup. rectus m.

② Lateral rectus m.

Br. of lacrimal a.

Zygomatic process of frontal bone

Ant. clinoid process

Supraorbital margin

⑪ Abducens n. [CN VI]

③ Trochlear n. [CN IV]

Zygomatic bone

⑩ Ophthalmic n. [CN V¹]

Br. of oculomotor n. to inf. oblique m.

Muscular br. of ophthalmic a.

Br. of ophthalmic v.

Orbital br. of pterygopalatine ganglion

Zygomaticofacial n. & a.

Zygomatic n.

Greater wing of sphenoid bone

Maxillary sinus ⑦

⑭ Sphenopalatine a.

Maxillary a.   Maxillary n. [CN V²] ⑤   Infraorbital a. ⑥   Buccal a.   Maxillary a.

LATERAL VIEWS OF RIGHT ORBIT

Olfactory tracts [CN I]

⑭ Levator palpebrae superioris m.

Br. of oculomotor n. to levator palpebrae superioris m.

Supraorbital n.

①

⑯ Optic n. [CN II]

Dural sheath of optic n. [CN II] ⑫

⑰ Sup. br. of oculomotor n. [CN III]

Short & long post. ciliary aa.

⑱ Inf. br. of oculomotor n. [CN III]

③

Frontal n.

Eyeball

㉒ Nasociliary n.

② (cut end)

④

⑪

Inf. oblique m. ⑳

⑬ Ophthalmic a.

⑥

Ciliary ganglion

Infraorbital n.

⑤

⑮ Pterygopalatine ganglion

⑨ Sphenopalatine a.   Short ciliary nn.   ⑧   ⑲ Inf. rectus m.   Infraorbital groove ㉑   Infraorbital n. ⑮

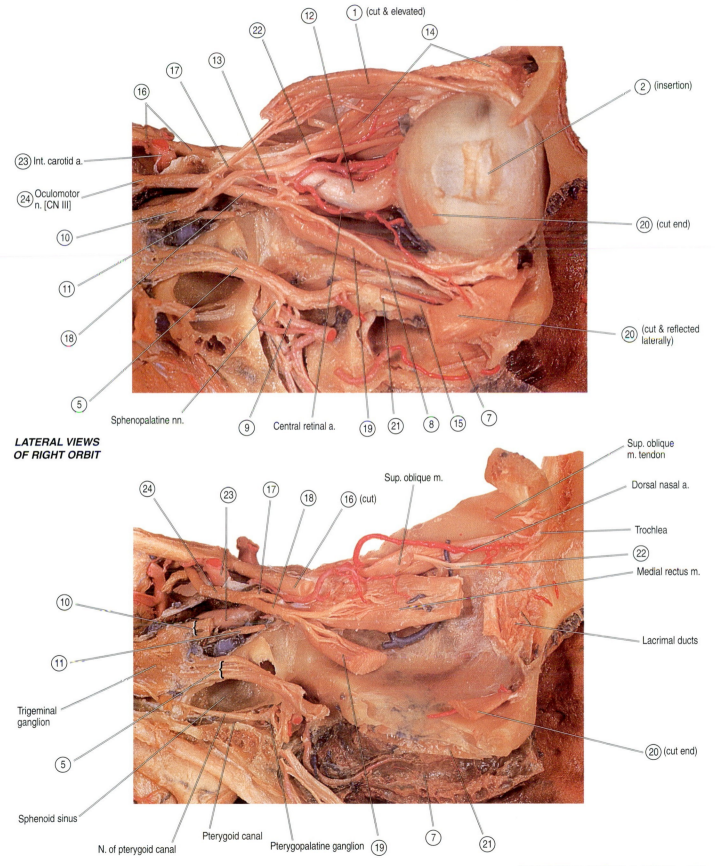

① (cut & elevated)

② (insertion)

⑫ ⑭

㉒

⑬ ⑰

⑯

㉓ Int. carotid a.

㉔ Oculomotor n. [CN III]

⑩

⑪

⑱

⑳ (cut end)

⑳ (cut & reflected laterally)

⑤

Sphenopalatine nn.

⑨ Central retinal a. ⑲ ㉑ ⑧ ⑮ ⑦

LATERAL VIEWS OF RIGHT ORBIT

Sup. oblique m. tendon

Sup. oblique m.

Dorsal nasal a.

Trochlea

㉒

Medial rectus m.

Lacrimal ducts

㉔ ㉓ ⑰ ⑱ ⑯ (cut)

⑩

⑪

Trigeminal ganglion

⑳ (cut end)

⑤

Sphenoid sinus

N. of pterygoid canal   Pterygoid canal   Pterygopalatine ganglion ⑲   ⑦ ㉑

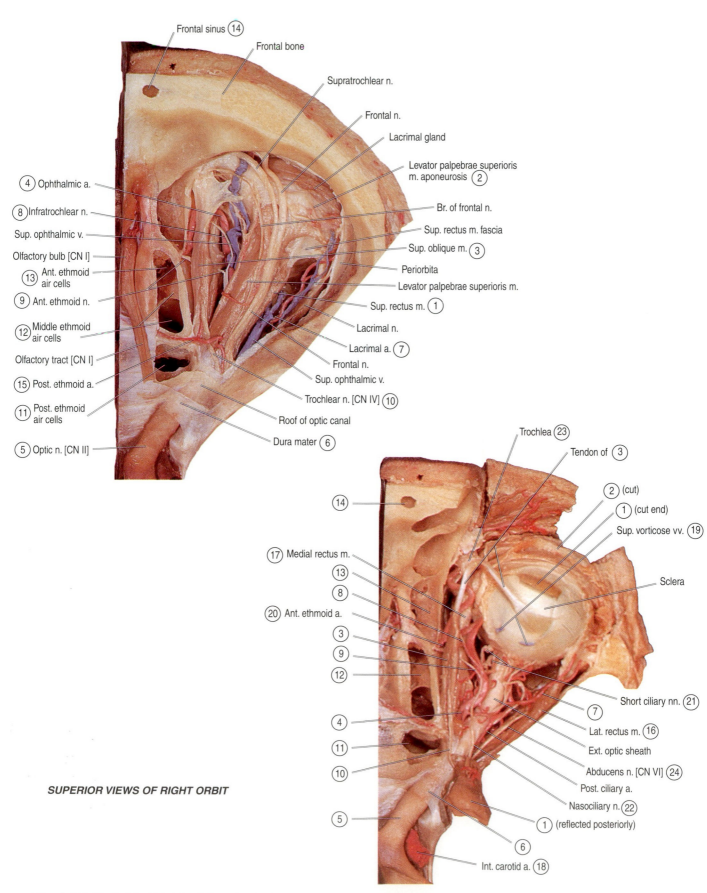

Frontal sinus (14)

Frontal bone

Supratrochlear n.

Frontal n.

Lacrimal gland

Levator palpebrae superioris
m. aponeurosis (2)

(4) Ophthalmic a.

(8) Infratrochlear n.

Sup. ophthalmic v.

Olfactory bulb [CN I]

(13) Ant. ethmoid
air cells

(9) Ant. ethmoid n.

(12) Middle ethmoid
air cells

Olfactory tract [CN I]

(15) Post. ethmoid a.

(11) Post. ethmoid
air cells

(5) Optic n. [CN II]

Br. of frontal n.

Sup. rectus m. fascia

Sup. oblique m. (3)

Periorbita

Levator palpebrae superioris m.

Sup. rectus m. (1)

Lacrimal n.

Lacrimal a. (7)

Frontal n.

Sup. ophthalmic v.

Trochlear n. [CN IV] (10)

Roof of optic canal

Dura mater (6)

Trochlea (23)

Tendon of (3)

(2) (cut)

(1) (cut end)

Sup. vorticose vv. (19)

(14)

(17) Medial rectus m.

(13)

(8)

(20) Ant. ethmoid a.

(3)

(9)

(12)

(4)

(11)

(10)

(5)

Sclera

Short ciliary nn. (21)

(7)

Lat. rectus m. (16)

Ext. optic sheath

Abducens n. [CN VI] (24)

Post. ciliary a.

Nasociliary n. (22)

(1) (reflected posteriorly)

(6)

Int. carotid a. (18)

SUPERIOR VIEWS OF RIGHT ORBIT

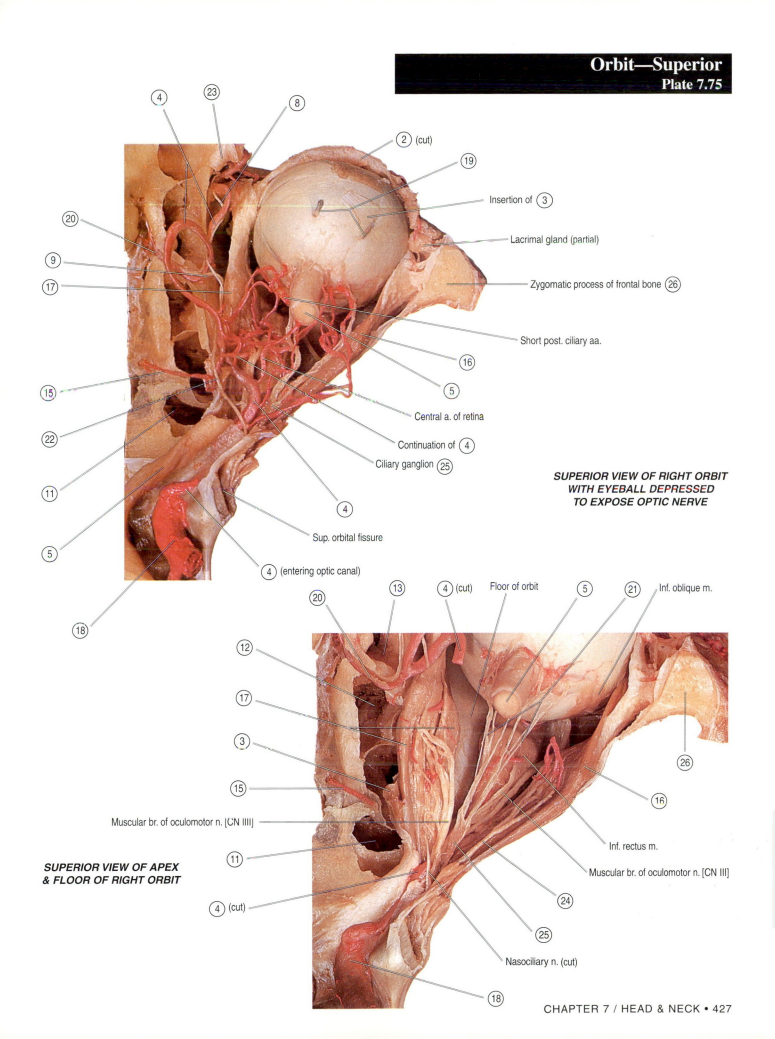

④ ㉓ ⑧

② (cut)

⑲

Insertion of ③

Lacrimal gland (partial)

⑳

⑨

⑰

Zygomatic process of frontal bone ㉖

Short post. ciliary aa.

⑯

⑤

⑮

Central a. of retina

㉒

Continuation of ④

Ciliary ganglion ㉕

⑪

*SUPERIOR VIEW OF RIGHT ORBIT
WITH EYEBALL DEPRESSED
TO EXPOSE OPTIC NERVE*

⑤

④

Sup. orbital fissure

⑱

④ (entering optic canal)

⑬ ④ (cut) Floor of orbit ⑤ ㉑ Inf. oblique m.

⑳

⑫

⑰

③

㉖

⑮

⑯

Muscular br. of oculomotor n. [CN IIII]

Inf. rectus m.

⑪

Muscular br. of oculomotor n. [CN III]

*SUPERIOR VIEW OF APEX
& FLOOR OF RIGHT ORBIT*

④ (cut)

㉔

㉕

Nasociliary n. (cut)

⑱

Infratemporal Fossa
Plate 7.76

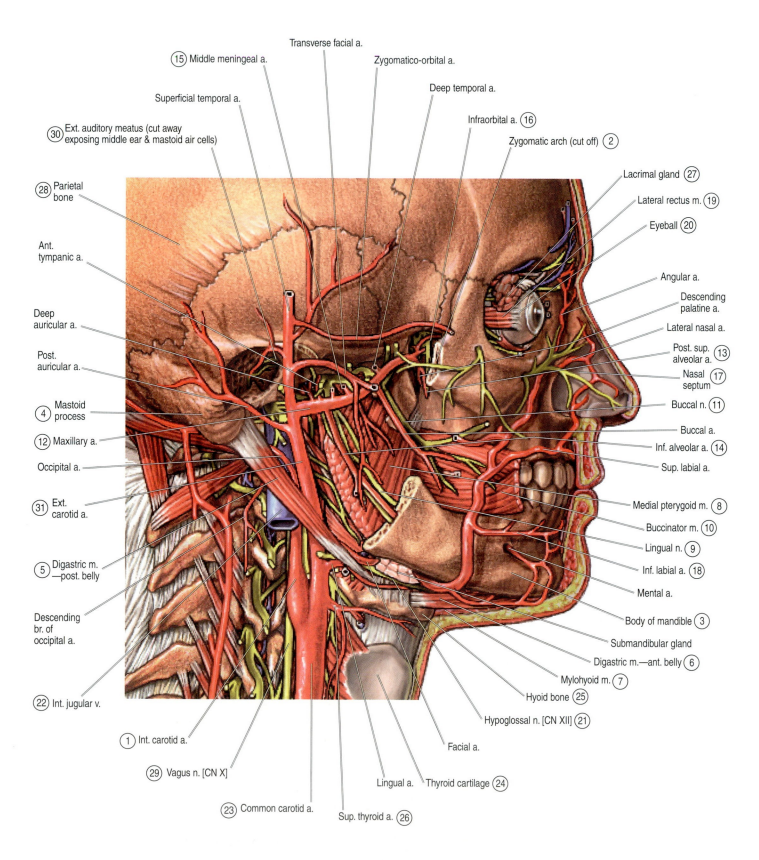

15 Middle meningeal a.

Transverse facial a.

Zygomatico-orbital a.

Deep temporal a.

Infraorbital a. 16

Superficial temporal a.

30 Ext. auditory meatus (cut away exposing middle ear & mastoid air cells)

Zygomatic arch (cut off) 2

Lacrimal gland 27

Lateral rectus m. 19

28 Parietal bone

Eyeball 20

Ant. tympanic a.

Angular a.

Descending palatine a.

Deep auricular a.

Lateral nasal a.

Post. auricular a.

Post. sup. alveolar a. 13

Nasal septum 17

Buccal n. 11

4 Mastoid process

Buccal a.

12 Maxillary a.

Inf. alveolar a. 14

Occipital a.

Sup. labial a.

Medial pterygoid m. 8

31 Ext. carotid a.

Buccinator m. 10

Lingual n. 9

5 Digastric m. —post. belly

Inf. labial a. 18

Mental a.

Descending br. of occipital a.

Body of mandible 3

Submandibular gland

22 Int. jugular v.

Digastric m.—ant. belly 6

Mylohyoid m. 7

Hyoid bone 25

1 Int. carotid a.

Hypoglossal n. [CN XII] 21

29 Vagus n. [CN X]

Facial a.

Lingual a.

Thyroid cartilage 24

23 Common carotid a.

Sup. thyroid a. 26

LATERAL VIEW

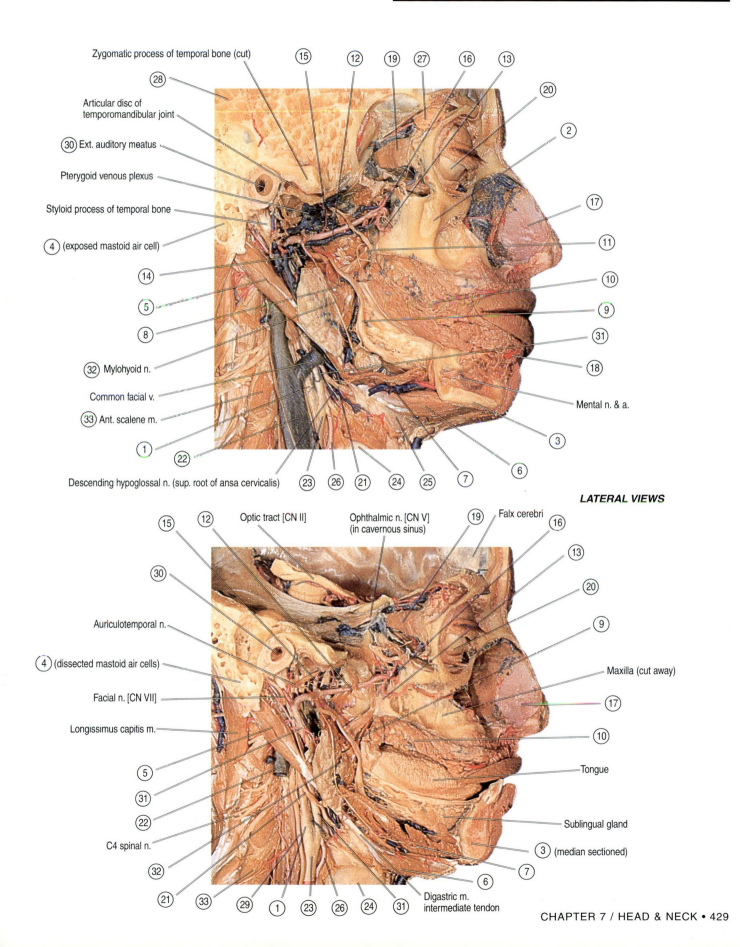

Zygomatic process of temporal bone (cut)
(28)
Articular disc of temporomandibular joint
(30) Ext. auditory meatus
Pterygoid venous plexus
Styloid process of temporal bone
(4) (exposed mastoid air cell)
(14)
(5)
(8)
(32) Mylohyoid n.
Common facial v.
(33) Ant. scalene m.
(1)
(22)
Descending hypoglossal n. (sup. root of ansa cervicalis)

(15) (12) (19) (27) (16) (13)
(20)
(2)
(17)
(11)
(10)
(9)
(31)
(18)
Mental n. & a.
(3)
(6)
(7)
(23) (26) (21) (24) (25)

LATERAL VIEWS

(15) (12) Optic tract [CN II] Ophthalmic n. [CN V] (in cavernous sinus) (19) Falx cerebri (16)
(13)
(30)
(20)
Auriculotemporal n.
(9)
(4) (dissected mastoid air cells)
Maxilla (cut away)
Facial n. [CN VII]
(17)
Longissimus capitis m.
(10)
(5)
Tongue
(31)
(22)
Sublingual gland
C4 spinal n.
(3) (median sectioned)
(32)
(7)
(21) (33) (29) (1) (23) (26) (24) (31)
(6)
Digastric m. intermediate tendon

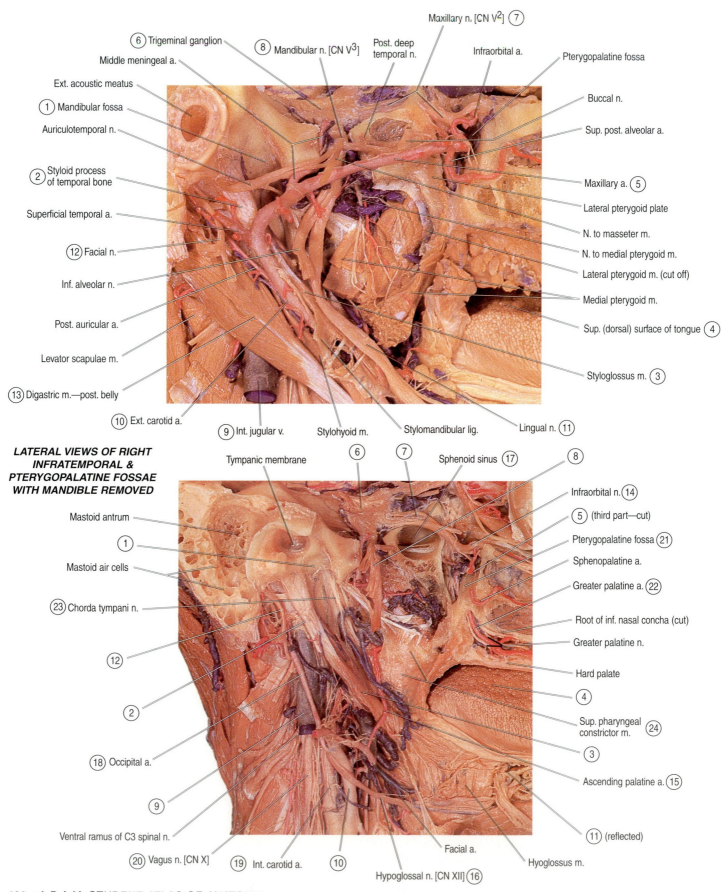

6 Trigeminal ganglion

Middle meningeal a.

Ext. acoustic meatus

1 Mandibular fossa

Auriculotemporal n.

2 Styloid process of temporal bone

Superficial temporal a.

12 Facial n.

Inf. alveolar n.

Post. auricular a.

Levator scapulae m.

13 Digastric m.—post. belly

10 Ext. carotid a.

9 Int. jugular v.

8 Mandibular n. [CN V³]

Post. deep temporal n.

Maxillary n. [CN V²] 7

Infraorbital a.

Pterygopalatine fossa

Buccal n.

Sup. post. alveolar a.

Maxillary a. 5

Lateral pterygoid plate

N. to masseter m.

N. to medial pterygoid m.

Lateral pterygoid m. (cut off)

Medial pterygoid m.

Sup. (dorsal) surface of tongue 4

Styloglossus m. 3

Stylohyoid m.

Stylomandibular lig.

Lingual n. 11

LATERAL VIEWS OF RIGHT INFRATEMPORAL & PTERYGOPALATINE FOSSAE WITH MANDIBLE REMOVED

Tympanic membrane

6

7

Sphenoid sinus 17

8

Mastoid antrum

1

Mastoid air cells

23 Chorda tympani n.

12

2

18 Occipital a.

9

Ventral ramus of C3 spinal n.

20 Vagus n. [CN X]

19 Int. carotid a.

10

Hypoglossal n. [CN XII] 16

Facial a.

Hyoglossus m.

Infraorbital n. 14

5 (third part—cut)

Pterygopalatine fossa 21

Sphenopalatine a.

Greater palatine a. 22

Root of inf. nasal concha (cut)

Greater palatine n.

Hard palate

4

Sup. pharyngeal constrictor m. 24

3

Ascending palatine a. 15

11 (reflected)

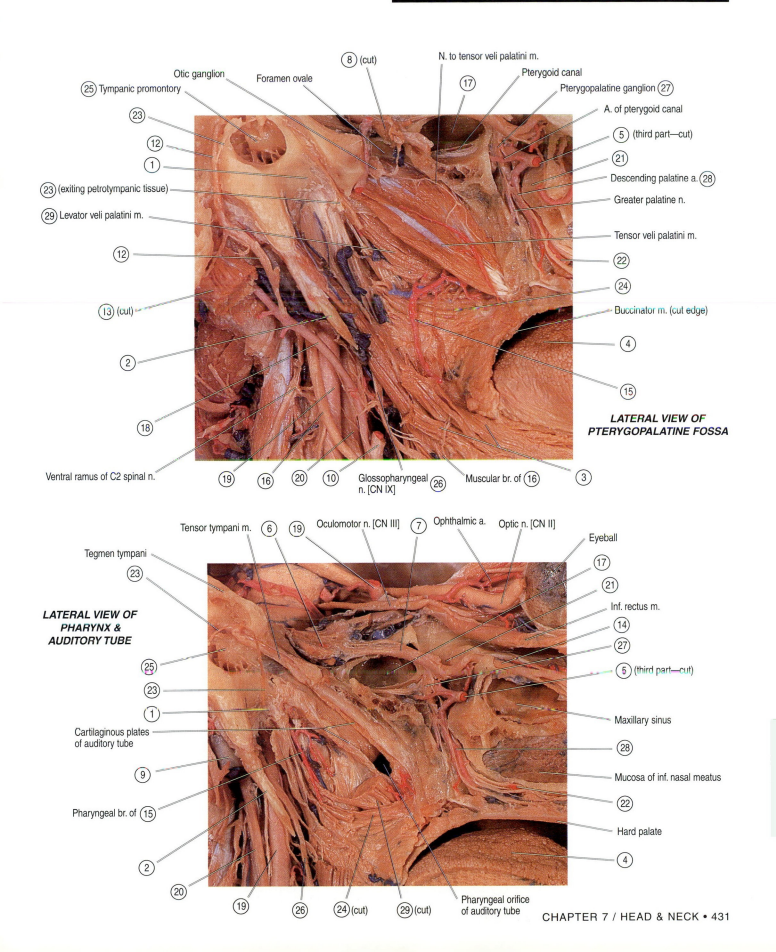

(8) (cut)

N. to tensor veli palatini m.

Otic ganglion

Foramen ovale

(17)

Pterygoid canal

(25) Tympanic promontory

Pterygopalatine ganglion (27)

A. of pterygoid canal

(23)

(12)

(5) (third part—cut)

(1)

(21)

(23) (exiting petrotympanic tissue)

Descending palatine a. (28)

Greater palatine n.

(29) Levator veli palatini m.

Tensor veli palatini m.

(12)

(22)

(24)

(13) (cut)

Buccinator m. (cut edge)

(2)

(4)

(15)

LATERAL VIEW OF PTERYGOPALATINE FOSSA

(18)

Ventral ramus of C2 spinal n.

(19) (16) (20) (10)

Glossopharyngeal n. [CN IX]

(26)

Muscular br. of (16)

(3)

Tensor tympani m.

(6) (19)

Oculomotor n. [CN III]

(7)

Ophthalmic a.

Optic n. [CN II]

Eyeball

Tegmen tympani

(17)

(23)

(21)

Inf. rectus m.

LATERAL VIEW OF PHARYNX & AUDITORY TUBE

(14)

(27)

(25)

(5) (third part—cut)

(23)

(1)

Maxillary sinus

Cartilaginous plates of auditory tube

(28)

(9)

Mucosa of inf. nasal meatus

Pharyngeal br. of (15)

(22)

(2)

Hard palate

(4)

(20)

(19)

(26)

(24) (cut)

(29) (cut)

Pharyngeal orifice of auditory tube

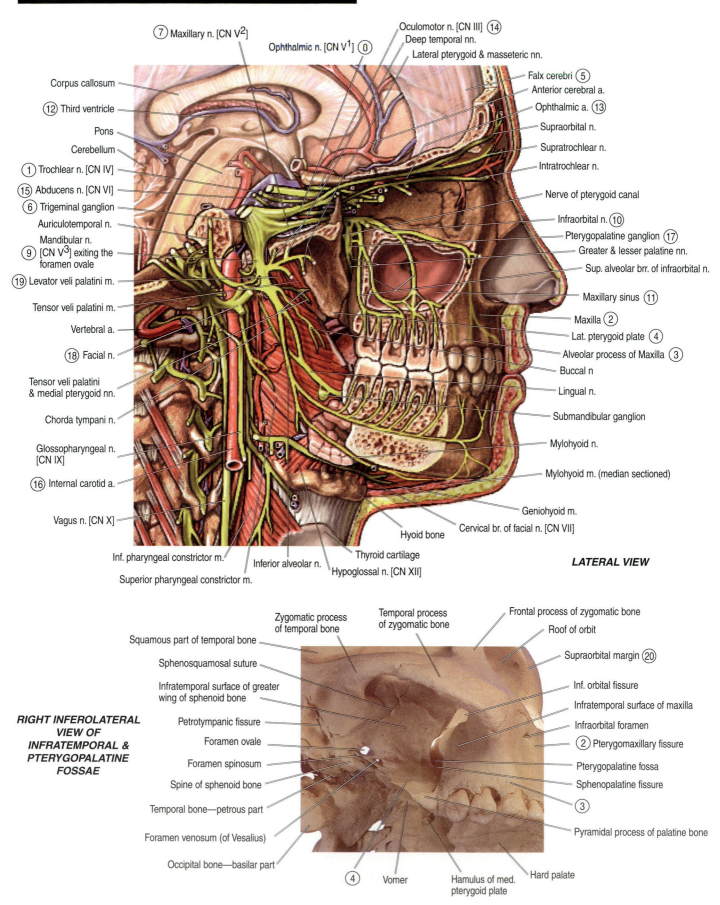

⑦ Maxillary n. [CN V²]

Ophthalmic n. [CN V¹] ⓪

Oculomotor n. [CN III] ⑭
Deep temporal nn.
Lateral pterygoid & masseteric nn.

Corpus callosum

⑫ Third ventricle

Pons

Cerebellum

① Trochlear n. [CN IV]

⑮ Abducens n. [CN VI]

⑥ Trigeminal ganglion

Auriculotemporal n.

Mandibular n.

⑨ [CN V³] exiting the foramen ovale

⑲ Levator veli palatini m.

Tensor veli palatini m.

Vertebral a.

⑱ Facial n.

Tensor veli palatini & medial pterygoid nn.

Chorda tympani n.

Glossopharyngeal n. [CN IX]

⑯ Internal carotid a.

Vagus n. [CN X]

Inf. pharyngeal constrictor m.

Inferior alveolar n.

Superior pharyngeal constrictor m.

Hypoglossal n. [CN XII]

Thyroid cartilage

Hyoid bone

Cervical br. of facial n. [CN VII]

Geniohyoid m.

Mylohyoid m. (median sectioned)

Mylohyoid n.

Submandibular ganglion

Lingual n.

Buccal n

Alveolar process of Maxilla ③

Lat. pterygoid plate ④

Maxilla ②

Maxillary sinus ⑪

Sup. alveolar brr. of infraorbital n.

Greater & lesser palatine nn.

Pterygopalatine ganglion ⑰

Infraorbital n. ⑩

Nerve of pterygoid canal

Intratrochlear n.

Supratrochlear n.

Supraorbital n.

Ophthalmic a. ⑬

Anterior cerebral a.

Falx cerebri ⑤

LATERAL VIEW

RIGHT INFEROLATERAL VIEW OF INFRATEMPORAL & PTERYGOPALATINE FOSSAE

Zygomatic process of temporal bone

Squamous part of temporal bone

Sphenosquamosal suture

Infratemporal surface of greater wing of sphenoid bone

Petrotympanic fissure

Foramen ovale

Foramen spinosum

Spine of sphenoid bone

Temporal bone—petrous part

Foramen venosum (of Vesalius)

Occipital bone—basilar part

Temporal process of zygomatic bone

Frontal process of zygomatic bone

Roof of orbit

Supraorbital margin ⑳

Inf. orbital fissure

Infratemporal surface of maxilla

Infraorbital foramen

② Pterygomaxillary fissure

Pterygopalatine fossa

Sphenopalatine fissure

③

Pyramidal process of palatine bone

Hard palate

Hamulus of med. pterygoid plate

Vomer

④

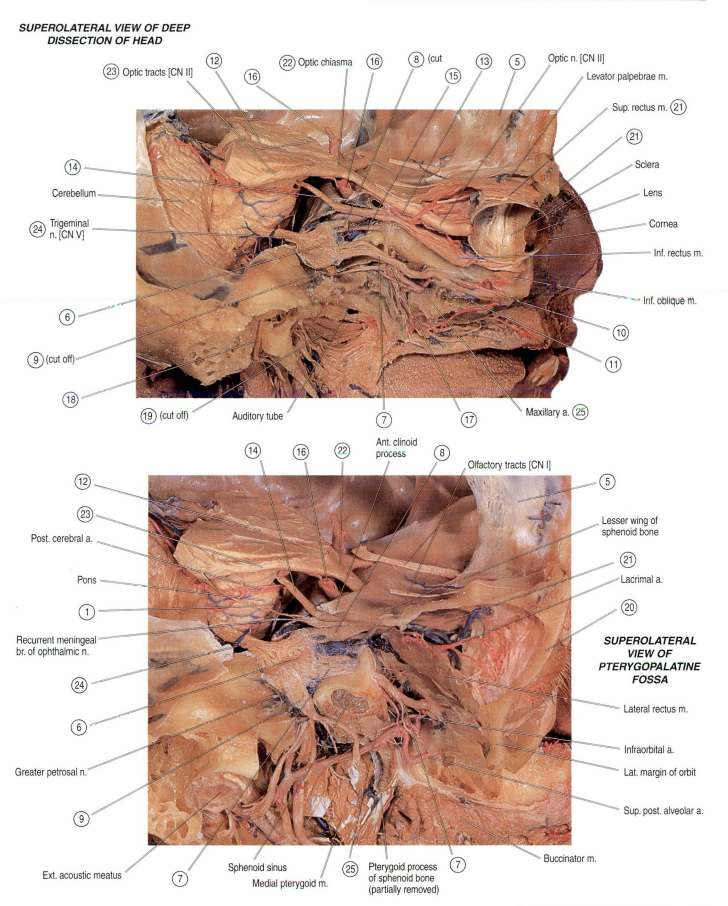

SUPEROLATERAL VIEW OF DEEP DISSECTION OF HEAD

(23) Optic tracts [CN II]
(12)
(16)
(22) Optic chiasma
(16)
(8) (cut
(15)
(13)
(5)
Optic n. [CN II]
Levator palpebrae m.
Sup. rectus m. (21)
(21)
Sclera
(14)
Lens
Cerebellum
Cornea
(24) Trigeminal n. [CN V]
Inf. rectus m.
Inf. oblique m.
(6)
(10)
(9) (cut off)
(11)
(18)
(19) (cut off)
Auditory tube
(7)
(17)
Maxillary a. (25)

(12)
(23)
(14)
(16)
(22)
Ant. clinoid process
(8)
Olfactory tracts [CN I]
(5)
Post. cerebral a.
Lesser wing of sphenoid bone
Pons
(21)
Lacrimal a.
(1)
(20)
Recurrent meningeal br. of ophthalmic n.
SUPEROLATERAL VIEW OF PTERYGOPALATINE FOSSA
(24)
(6)
Lateral rectus m.
Greater petrosal n.
Infraorbital a.
Lat. margin of orbit
(9)
Sup. post. alveolar a.
Ext. acoustic meatus
(7)
Sphenoid sinus
(25)
Pterygoid process of sphenoid bone (partially removed)
(7)
Buccinator m.
Medial pterygoid m.

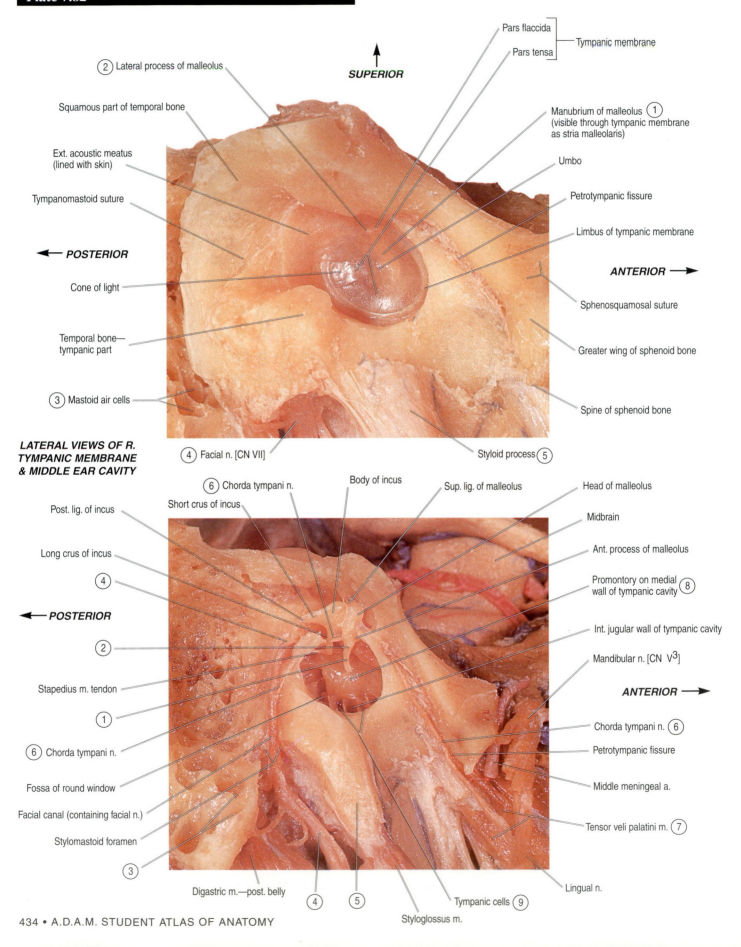

Pars flaccida — Tympanic membrane
Pars tensa

SUPERIOR

2 Lateral process of malleolus

Squamous part of temporal bone

Manubrium of malleolus 1
(visible through tympanic membrane
as stria malleolaris)

Ext. acoustic meatus
(lined with skin)

Umbo

Tympanomastoid suture

Petrotympanic fissure

POSTERIOR

Limbus of tympanic membrane

Cone of light

ANTERIOR

Sphenosquamosal suture

Temporal bone—
tympanic part

Greater wing of sphenoid bone

3 Mastoid air cells

Spine of sphenoid bone

LATERAL VIEWS OF R.
TYMPANIC MEMBRANE
& MIDDLE EAR CAVITY

4 Facial n. [CN VII]

Styloid process 5

6 Chorda tympani n.

Body of incus

Sup. lig. of malleolus

Head of malleolus

Post. lig. of incus

Short crus of incus

Midbrain

Long crus of incus

Ant. process of malleolus

4

Promontory on medial
wall of tympanic cavity 8

POSTERIOR

Int. jugular wall of tympanic cavity

2

Mandibular n. [CN V³]

Stapedius m. tendon

ANTERIOR

1

Chorda tympani n. 6

6 Chorda tympani n.

Petrotympanic fissure

Fossa of round window

Middle meningeal a.

Facial canal (containing facial n.)

Stylomastoid foramen

Tensor veli palatini m. 7

3

Lingual n.

Digastric m.—post. belly

4

5

Tympanic cells 9

Styloglossus m.

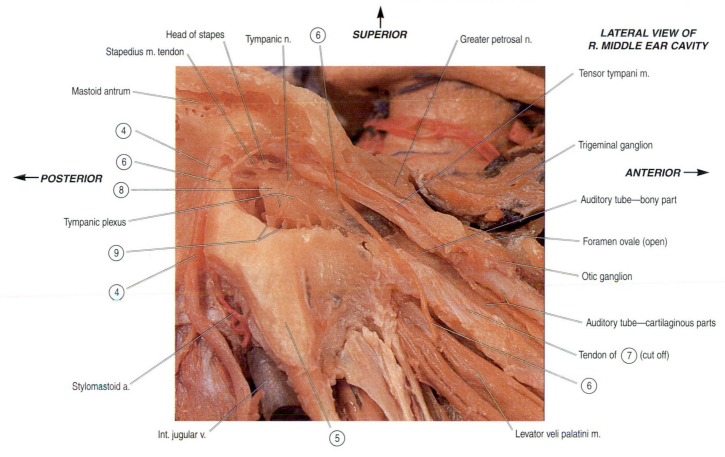

LATERAL VIEW OF R. MIDDLE EAR CAVITY

SUPERIOR

POSTERIOR ← → ANTERIOR

Head of stapes
Stapedius m. tendon
Tympanic n.
(6)
Greater petrosal n.
Mastoid antrum
Tensor tympani m.
(4)
(6)
(8)
Trigeminal ganglion
Tympanic plexus
Auditory tube—bony part
(9)
Foramen ovale (open)
(4)
Otic ganglion
Auditory tube—cartilaginous parts
Tendon of (7) (cut off)
(6)
Stylomastoid a.
Int. jugular v.
(5)
Levator veli palatini m.

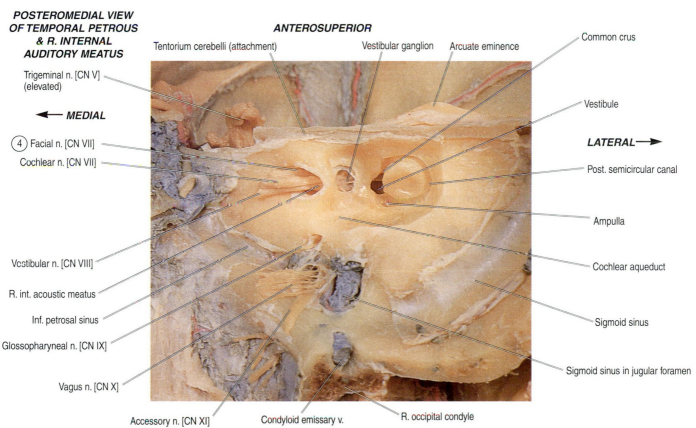

POSTEROMEDIAL VIEW OF TEMPORAL PETROUS & R. INTERNAL AUDITORY MEATUS

ANTEROSUPERIOR

MEDIAL ← → LATERAL

Tentorium cerebelli (attachment)
Vestibular ganglion
Arcuate eminence
Common crus
Trigeminal n. [CN V] (elevated)
Vestibule
(4) Facial n. [CN VII]
Cochlear n. [CN VII]
Post. semicircular canal
Ampulla
Vestibular n. [CN VIII]
R. int. acoustic meatus
Cochlear aqueduct
Inf. petrosal sinus
Glossopharyneal n. [CN IX]
Sigmoid sinus
Vagus n. [CN X]
Sigmoid sinus in jugular foramen
Accessory n. [CN XI]
Condyloid emissary v.
R. occipital condyle

Cranial and Autonomic Nerves

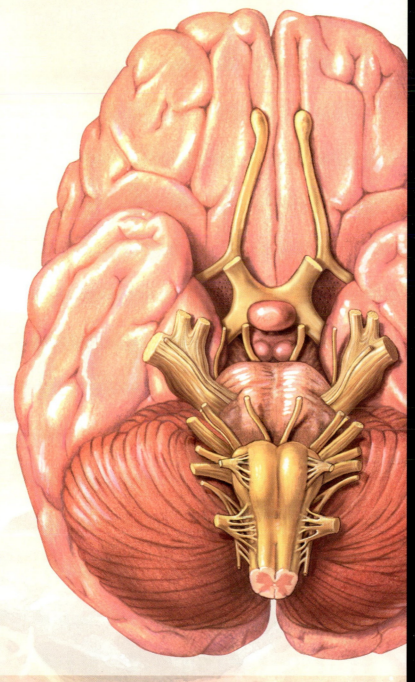

Chapter **8**

Cranial Nerve Functions
Table 8.1

Overview of Cranial Nerves

Nerve	Efferent or Motor			Afferent or Sensory		
	Striated Muscles	Smooth & Cardiac Muscles & Glands	Skin	Mucous Membranes & Organs	Special Senses
CN I					Olfaction or sensation of smell
CN II					Vision or sight
CN III	Supplies all muscles of eyeball except lateral rectus	Parasympathetic to ciliary m. (lens) & sphincter m. of iris of eye		Proprioceptive fibers from eye m.	
CN IV	Supplies superior oblique mm. of eyeball			Proprioceptive fibers from eye m.	
CN V	Supplies muscles of mastication & tensors of tympanic membrane & palate & mylohyoid m. ant. belly of digastric m.	Carries parasympathetic preganglionic nerve fibers of CN, III, VII & IX	Face & ant. part of scalp	Teeth, mucous membrane of mouth, nose & eye, general sensory from anterior two-thirds of tongue	Taste (fibers from chorda tympani) from ant. two-thirds of tongue
CN VI	Supplies lateral rectus m. of eyeball			Proprioceptive fibers from lateral rectus m.	
CN VII	Supplies muscles of facial expression, stapedius m., stylohyoid m., & post. belly of digastric m.	Parasympathetic nervus intermedius; glands of mouth, nose & palate; lacrimal gland; submandibular & sublingual glands	Ext. ear	Proprioceptive fibers from muscles of facial expression	Nervus intermedius, taste, ant. two-thirds of tongue
CN VIII					Hearing & equilibrium
CN IX	Supplies stylopharyngeus m.	Parasympathetic to parotid gland		Internal surface of tympanic membrane, middle ear, pharynx & general sensory from tongue (post. one-third)	Taste from post. one-third of tongue
CN X	Supplies muscles of pharynx & larynx	Parasympathetic to organs in neck, thorax & abdomen	Ext. acoustic meatus & tympanic membrane	Organs in neck, thorax & abdomen, general sensory from root of tongue	Taste, epiglottis
CN XI	Supplies muscles of soft palate, pharynx, larynx (from cranial root & distributed in vagus n.) & sternocleidomastoid & trapezius m.				
CN XII	Supplies extrinsic & intrinsic mm. of tongue except palatoglossus m. (from cranial root distributed in vagus n.)				

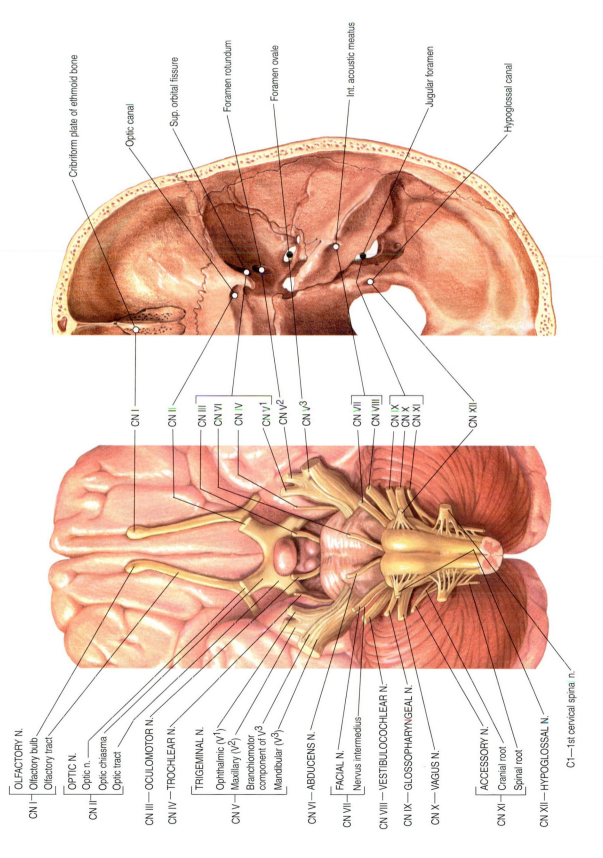

Cribriform plate of ethmoid bone

Optic canal

Sup. orbital fissure

Foramen rotundum

Foramen ovale

Int. acoustic meatus

Jugular foramen

Hypoglossal canal

CN I
CN II
CN III
CN VI
CN IV
CN V¹
CN V²
CN V³
CN VII
CN VIII
CN IX
CN X
CN XI
CN XII

CN I ⎡ OLFACTORY N.
⎢ Olfactory bulb
⎣ Olfactory tract

CN II ⎡ OPTIC N.
⎢ Optic n.
⎢ Optic chiasma
⎣ Optic tract

CN III — OCULOMOTOR N.

CN IV — TROCHLEAR N.

CN V ⎡ TRIGEMINAL N.
⎢ Ophthalmic (V¹)
⎢ Maxillary (V²)
⎢ Branchiomotor
⎢ component of V³
⎣ Mandibular (V³)

CN VI — ABDUCENS N.

CN VII ⎡ FACIAL N.
⎣ Nervus intermedius

CN VIII — VESTIBULOCOCHLEAR N.

CN IX — GLOSSOPHARYNGEAL N.

CN X — VAGUS N.

CN XI ⎡ ACCESSORY N.
⎢ Cranial root
⎣ Spinal root

CN XII — HYPOGLOSSAL N.

C1—1st cervical spinal n.

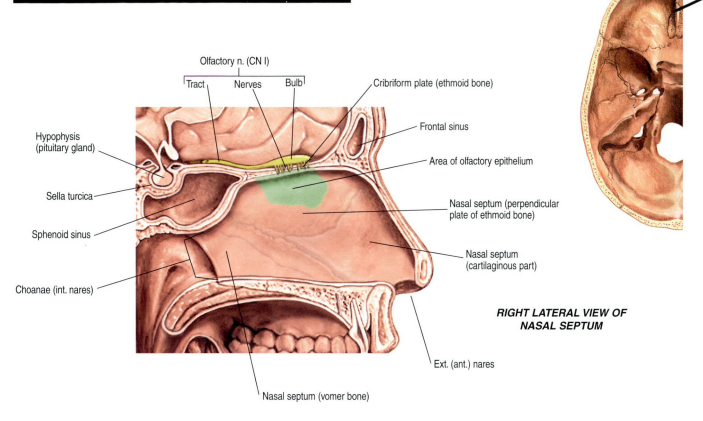

Olfactory n. (CN I)

Tract — Nerves — Bulb

Cribriform plate (ethmoid bone)

Hypophysis (pituitary gland)

Frontal sinus

Area of olfactory epithelium

Sella turcica

Sphenoid sinus

Nasal septum (perpendicular plate of ethmoid bone)

Nasal septum (cartilaginous part)

Choanae (int. nares)

Nasal septum (vomer bone)

Ext. (ant.) nares

RIGHT LATERAL VIEW OF NASAL SEPTUM

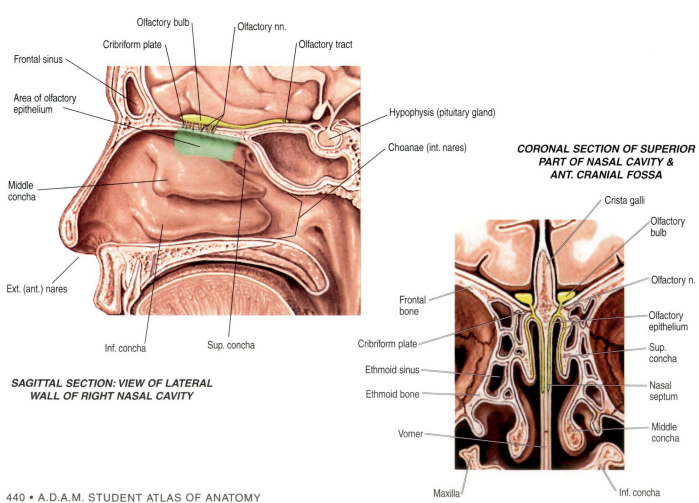

Olfactory bulb

Olfactory nn.

Cribriform plate

Olfactory tract

Frontal sinus

Area of olfactory epithelium

Hypophysis (pituitary gland)

Choanae (int. nares)

Middle concha

CORONAL SECTION OF SUPERIOR PART OF NASAL CAVITY & ANT. CRANIAL FOSSA

Ext. (ant.) nares

Inf. concha

Sup. concha

Crista galli

Olfactory bulb

Olfactory n.

Frontal bone

Cribriform plate

Olfactory epithelium

Ethmoid sinus

Sup. concha

Ethmoid bone

Nasal septum

Vomer

Middle concha

SAGITTAL SECTION: VIEW OF LATERAL WALL OF RIGHT NASAL CAVITY

Maxilla

Inf. concha

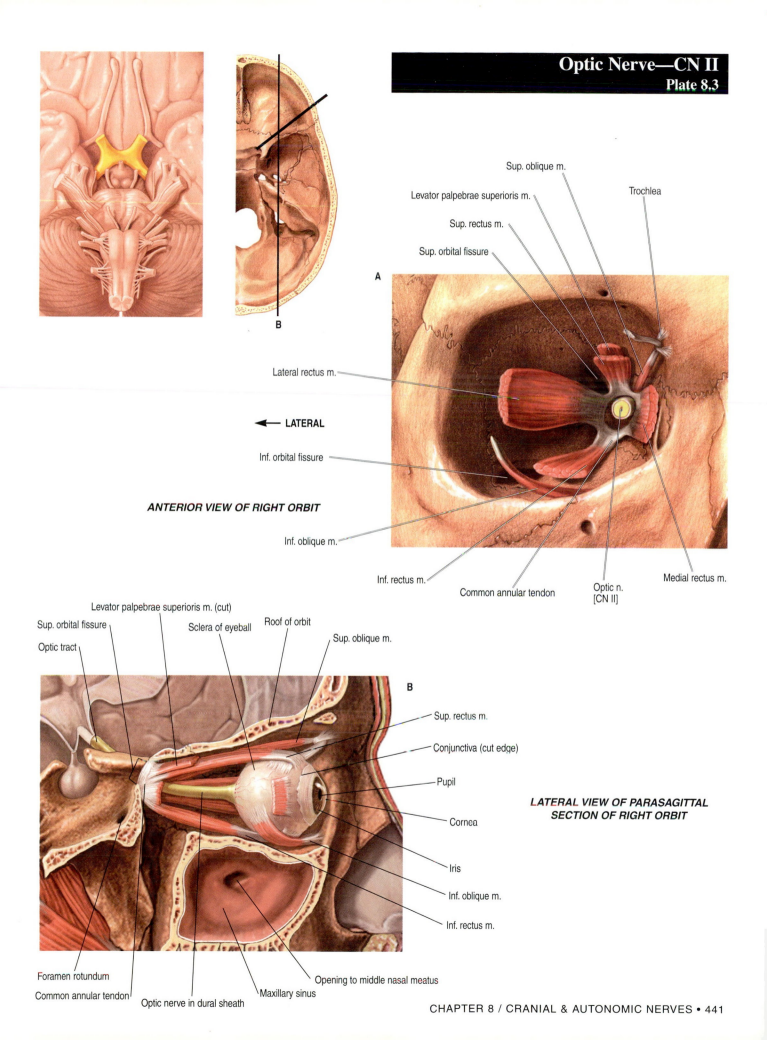

Sup. oblique m.

Levator palpebrae superioris m.

Trochlea

Sup. rectus m.

Sup. orbital fissure

A

Lateral rectus m.

← LATERAL

Inf. orbital fissure

ANTERIOR VIEW OF RIGHT ORBIT

Inf. oblique m.

Inf. rectus m.

Common annular tendon

Optic n.
[CN II]

Medial rectus m.

Sup. orbital fissure

Levator palpebrae superioris m. (cut)

Sclera of eyeball

Roof of orbit

Sup. oblique m.

Optic tract

B

Sup. rectus m.

Conjunctiva (cut edge)

Pupil

**LATERAL VIEW OF PARASAGITTAL
SECTION OF RIGHT ORBIT**

Cornea

Iris

Inf. oblique m.

Inf. rectus m.

Foramen rotundum

Common annular tendon

Optic nerve in dural sheath

Maxillary sinus

Opening to middle nasal meatus

Oculomotor Nerve—CN III
Plate 8.4

Levator palpebrae superioris m.

Sup. orbital fissure

Ciliary ganglion

Lateral rectus m.

Sup. rectus m.

Sup. oblique m.

Trochlea

Sup. division of CN III

Oculomotor n. [CN III]

Medial rectus m.

Inf. division of CN III

A

MEDIAL ⟶

Inf. orbital fissure

Inf. oblique m.

Inf. rectus m.

Common annular tendon

ANTERIOR VIEW OF RIGHT ORBIT

Sup. rectus m.

Sclera

Sup. oblique m.

Levator palpebrae superioris m.

Sup. division of CN III

Common annular tendon

Oculomotor n. [CN III]

Inf. division of CN III

B

**PARASAGITTAL SECTION
THROUGH RIGHT ORBIT**

Ciliary ganglion

Parasympathetic root of ciliary ganglion

Short ciliary nn.

Inf. oblique m.

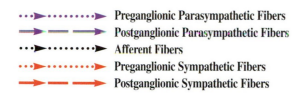

- •••▸•••▸ Preganglionic Parasympathetic Fibers
- ━─━▸ Postganglionic Parasympathetic Fibers
- •••▸•••▸ Afferent Fibers
- •••▸•••▸ Preganglionic Sympathetic Fibers
- ━─━▸ Postganglionic Sympathetic Fibers

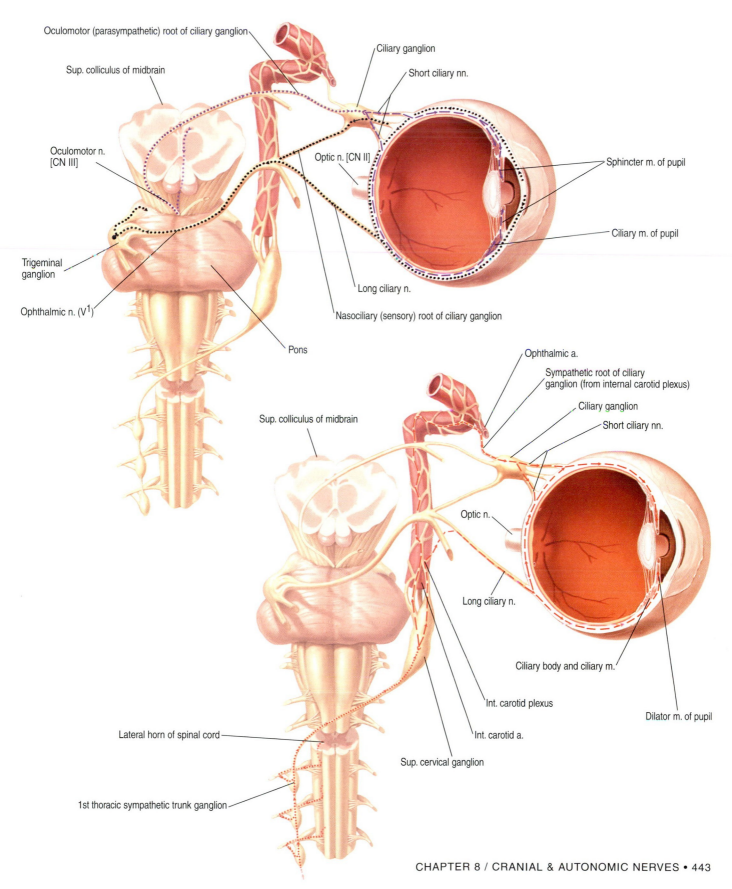

Oculomotor (parasympathetic) root of ciliary ganglion

Sup. colliculus of midbrain

Ciliary ganglion

Short ciliary nn.

Oculomotor n. [CN III]

Optic n. [CN II]

Sphincter m. of pupil

Trigeminal ganglion

Ciliary m. of pupil

Ophthalmic n. (V¹)

Long ciliary n.

Pons

Nasociliary (sensory) root of ciliary ganglion

Sup. colliculus of midbrain

Ophthalmic a.

Sympathetic root of ciliary ganglion (from internal carotid plexus)

Ciliary ganglion

Short ciliary nn.

Optic n.

Long ciliary n.

Ciliary body and ciliary m.

Lateral horn of spinal cord

Int. carotid plexus

Int. carotid a.

Dilator m. of pupil

Sup. cervical ganglion

1st thoracic sympathetic trunk ganglion

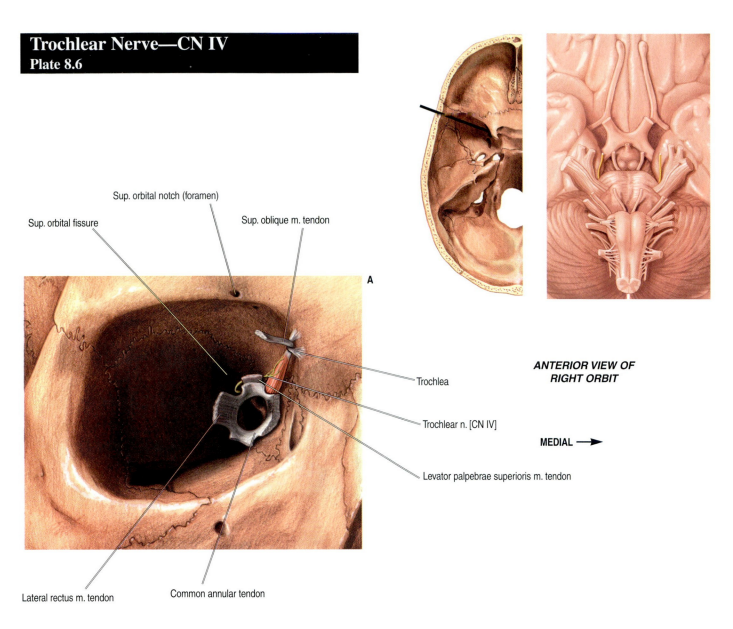

Sup. orbital fissure

Sup. orbital notch (foramen)

Sup. oblique m. tendon

A

Trochlea

Trochlear n. [CN IV]

Levator palpebrae superioris m. tendon

Lateral rectus m. tendon

Common annular tendon

ANTERIOR VIEW OF RIGHT ORBIT

MEDIAL ⟶

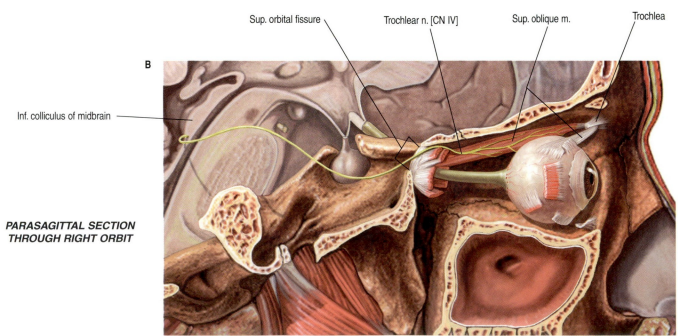

B

Sup. orbital fissure

Trochlear n. [CN IV]

Sup. oblique m.

Trochlea

Inf. colliculus of midbrain

PARASAGITTAL SECTION THROUGH RIGHT ORBIT

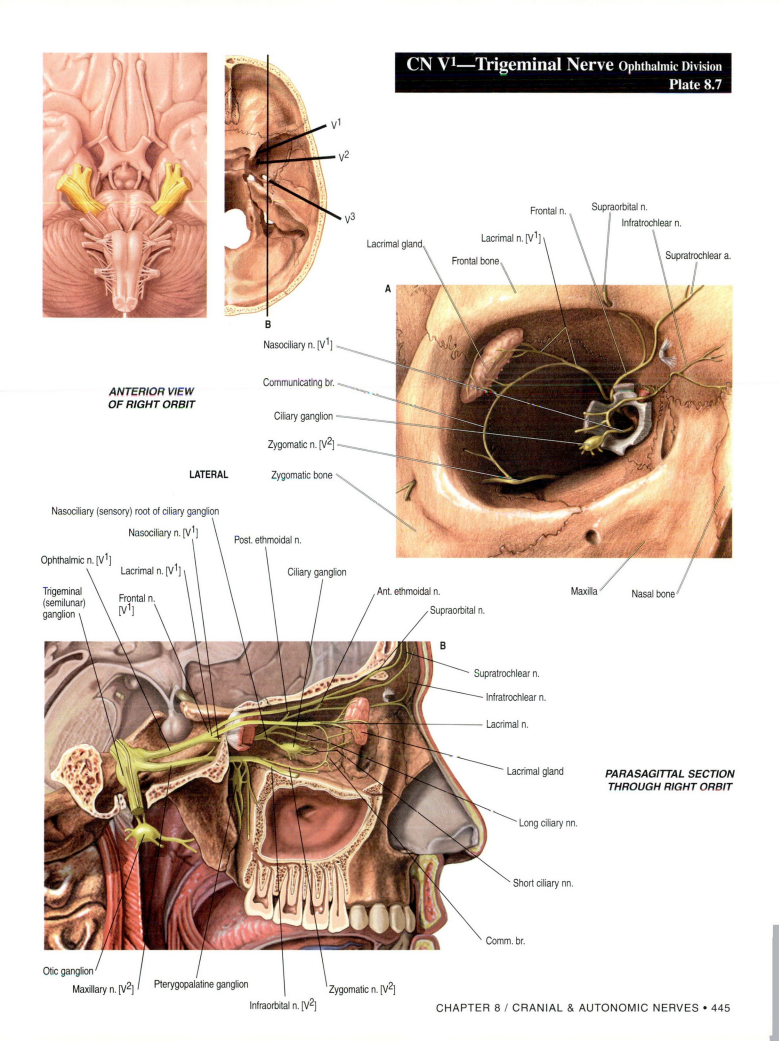

ANTERIOR VIEW OF RIGHT ORBIT

V¹

V²

V³

B

A

Lacrimal gland

Frontal bone

Lacrimal n. [V¹]

Frontal n.

Supraorbital n.

Infratrochlear n.

Supratrochlear a.

Nasociliary n. [V¹]

Communicating br.

Ciliary ganglion

Zygomatic n. [V²]

Zygomatic bone

Maxilla

Nasal bone

LATERAL

Nasociliary (sensory) root of ciliary ganglion

Nasociliary n. [V¹]

Post. ethmoidal n.

Ophthalmic n. [V¹]

Lacrimal n. [V¹]

Ciliary ganglion

Ant. ethmoidal n.

Supraorbital n.

Trigeminal (semilunar) ganglion

Frontal n. [V¹]

B

Supratrochlear n.

Infratrochlear n.

Lacrimal n.

Lacrimal gland

PARASAGITTAL SECTION THROUGH RIGHT ORBIT

Long ciliary nn.

Short ciliary nn.

Comm. br.

Otic ganglion

Maxillary n. [V²]

Pterygopalatine ganglion

Infraorbital n. [V²]

Zygomatic n. [V²]

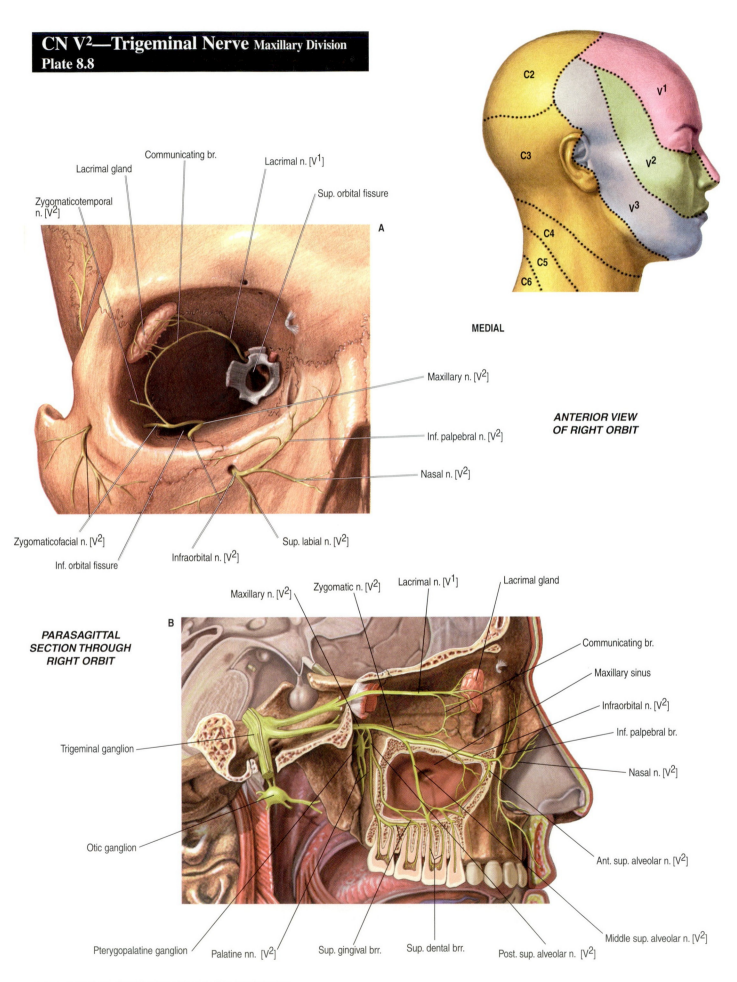

Communicating br.

Lacrimal gland

Zygomaticotemporal n. [V²]

Lacrimal n. [V¹]

Sup. orbital fissure

A

Maxillary n. [V²]

Inf. palpebral n. [V²]

Nasal n. [V²]

Zygomaticofacial n. [V²]

Inf. orbital fissure

Infraorbital n. [V²]

Sup. labial n. [V²]

MEDIAL

ANTERIOR VIEW OF RIGHT ORBIT

C2

C3

C4

C5

C6

V¹

V²

V³

PARASAGITTAL SECTION THROUGH RIGHT ORBIT

B

Maxillary n. [V²]

Zygomatic n. [V²]

Lacrimal n. [V¹]

Lacrimal gland

Communicating br.

Maxillary sinus

Infraorbital n. [V²]

Inf. palpebral br.

Nasal n. [V²]

Trigeminal ganglion

Otic ganglion

Ant. sup. alveolar n. [V²]

Middle sup. alveolar n. [V²]

Pterygopalatine ganglion

Palatine nn. [V²]

Sup. gingival brr.

Sup. dental brr.

Post. sup. alveolar n. [V²]

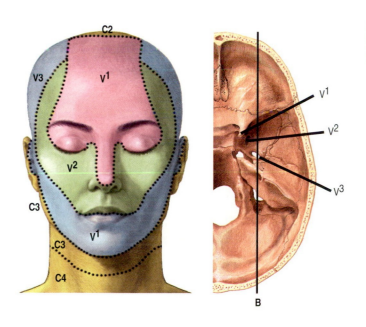

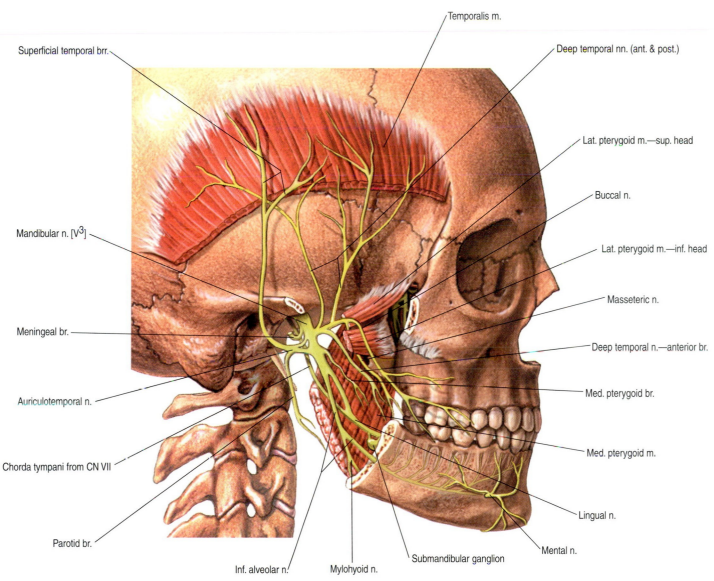

Temporalis m.

Deep temporal nn. (ant. & post.)

Superficial temporal brr.

Lat. pterygoid m.—sup. head

Buccal n.

Mandibular n. [V³]

Lat. pterygoid m.—inf. head

Masseteric n.

Deep temporal n.—anterior br.

Meningeal br.

Med. pterygoid br.

Auriculotemporal n.

Med. pterygoid m.

Chorda tympani from CN VII

Lingual n.

Mental n.

Parotid br.

Submandibular ganglion

Inf. alveolar n.

Mylohyoid n.

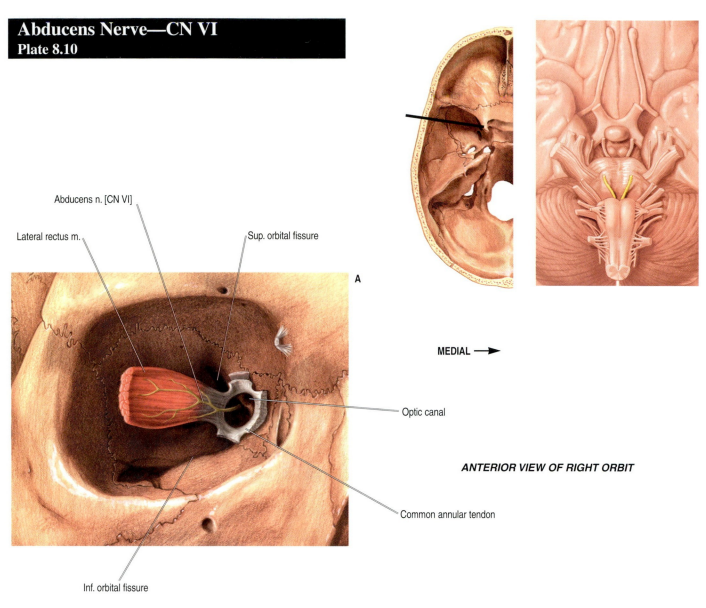

Abducens n. [CN VI]

Lateral rectus m.

Sup. orbital fissure

A

MEDIAL ⟶

Optic canal

ANTERIOR VIEW OF RIGHT ORBIT

Common annular tendon

Inf. orbital fissure

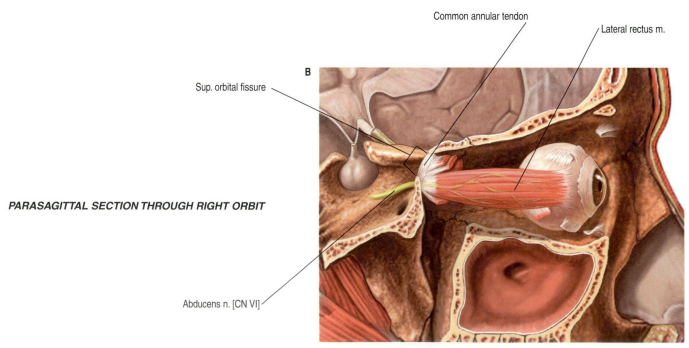

Common annular tendon

Lateral rectus m.

B

Sup. orbital fissure

PARASAGITTAL SECTION THROUGH RIGHT ORBIT

Abducens n. [CN VI]

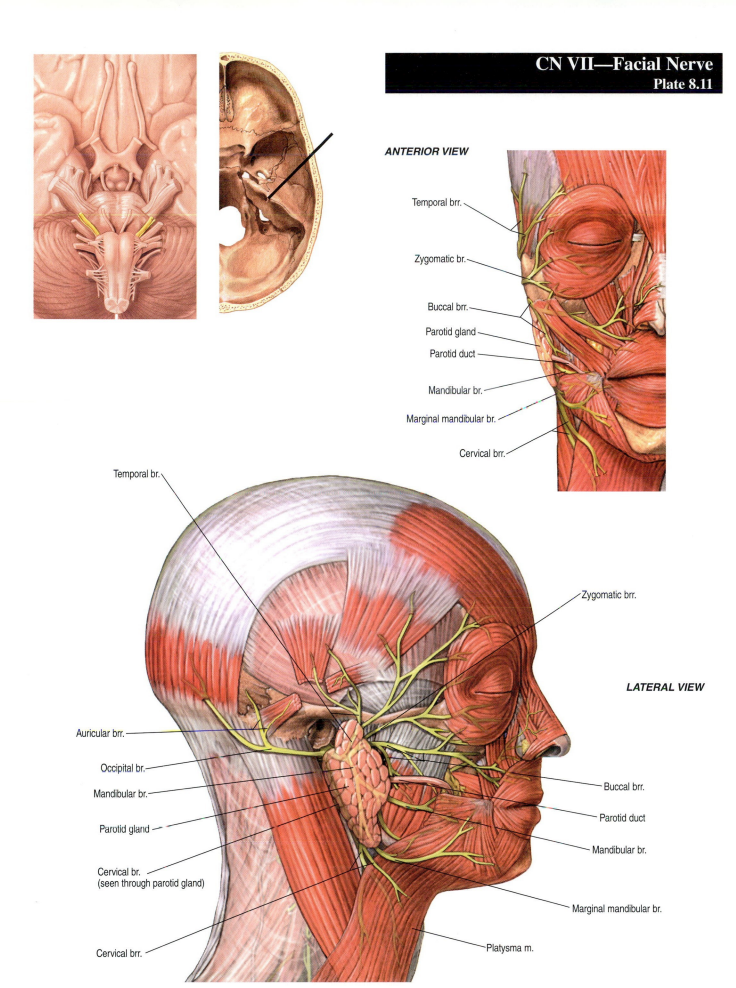

ANTERIOR VIEW

Temporal brr.

Zygomatic br.

Buccal brr.

Parotid gland

Parotid duct

Mandibular br.

Marginal mandibular br.

Cervical brr.

Temporal br.

Zygomatic brr.

LATERAL VIEW

Auricular brr.

Occipital br.

Mandibular br.

Parotid gland

Cervical br.
(seen through parotid gland)

Cervical brr.

Buccal brr.

Parotid duct

Mandibular br.

Marginal mandibular br.

Platysma m.

Pterygopalatine Ganglion
Plate 8.12

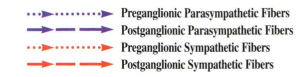

··▶·······▶ Preganglionic Parasympathetic Fibers
──▶── ── ──▶ Postganglionic Parasympathetic Fibers
··▶·······▶ Preganglionic Sympathetic Fibers
──▶── ── ──▶ Postganglionic Sympathetic Fibers

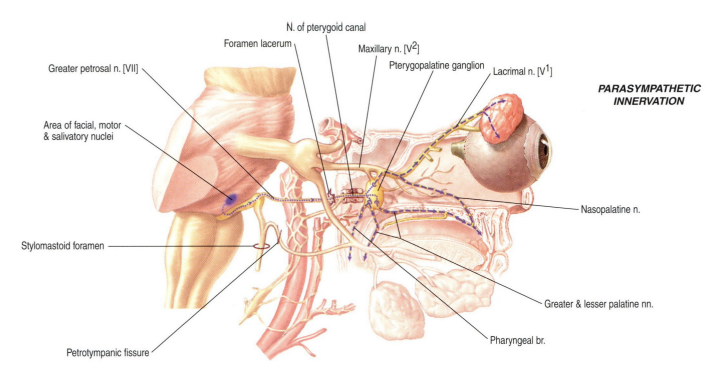

N. of pterygoid canal

Foramen lacerum

Maxillary n. [V²]

Pterygopalatine ganglion

Lacrimal n. [V¹]

Greater petrosal n. [VII]

PARASYMPATHETIC INNERVATION

Area of facial, motor & salivatory nuclei

Nasopalatine n.

Stylomastoid foramen

Greater & lesser palatine nn.

Pharyngeal br.

Petrotympanic fissure

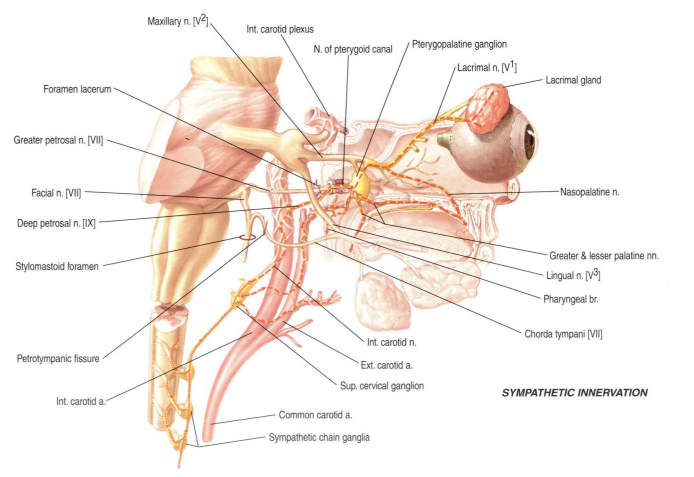

Maxillary n. [V²]

Int. carotid plexus

N. of pterygoid canal

Pterygopalatine ganglion

Lacrimal n. [V¹]

Lacrimal gland

Foramen lacerum

Greater petrosal n. [VII]

Facial n. [VII]

Nasopalatine n.

Deep petrosal n. [IX]

Greater & lesser palatine nn.

Stylomastoid foramen

Lingual n. [V³]

Pharyngeal br.

Chorda tympani [VII]

Petrotympanic fissure

Int. carotid n.

Ext. carotid a.

Int. carotid a.

Sup. cervical ganglion

SYMPATHETIC INNERVATION

Common carotid a.

Sympathetic chain ganglia

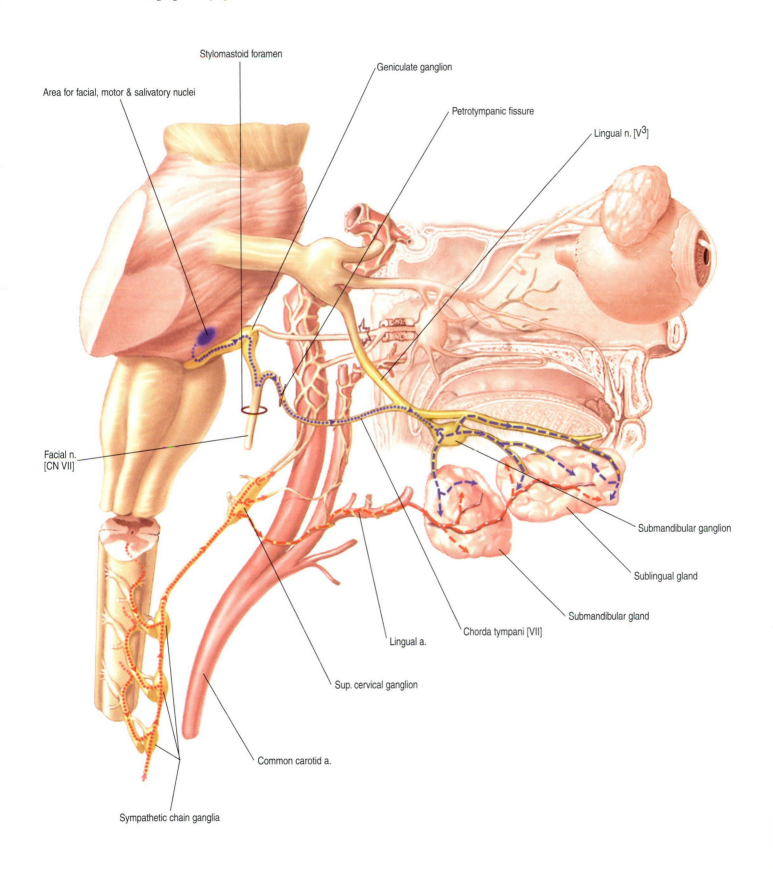

Preganglionic Parasympathetic Fibers
Postganglionic Parasympathetic Fibers
Preganglionic Sympathetic Fibers
Postganglionic Sympathetic Fibers

Stylomastoid foramen

Area for facial, motor & salivatory nuclei

Geniculate ganglion

Petrotympanic fissure

Lingual n. [V³]

Facial n.
[CN VII]

Submandibular ganglion

Sublingual gland

Submandibular gland

Chorda tympani [VII]

Lingual a.

Sup. cervical ganglion

Common carotid a.

Sympathetic chain ganglia

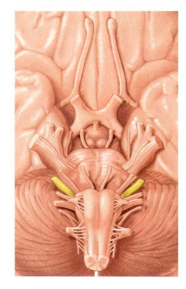

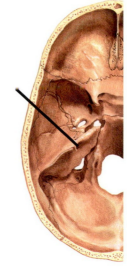

*HORIZONTAL SECTION THROUGH TEMPORAL BONE
AND CHAMBERS OF THE EAR*

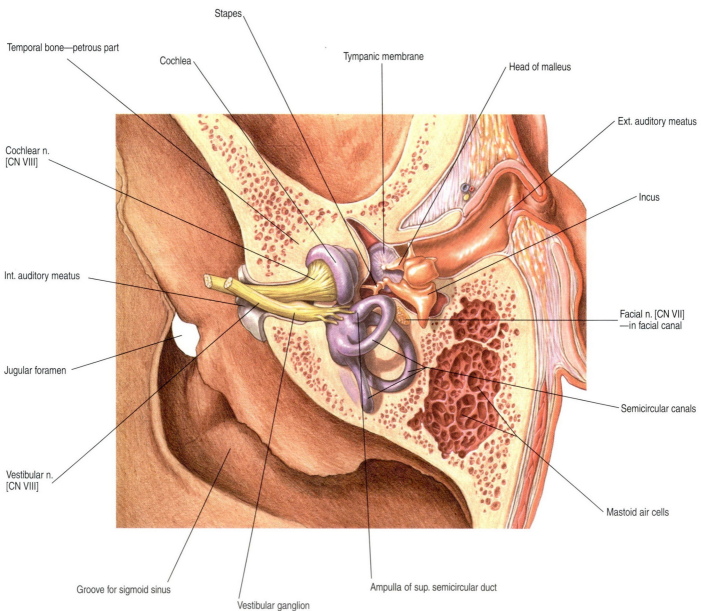

Stapes

Temporal bone—petrous part

Cochlea

Tympanic membrane

Head of malleus

Ext. auditory meatus

Cochlear n.
[CN VIII]

Incus

Int. auditory meatus

Facial n. [CN VII]
—in facial canal

Jugular foramen

Semicircular canals

Vestibular n.
[CN VIII]

Mastoid air cells

Groove for sigmoid sinus

Vestibular ganglion

Ampulla of sup. semicircular duct

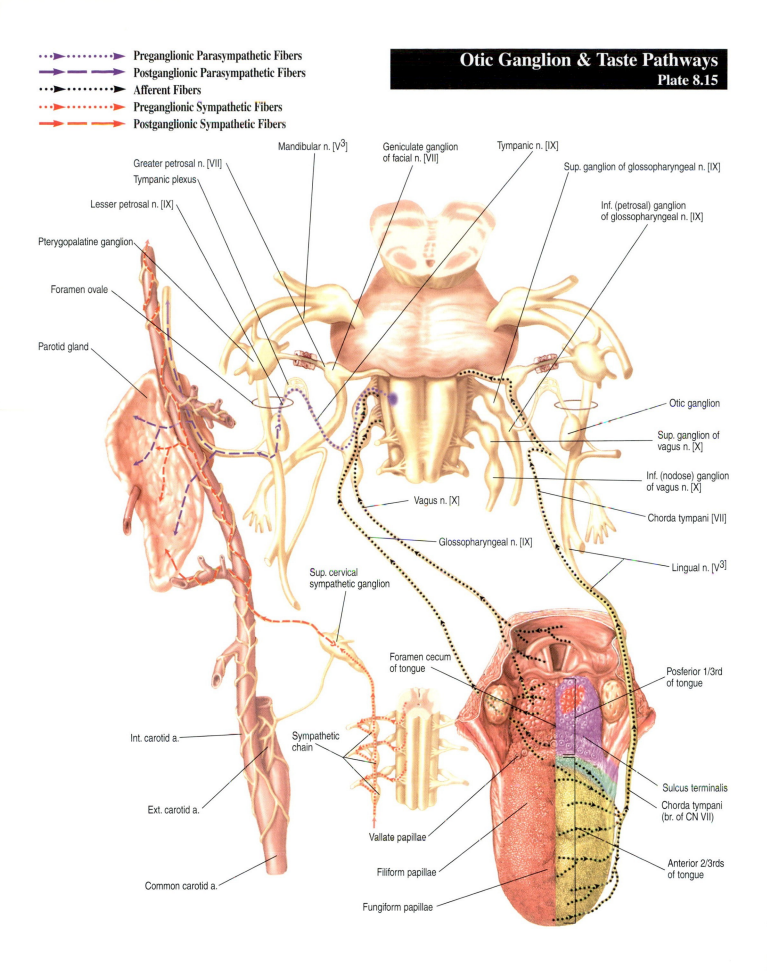

Preganglionic Parasympathetic Fibers
Postganglionic Parasympathetic Fibers
Afferent Fibers
Preganglionic Sympathetic Fibers
Postganglionic Sympathetic Fibers

Greater petrosal n. [VII]
Tympanic plexus
Lesser petrosal n. [IX]
Pterygopalatine ganglion
Foramen ovale
Parotid gland

Mandibular n. [V³]
Geniculate ganglion of facial n. [VII]
Tympanic n. [IX]
Sup. ganglion of glossopharyngeal n. [IX]
Inf. (petrosal) ganglion of glossopharyngeal n. [IX]

Otic ganglion
Sup. ganglion of vagus n. [X]
Inf. (nodose) ganglion of vagus n. [X]
Chorda tympani [VII]
Lingual n. [V³]

Vagus n. [X]
Glossopharyngeal n. [IX]

Sup. cervical sympathetic ganglion
Foramen cecum of tongue
Posferior 1/3rd of tongue
Sulcus terminalis
Chorda tympani (br. of CN VII)
Anterior 2/3rds of tongue

Int. carotid a.
Sympathetic chain
Ext. carotid a.
Vallate papillae
Filiform papillae
Common carotid a.
Fungiform papillae

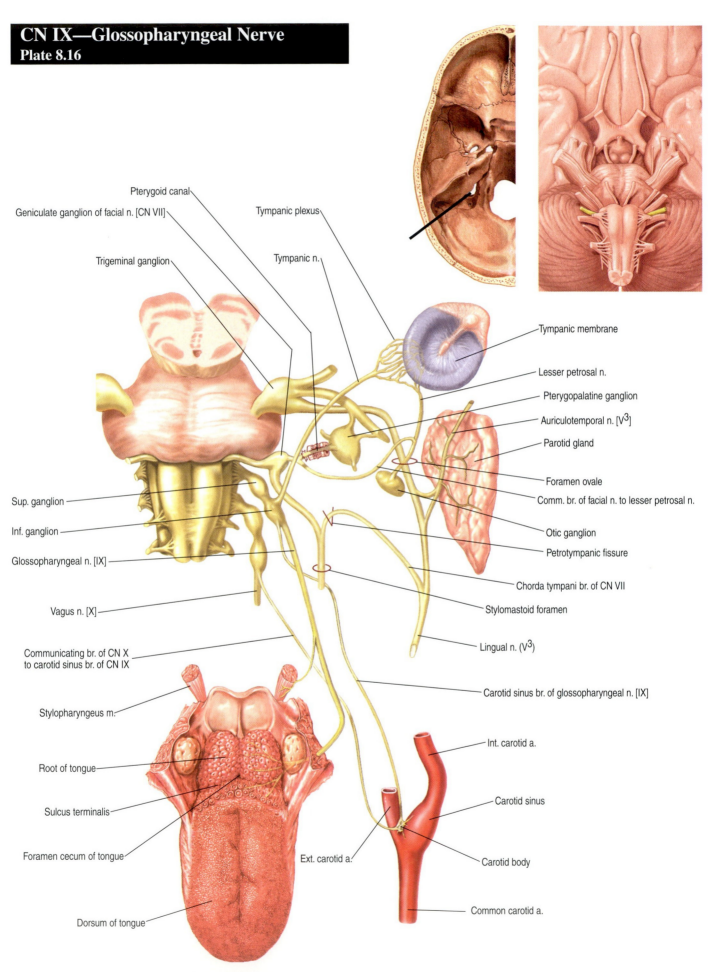

Pterygoid canal

Geniculate ganglion of facial n. [CN VII]

Trigeminal ganglion

Tympanic plexus

Tympanic n.

Tympanic membrane

Lesser petrosal n.

Pterygopalatine ganglion

Auriculotemporal n. [V³]

Parotid gland

Foramen ovale

Comm. br. of facial n. to lesser petrosal n.

Sup. ganglion

Inf. ganglion

Otic ganglion

Glossopharyngeal n. [IX]

Petrotympanic fissure

Chorda tympani br. of CN VII

Vagus n. [X]

Stylomastoid foramen

Communicating br. of CN X
to carotid sinus br. of CN IX

Lingual n. (V³)

Carotid sinus br. of glossopharyngeal n. [IX]

Stylopharyngeus m.

Root of tongue

Int. carotid a.

Sulcus terminalis

Carotid sinus

Foramen cecum of tongue

Ext. carotid a.

Carotid body

Dorsum of tongue

Common carotid a.

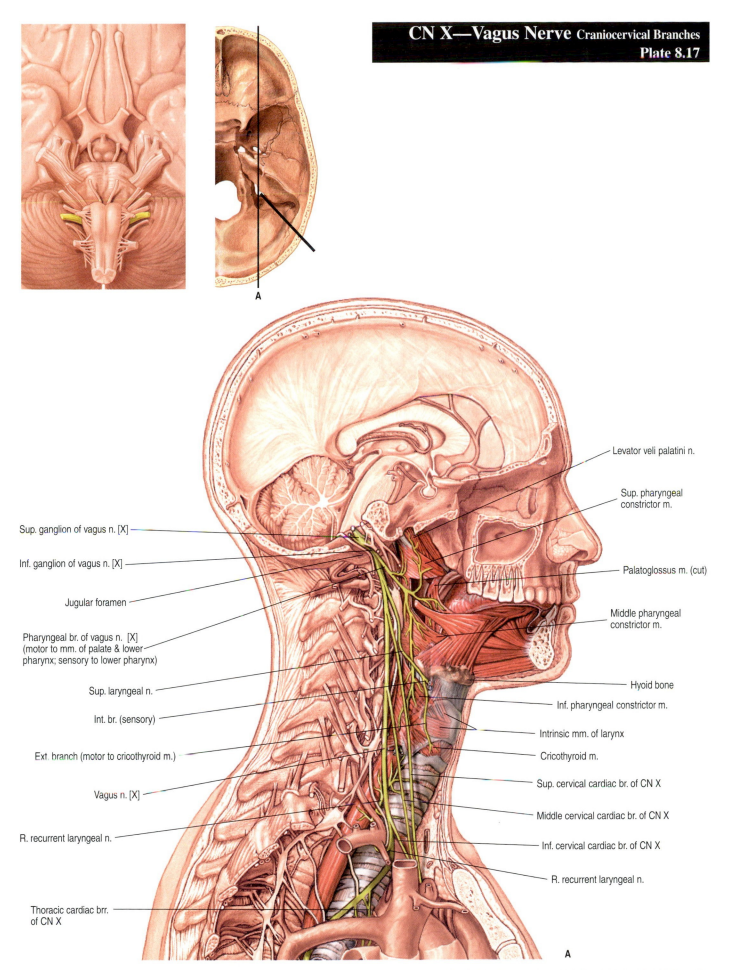

A

Levator veli palatini n.

Sup. pharyngeal constrictor m.

Sup. ganglion of vagus n. [X]

Inf. ganglion of vagus n. [X]

Palatoglossus m. (cut)

Jugular foramen

Middle pharyngeal constrictor m.

Pharyngeal br. of vagus n. [X]
(motor to mm. of palate & lower
pharynx; sensory to lower pharynx)

Sup. laryngeal n.

Hyoid bone

Inf. pharyngeal constrictor m.

Int. br. (sensory)

Intrinsic mm. of larynx

Cricothyroid m.

Ext. branch (motor to cricothyroid m.)

Sup. cervical cardiac br. of CN X

Vagus n. [X]

Middle cervical cardiac br. of CN X

Inf. cervical cardiac br. of CN X

R. recurrent laryngeal n.

R. recurrent laryngeal n.

Thoracic cardiac brr.
of CN X

A

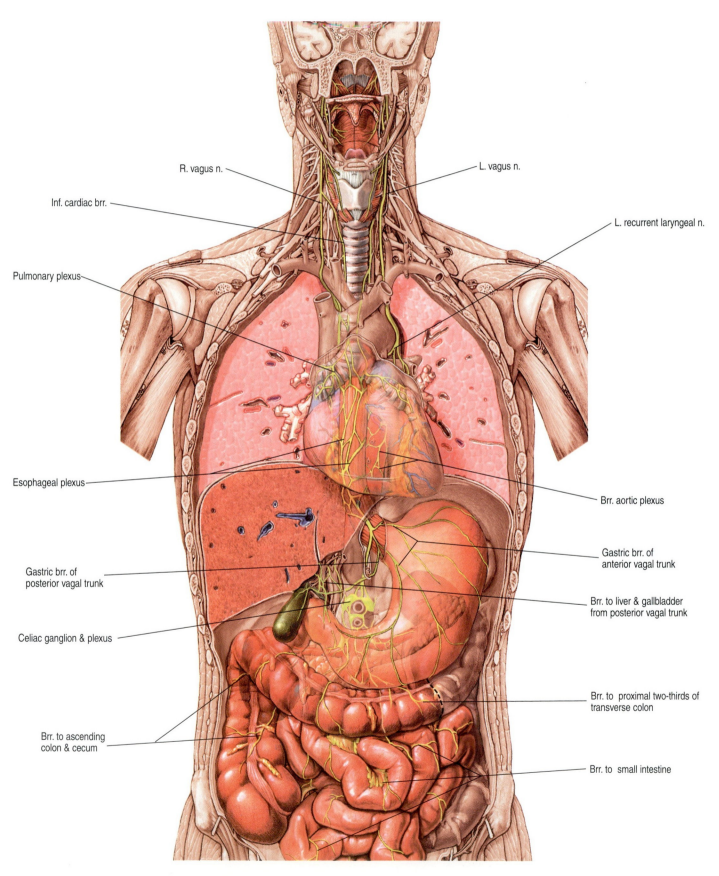

R. vagus n.

L. vagus n.

Inf. cardiac brr.

L. recurrent laryngeal n.

Pulmonary plexus

Esophageal plexus

Brr. aortic plexus

Gastric brr. of
anterior vagal trunk

Gastric brr. of
posterior vagal trunk

Brr. to liver & gallbladder
from posterior vagal trunk

Celiac ganglion & plexus

Brr. to proximal two-thirds of
transverse colon

Brr. to ascending
colon & cecum

Brr. to small intestine

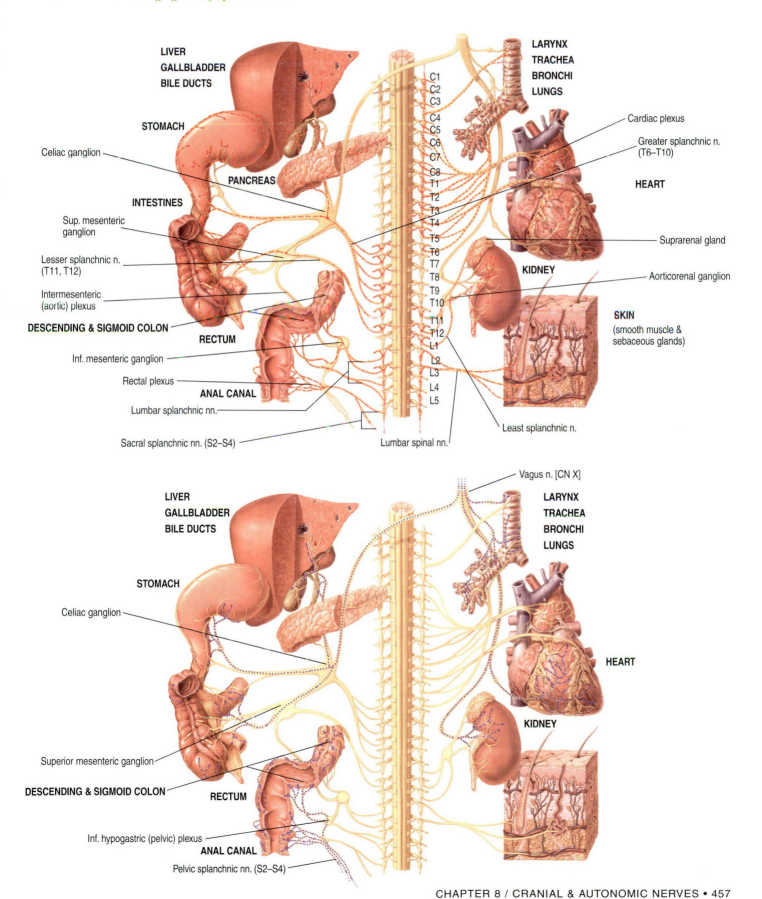

········▶ Preganglionic Parasympathetic Fibers
──▶──── Postganglionic Parasympathetic Fibers
········▶ Preganglionic Sympathetic Fibers
──▶──── Postganglionic Sympathetic Fibers

LIVER
GALLBLADDER
BILE DUCTS

STOMACH

Celiac ganglion

PANCREAS

INTESTINES

Sup. mesenteric ganglion

Lesser splanchnic n. (T11, T12)

Intermesenteric (aortic) plexus

DESCENDING & SIGMOID COLON

RECTUM

Inf. mesenteric ganglion

Rectal plexus

ANAL CANAL

Lumbar splanchnic nn.

Sacral splanchnic nn. (S2–S4)

Lumbar spinal nn.

C1
C2
C3
C4
C5
C6
C7
C8
T1
T2
T3
T4
T5
T6
T7
T8
T9
T10
T11
T12
L1
L2
L3
L4
L5

LARYNX
TRACHEA
BRONCHI
LUNGS

Cardiac plexus

Greater splanchnic n. (T6–T10)

HEART

Suprarenal gland

KIDNEY

Aorticorenal ganglion

SKIN
(smooth muscle & sebaceous glands)

Least splanchnic n.

Vagus n. [CN X]

LIVER
GALLBLADDER
BILE DUCTS

STOMACH

Celiac ganglion

LARYNX
TRACHEA
BRONCHI
LUNGS

HEART

KIDNEY

Superior mesenteric ganglion

DESCENDING & SIGMOID COLON

RECTUM

Inf. hypogastric (pelvic) plexus

ANAL CANAL

Pelvic splanchnic nn. (S2–S4)

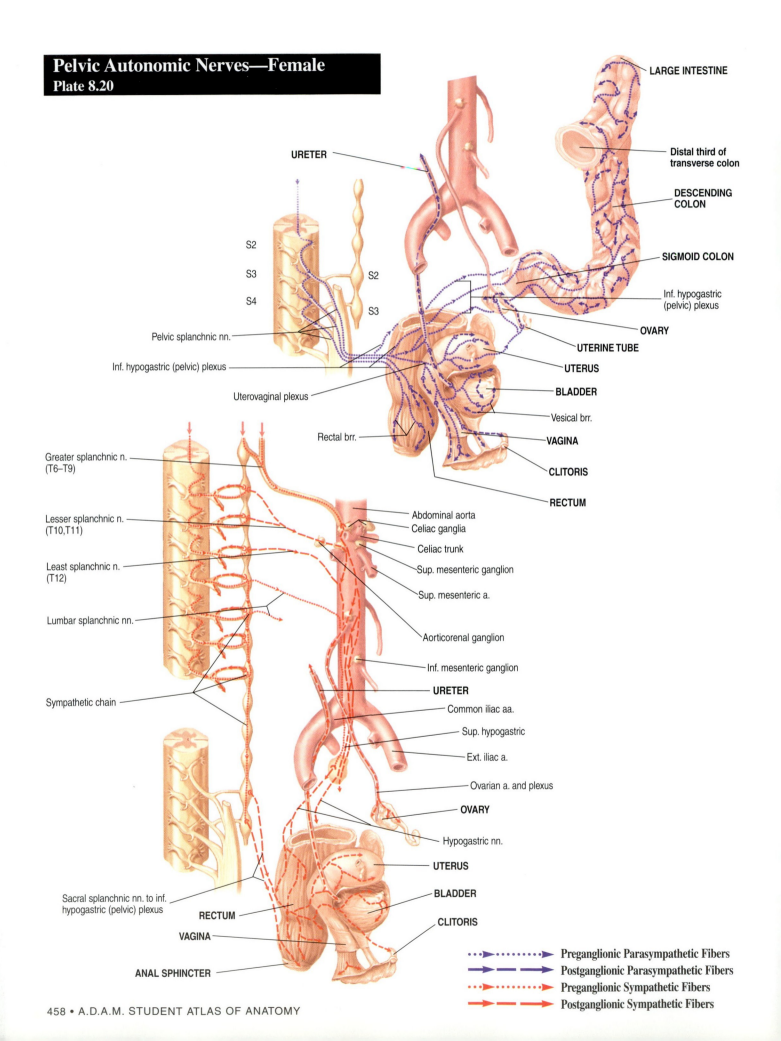

URETER

LARGE INTESTINE

Distal third of
transverse colon

DESCENDING
COLON

S2
S3
S4

S2

S3

SIGMOID COLON

Inf. hypogastric
(pelvic) plexus

OVARY

UTERINE TUBE

UTERUS

BLADDER

Pelvic splanchnic nn.

Inf. hypogastric (pelvic) plexus

Uterovaginal plexus

Vesical brr.

VAGINA

Rectal brr.

CLITORIS

RECTUM

Greater splanchnic n.
(T6–T9)

Abdominal aorta

Celiac ganglia

Celiac trunk

Lesser splanchnic n.
(T10,T11)

Sup. mesenteric ganglion

Sup. mesenteric a.

Least splanchnic n.
(T12)

Aorticorenal ganglion

Lumbar splanchnic nn.

Inf. mesenteric ganglion

URETER

Common iliac aa.

Sympathetic chain

Sup. hypogastric

Ext. iliac a.

Ovarian a. and plexus

OVARY

Hypogastric nn.

UTERUS

BLADDER

Sacral splanchnic nn. to inf.
hypogastric (pelvic) plexus

CLITORIS

RECTUM

VAGINA

ANAL SPHINCTER

Preganglionic Parasympathetic Fibers
Postganglionic Parasympathetic Fibers
Preganglionic Sympathetic Fibers
Postganglionic Sympathetic Fibers

Preganglionic Parasympathetic Fibers
Postganglionic Parasympathetic Fibers
Preganglionic Sympathetic Fibers
Postganglionic Sympathetic Fibers

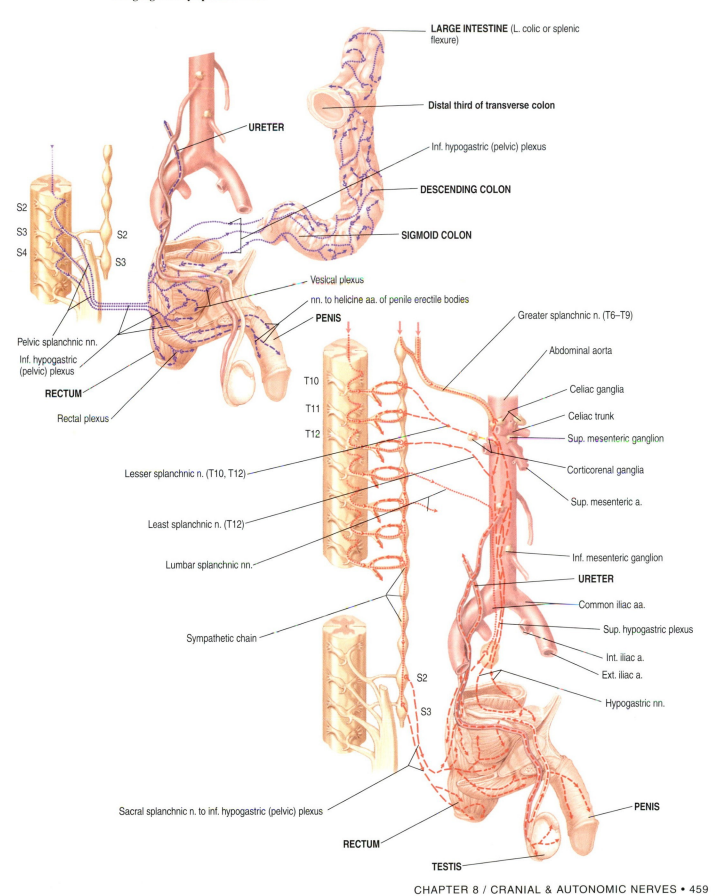

LARGE INTESTINE (L. colic or splenic flexure)

Distal third of transverse colon

Inf. hypogastric (pelvic) plexus

DESCENDING COLON

SIGMOID COLON

URETER

Vesical plexus

nn. to helicine aa. of penile erectile bodies

PENIS

Greater splanchnic n. (T6–T9)

Abdominal aorta

Celiac ganglia

Celiac trunk

Sup. mesenteric ganglion

Corticorenal ganglia

Sup. mesenteric a.

Inf. mesenteric ganglion

URETER

Common iliac aa.

Sup. hypogastric plexus

Int. iliac a.

Ext. iliac a.

Hypogastric nn.

S2

S3

S4

S2

S3

Pelvic splanchnic nn.

Inf. hypogastric (pelvic) plexus

RECTUM

Rectal plexus

T10

T11

T12

Lesser splanchnic n. (T10, T12)

Least splanchnic n. (T12)

Lumbar splanchnic nn.

Sympathetic chain

S2

S3

Sacral splanchnic n. to inf. hypogastric (pelvic) plexus

RECTUM

TESTIS

PENIS

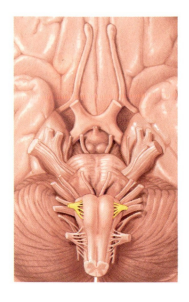

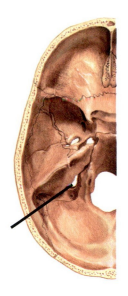

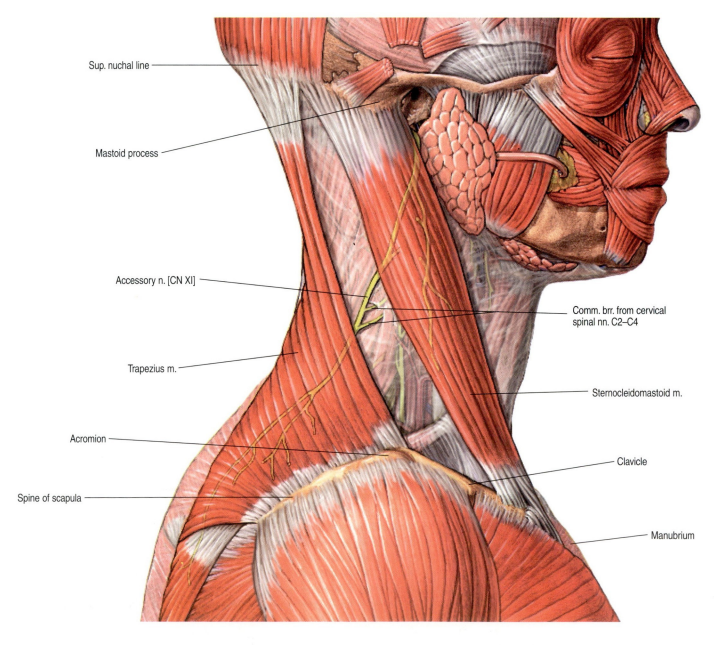

Sup. nuchal line

Mastoid process

Accessory n. [CN XI]

Comm. brr. from cervical spinal nn. C2–C4

Trapezius m.

Sternocleidomastoid m.

Acromion

Clavicle

Spine of scapula

Manubrium

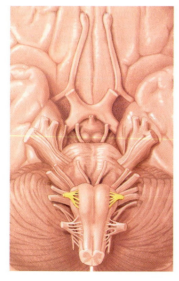

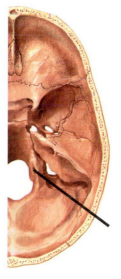

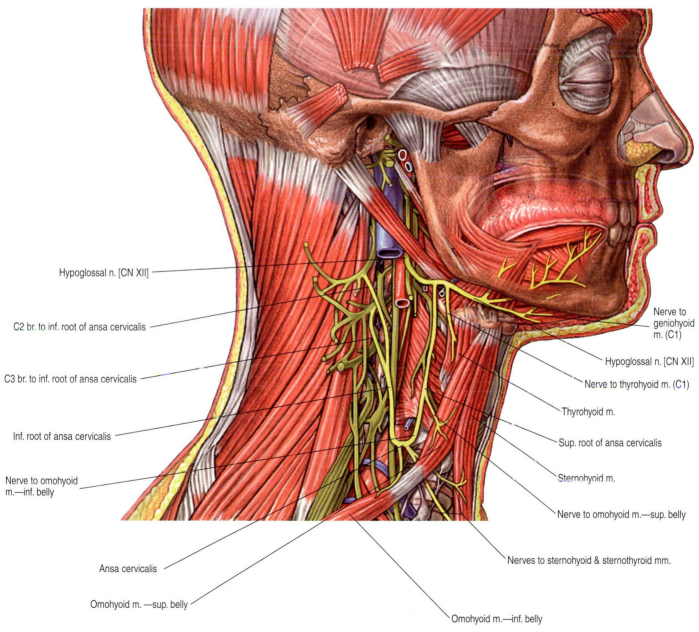

Hypoglossal n. [CN XII]

C2 br. to inf. root of ansa cervicalis

C3 br. to inf. root of ansa cervicalis

Inf. root of ansa cervicalis

Nerve to omohyoid m.—inf. belly

Ansa cervicalis

Omohyoid m. —sup. belly

Omohyoid m.—inf. belly

Nerve to geniohyoid m. (C1)

Hypoglossal n. [CN XII]

Nerve to thyrohyoid m. (C1)

Thyrohyoid m.

Sup. root of ansa cervicalis

Sternohyoid m.

Nerve to omohyoid m.—sup. belly

Nerves to sternohyoid & sternothyroid mm.

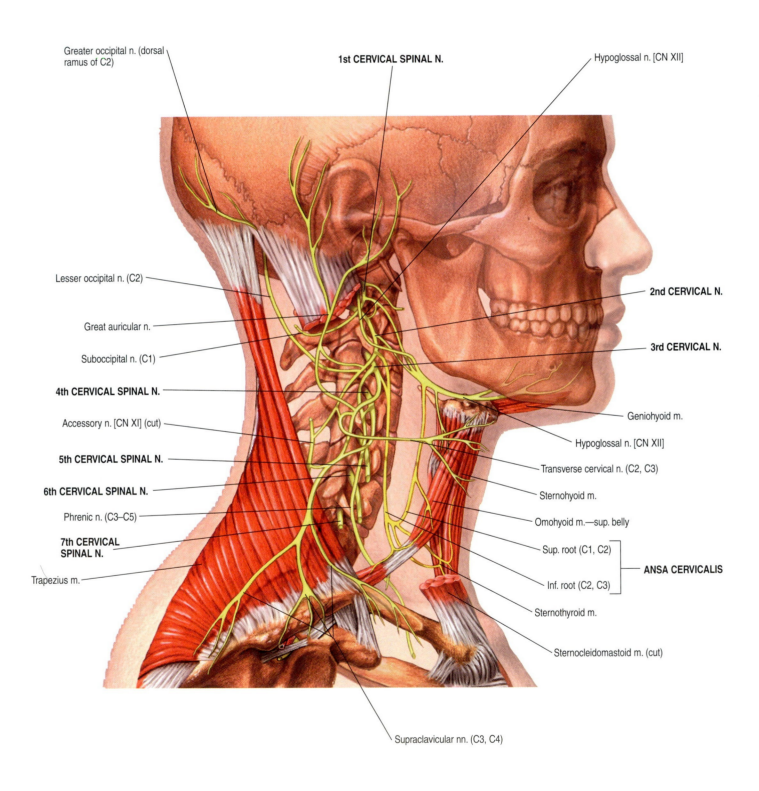

Greater occipital n. (dorsal ramus of C2)

1st CERVICAL SPINAL N.

Hypoglossal n. [CN XII]

Lesser occipital n. (C2)

Great auricular n.

Suboccipital n. (C1)

4th CERVICAL SPINAL N.

Accessory n. [CN XI] (cut)

5th CERVICAL SPINAL N.

6th CERVICAL SPINAL N.

Phrenic n. (C3–C5)

7th CERVICAL SPINAL N.

Trapezius m.

2nd CERVICAL N.

3rd CERVICAL N.

Geniohyoid m.

Hypoglossal n. [CN XII]

Transverse cervical n. (C2, C3)

Sternohyoid m.

Omohyoid m.—sup. belly

Sup. root (C1, C2)

Inf. root (C2, C3)

ANSA CERVICALIS

Sternothyroid m.

Sternocleidomastoid m. (cut)

Supraclavicular nn. (C3, C4)

Overview of Cranial Nerves

Nerve	Efferent or Motor		Skin	Afferent or Sensory	
	Striated Muscles	Smooth & Cardiac Muscles & Glands		Mucous Membranes & Organs	Special Senses
CN I					Olfaction or sensation of smell
CN II					Vision or sight
CN III	Supplies all muscles of eyeball except lateral rectus & superior oblique mm.	Parasympathetic to ciliary m. (lens) & sphincter m. of iris of eye		Proprioceptive fibers from eye m.	
CN IV	Supplies superior oblique m. of eyeball			Proprioceptive fibers from eye m.	
CN V	Supplies muscles of mastication, tensors of tympanic membrane, palate, mylohyoid m. & ant. belly of digastric m.	Carries parasympathetic preganglionic nerve fibers of CN, III, VII & IX	Face & ant. part of scalp	Teeth, mucous membrane of mouth, nose & eye, general sensory from ant. two-thirds of tongue	Taste (fibers from chorda tympani) from ant. two-thirds of tongue
CN VI	Supplies lateral rectus m. of eyeball			Proprioceptive fibers from lateral rectus m.	
CN VII	Supplies muscles of facial expression, stapedius m., stylohyoid m. & post. belly of digastric m.	Parasympathetic nervus intermedius; glands of mouth, nose & palate; lacrimal gland; submandibular & sublingual glands	Ext. ear	Proprioceptive fibers from muscles of facial expression	Nervus intermedius, taste, ant. two-thirds of tongue
CN VIII					Hearing & equilibrium
CN IX	Supplies stylopharyngeus m.	Parasympathetic to parotid gland		Internal surface of tympanic membrane, middle ear, pharynx & general sensory from tongue (post. third)	Taste, from post. third of tongue
CN X	Supplies muscles of pharynx and larynx	Parasympathetic to organs in neck, thorax & abdomen	Ext. acoustic meatus & tympanic membrane	Organs in neck, thorax & abdomen, general sensory from root of tongue	Taste, epiglottis
CN XI	Supplies muscles of soft palate, pharynx, larynx (from cranial root & distributed in vagus n.)& sternocleidomastoid & trapezius m.				
CN XII	Supplies extrinsic & intrinsic mm. of tongue except palatoglossus m.				

Index